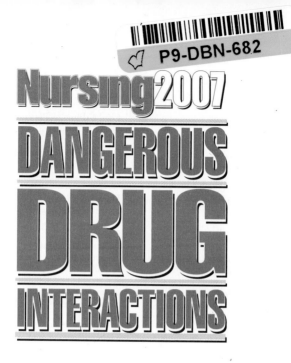

Nursing2007
DANGEROUS
DRUG
INTERACTIONS

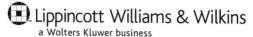

Lippincott Williams & Wilkins
a Wolters Kluwer business

Philadelphia · Baltimore · New York · London
Buenos Aires · Hong Kong · Sydney · Tokyo

Staff

publisher to instructors whose schools have adopted its accompanying textbook. Printed in the United States of America. For information, write Lippincott Williams & Wilkins, 323 Norristown Road, Suite 200, Ambler, PA 19002-2756.

DDI010306

Library of Congress Cataloging-in-Publication Data
Nursing2007 dangerous drug interactions.
    p. ; cm.
    ISBN 1-58255-615-6 (alk. paper)
    1. Pharmacology—Handbooks, manuals, etc. 2. Nursing—Handbooks, manuals, etc. 3. Drug interactions—Handbooks, manuals, etc. 4. Drugs—Safety measures—Handbooks, manuals, etc. I. Lippincott Williams & Wilkins. II. Title: Dangerous drug interactions. III. Title: Nursing 2007 dangerous drug interactions.
    [DNLM: 1. Drug Interactions—Handbooks. 2. Nursing Process—Handbooks. 3. Pharmaceutical Preparations—adverse effects—Handbooks. WY 49 N9765 2006]
RM302.N87 2006
615'.7045—dc22   2005034582

Contents

Contributors and consultants

Special thanks to David S. Tatro, PharmD, Editor, *Drug Interaction Facts*.

Frances Davis Baldwin, RN, MSN
Consultant
Charlotte, N.C.

Dana Bartlett, RN, MSN
Poison Information Specialist
Philadelphia Poison Control
    Center

Jennalie E. Blackwood, PharmD
Clinical Infusion Pharmacist
Interlock Pharmacy
Florissant, Mo.

Lisa Colodny, MBA, PharmD, BCNSP
Pharmacy Director
Coral Springs (Fla.) Medical
    Center

Jennifer J. Gorrell, PharmD
Director of Pharmacy
Charleston (W.Va.) Area
    Medical Center
Women & Childrens Hospital

Theresa R. Howard, RN
Trauma Nurse Coordinator
Limestone Medical Center
Groesbeck, Tex.

Julia N. Kleckner, PharmD
Clinical Coordinator
Mercy Fitzgerald Hospital
Darby, Pa.

Caroline Kramer, RN
Staff Nurse
North Hill Home Health
Needham, Mass.

Phyllis Magaletto, RN, MSN, BC
Instructor, Medical-Surgical
    Nursing
Cochran School of Nursing
Yonkers, N.Y.

Jeffrey B. Purcell, PharmD
Clinical Lead Pharmacist
Harborview Medical Center
Clinical Associate Professor
University of Washington
    School of Pharmacy
Seattle, Wash.

How to use this book

Dangerous Drug Interactions is an easy-to-use resource to help you avoid thousands of unintended drug interactions as quickly and conveniently as possible.

You can use this book in two ways. With its A-to-Z organization, you can flip quickly to the generic name of the drug you plan to give. There you'll find, in alphabetical order, the drugs, drug classes, herbs, and foods that may interact with it. Or you can turn first to the book's comprehensive index, find the drug you plan to give, and scan the list of drugs and drug classes it may interact with.

Format

Each entry follows a standard format, making it easy for you to find key information fast. An entry starts with an interacting pair. The pair may be drug-drug, drug-class, drug-herb, or drug-food. Just below the interacting pair, as appropriate, you'll find a selection of common names. If the interacting element is a generic drug, the monograph typically provides common trade names. If the interacting element is a drug class, the monograph provides the generic names of applicable drugs in that class.

Risk rating. The risk rating gives you a quick idea of the overall importance of an interaction. The rating is based on the combined influence of the interaction's severity, onset, and likelihood. Because this book focuses only on potentially dangerous interactions, you'll find either a 1 or a 2 as the risk rating.

Severity. The severity of a drug interaction may be major, moderate, or minor. A major interaction is one that may be life-threatening or cause permanent damage. A moderate interaction is one that may worsen the patient's condition. A minor interaction may be bothersome or cause little effect. Because this book focuses on dangerous drug interactions, it includes only those considered major or moderate.

Onset. A drug interaction with a rapid onset starts within 24 hours of combined use. An interaction with a delayed onset starts days to weeks after the start of combined use.

Likelihood. In this section you'll get an idea of the likelihood that an interaction may occur. An established interaction is one that well-controlled clinical trials have proven can occur. A probable interaction is a very likely possibility but not proven clinically. And a suspected interaction is one that's supported by some reliable evidence but still needs more study. Interactions that are merely possible or unlikely aren't included in this book.

Cause. Next you'll find a brief description of the mechanism by which the interaction occurs.

Effect. This section reviews the main clinical effect of the interaction, usually in a single quick-read sentence.

Nursing considerations. Finally, each entry includes key information about drug usage, patient care, and patient teaching. This section also includes a special, in-text ◣**ALERT** logo to direct your attention to especially important information.

Index

The comprehensive index for *Dangerous Drug Interactions* includes generic drug names, common trade names, and drug classes. The index provides a full, book-wide look at the potentially dangerous interactions for each drug included in this handy volume.

Guide to abbreviations

ACE	angiotensin-converting enzyme	D$_5$W	dextrose 5% in water
ADH	antidiuretic hormone	DIC	disseminated intravascular coagulation
AIDS	acquired immunodeficiency syndrome	dl	deciliter
		DNA	deoxyribonucleic acid
ALT	alanine transaminase	ECG	electrocardiogram
APTT	activated partial thromboplastin time	EEG	electroencephalo-gram
		EENT	eyes, ears, nose, throat
AST	aspartate transaminase	FDA	Food and Drug Administration
AV	atrioventricular	g	gram
b.i.d.	twice daily	G	gauge
BPH	benign prostatic hypertrophy	GGT	gamma-glutamyltransferase
BSA	body surface area	GI	gastrointestinal
BUN	blood urea nitrogen	gtt	drops
cAMP	cyclic 3', 5' adenosine monophosphate	GU	genitourinary
		G6PD	glucose-6-phosphate dehy-drogenase
CBC	complete blood count		
CK	creatine kinase	H$_1$	histamine$_1$
CMV	cytomegalovirus	H$_2$	histamine$_2$
CNS	central nervous system	HDL	high-density lipoprotein
COPD	chronic obstructive pulmonary disease	HIV	human immuno-deficiency virus
CSF	cerebrospinal fluid	HMG-CoA	3-hydroxy-3-methylglutaryl coenzyme A
CV	cardiovascular		
CVA	cerebrovascular accident	h.s.	at bedtime
CYP	cytochrome P-450	5-HT	5-hydroxytryp-tamine

I.D.	intradermal	PTT	partial thrombo-plastin time
I.M.	intramuscular		
INR	International Normalized Ratio	PVC	premature ventric-ular contraction
IPPB	intermittent positive-pressure breathing	q	every
		q.i.d.	four times daily
		RBC	red blood cell
IU	international unit	RDA	recommended daily allowance
I.V.	intravenous		
kg	kilogram	REM	rapid eye movement
L	liter		
lb	pound	RNA	ribonucleic acid
LDH	lactate dehydrogenase	RSV	respiratory syncytial virus
LDL	low-density lipoprotein	SA	sinoatrial
		S.C.	subcutaneous
M	molar	sec	second
m^2	square meter	SIADH	syndrome of inappropriate antidiuretic hormone
MAO	monoamine oxidase		
mcg	microgram		
mEq	milliequivalent	S.L.	sublingual
mg	milligram	SSRI	selective serotonin reuptake inhibitor
MI	myocardial infarction		
		T_3	triiodothyronine
min	minute	T_4	thyroxine
ml	milliliter	t.i.d.	three times daily
mm^3	cubic millimeter	TSH	thyroid-stimulating hormone
NSAID	nonsteroidal anti-inflammatory drug		
		tsp	teaspoon
OTC	over-the-counter	USP	United States Pharmacopeia
PABA	para-aminobenzoic acid		
		UTI	urinary tract infection
PCA	patient-controlled analgesia		
		WBC	white blood cell
P.O.	by mouth	wk	week
P.R.	by rectum		
p.r.n.	as needed		
PT	prothrombin time		

acebutolol ▶◀ NSAIDs
Sectral

ibuprofen, indomethacin, naproxen, piroxicam

Risk rating: 2
Severity: Moderate **Onset: Delayed** **Likelihood: Probable**

Cause
NSAIDs may inhibit renal prostaglandin synthesis, allowing pressor systems to be unopposed.

Effect
Acebutolol and other beta blockers may not be able to lower blood pressure.

Nursing considerations
- Avoid using these drugs together if possible.
- Monitor blood pressure and other evidence of hypertension closely.
- Talk with prescriber about ways to minimize or eliminate interaction, such as adjusting beta blocker dosage or switching to sulindac as the NSAID.
- Explain the risks of using these drugs together, and teach patient how to monitor his own blood pressure.
- Other NSAIDs may interact with beta blockers. If you suspect an interaction, consult prescriber or pharmacist.

acebutolol ▶◀ prazosin
Sectral

Minipress

Risk rating: 2
Severity: Moderate **Onset: Rapid** **Likelihood: Probable**

Cause
The mechanism of this interaction is unknown.

Effect
Risk of orthostatic hypotension increases.

Nursing considerations
- Assess patient's lying, sitting, and standing blood pressures closely, especially when combined therapy starts.
- Adjust dosages of either drug, as needed.
- To minimize effects of orthostatic hypotension, teach patient to change positions slowly.
- Interaction is confirmed only with propranolol but may occur with other beta blockers as well.

acebutolol ▶◀ salicylates

Sectral

aspirin, bismuth subsalicylate, choline salicylate, magnesium salicylate, salsalate, sodium salicylate, sodium thiosalicylate

Risk rating: 2
Severity: Moderate   **Onset: Rapid**   **Likelihood: Suspected**

Cause
Salicylates inhibit synthesis of prostaglandins, which acebutolol and other beta blockers need to reduce blood pressure. In patients with heart failure, the mechanism of this interaction is unknown.

Effect
Beta blocker effect decreases.

Nursing considerations
■ Watch closely for signs of heart failure and hypertension; notify prescriber if they occur.
■ Talk with prescriber about switching patient to a different antihypertensive or antiplatelet drug.
■ Other beta blockers may interact with salicylates. If you suspect an interaction, consult prescriber or pharmacist.
■ Explain signs and symptoms of heart failure, and tell patient when to contact prescriber.

acebutolol ▶◀ verapamil

Sectral   Calan

Risk rating: 1
Severity: Major   **Onset: Rapid**   **Likelihood: Probable**

Cause
Verapamil may inhibit metabolism of acebutolol and other beta blockers.

Effect
Effects of both drugs may increase.

Nursing considerations
■ Combined therapy is common in hypertension and unstable angina.
◪ ALERT Combined use increases risk of adverse effects, including heart failure, conduction disturbances, arrhythmias, and hypotension.
■ Assess patient for adverse effects, including left ventricular dysfunction and AV conduction defects.

- Risk of interaction is greater when drugs are given I.V.
- Monitor cardiac function.
- Dosages of both drugs may need to be decreased.

---

acetaminophen ◄► alcohol
Acephen, Neopap,
Tylenol

Risk rating: 2
Severity: Moderate   **Onset: Delayed**   **Likelihood: Suspected**

Cause
Long-term alcohol use and acetaminophen-induced hepatotoxicity may induce hepatic microsomal enzymes.

Effect
Risk of liver damage increases.

Nursing considerations
- Monitor liver function tests as needed.
- If patient drinks alcohol often or excessively, urge him to avoid regular or excessive use of acetaminophen.
- If patient is an alcoholic, explain that even moderate use of acetaminophen may cause significant hepatotoxicity.
- Tell patient to report abdominal pain, yellow skin, or dark urine.

---

acetaminophen ◄► phenytoin
Acephen, Neopap,   Dilantin
Tylenol

Risk rating: 2
Severity: Moderate   **Onset: Delayed**   **Likelihood: Suspected**

Cause
Phenytoin, a hydantoin, may induce hepatic microsomal enzymes, accelerating acetaminophen metabolism.

Effect
Hepatotoxic metabolites and risk of hepatic impairment may increase.

Nursing considerations
- Other hydantoins may interact with acetaminophen. If you suspect an interaction, consult prescriber or pharmacist.
- If patient takes phenytoin, warn against regular acetaminophen use.
- ◤ **ALERT** After acetaminophen overdose, risk of hepatotoxicity is highest in a patient who takes phenytoin regularly.

■ At usual therapeutic dosages, no special monitoring or dosage adjustment is needed.
■ Tell patient to notify prescriber if he has abdominal pain, yellowing of skin or eyes, or dark urine.

---

acetaminophen ➤◀ sulfinpyrazone
Acephen, Neopap,   Anturane
Tylenol

Risk rating: 2
Severity: Moderate   **Onset: Delayed**   **Likelihood: Suspected**

Cause
Sulfinpyrazone may induce hepatic microsomal enzymes, accelerating acetaminophen metabolism.

Effect
Hepatotoxic metabolites and risk of hepatic impairment may increase.

Nursing considerations
■ If patient takes sulfinpyrazone, advise against regular use of acetaminophen.
◄ ALERT After acetaminophen overdose, risk of hepatotoxicity is highest in a patient who takes sulfinpyrazone regularly.
■ At usual therapeutic dosages, no special monitoring or dosage adjustment is needed.
■ Tell patient to notify prescriber if he has abdominal pain, yellowing of skin or eyes, or dark urine.

---

acetaminophen ➤◀ warfarin
Acephen, Neopap,   Coumadin
Tylenol

Risk rating: 2
Severity: Moderate   **Onset: Delayed**   **Likelihood: Suspected**

Cause
Acetaminophen or one of its metabolites may antagonize vitamin K.

Effect
Antithrombotic effect of warfarin may increase.

Nursing considerations
◄ ALERT The effects of this interaction seem to be dose related. Daily acetaminophen use at 325 to 650 mg may increase INR 3.5-fold. Daily ingestion of 1,250 mg may increase INR 10-fold.

- At low acetaminophen doses (up to six 325-mg tablets weekly), interaction may have little significance.
- When starting or stopping acetaminophen, monitor coagulation studies once or twice weekly.
- Other risk factors may place patient at a higher risk, including diarrhea and conditions that affect acetaminophen metabolism.

acetohexamide ▬▶◀▬ chloramphenicol
Chloromycetin

Risk rating: 2
Severity: Moderate   Onset: Delayed   Likelihood: Suspected

Cause
Chloramphenicol reduces hepatic clearance of sulfonylureas, such as acetohexamide.

Effect
Because sulfonylurea level is prolonged, hypoglycemia may occur.

Nursing considerations
- Monitor patient for hypoglycemia.
- Describe signs and symptoms of hypoglycemia, including diaphoresis, fatigue, headache, hunger, irritability, malaise, nervousness, rapid heart rate, tension, and trembling.
- Instruct patient to eat a small carbohydrate snack or meal if hypoglycemia develops, preferably after checking blood glucose level.

acetohexamide ▬▶◀▬ diazoxide
Hyperstat, Proglycem

Risk rating: 2
Severity: Moderate   Onset: Delayed   Likelihood: Probable

Cause
Diazoxide may decrease insulin release or stimulate release of glucose and free fatty acids.

Effect
The risk of hyperglycemia increases if a patient stabilized on a sulfonylurea, such as acetohexamide, starts diazoxide.

Nursing considerations
- Use these drugs together cautiously.
- Monitor blood glucose level regularly, and consult prescriber about adjustments to either drug to maintain stable glucose level.

■ Tell patient to stay alert for evidence of high blood glucose level, such as increased fatigue, thirst, appetite, or urination and possible blurred vision or dry skin and mucous membranes.

acetohexamide ►◄ MAO inhibitors
isocarboxazid, phenelzine, tranylcypromine

Risk rating: 2
Severity: Moderate   **Onset: Rapid**   **Likelihood: Suspected**

Cause
The mechanism of this interaction is unknown.

Effect
MAO inhibitors increase the hypoglycemic effects of sulfonylureas, such as acetohexamide.

Nursing considerations
■ Monitor patient for hypoglycemia.
■ Consult prescriber about adjustments to either drug to control glucose level and mental status.
■ Describe evidence of hypoglycemia, including diaphoresis, fatigue, headache, hunger, irritability, malaise, nervousness, rapid heart rate, tension, and trembling.
■ Instruct patient to eat a small carbohydrate snack or meal if hypoglycemia develops, preferably after checking blood glucose level.

acetohexamide ►◄ rifamycins
rifabutin, rifampin, rifapentine

Risk rating: 2
Severity: Moderate   **Onset: Delayed**   **Likelihood: Probable**

Cause
Rifamycins may increase hepatic metabolism of certain sulfonylureas, such as acetohexamide.

Effect
Risk of hyperglycemia increases.

Nursing considerations
■ Use these drugs together cautiously.
■ Monitor patient's blood glucose level regularly, and consult prescriber about adjustments to either drug to maintain stable glucose level.

■ Tell patient to stay alert for evidence of high blood glucose level, such as increased fatigue, thirst, eating, or urination and possible blurred vision or dry skin and mucous membranes.

acetohexamide ▸◂ salicylates
aspirin, choline salicylate, magnesium salicylate, salsalate, sodium salicylate, sodium thiosalicylate

Risk rating: 2
Severity: Moderate   Onset: Delayed   Likelihood: Probable

Cause
Salicylates reduce glucose level and promote insulin secretion.

Effect
Hypoglycemic effects of sulfonylureas, such as acetohexamide, increase.

Nursing considerations
■ Monitor patient for hypoglycemia.
■ Consult prescriber about possibly replacing a salicylate with acetaminophen or an NSAID.
■ Describe evidence of hypoglycemia, including diaphoresis, fatigue, headache, hunger, irritability, malaise, nervousness, rapid heart rate, tension, and trembling.
■ Instruct patient to eat a small carbohydrate snack or meal if hypoglycemia develops, preferably after checking blood glucose level.

acetohexamide ▸◂ sulfonamides
sulfasalazine, sulfisoxazole

Risk rating: 2
Severity: Moderate   Onset: Delayed   Likelihood: Suspected

Cause
Sulfonamides may hinder hepatic metabolism of certain sulfonylureas, such as acetohexamide.

Effect
Prolonged sulfonylurea level increases the risk of hypoglycemia.

Nursing considerations
■ Monitor patient for hypoglycemia.

■ Monitor patient's blood glucose level, and consult prescriber about adjustments to either drug to maintain stable glucose level.
■ Glyburide doesn't interact and may be a good alternative to other sulfonylureas.
■ Describe evidence of hypoglycemia, including diaphoresis, fatigue, headache, hunger, irritability, malaise, nervousness, rapid heart rate, tension, and trembling.
■ Instruct patient to eat a small carbohydrate snack or meal if hypoglycemia develops, preferably after checking blood glucose level.

---

acetohexamide ➤◄ thiazide diuretics
chlorothiazide, hydrochlorothiazide, indapamide, metolazone

Risk rating: 2
Severity: Moderate   **Onset: Delayed**   **Likelihood: Probable**

Cause
Thiazide diuretics may decrease insulin secretion and tissue sensitivity to insulin, and they may increase sodium loss.

Effect
Risk of hyperglycemia and hyponatremia may increase.

Nursing considerations
■ Use these drugs together cautiously.
■ Check blood glucose and sodium levels regularly, and consult prescriber about adjustments to either drug to maintain stable levels.
■ Interaction may occur several days to many months after dual therapy starts but is readily reversible when the diuretic stops.
■ Describe evidence of hypoglycemia, including diaphoresis, fatigue, headache, hunger, irritability, malaise, nervousness, rapid heart rate, tension, and trembling.
■ Instruct patient to eat a small carbohydrate snack or meal if hypoglycemia develops, preferably after checking blood glucose level.

---

acyclovir ➤◄ theophyllines
Zovirax   aminophylline, theophylline

Risk rating: 2
Severity: Moderate   **Onset: Delayed**   **Likelihood: Suspected**

Cause
Acyclovir may inhibit oxidative metabolism of theophyllines.

Effect
Theophylline level, adverse effects, and toxicity may increase.

Nursing considerations
■ Monitor serum theophylline level closely. Normal therapeutic range is 10 to 20 mcg/ml for adults and 5 to 15 mcg/ml for children.
■ Theophylline dosage may need to be decreased while patient takes acyclovir.
■ Watch for increased adverse effects of theophylline, such as tachycardia, anorexia, nausea, vomiting, diarrhea, seizures, restlessness, irritability, and headache.
■ Describe adverse effects of theophylline and signs of toxicity, and tell patient to report them immediately to prescriber.

---

allopurinol ▶◀ **ampicillin**
Aloprim, Zyloprim   Principen

Risk rating: 2
Severity: Moderate   Onset: Delayed   Likelihood: Suspected

Cause
The mechanism of this interaction is unknown.

Effect
Risk of ampicillin-induced rash increases.

Nursing considerations
■ Allopurinol may increase hypersensitivity to ampicillin, a penicillin.
■ Other penicillins may interact with allopurinol. If you suspect an interaction, consult prescriber or pharmacist.
◣ ALERT Notify prescriber if rash appears. Patient may need a lower allopurinol dose or a different drug.
■ Instruct patient to watch for skin changes.

---

almotriptan ▶◀ **azole antifungals**
Axert   itraconazole, ketoconazole

Risk rating: 2
Severity: Moderate   Onset: Delayed   Likelihood: Suspected

Cause
Azole antifungals inhibit CYP3A4 metabolism of certain 5-HT$_1$ receptor agonists, such as almotriptan.

Effect
Selective 5-HT$_1$ receptor agonist level and adverse effects may increase.

Nursing considerations
◪ ALERT Don't give almotriptan within 7 days of itraconazole or ketoconazole.
■ Adverse effects of selective 5-HT$_1$ receptor agonists may include coronary artery vasospasm, dizziness, nausea, paresthesia, and somnolence.
■ To help avoid interactions, urge patient to tell prescribers about all drugs and supplements he takes.

---

almotriptan ▶◀ **serotonin reuptake inhibitors**
Axert

citalopram, fluoxetine, fluvoxamine, nefazodone, paroxetine, sertraline, venlafaxine

---

Risk rating: **1**
Severity: **Major**   Onset: **Rapid**   Likelihood: **Suspected**

Cause
Serotonin may accumulate rapidly in the CNS.

Effect
Risk of serotonin syndrome increases.

Nursing considerations
◪ ALERT Avoid combined use of these drugs.
■ If combined use can't be avoided, start with lowest dosages possible and assess patient closely.
■ Stop almotriptan, a selective 5-HT$_1$ receptor agonist, at first sign of interaction and start an antiserotonergic.
■ In some patients, migraine frequency may increase and antimigraine drug efficacy may decrease when therapy with a serotonin reuptake inhibitor starts.
■ Describe the traits of serotonin syndrome, including CNS irritability, motor weakness, shivering, muscle twitching, and altered consciousness.
■ Explain that serotonin-induced symptoms can be fatal if not treated immediately.

alprazolam ◀▶ alcohol
Xanax

Risk rating: 2
Severity: Moderate **Onset: Rapid** **Likelihood: Established**

Cause
Alcohol inhibits hepatic enzymes, which decreases clearance and increases peak level of benzodiazepines, such as alprazolam.

Effect
Risk of additive or synergistic effects increases.

Nursing considerations
- Advise against consuming alcohol while taking alprazolam.
- Before therapy starts, assess patient thoroughly for history or evidence of alcohol use.
- Watch for additive CNS effects, which may suggest benzodiazepine overdose.
- Other benzodiazepines interact with alcohol. If you suspect an interaction, consult prescriber or pharmacist.

alprazolam ◀▶ azole antifungals
Xanax   fluconazole, itraconazole,
                              ketoconazole, miconazole

Risk rating: 2
Severity: Moderate **Onset: Rapid** **Likelihood: Established**

Cause
Azole antifungals decrease CYP3A4 metabolism of certain benzodiazepines, such as alprazolam.

Effect
Benzodiazepine effects are increased and prolonged, which may cause CNS depression and psychomotor impairment.

Nursing considerations
◤ **ALERT** Use of alprazolam with itraconazole or ketoconazole is contraindicated.
- Various benzodiazepine–azole antifungal combinations may interact. If you suspect an interaction, consult prescriber or pharmacist.
- If patient takes fluconazole or miconazole, talk with prescriber about giving a lower benzodiazepine dose or a related drug not metabolized by CYP3A4, such as temazepam or lorazepam.

■ Caution that the effects of this interaction may last several days after stopping the azole antifungal.
■ Explain that taking these drugs together may increase sedative effects; tell patient to report such effects promptly.

---

alprazolam ▸◂ macrolide antibiotics
Xanax   clarithromycin, erythromycin

Risk rating: 2
Severity: Moderate   Onset: Rapid   Likelihood: Suspected

Cause
Macrolide antibiotics may decrease the metabolism of certain benzodiazepines, such as alprazolam.

Effect
Sedative effects of benzodiazepines may be increased or prolonged.

Nursing considerations
■ Talk with prescriber about decreasing benzodiazepine dosage during antibiotic therapy.
■ Lorazepam, oxazepam, and temazepam probably don't interact with macrolide antibiotics; substitution may be possible.
■ Urge patient to promptly report oversedation.

---

alprazolam ▸◂ nonnucleoside reverse-transcriptase inhibitors
Xanax   delavirdine, efavirenz

Risk rating: 2
Severity: Moderate   Onset: Delayed   Likelihood: Suspected

Cause
Nonnucleoside reverse-transcriptase inhibitors may inhibit CYP3A4 metabolism of certain benzodiazepines, such as alprazolam.

Effect
Sedative effects of benzodiazepines may be increased or prolonged, leading to respiratory depression.

Nursing considerations
⚡ **ALERT** Don't combine alprazolam with delavirdine or efavirenz.
■ Other benzodiazepines and nonnucleoside reverse-transcriptase inhibitors may interact. If you suspect an interaction, consult prescriber or pharmacist.
■ Explain the risk of oversedation and respiratory depression.

alprazolam ▄▄▄▄▄▶◀▄▄▄▄ protease inhibitors
Xanax

amprenavir, atazanavir, indinavir, lopinavir-ritonavir, nelfinavir, ritonavir, saquinavir

Risk rating: 2
Severity: Moderate   **Onset: Delayed**   **Likelihood: Suspected**

Cause
Protease inhibitors may inhibit CYP3A4 metabolism of certain benzodiazepines, such as alprazolam.

Effect
Sedative effects of benzodiazepines may be increased and prolonged, leading to severe respiratory depression.

Nursing considerations
▪ **ALERT** Don't combine alprazolam with protease inhibitors.
▪ If patient takes any benzodiazepine–protease inhibitor combination, notify prescriber. Interaction could involve other drugs in the class.
▪ Watch for evidence of oversedation and respiratory depression.
▪ Teach patient and family about the risks of using these drugs together.

alprazolam ▄▄▄▄▄▶◀▄▄▄▄ rifamycins
Xanax

rifabutin, rifampin, rifapentine

Risk rating: 2
Severity: Moderate   **Onset: Delayed**   **Likelihood: Suspected**

Cause
Rifamycins may increase CYP3A4 metabolism of benzodiazepines, such as alprazolam.

Effect
Antianxiety, sedative, and sleep-inducing effects of benzodiazepines may decrease.

Nursing considerations
▪ Watch for expected benzodiazepine effects and lack of efficacy.
▪ Other benzodiazepines may interact with rifamycins. If you suspect an interaction, consult prescriber or pharmacist.
▪ For insomnia, temazepam may be more effective than alprazolam because it doesn't undergo CYP3A4 metabolism.

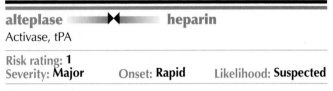

alteplase ◄► heparin
Activase, tPA

Risk rating: 1
Severity: **Major**   Onset: **Rapid**   Likelihood: **Suspected**

Cause
The combined effect of these drugs may be greater than the sum of their individual effects.

Effect
Risk of serious bleeding increases.

Nursing considerations
⚑ ALERT Use of heparin with alteplase is contraindicated.
⚑ ALERT Alteplase is contraindicated for acute ischemic stroke when patient has a bleeding diathesis, including the use of heparin within 48 hours before onset of stroke and when APTT is elevated. This increases risk of bleeding, disability, and death.

alteplase ◄► nitroglycerin
Activase, tPA   Minitran, Nitro-Bid, Nitro-Dur, NitroQuick, Nitrostat, Nitrotab

Risk rating: 1
Severity: **Major**   Onset: **Rapid**   Likelihood: **Probable**

Cause
Nitroglycerin may enhance hepatic blood flow, thereby increasing alteplase metabolism.

Effect
Alteplase level may decrease, interfering with thrombolytic effect.

Nursing considerations
▪ Don't use together, if possible.
▪ If use together is unavoidable, give nitroglycerin at the lowest effective dose.
▪ Monitor patient for inadequate thrombolytic effects.

alteplase ▶◀ warfarin
Activase, tPA   Coumadin

Risk rating: 1
Severity: Major   **Onset: Rapid**   **Likelihood: Suspected**

Cause
The combined effect of these drugs may be greater than the sum of their individual effects.

Effect
Risk of serious bleeding increases.

Nursing considerations
⚠ **ALERT** Alteplase is contraindicated for acute ischemic stroke when patient has a bleeding diathesis, including the use of oral anticoagulants. This increases risk of bleeding, disability, and death.
■ Alert prescriber that patient is also taking warfarin and use together is contraindicated.

aluminum salts ▶◀ penicillamine
aluminum carbonate,   Cuprimine, Depen
aluminum hydroxide,
attapulgite, kaolin,
magaldrate, sucralfate

Risk rating: 2
Severity: Moderate   **Onset: Delayed**   **Likelihood: Probable**

Cause
Formation of a physical or chemical complex with aluminum may decrease GI absorption of penicillamine.

Effect
Penicillamine efficacy may be reduced.

Nursing considerations
■ Separate administration times.
■ If patient must take these drugs together, notify prescriber. Penicillamine dose may need adjustment.
■ Help patient develop a daily plan to ensure proper intervals between drug doses.

aluminum salts ▬▶◀▬ tetracyclines

aluminum carbonate,
aluminum hydroxide,
attapulgite, kaolin,
magaldrate, sucralfate

doxycycline, minocycline,
tetracycline

Risk rating: 2
Severity: **Moderate**   Onset: **Delayed**   Likelihood: **Probable**

Cause
Formation of an insoluble chelate with aluminum may decrease
tetracycline absorption.

Effect
Tetracycline level may decline more than 50%, reducing efficacy.

Nursing considerations
■ Separate doses by at least 3 hours.
■ Monitor patient for reduced anti-infective response, including in-
fection flare-up, fever, and malaise.
■ Other tetracyclines may interact with aluminum salts. If you suspect
an interaction, consult prescriber or pharmacist.
■ Help patient develop a daily plan to ensure proper dosing intervals.

amikacin ▬▶◀▬ cephalosporins

Amikin

cefazolin, cefoperazone,
cefotaxime, cefotetan,
cefoxitin, ceftazidime,
ceftizoxime, ceftriaxone,
cefuroxime, cephradine

Risk rating: 2
Severity: **Moderate**   Onset: **Delayed**   Likelihood: **Suspected**

Cause
The mechanism of this interaction is unknown.

Effect
Bactericidal activity may increase against some organisms, but the
risk of nephrotoxicity also may increase.

Nursing considerations
◣ ALERT Check peak and trough aminoglycoside level after third
dose of amikacin. For peak level, draw blood 30 minutes after I.V. or
60 minutes after I.M. dose. For trough level, draw blood just before
a dose.

- Assess BUN and creatinine levels.
- Monitor urine output, and check urine for increased protein, cell, or cast levels.
- If renal insufficiency develops, notify prescriber. Dosage may need to be reduced, or drugs may need to be stopped.
- Other aminoglycosides may interact with cephalosporins. If you suspect an interaction, consult prescriber or pharmacist.

---

amikacin ▶◀ loop diuretics

Amikin

bumetanide, ethacrynic acid, furosemide, torsemide

Risk rating: 1
Severity: **Major**   Onset: **Rapid**   Likelihood: **Suspected**

Cause
The mechanism of the interaction is unknown.

Effect
Synergistic ototoxicity may cause hearing loss of varying degrees, possibly permanent.

Nursing considerations
- Permanent hearing loss is more likely with this combination than with either drug used alone.
- ⚡ **ALERT** Renal insufficiency increases the risk of ototoxicity.
- Perform baseline and periodic hearing function tests.
- Aminoglycosides other than amikacin may interact with loop diuretics. If you suspect an interaction, consult prescriber or pharmacist.
- Tell patient to immediately report ringing or roaring in the ears, muffled sounds, or any noticeable changes in hearing.
- Advise family members to stay alert for evidence of hearing loss.

---

amikacin ▶◀ nondepolarizing muscle relaxants

Amikin

atracurium, mivacurium, pancuronium, rocuronium, vecuronium

Risk rating: 1
Severity: **Major**   Onset: **Rapid**   Likelihood: **Probable**

Cause
These drugs may be synergistic.

Effect
Effects of nondepolarizing muscle relaxants may increase.

Nursing considerations
■ The nondepolarizing muscle relaxant dose may need adjustment based on neuromuscular response.
■ Monitor patient for prolonged respiratory depression.
■ Provide ventilatory support as needed.

---

amikacin ►◄	NSAIDs
Amikin	diclofenac, etodolac, fenoprofen, flurbiprofen, ibuprofen, indomethacin, ketoprofen, ketorolac, nabumetone, naproxen, oxaprozin, piroxicam, sulindac, tolmetin

Risk rating: 2
Severity: **Moderate**   Onset: **Delayed**   Likelihood: **Suspected**

Cause
NSAIDs may reduce glomerular filtration rate (GFR), causing aminoglycosides, such as amikacin, to accumulate.

Effect
Aminoglycoside level in premature infants may increase.

Nursing considerations
■ Before NSAID therapy starts, aminoglycoside dose should be reduced.
⚡ ALERT Check peak and trough aminoglycoside level after third dose. For peak level, draw blood 30 minutes after I.V. or 60 minutes after I.M. dose. For trough level, draw blood just before a dose.
■ Monitor patient's renal function.
■ Although only indomethacin is known to interact with aminoglycosides, other NSAIDs probably do as well. If you suspect an interaction, consult prescriber or pharmacist.
■ Other drugs cleared by GFR may have a similar interaction.

amikacin ━━━▶◀━━━ penicillins

Amikin

ampicillin, oxacillin, nafcillin, penicillin G, piperacillin, ticarcillin

Risk rating: 2
Severity: Moderate   **Onset: Delayed**   **Likelihood: Probable**

Cause
The mechanism of this interaction is unknown.

Effect
Penicillins may inactivate certain aminoglycosides, such as amikacin, decreasing their therapeutic effects.

Nursing considerations
◪ ALERT Check peak and trough aminoglycoside level after third dose. For peak level, draw blood 30 minutes after I.V. or 60 minutes after I.M. dose. For trough level, draw blood just before a dose.
■ Monitor patient's renal function.
■ Other aminoglycosides may interact with penicillins. If you suspect an interaction, consult prescriber or pharmacist.
■ Penicillins affect gentamicin and tobramycin more than amikacin.

amikacin ━━━▶◀━━━ succinylcholine

Amikin

Anectine, Quelicin

Risk rating: 2
Severity: Moderate   **Onset: Rapid**   **Likelihood: Probable**

Cause
Aminoglycosides, such as amikacin, may stabilize the postjunctional membrane and disrupt prejunctional calcium influx and acetylcholine output, thereby causing a synergistic interaction with succinylcholine.

Effect
Neuromuscular effects of succinylcholine increase.

Nursing considerations
◪ ALERT Patients with renal impairment and those receiving aminoglycosides by peritoneal instillation have an increased risk of prolonged neuromuscular blockade.
■ After succinylcholine use, delay aminoglycoside delivery as long as possible after adequate respirations return.
■ If drugs must be given together, use extreme caution and monitor respiratory status closely.

■ If respiratory depression occurs, patient may need mechanical ventilation. Give I.V. calcium or a cholinesterase inhibitor if needed.

---

amiloride ▬▬►◄▬▬ ACE inhibitors

Midamor

benazepril, captopril, enalapril, fosinopril, lisinopril, moexipril, perindopril, quinapril, ramipril, trandolapril

Risk rating: 1
Severity: Major   **Onset: Delayed**   **Likelihood: Probable**

Cause
The mechanism of this interaction is unknown.

Effect
Serum potassium level may increase.

Nursing considerations
■ Use cautiously in patients at high risk for hyperkalemia, especially those with renal impairment.
■ Monitor BUN, creatinine, and serum potassium levels as needed.
■ Other ACE inhibitors may interact with potassium-sparing diuretics, such as amiloride. If you suspect an interaction, consult prescriber or pharmacist.
■ Urge patient to immediately report an irregular heart beat, a slow pulse, weakness, and other evidence of hyperkalemia.

---

amiloride ▬▬►◄▬▬ angiotensin II receptor antagonists

Midamor

candesartan, eprosartan, irbesartan, losartan, olmesartan, telmisartan, valsartan

Risk rating: 1
Severity: Major   **Onset: Delayed**   **Likelihood: Suspected**

Cause
Both angiotensin II receptor antagonists and potassium-sparing diuretics, such as amiloride, may increase serum potassium level.

Effect
Risk of hyperkalemia may increase, especially among high-risk patients.

Nursing considerations

■ High-risk patients include elderly people and those with renal impairment, type 2 diabetes, or decreased renal perfusion; monitor these patients closely.

■ Check serum potassium, BUN, and creatinine levels regularly. If they increase, notify prescriber.

■ Advise patient to immediately report an irregular heart beat, slow pulse, weakness, or other evidence of hyperkalemia.

■ Give patient a list of foods high in potassium; stress the need to eat only moderate amounts.

---

amiloride ▸◂ potassium preparations

Midamor

potassium acetate, potassium bicarbonate, potassium chloride, potassium citrate, potassium gluconate, potassium iodine, potassium phosphate

Risk rating: 1
Severity: Major   Onset: **Delayed**   Likelihood: **Established**

Cause
This interaction reduces renal elimination of potassium ions.

Effect
Risk of severe hyperkalemia increases.

Nursing considerations
⚑ ALERT Don't use this combination unless patient has severe hypokalemia that isn't responding to either drug class alone.

■ To avoid hyperkalemia, monitor potassium level when therapy starts and often thereafter.

■ Tell patient to avoid high-potassium foods, such as citrus juices, bananas, spinach, broccoli, beans, potatoes, and salt substitutes.

■ Urge patient to immediately report palpitations, chest pain, nausea, vomiting, paresthesias, muscle weakness, and other signs of potassium overload.

amiodarone ➤◄ cyclosporine

Cordarone, Pacerone Gengraf, Neoral, Sandimmune

Risk rating: 2
Severity: Moderate   **Onset: Delayed**   **Likelihood: Suspected**

Cause
Amiodarone probably inhibits cyclosporine metabolism.

Effect
Cyclosporine level and risk of nephrotoxicity may increase.

Nursing considerations
■ Closely monitor cyclosporine level when amiodarone is started, stopped, or the dose is changed.
■ Because amiodarone has a long half-life, monitor cyclosporine level for several weeks after dosage changes.
■ Dosage reductions of cyclosporine (up to 50% in some cases) may be needed to keep cyclosporine level in the desired range.
■ Monitor BUN and creatinine levels and urine output.

amiodarone ➤◄ digoxin

Cordarone, Pacerone Lanoxin

Risk rating: 1
Severity: Major   **Onset: Delayed**   **Likelihood: Probable**

Cause
The mechanism of this interaction is unknown.

Effect
Digoxin level and risk of toxicity may increase.

Nursing considerations
■ Watch for evidence of digoxin toxicity, such as arrhythmias, nausea, vomiting, and agitation.
■ Monitor digoxin level.
■ Digoxin dosage may need reduction during amiodarone treatment.
■ Because amiodarone has a long half-life, the effects of the interaction may persist after amiodarone is stopped.

amiodarone ▶◀ fentanyl

Cordarone, Pacerone   Sublimaze

Risk rating: 1
Severity: Major   **Onset: Rapid**   **Likelihood: Suspected**

Cause
The mechanism of this interaction is unknown.

Effect
Patient may develop profound bradycardia, sinus arrest, and hypotension.

Nursing considerations
■ It isn't known if these effects are related to fentanyl anesthesia or anesthesia in general; use together cautiously.
■ Monitor hemodynamic function.
■ Keep inotropic, chronotropic, and pressor support available.
◼ **ALERT** The bradycardia caused by this interaction usually doesn't respond to atropine.

amiodarone ▶◀ hydantoins

Cordarone, Pacerone   ethotoin, fosphenytoin,
                             phenytoin

Risk rating: 2
Severity: Moderate   **Onset: Delayed**   **Likelihood: Probable**

Cause
Hydantoin metabolism may decrease. Amiodarone metabolism may increase.

Effect
Serum hydantoin level and risk of toxicity increases, and amiodarone level decreases.

Nursing considerations
■ The therapeutic range of phenytoin is 10 to 20 mcg/ml. Patients with decreased protein binding may show signs of toxicity despite a "normal" phenytoin level. Free phenytoin level is a better indicator in these patients (range: 1 to 2 mcg/ml).
◼ **ALERT** Signs and symptoms of toxicity may progress in the following manner: nystagmus, ataxia, slurred speech, nausea, vomiting, lethargy, confusion, seizures, and coma.
■ After adjusting dosage of either drug, patient will need long-term monitoring because effects may be delayed several weeks.

■ Watch for loss of amiodarone effect, including palpitations, shortness of breath, dizziness, and chest pain.

---

amiodarone ▶◀ protease inhibitors

Cordarone, Pacerone

amprenavir, atazanavir, indinavir, lopinavir-ritonavir, nelfinavir, ritonavir, saquinavir

Risk rating: 1
Severity: Major   **Onset: Delayed**   **Likelihood: Suspected**

Cause
Protease inhibitors inhibit the CYP3A4 metabolism of amiodarone.

Effect
Amiodarone level increases, increasing the risk of toxicity.

Nursing considerations
◢ **ALERT** Ritonavir and nelfinavir are contraindicated for use with amiodarone because of large increase in amiodarone level.
■ Use other protease inhibitors cautiously; they may have a similar effect.
■ Increased amiodarone level may prolong the QT interval and cause life-threatening arrhythmias.
■ Monitor ECG and QTc interval closely during combined therapy.
■ Tell patient to immediately report slowed pulse or fainting.

---

amiodarone ▶◀ quinolones

Cordarone, Pacerone

gatifloxacin, levofloxacin, moxifloxacin, sparfloxacin

Risk rating: 1
Severity: Major   **Onset: Delayed**   **Likelihood: Suspected**

Cause
The mechanism of this interaction is unknown.

Effect
Risk of life-threatening arrhythmias, including torsades de pointes, increases.

Nursing considerations
◢ **ALERT** Use of sparfloxacin with an antiarrhythmic, such as amiodarone, is contraindicated.
■ Quinolones that aren't metabolized by CYP3A4 isoenzymes or that don't prolong the QT interval may be given with antiarrhythmics.

■ Avoid giving class IA or class III antiarrhythmics with gatifloxacin, levofloxacin, and moxifloxacin.

■ Tell patient to report a rapid heart rate, shortness of breath, dizziness, fainting, and chest pain.

---

amiodarone ◄►► vardenafil
Cordarone, Pacerone   Levitra

Risk rating: 1
Severity: Major   **Onset: Rapid**   **Likelihood: Suspected**

Cause
The mechanism of this interaction is unknown.

Effect
The QTc interval may be prolonged, particularly in patients with previous QT-interval prolongation, increasing the risk of such life-threatening cardiac arrhythmias as torsades de pointes.

Nursing considerations
⚑ ALERT Use of vardenafil with amiodarone or another class IA or class III antiarrhythmic is contraindicated.

■ Monitor patient's ECG before and periodically after patient starts taking vardenafil.

■ Urge patient to report light-headedness, faintness, palpitations, and chest pain or pressure while taking vardenafil.

■ To reduce risk of adverse effects, patients age 65 and older should start with 5 mg vardenafil, half the usual starting dose.

---

amiodarone ◄►► warfarin
Cordarone, Pacerone   Coumadin

Risk rating: 1
Severity: Major   **Onset: Delayed**   **Likelihood: Established**

Cause
Amiodarone inhibits CYP1A2 and CYP2C9 metabolism of warfarin.

Effect
Anticoagulant effects increase.

Nursing considerations
■ Monitor patient closely for bleeding. Urge compliance with required blood tests.

⚑ ALERT Check INR closely during first 6 to 8 weeks of amiodarone therapy. Warfarin dosage reduction depends on escalating

amiodarone dosage. Typically, warfarin dose needs 30% to 50% reduction.
- If amiodarone is stopped, these effects may persist up to 4 months, requiring continual warfarin adjustment.
- Tell patient and family to watch for signs of bleeding or abnormal bruising and to call prescriber at once if they occur.
- Advise the use of an electric razor and a soft toothbrush.
- Tell patient to wear or carry medical identification that says he takes an anticoagulant.

---

amitriptyline ➤◀ azole antifungals
fluconazole, ketoconazole

Risk rating: 2
Severity: **Moderate**   Onset: **Delayed**   Likelihood: **Suspected**

Cause
Azole antifungals may inhibit metabolism of tricyclic antidepressants (TCAs), such as amitriptyline, by cytochrome P-450 pathways.

Effect
Serum TCA level and risk of toxicity may increase.

Nursing considerations
- When starting or stopping an azole antifungal, monitor serum TCA level and adjust dosage as needed.
- After starting an azole antifungal, check sitting and standing blood pressure for changes.
- If patient takes a TCA and an azole antifungal, assess symptoms and behavior for evidence of adverse reactions, such as increased drowsiness, dizziness, confusion, heart rate or rhythm changes, and urine retention.

---

amitriptyline ➤◀ fluoxetine
Prozac, Sarafem

Risk rating: 2
Severity: **Moderate**   Onset: **Delayed**   Likelihood: **Probable**

Cause
Fluoxetine may inhibit hepatic metabolism of tricyclic antidepressants (TCAs), such as amitriptyline.

Effect
Serum TCA level and toxicity may increase.

Nursing considerations
■ Monitor TCA level; watch for evidence of toxicity, such as increased anticholinergic effects, delirium, dizziness, drowsiness, and psychosis.
■ If TCA starts when patient already takes fluoxetine, TCA dosage may need to be decreased by up to 75% to avoid interaction.
■ Other TCAs may interact with fluoxetine. If you suspect an interaction, consult prescriber or pharmacist.

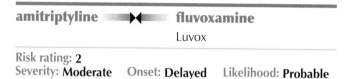

amitriptyline ▶◀ fluvoxamine
Luvox

Risk rating: 2
Severity: Moderate   **Onset: Delayed**   **Likelihood: Probable**

Cause
Fluvoxamine may inhibit oxidative metabolism of tricyclic antidepressants (TCAs), such as amitriptyline, via the CYP2D6 pathway.

Effect
TCA level and risk of toxicity increase.

Nursing considerations
■ When starting or stopping fluvoxamine, monitor serum TCA level.
■ Inhibitory effects of fluvoxamine may take up to 2 weeks to dissipate after drug is stopped.
■ Using desipramine may avoid this interaction.
■ Urge patient and family to watch for and report increased anticholinergic effects, dizziness, drowsiness, and psychosis.

amitriptyline ▶◀ MAO inhibitors
isocarboxazid, phenelzine, tranylcypromine

Risk rating: 1
Severity: Major   **Onset: Rapid**   **Likelihood: Suspected**

Cause
The mechanism of this interaction is unknown.

Effect
The risk of hyperpyretic crisis, seizures, and death increase.

Nursing considerations
⚡ **ALERT** Don't give a tricyclic antidepressant (TCA), such as amitriptyline, with or within 2 weeks of an MAO inhibitor.

■ Watch for adverse effects, including confusion, hyperexcitability, rigidity, seizures, increased temperature, increased pulse, increased respiration, sweating, mydriasis, flushing, headache, coma, and DIC.

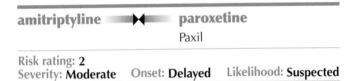

amitriptyline ▶◀ paroxetine
Paxil

Risk rating: 2
Severity: **Moderate**   Onset: **Delayed**   Likelihood: **Suspected**

Cause
Paroxetine may decrease metabolism of tricyclic antidepressants (TCAs), such as amitriptyline, in some people and increase it in others.

Effect
Therapeutic and toxic effects of certain TCAs may increase.

Nursing considerations
■ When starting or stopping paroxetine, monitor TCA level and adjust dosage as needed.
■ If patient takes a TCA and paroxetine, assess symptoms and behavior for adverse reactions, such as increased drowsiness, dizziness, confusion, heart rate or rhythm changes, and urine retention.
■ Watch closely for evidence of serotonin syndrome, such as delirium, bizarre movements, and tachycardia. Alert prescriber if they occur.

amitriptyline ▶◀ quinolones
gatifloxacin, levofloxacin, moxifloxacin, sparfloxacin

Risk rating: 1
Severity: **Major**   Onset: **Delayed**   Likelihood: **Suspected**

Cause
The mechanism of this interaction is unknown.

Effect
Life-threatening cardiac arrhythmias, including torsades de pointes, may increase when certain of these drugs are used together.

Nursing considerations
⚡ ALERT Sparfloxacin is contraindicated in patients taking a tricyclic antidepressant (TCA), such as amitriptyline, because QTc interval may be prolonged.

⚡ **ALERT** Avoid giving levofloxacin with a TCA.
■ Use gatifloxacin and moxifloxacin cautiously with TCAs.
■ If possible, use other quinolone antibiotics that don't prolong the QTc interval or aren't metabolized by the CYP3A4 isoenzyme.

---

amitriptyline ▶◀ rifamycins
rifabutin, rifampin

Risk rating: 2
Severity: Moderate   **Onset: Delayed**   **Likelihood: Suspected**

Cause
Metabolism of tricyclic antidepressants (TCAs), such as amitriptyline, in the liver may increase.

Effect
TCA level and efficacy may decrease.

Nursing considerations
■ When starting, stopping, or changing the dosage of a rifamycin, monitor serum TCA level to maintain therapeutic range.
■ Watch for resolution of depression as TCA dosage is adjusted to therapeutic level during rifamycin therapy.
■ Urge patient and family to watch for adverse reactions, including increased drowsiness and dizziness, for several weeks after rifamycin stops. Tell them to notify prescriber promptly.
■ Other TCAs may interact with rifamycins. If you suspect an interaction, consult prescriber or pharmacist.

---

amitriptyline ▶◀ sertraline
Zoloft

Risk rating: 2
Severity: Moderate   **Onset: Delayed**   **Likelihood: Suspected**

Cause
Hepatic metabolism of tricyclic antidepressants (TCAs), such as amitriptyline, by CYP2D6 may be inhibited.

Effect
Therapeutic and toxic effects of certain TCAs may increase.

Nursing considerations
■ If possible, avoid this drug combination.
■ If these drugs must be used together, watch for evidence of TCA toxicity and serotonin syndrome.

- Signs of serotonin syndrome include delirium, bizarre movements, and tachycardia.
- Monitor serum TCA levels when starting or stopping sertraline.
- If abnormalities occur, decrease TCA dosage or stop drug.

---

amitriptyline ▶◀ sympathomimetics

direct: dobutamine, epinephrine, norepinephrine, phenylephrine
mixed: dopamine, ephedrine

Risk rating: 2
Severity: Moderate   Onset: Rapid   Likelihood: Established

Cause
Tricyclic antidepressants (TCAs), such as amitriptyline, increase the effects of direct-acting sympathomimetics and decrease the effects of indirect-acting sympathomimetics.

Effect
When sympathomimetic effects increase, the risk of hypertension and arrhythmias increases. When sympathomimetic effects decrease, blood pressure control decreases.

Nursing considerations
- If possible, avoid using these drugs together.
- Watch patient closely for hypertension and heart rhythm changes; they may warrant reduction of sympathomimetic dosage.
- If patient takes a mixed-acting sympathomimetic, watch for negative effects; dosage may need to be altered.
- Other TCAs and sympathomimetics may interact. If you suspect an interaction, consult prescriber or pharmacist.

---

amitriptyline ▶◀ valproic acid

divalproex sodium, valproate sodium, valproic acid

Risk rating: 2
Severity: Moderate   Onset: Delayed   Likelihood: Suspected

Cause
Valproic acid may inhibit hepatic metabolism of tricyclic antidepressants (TCAs), such as amitriptyline.

Effect
Level and adverse effects of TCAs may increase.

Nursing considerations
- Use these drugs together cautiously.
- If patient is stable on valproic acid, start TCA at reduced dosage and adjust upward slowly to address symptoms and serum level.
- If patient is stable on a TCA, monitor serum level and patient status closely when starting or stopping valproic acid.
- Explain signs and symptoms to watch for.
- Other TCAs may interact with valproic acid. If you suspect an interaction, consult prescriber or pharmacist.

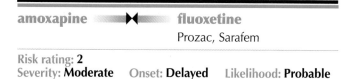

amoxapine ◄► **fluoxetine**
Prozac, Sarafem

Risk rating: 2
Severity: Moderate   **Onset: Delayed**   **Likelihood: Probable**

Cause
Fluoxetine may inhibit hepatic metabolism of tricyclic antidepressants (TCAs), such as amoxapine.

Effect
Serum TCA level and toxicity may increase.

Nursing considerations
- Monitor serum TCA level and watch closely for evidence of toxicity, such as increased anticholinergic effects, delirium, dizziness, drowsiness, and psychosis.
- If TCA starts in patient who already takes fluoxetine, TCA dosage may need to be decreased by up to 75% to avoid interaction.
- Other TCAs may interact with fluoxetine. If you suspect an interaction, consult prescriber or pharmacist.

amoxapine ◄► **MAO inhibitors**
isocarboxazid, phenelzine, tranylcypromine

Risk rating: 1
Severity: Major   **Onset: Rapid**   **Likelihood: Suspected**

Cause
The mechanism of this interaction is unknown.

Effect
The risk of hyperpyretic crisis, seizures, and death increases.

Nursing considerations

🔌 ALERT Don't give a tricyclic antidepressant (TCA), such as amoxapine, with or within 2 weeks of an MAO inhibitor.

■ Watch for adverse effects, including confusion, hyperexcitability, rigidity, seizures, increased temperature, increased pulse, increased respiration, sweating, mydriasis, flushing, headache, coma, and DIC.

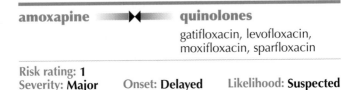

amoxapine ◀▶ **quinolones**
gatifloxacin, levofloxacin, moxifloxacin, sparfloxacin

Risk rating: 1
Severity: Major   **Onset: Delayed**   **Likelihood: Suspected**

Cause
The mechanism of this interaction is unknown.

Effect
Risk of life-threatening arrhythmias, including torsades de pointes, may increase when certain of these drugs are used together.

Nursing considerations
🔌 ALERT Sparfloxacin is contraindicated in patients taking a tricyclic antidepressant (TCA), such as amoxapine, because QTc interval may be prolonged.

🔌 ALERT Avoid giving levofloxacin with a TCA.

■ Use gatifloxacin and moxifloxacin cautiously with TCAs.

■ If possible, use other quinolone antibiotics that don't prolong the QTc interval or aren't metabolized by the CYP3A4 isoenzyme.

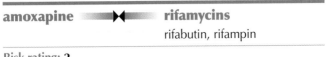

amoxapine ◀▶ **rifamycins**
rifabutin, rifampin

Risk rating: 2
Severity: Moderate   **Onset: Delayed**   **Likelihood: Suspected**

Cause
Metabolism of tricyclic antidepressants (TCAs), such as amoxapine, in the liver may increase.

Effect
TCA level and efficacy may decrease.

Nursing considerations
■ When starting, stopping, or changing the dosage of a rifamycin, monitor serum TCA level to maintain therapeutic range.
■ Watch for resolution of depression as TCA dosage is adjusted to therapeutic level during rifamycin therapy.
■ Urge patient and family to watch for adverse reactions, including increased drowsiness and dizziness, for several weeks after rifamycin stops. Tell them to notify prescriber promptly.
■ Other TCAs may interact with rifamycins. If you suspect an interaction, consult prescriber or pharmacist.

---

amoxapine ■━━►◄━━ sertraline
Zoloft

Risk rating: 2
Severity: Moderate   **Onset: Delayed**   **Likelihood: Suspected**

Cause
Hepatic metabolism of tricyclic antidepressants (TCAs), such as amoxapine, by CYP2D6 may be inhibited.

Effect
Therapeutic and toxic effects of certain TCAs may increase.

Nursing considerations
■ If possible, avoid this drug combination.
■ Watch for evidence of TCA toxicity and serotonin syndrome.
■ Signs of serotonin syndrome include delirium, bizarre movements, and tachycardia.
■ Monitor serum TCA level when starting or stopping sertraline.

---

amoxapine ■━━►◄━━ sympathomimetics
direct: dobutamine, epinephrine, norepinephrine, phenylephrine
mixed: dopamine, ephedrine

Risk rating: 2
Severity: Moderate   **Onset: Rapid**   **Likelihood: Established**

Cause
Tricyclic antidepressants (TCAs), such as amoxapine, increase the effects of direct-acting sympathomimetics and decrease the effects of indirect-acting sympathomimetics.

Effect
When sympathomimetic effects increase, the risk of hypertension and arrhythmias increases. When sympathomimetic effects decrease, blood pressure control decreases.

Nursing considerations
- If possible, avoid using these drugs together.
- Watch patient closely for hypertension and heart rhythm changes; they may warrant reduction of sympathomimetic dosage.
- If patient takes a mixed-acting sympathomimetic, watch for negative effects; dosage may need to be altered.
- Other TCAs and sympathomimetics may interact. If you suspect an interaction, consult prescriber or pharmacist.

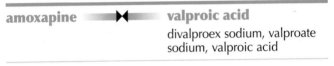

amoxapine ▶◀ valproic acid
divalproex sodium, valproate sodium, valproic acid

Risk rating: 2
Severity: Moderate   **Onset: Delayed**   **Likelihood: Suspected**

Cause
Valproic acid may inhibit hepatic metabolism of tricyclic antidepressants (TCAs), such as amoxapine.

Effect
Level and adverse effects of TCAs may increase.

Nursing considerations
- Use these drugs together cautiously.
- If patient is stable on a TCA, monitor serum level and patient status closely when starting or stopping valproic acid.
- Explain signs and symptoms to watch for.
- Other TCAs may interact with valproic acid. If you suspect an interaction, consult prescriber or pharmacist.

amoxicillin ▶◀ tetracyclines
Amoxil
demeclocycline, doxycycline, minocycline, tetracycline

Risk rating: 1
Severity: Major   **Onset: Delayed**   **Likelihood: Suspected**

Cause
Tetracyclines may disrupt bactericidal activity of penicillins, such as amoxicillin.

Effect
Penicillin efficacy may be reduced.

Nursing considerations
- If possible, avoid giving tetracyclines with penicillins.
- Monitor patient closely for lack of penicillin effect.

---

amphetamine ▶◀ MAO inhibitors
Adderall   phenelzine, tranylcypromine

Risk rating: 1
Severity: **Major**   Onset: **Rapid**   Likelihood: **Suspected**

Cause
This interaction probably stems from increased norepinephrine level at the synaptic cleft.

Effect
Anorexiant effects increase.

Nursing considerations
- If possible, avoid giving these drugs together.
- Headache and severe hypertension may occur rapidly if amphetamine is given to patient who takes an MAO inhibitor.
- ⚠ ALERT Several deaths have resulted from hypertensive crisis and resulting cerebral hemorrhage.
- Monitor patient for hypotension, hyperpyrexia, and seizures.
- Hypertensive reaction may occur for several weeks after stopping an MAO inhibitor.

---

amphetamine ▶◀ serotonin reuptake inhibitors
Adderall   fluoxetine, fluvoxamine, paroxetine, sertraline

Risk rating: 1
Severity: **Major**   Onset: **Rapid**   Likelihood: **Suspected**

Cause
The mechanism of this interaction is unknown.

Effect
Sympathomimetic effects and the risk of serotonin syndrome increase.

Nursing considerations
- If these drugs must be used together, watch closely for increased CNS effects, such as anxiety, jitteriness, agitation, and restlessness.
- Mild serotonin-like symptoms may develop, including confuson, diaphoresis, restlessness, tremor, and muscle twitching.
- Inform patient of the risk of interaction.
- Describe the traits of serotonin syndrome, including confusion, restlessness, incoordination, muscle rigidity, fever, sweating, and tremors.

---

amphetamine ▶◀ urine alkalinizers
Adderall

potassium citrate, sodium acetate, sodium bicarbonate, sodium citrate, sodium lactate, tromethamine

Risk rating: 2
Severity: Moderate   **Onset: Rapid**   **Likelihood: Established**

Cause
When urine is alkaline, amphetamine clearance is prolonged.

Effect
In amphetamine overdose, the toxic period will be extended, increasing the risk of injury.

Nursing considerations
- **ALERT** Avoid drugs that may alkalinize the urine, particularly during amphetamine overdose.
- Watch for evidence of amphetamine toxicity, such as dermatoses, marked insomnia, irritability, hyperactivity, and personality changes.
- If patient takes an anorexiant, advise against excessive use of sodium bicarbonate as an antacid.

---

ampicillin ▶◀ allopurinol
Principen

Aloprim, Zyloprim

Risk rating: 2
Severity: Moderate   **Onset: Delayed**   **Likelihood: Suspected**

Cause
The mechanism of this interaction is unknown.

Effect
Risk of ampicillin-induced rash increases.

Nursing considerations
■ Penicillins other than ampicillin may have a similar interaction with allopurinol. Discuss any concerns with prescriber or pharmacist.
◤ ALERT Notify prescriber if a rash appears. A lower dose of allopurinol or a different drug may be needed.
■ Inform patient of this interaction so he can watch for skin changes.

---

ampicillin ◄►◄ aminoglycosides
Principen

amikacin, gentamicin, kanamycin, streptomycin, tobramycin

Risk rating: 2
Severity: Moderate   **Onset: Delayed**   **Likelihood: Probable**

Cause
The mechanism of this interaction is unknown.

Effect
Penicillins, such as ampicillin, may inactivate certain aminoglycosides, decreasing their therapeutic effects.

Nursing considerations
◤ ALERT Check peak and trough aminoglycoside level after third dose. For peak level, draw blood 30 minutes after I.V. or 60 minutes after I.M. dose. For trough level, draw blood just before a dose.
■ Monitor patient's renal function.
■ Other aminoglycosides may interact with penicillins. If you suspect an interaction, consult prescriber or pharmacist.
■ Penicillins affect gentamicin and tobramycin more than amikacin.

---

ampicillin ◄►◄ atenolol
Principen

Tenormin

Risk rating: 2
Severity: Moderate   **Onset: Rapid**   **Likelihood: Suspected**

Cause
Ampicillin may impair GI absorption of atenolol.

Effect
Usual blood pressure lowering and antianginal effects of atenolol may be decreased.

Nursing considerations
■ Beta blockers other than atenolol and penicillins other than ampi-

cillin may have this interaction. If you suspect a drug interaction, consult prescriber or pharmacist.
- Suggest that patient separate doses to decrease GI interaction.
- Notify prescriber if blood pressure increases; atenolol dosage may be increased or ampicillin broken into smaller, more frequent doses.
- Teach patient to report increased episodes or severity of chest pain to prescriber immediately.

ampicillin ▶◀ food

Principen

Risk rating: 2
Severity: Moderate   Onset: Delayed   Likelihood: Suspected

Cause
Food may delay or reduce GI absorption of certain penicillins, such as ampicillin.

Effect
Penicillin efficacy may decrease.

Nursing considerations
- Food may affect penicillin absorption and peak level.
- If patient took ampicillin with food, watch for lack of drug efficacy.
- Tell patient to take penicillin 1 hour before or 2 hours after a meal.
- Other penicillins may interact with food. If you suspect an interaction, consult prescriber or pharmacist.

ampicillin ▶◀ tetracyclines

Principen   demeclocycline, doxycycline, minocycline, tetracycline

Risk rating: 1
Severity: Major   Onset: Delayed   Likelihood: Suspected

Cause
Tetracyclines may disrupt bactericidal activity of penicillins, such as ampicillin.

Effect
Penicillin efficacy may be reduced.

Nursing considerations
- If possible, avoid giving tetracyclines with penicillins.
- Monitor patient closely for lack of penicillin effect.

amprenavir ▶◀ azole antifungals

Agenerase

fluconazole, itraconazole,
ketoconazole

Risk rating: 2
Severity: Moderate **Onset: Delayed** **Likelihood: Suspected**

Cause
Azole antifungals may inhibit metabolism of protease inhibitors, such
as amprenavir.

Effect
Protease inhibitor plasma level may increase.

Nursing considerations
- Protease inhibitor dosage may be decreased when therapy starts.
- Monitor patient for increased protease inhibitor effects, including
hyperglycemia, rash, GI complaints, and altered liver function tests.
- Advise patient to report increased hunger or thirst, frequent urina-
tion, fatigue, and dry, itchy skin.
- Tell patient not to change dosage or stop either drug without con-
sulting prescriber.
- To help avoid interactions, urge patient to tell prescribers about all
drugs and supplements he takes.

amprenavir ▶◀ benzodiazepines

Agenerase

alprazolam, chlordiazepoxide,
clonazepam, clorazepate,
diazepam, estazolam,
flurazepam, midazolam,
quazepam, triazolam

Risk rating: 2
Severity: Moderate **Onset: Delayed** **Likelihood: Suspected**

Cause
Protease inhibitors, such as amprenavir, may inhibit CYP3A4 metabolism of certain benzodiazepines.

Effect
Sedative effects of benzodiazepines may be increased and prolonged,
leading to severe respiratory depression.

Nursing considerations
◼ ALERT Don't combine listed benzodiazepines with protease inhibitors.

- If patient takes any benzodiazepine–protease inhibitor combination, notify prescriber. Interaction could involve other drugs in the class.
- Watch for evidence of oversedation and respiratory depression.
- Explain the risks of using these drugs together.

---

amprenavir ►◄ delavirdine

Agenerase   Rescriptor

Risk rating: 2
Severity: Moderate   Onset: Delayed   Likelihood: Suspected

Cause
Amprenavir may induce CYP3A4 metabolism of delavirdine. Delavirdine may inhibit CYP3A4 metabolism of amprenavir.

Effect
Amprenavir level may increase. Delavirdine level may decrease.

Nursing considerations
- Monitor patient for a decreased response to delavirdine.
- Tell patient the most common adverse reactions from this interaction are headache, fatigue, rash, and GI complaints.
- Caution patient to notify prescriber if side effects are bothersome and to not alter his treatment regimen without medical consent.
- To help avoid interactions, urge patient to tell prescribers about all drugs and supplements he takes.

---

amprenavir ►◄ ergot derivatives

Agenerase   dihydroergotamine, ergonovine, ergotamine, methylergonovine

Risk rating: 1
Severity: Major   Onset: Delayed   Likelihood: Probable

Cause
Protease inhibitors, such as amprenavir, may interfere with CYP3A4 metabolism of ergot derivatives.

Effect
Risk of ergot-induced peripheral vasospasm and ischemia may increase.

Nursing considerations
⚑ ALERT Use of ergot derivatives with protease inhibitors is contraindicated.

■ Monitor patient for evidence of peripheral ischemia, including pain in limb muscles while exercising and later at rest; numbness and tingling of fingers and toes; cool, pale, or cyanotic limbs; red or violet blisters on hands or feet; and gangrene.

■ Sodium nitroprusside may be used to treat ergot-induced vasospasm.

■ If patient takes a protease inhibitor, consult prescriber and pharmacist about alternative migraine treatments.

■ Advise patient to tell prescriber about all drugs and supplements he takes and any increase in adverse effects.

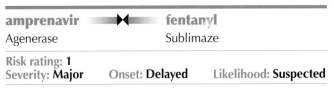

amprenavir ▶◀ fentanyl
Agenerase   Sublimaze

Risk rating: 1
Severity: Major   **Onset: Delayed**   **Likelihood: Suspected**

Cause
Metabolism of fentanyl in the GI tract and liver may be inhibited.

Effect
Fentanyl level may increase and half-life may lengthen.

Nursing considerations
⚡ ALERT If patient takes a protease inhibitor, such as amprenavir, watch closely for respiratory depression if fentanyl is added.

■ Because fentanyl half-life may be prolonged, monitoring period should be extended, even after fentanyl is stopped.

■ Keep naloxone available to treat respiratory depression.

■ If fentanyl is continuously infused, dosage should be decreased.

amprenavir ▶◀ HMG-CoA reductase inhibitors
Agenerase

atorvastatin, lovastatin, simvastatin

Risk rating: 1 lovastatin, simvastatin
              2 atorvastatin
Severity: Major   **Onset: Delayed**   **Likelihood: Suspected**
          lovastatin,
          simvastatin
          Moderate
          atorvastatin

Cause
Metabolism of HMG-CoA reductase inhibitors may be inhibited.

Effect
HMG-CoA reductase inhibitor level may increase.

Nursing considerations
■ Monitor patient closely if a protease inhibitor, such as amprenavir, is added to HMG-CoA reductase inhibitor therapy.

◣ ALERT Watch for evidence of rhabdomyolysis, including dark or red urine, muscle weakness, and myalgia.

■ Tell patient to immediately report unexplained muscle weakness.

■ To help avoid interactions, urge patient to tell prescribers about all drugs and supplements he takes.

---

amprenavir ▶◀ nevirapine
Agenerase   Viramune

Risk rating: 2
Severity: Major   **Onset: Delayed**   **Likelihood: Suspected**

Cause
Nevirapine may increase hepatic metabolism of protease inhibitors, such as amprenavir.

Effect
Protease inhibitor level and effects decrease.

Nursing considerations
■ If nevirapine is started or stopped, monitor protease inhibitor level closely.

■ Protease inhibitor dosage may need adjustment.

■ Monitor CD4+ and T-cell counts; tell prescriber if they decrease.

■ Urge patient to report opportunistic infections.

■ Tell patient not to change an HIV regimen without consulting prescriber.

---

amprenavir ▶◀ rifamycins
Agenerase   rifabutin, rifampin, rifapentine

Risk rating: 2
Severity: Moderate   **Onset: Delayed**   **Likelihood: Suspected**

Cause
Amprenavir may decrease CYP3A4 metabolism of rifabutin. Rifampin may increase CYP3A4 metabolism of amprenavir.

Effect
Amprenavir level, effects, and risk of adverse effects may increase.

Nursing considerations

⚠ ALERT Use of amprenavir with rifampin is contraindicated.

■ If patient takes amprenavir with rifabutin or rifapentine, watch for adverse reactions.

■ Tell patient he may develop diarrhea, fever, headache, muscle pain, or nausea, but not to alter regimen without consulting prescriber.

■ To minimize interactions, urge patient to tell prescriber about all drugs and supplements he takes.

---

amprenavir 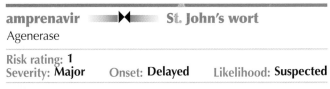 **sildenafil**
Agenerase   Viagra

Risk rating: 1
Severity: Major   **Onset: Rapid**   **Likelihood: Suspected**

Cause
Sildenafil metabolism is inhibited.

Effect
Sildenafil level may increase, possibly leading to fatal hypotension.

Nursing considerations
⚠ ALERT Tell patient to take sildenafil exactly as prescribed.

■ Dosage of sildenafil may be reduced to 25 mg and an interval of at least 48 hours may be needed.

■ Warn patient about potentially fatal low blood pressure if these drugs are taken together.

■ Tell patient to notify his prescriber if he has dizziness, fainting, or chest pain during use together.

---

amprenavir **St. John's wort**
Agenerase

Risk rating: 1
Severity: Major   **Onset: Delayed**   **Likelihood: Suspected**

Cause
Hepatic metabolism of protease inhibitor, such as amprenavir, may increase.

Effect
Protease inhibitor level and effects may decrease.

Nursing considerations
■ If patient starts or stops taking St. John's wort, monitor protease inhibitor level closely.

■ Tell patient not to alter HIV regimen without consulting prescriber.
■ To help avoid interactions, urge patient to tell prescribers about all drugs, supplements, and alternative therapies he uses.

amyl nitrite ▶◀ dihydroergotamine
D.H.E. 45

Risk rating: 2
Severity: Moderate   **Onset: Rapid**   **Likelihood: Suspected**

Cause
Metabolism of dihydroergotamine decreases, increasing its availability, which antagonizes nitrate-induced coronary vasodilation.

Effect
Increased dihydroergotamine availability may increase systolic blood pressure and decrease antianginal effects.

Nursing considerations
■ Use these drugs together cautiously in patients with angina.
■ I.V. dihydroergotamine may antagonize coronary vasodilation.
■ Monitor patient for evidence of ergotism, such as peripheral ischemia, paresthesia, headache, nausea, and vomiting.
■ Teach patient to immediately report indicators of peripheral ischemia, such as numbness or tingling in fingers and toes or red blisters on hands or feet. Dihydroergotamine dosage may need to be decreased.

amyl nitrite ▶◀ phosphodiesterase-5 inhibitors
sildenafil, tadalafil, vardenafil

Risk rating: 1
Severity: Major   **Onset: Rapid**   **Likelihood: Suspected**

Cause
Phosphodiesterase-5 (PDE-5) inhibitors potentiate the hypotensive effects of nitrates, such as amyl nitrate.

Effect
Risk of severe hypotension increases.

Nursing considerations
◼ **ALERT** Use of nitrates with PDE-5 inhibitors is contraindicated.
■ Carefully screen patient for PDE-5 inhibitor use before giving a nitrate.
■ Even during an emergency, before you give a nitrate, find out if a

patient with chest pain has taken an erectile dysfunction drug during the previous 24 hours.
- Monitor patient for orthostatic hypotension, dizziness, sweating, and headache.

---

angiotensin II receptor antagonists ▶◀ potassium-sparing diuretics

candesartan, eprosartan, irbesartan, losartan, olmesartan, telmisartan, valsartan

amiloride, spironolactone, triamterene

Risk rating: 1
Severity: Major   **Onset: Delayed**   **Likelihood: Suspected**

Cause
Both angiotensin II receptor antagonists and potassium-sparing diuretics may increase serum potassium level.

Effect
Risk of hyperkalemia may increase, especially in high-risk patients.

Nursing considerations
- High-risk patients include elderly people and those with renal impairment, type 2 diabetes, or decreased renal perfusion; monitor these patients closely.
- Check serum potassium, BUN, and creatinine levels regularly. If they increase, notify prescriber.
- Advise patient to immediately report an irregular heartbeat, slow pulse, weakness, or other evidence of hyperkalemia.

---

aprepitant ▶◀ cisapride

Emend

Propulsid

Risk rating: 1
Severity: Major   **Onset: Delayed**   **Likelihood: Suspected**

Cause
Aprepitant may inhibit CYP3A4 metabolism of cisapride.

Effect
Risk of life-threatening arrhythmias may increase.

Nursing considerations
- ALERT Use of aprepitant with cisapride is contraindicated.

■ Patients taking cisapride with drugs that inhibit the CYP3A4 isoenzyme may develop prolonged QT interval, torsades de pointes, other life-threatening arrhythmias, cardiac arrest, or sudden death.
■ Cisapride is only available through a limited access program to patients who don't respond to other standard treatments and who meet strict eligibility criteria.

---

aprepitant ━━━━━▶◀━━━ corticosteroids

Emend

dexamethasone, hydrocortisone, methylprednisolone

Risk rating: 2
Severity: Moderate   Onset: Delayed   Likelihood: Suspected

Cause
Aprepitant may inhibit first-pass metabolism of certain corticosteroids.

Effect
Corticosteroid level may be increased and the half-life prolonged.

Nursing considerations
■ Corticosteroid dosage may need to be decreased.
■ When starting or stopping aprepitant, adjust corticosteroid dosage as needed.
■ Watch closely for evidence of increased corticosteroid level, such as insomnia, euphoria, increased appetite, mood changes, and increased blood glucose level.
■ Tell patient to report symptoms of increased blood glucose level, including increased thirst or hunger and increased frequency of urination.

---

aspirin ━━━━━▶◀━━━ ACE inhibitors

Bayer

benazepril, captopril, enalapril, fosinopril, lisinopril, moexipril, perindopril, quinapril, ramipril, trandolapril

Risk rating: 2
Severity: Moderate   Onset: Rapid   Likelihood: Suspected

Cause
Salicylates, such as aspirin, inhibit synthesis of prostaglandins, which ACE inhibitors need to lower blood pressure.

Effect
The ACE inhibitor's hypotensive effect will be reduced.

Nursing considerations
■ This interaction is more likely in people with hypertension, coronary artery disease, or possibly heart failure.
■ At doses less than 100 mg daily, aspirin is less likely to interact.

aspirin ━━━━◄►	beta blockers
Bayer	acebutolol, atenolol, betaxolol, bisoprolol, carteolol, carvedilol, metoprolol, nadolol, penbutolol, pindolol, propranolol, timolol

Risk rating: 2
Severity: **Moderate**   Onset: **Rapid**   Likelihood: **Suspected**

Cause
Salicylates, such as aspirin, inhibit synthesis of prostaglandins, which beta blockers need to lower blood pressure. In patients with heart failure, the mechanism of this interaction is unknown.

Effect
Beta blocker effects will decrease.

Nursing considerations
■ Watch closely for signs of heart failure and hypertension.
■ Beta blockers may interact with other salicylates. If you suspect an interaction, consult prescriber or pharmacist.
■ Explain signs and symptoms of heart failure, and tell patient when to contact prescriber.

aspirin ━━━━◄►	carbonic anhydrase inhibitors
Bayer	acetazolamide, dichlorphen-amide, methazolamide

Risk rating: 2
Severity: **Moderate**   Onset: **Delayed**   Likelihood: **Suspected**

Cause
Aspirin displaces the carbonic anhydrase inhibitor from protein-binding sites and inhibits renal clearance. As a result, carbonic anhy-

drase inhibitor accumulates, causing acidosis and increased risk of salicylate penetration into the CNS.

Effect
Carbonic anhydrase inhibitor level and risk of toxicity increase.

Nursing considerations
■ Minimize or avoid using a salicylate, such as aspirin, with a carbonic anhydrase inhibitor.
■ If drugs must be given together, monitor patient for evidence of toxicity, including lethargy, confusion, fatigue, anorexia, urinary incontinence, tachypnea, and hyperchloremic metabolic acidosis.
■ Chronic salicylate values higher than 15 mg/dl may produce toxicity. Symptoms may appear in days to weeks.
■ Elderly patients and those with renal impairment are at greatest risk of toxic effects.

aspirin ▶◀	corticosteroids
Bayer	betamethasone, cortisone, dexamethasone, fludrocortisone, hydrocortisone, methylprednisolone, prednisolone, prednisone, triamcinolone

Risk rating: 2
Severity: **Moderate**　　Onset: **Delayed**　　Likelihood: **Probable**

Cause
Corticosteroids stimulate hepatic metabolism of salicylates, such as aspirin, and may increase renal excretion.

Effect
Salicylate level and effects decrease.

Nursing considerations
■ Monitor salicylate level; dosage may need adjustment.
◣ ALERT Giving a salicylate while tapering a corticosteroid may result in salicylate toxicity.
■ Watch for evidence of salicylate toxicity, including diaphoresis, nausea, vomiting, tinnitus, hyperventilation, and CNS depression.
■ Patients with renal impairment may be at greater risk.

aspirin ▶◀ heparin sodium

Bayer

Risk rating: 2
Severity: Moderate   **Onset: Rapid**   **Likelihood: Probable**

Cause
Aspirin may inhibit platelet aggregation and cause bleeding, adding to heparin's anticoagulation effects.

Effect
Risk of bleeding increases.

Nursing considerations
■ Monitor patient for signs of bleeding, including bleeding gums, bruises on arms or legs, petechiae, epistaxis, melena, hematuria, and hematemesis.
■ Urge patient to tell prescriber about all drugs and supplements he takes and about any increase in adverse effects.

aspirin ▶◀ ketorolac

Bayer   Toradol

Risk rating: 1
Severity: Major   **Onset: Delayed**   **Likelihood: Suspected**

Cause
Aspirin may displace ketorolac from protein-binding sites, increasing the level of unbound ketorolac.

Effect
Risk of serious ketorolac-related adverse effects increases.

Nursing considerations
⚠ **ALERT** Ketorolac is contraindicated in patients taking aspirin.
■ Watch for adverse effects, such as GI bleeding, neurotoxicity, renal failure, blood dyscrasias, and hepatotoxicity.
■ Urge patient to tell prescriber and pharmacist about all drugs and supplements he takes.

aspirin 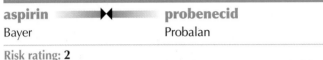 probenecid
Bayer   Probalan

Risk rating: 2
Severity: Moderate   Onset: Delayed   Likelihood: Probable

Cause
The mechanism of this interaction is unknown. It may stem from altered renal filtration of uric acid.

Effect
Uricosuric action of both drugs is inhibited.

Nursing considerations
■ Typically, giving probenecid with a salicylate, such as aspirin, is contraindicated.
■ Occasional use of aspirin at low doses may not interfere with the uricosuric action of probenecid.
■ Monitor serum urate level; the usual goal of probenecid therapy is about 6 mg/dl.
◤ ALERT Remind patient to carefully read the labels of OTC medicines because many contain salicylates.
■ If an analgesic or antipyretic is needed during probenecid therapy, suggest acetaminophen.
■ Advise adequate fluid intake to prevent uric acid kidney stones.

aspirin ◀▶ sulfinpyrazone
Bayer   Anturane

Risk rating: 2
Severity: Moderate   Onset: Delayed   Likelihood: Established

Cause
Salicylates, such as aspirin, block the effect of sulfinpyrazone on tubular reabsorption of uric acid, and they displace sulfinpyrazone from plasma protein-binding sites, decreasing sulfinpyrazone level.

Effect
Uricosuric effects of sulfinpyrazone are inhibited.

Nursing considerations
■ Typically, giving sulfinpyrazone with a salicylate is contraindicated.
■ Monitor serum urate level; the usual goal of sulfinpyrazone therapy is about 6 mg/dl.
◤ ALERT Remind patient to carefully read the labels of OTC medicines because many contain salicylates.
■ Encourage adequate fluid intake to prevent uric acid kidney stones.

aspirin　▶◀　sulfonylureas

Bayer

acetohexamide,
chlorpropamide, glimepiride,
glipizide, glyburide,
tolazamide, tolbutamide

Risk rating: 2
Severity: Moderate   Onset: Delayed   Likelihood: Probable

Cause
Salicylates, such as aspirin, reduce glucose level and promote insulin secretion.

Effect
Hypoglycemic effects of sulfonylureas increase.

Nursing considerations
■ If patient takes a sulfonylurea, start salicylate carefully, monitoring patient for hypoglycemia.
■ Consult prescriber and patient about possibly replacing a salicylate with acetaminophen or an NSAID.
■ Describe signs and symptoms of hypoglycemia, including diaphoresis, fatigue, headache, hunger, irritability, malaise, nervousness, rapid heart rate, tension, and trembling.
■ Instruct patient to eat a small carbohydrate snack or meal if hypoglycemia develops, preferably after checking blood glucose level.

atazanavir　▶◀　azole antifungals

Reyataz

fluconazole, itraconazole,
ketoconazole

Risk rating: 2
Severity: Moderate   Onset: Delayed   Likelihood: Suspected

Cause
Azole antifungals may inhibit metabolism of protease inhibitors, such as atazanavir.

Effect
Protease inhibitor level may increase.

Nursing considerations
■ Monitor patient for increased protease inhibitor effects, including hyperglycemia, rash, and GI complaints.
■ Advise patient to report increased hunger or thirst, frequent urination, fatigue, and dry, itchy skin.

- Tell patient not to change dosage or stop either drug without consulting prescriber.
- To help avoid interactions, urge patient to tell prescribers about all drugs and supplements he takes.

atazanavir ▶◀	benzodiazepines
Reyataz	alprazolam, chlordiazepoxide, clonazepam, clorazepate, diazepam, estazolam, flurazepam, midazolam, quazepam, triazolam

Risk rating: 2
Severity: Moderate   Onset: Delayed   Likelihood: Suspected

Cause
Protease inhibitors, such as atazanavir, may inhibit CYP3A4 metabolism of certain benzodiazepines.

Effect
Sedative effects of benzodiazepines may be increased and prolonged, leading to severe respiratory depression.

Nursing considerations
⚠ ALERT Don't combine a protease inhibitor with alprazolam, chlordiazepoxide, clonazepam, clorazepate, diazepam, estazolam, flurazepam, midazolam, quazepam, or triazolam.
- If patient takes any benzodiazepine–protease inhibitor combination, notify prescriber. Interaction could involve other drugs in the class.

atazanavir ▶◀	ergot derivatives
Reyataz	dihydroergotamine, ergonovine, ergotamine, methylergonovine

Risk rating: 1
Severity: Major   Onset: Delayed   Likelihood: Probable

Cause
Protease inhibitors, such as atazanavir, may interfere with CYP3A4 metabolism of ergot derivatives.

Effect
Risk of ergot-induced peripheral vasospasm and ischemia may increase.

Nursing considerations
◤ ALERT Use of ergot derivatives with protease inhibitors is contraindicated.

■ Monitor patient for evidence of peripheral ischemia, including pain in limb muscles while exercising and later at rest; numbness and tingling of fingers and toes; cool, pale, or cyanotic limbs; red or violet blisters on hands or feet; and gangrene.

■ Sodium nitroprusside may be given for ergot-induced vasospasm.

■ If patient takes a protease inhibitor, consult prescriber or pharmacist about alternative treatments for migraine pain.

■ Advise patient to tell prescriber about all drugs and supplements he takes and any increase in adverse effects.

---

atazanavir ▶◀ simvastatin
Reyataz   Zocor

Risk rating: 1
Severity: Major   **Onset: Delayed**   **Likelihood: Suspected**

Cause
Atazanavir may inhibit first-pass metabolism of simvastatin by CYP3A4 in the GI tract.

Effect
Simvastatin level may increase.

Nursing considerations
■ If a protease inhibitor, such as atazanavir, is added to regimen that includes simvastatin, monitor patient closely.

◤ ALERT Watch for evidence of rhabdomyolysis, including dark or red urine, muscle weakness, and myalgia.

■ Urge patient to immediately report unexplained muscle weakness.

---

atazanavir ▶◀ St. John's wort
Reyataz

Risk rating: 1
Severity: Major   **Onset: Delayed**   **Likelihood: Suspected**

Cause
Hepatic metabolism of protease inhibitor, such as atazanavir, may increase.

Effect
Protease inhibitor level and effects may decrease.

Nursing considerations
■ If patient starts or stops taking St. John's wort, monitor protease inhibitor level closely.
■ Monitor CD4+ and T-cell counts; tell prescriber if they decrease.
■ Urge patient to report opportunistic infections.
■ Tell patient not to change an HIV regimen without consulting prescriber.
■ To help avoid interactions, urge patient to tell prescribers about all drugs, supplements, and alternative therapies he uses.

---

atenolol ▶◀ ampicillin
Tenormin   Principen

Risk rating: 2
Severity: Moderate   **Onset: Rapid**   **Likelihood: Suspected**

Cause
Ampicillin may impair GI absorption of atenolol.

Effect
Blood-pressure lowering and antianginal effects of atenolol may decrease.

Nursing considerations
■ Beta blockers other than atenolol and penicillins other than ampicillin may interact. If you suspect an interaction, consult prescriber or pharmacist.
■ Monitor patient's blood pressure, and assess for anginal symptoms during ampicillin therapy.
■ Suggest that patient separate doses to decrease GI interaction.
■ Notify prescriber if blood pressure increases; atenolol dosage may be increased or ampicillin broken into smaller, more frequent doses.
■ Teach patient to tell prescriber immediately about increased episodes or severity of chest pain.

atenolol ▸◂ lidocaine

Tenormin

Risk rating: 2
Severity: Moderate   **Onset: Rapid**   **Likelihood: Established**

Cause
Beta blockers, such as atenolol, reduce hepatic metabolism of lidocaine.

Effect
Lidocaine level and risk of toxicity may increase.

Nursing considerations
■ Check for normal therapeutic level of lidocaine: 2 to 5 mcg/ml.
■ Watch closely for evidence of lidocaine toxicity, including dizziness, somnolence, confusion, paresthesias, and seizures.
■ Slow the I.V. bolus rate to decrease the risk of high peak level and toxic reactions.
■ Explain the warning signs of toxicity to patient and family, and tell them to contact prescriber if they have concerns.

atenolol ▸◂ NSAIDs

Tenormin   ibuprofen, indomethacin, naproxen, piroxicam

Risk rating: 2
Severity: Moderate   **Onset: Delayed**   **Likelihood: Probable**

Cause
NSAIDs may inhibit renal prostaglandin synthesis, allowing pressor systems to be unopposed.

Effect
Beta blocker, such as atenolol, may not be able to lower blood pressure.

Nursing considerations
■ Avoid using these drugs together, if possible.
■ Monitor blood pressure and other evidence of hypertension closely.
■ Consult prescriber about ways to reduce interaction, such as adjusting beta blocker dosage or switching to sulindac as the NSAID.
■ Explain the risks of using these drugs together, and teach patient how to monitor his own blood pressure.
■ Other NSAIDs may interact with beta blockers. If you suspect an interaction, consult prescriber or pharmacist.

atenolol 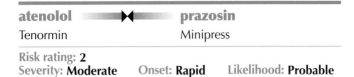 prazosin

Tenormin   Minipress

Risk rating: 2
Severity: Moderate   Onset: Rapid   Likelihood: Probable

Cause
The mechanism of this interaction is unknown.

Effect
Risk of orthostatic hypotension increases.

Nursing considerations
■ Assess patient's lying, sitting, and standing blood pressures closely, especially when combined therapy starts.
■ To minimize effects of orthostatic hypotension, teach patient to change positions slowly.
■ Interaction is confirmed only with propranolol but also may occur with other beta blockers, such as atenolol.

atenolol 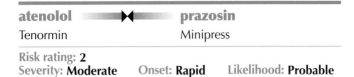 quinidine

Tenormin

Risk rating: 2
Severity: Moderate   Onset: Rapid   Likelihood: Suspected

Cause
Quinidine may inhibit metabolism of certain beta blockers, such as atenolol, in those who are extensive metabolizers of debrisoquin.

Effect
Beta blocker effects may be increased.

Nursing considerations
■ Monitor pulse and blood pressure more often.
■ If pulse slows or blood pressure falls, consult prescriber. Beta blocker dosage may need to be decreased.
■ Teach patient how to check blood pressure and pulse rate; tell him to do so regularly.

atenolol ━━━━◄► salicylates

Tenormin

aspirin, bismuth subsalicylate, choline salicylate, magnesium salicylate, salsalate, sodium salicylate, sodium thiosalicylate

Risk rating: 2
Severity: Moderate **Onset: Rapid** **Likelihood: Suspected**

Cause
Salicylates inhibit synthesis of prostaglandins, which atenolol and other beta blockers need to lower blood pressure. In patients with heart failure, the mechanism of this interaction is unknown.

Effect
Beta blocker effects decrease.

Nursing considerations
■ Watch closely for signs of heart failure and hypertension, and notify prescriber if they occur.
■ Consult prescriber about switching patient to a different antihypertensive or antiplatelet drug.
■ Other beta blockers may interact with salicylates. If you suspect an interaction, consult prescriber or pharmacist.
■ Explain evidence of heart failure and when to contact prescriber.

atenolol ━━━━◄► verapamil

Tenormin Calan

Risk rating: 1
Severity: Major **Onset: Rapid** **Likelihood: Probable**

Cause
Verapamil may inhibit metabolism of beta blockers, such as atenolol.

Effect
Effects of both drugs may increase.

Nursing considerations
■ Combination therapy is common in patients with hypertension and unstable angina.
◤ **ALERT** Risk of adverse effects increases, including heart failure, conduction disturbances, arrhythmias, and hypotension.
■ Monitor patient for adverse effects, including left ventricular dysfunction and AV conduction defects.

- Risk of interaction is greater when drugs are given I.V.
- Dosages of both drugs may need to be decreased.

atomoxetine ▶◀ MAO inhibitors

Strattera

isocarboxazid, phenelzine, tranylcypromine

Risk rating: 1
Severity: Major   Onset: **Rapid**   Likelihood: **Suspected**

Cause
Level of monoamine in the brain may change.

Effect
Risk of serious or fatal reaction resembling neuroleptic malignant syndrome may increase.

Nursing considerations
⚡ **ALERT** Use of atomoxetine and an MAO inhibitor together or within 2 weeks of each other is contraindicated.
- Before starting atomoxetine, ask patient when he last took an MAO inhibitor. Before starting an MAO inhibitor, ask patient when he last took atomoxetine.
- Monitor patient for hyperthermia, rapid changes in vital signs, rigidity, muscle twitching, and mental status changes.

atorvastatin ▶◀ azole antifungals

Lipitor

fluconazole, itraconazole, ketoconazole, voriconazole

Risk rating: 2
Severity: Moderate   Onset: **Rapid**   Likelihood: **Probable**

Cause
Azole antifungals may inhibit hepatic metabolism of HMG-CoA reductase inhibitors, such as atorvastatin.

Effect
HMG-CoA reductase inhibitor level and adverse effects may increase.

Nursing considerations
- If possible, avoid use together.
- If drugs must be taken together, HMG-CoA reductase inhibitor dosage may need to be decreased.

■ Monitor serum cholesterol and lipid levels to assess patient's response to therapy.

■ ALERT Assess patient for evidence of rhabdomyolysis, including fatigue; muscle aches and weakness; joint pain; dark, red, or cola-colored urine; weight gain; seizures; and greatly increased serum CK level.

■ Pravastatin is least affected by this interaction and may be preferable for use with an azole antifungal, if needed.

atorvastatin ▶◀ bile acid sequestrants
Lipitor   cholestyramine, colestipol

Risk rating: 2
Severity: **Moderate**   Onset: **Delayed**   Likelihood: **Suspected**

Cause
GI absorption of HMG-CoA reductase inhibitor, such as atorvastatin, may decrease.

Effect
HMG-CoA reductase inhibitor effects may decrease.

Nursing considerations
■ ALERT Separate doses of HMG-CoA reductase inhibitor and bile acid sequestrant by at least 4 hours.

■ If possible, give bile acid sequestrant before meals and HMG-CoA reductase inhibitor in the evening.

■ Monitor serum cholesterol and lipid levels to assess patient's response to therapy.

atorvastatin ▶◀ carbamazepine
Lipitor   Carbatrol, Epitol, Equetro, Tegretol

Risk rating: 2
Severity: **Moderate**   Onset: **Delayed**   Likelihood: **Suspected**

Cause
Carbamazepine may increase CYP3A4 metabolism of HMG-CoA reductase inhibitors, such as atorvastatin.

Effect
HMG-CoA reductase inhibitor effects may be reduced.

Nursing considerations
■ If possible, avoid use together.

■ If use together can't be avoided, monitor serum cholesterol and lipid levels to assess patient's response to therapy.
■ Pravastatin and rosuvastatin may be less likely to interact with carbamazepine and may be better choices than other HMG-CoA reductase inhibitors.

---

atorvastatin ▶◀ cyclosporine
Lipitor   Neoral

Risk rating: 1
Severity: Major   **Onset: Delayed**   **Likelihood: Probable**

Cause
Metabolism of certain HMG-CoA reductase inhibitors, such as atorvastatin, may decrease.

Effect
HMG-CoA reductase inhibitor level and adverse effects may increase.

Nursing considerations
■ If possible, avoid use together.
■ If used together, HMG-CoA reductase inhibitor dosage may need to be decreased.
■ Monitor serum cholesterol level, lipid levels, and liver function tests to assess patient's response to therapy and possible adverse effects.
◪ ALERT Assess patient for evidence of rhabdomyolysis, including fatigue; muscle aches and weakness; joint pain; dark, red, or cola-colored urine; weight gain; seizures; and greatly increased serum CK level.
■ Urge patient to report unexplained muscle pain, tenderness, or weakness to prescriber.

---

atorvastatin ▶◀ diltiazem
Lipitor   Cardizem

Risk rating: 2
Severity: Moderate   **Onset: Delayed**   **Likelihood: Probable**

Cause
CYP3A4 metabolism of certain HMG-CoA reductase inhibitors, such as atorvastatin, may be inhibited.

Effect
HMG-CoA reductase inhibitor level may increase, raising the risk of toxicity, including myositis and rhabdomyolysis.

Nursing considerations
▪ If possible, avoid use together.
▪ **ALERT** Assess patient for evidence of rhabdomyolysis, including fatigue; muscle aches and weakness; joint pain; dark, red, or cola-colored urine; weight gain; seizures; and greatly increased serum CK level.
▪ If patient may have rhabdomyolysis, notify prescriber and obtain renal function tests and serum potassium, sodium, calcium, lactic acid, and myoglobin levels.
▪ Pravastatin is less likely to interact with diltiazem than other HMG-CoA reductase inhibitors and may be best choice for combined use.
▪ Urge patient to report unexplained muscle pain, tenderness, or weakness to prescriber.

---

atorvastatin ▶◀ gemfibrozil
Lipitor   Lopid

Risk rating: 1
Severity: Major   **Onset: Delayed**   **Likelihood: Suspected**

Cause
The mechanism of this interaction is unknown.

Effect
Severe myopathy or rhabdomyolysis may occur.

Nursing considerations
▪ Avoid use together.
▪ If patient has severe hyperlipidemia, combined therapy may be an option, but only with careful monitoring.
▪ **ALERT** Assess patient for evidence of rhabdomyolysis, including fatigue; muscle aches and weakness; joint pain; dark, red, or cola-colored urine; weight gain; seizures; and greatly increased serum CK level.
▪ Watch for evidence of acute renal failure, including decreased urine output, elevated BUN and creatinine levels, edema, dyspnea, tachycardia, distended neck veins, nausea, vomiting, poor appetite, weakness, fatigue, confusion, and agitation.
▪ Urge patient to report unexplained muscle pain, tenderness, or weakness to prescriber.

atorvastatin ▸◀ grapefruit juice
Lipitor

Risk rating: 2
Severity: Moderate   **Onset: Rapid**   **Likelihood: Suspected**

Cause
Grapefruit juice may inhibit CYP3A4 metabolism of certain HMG-CoA reductase inhibitors, such as atorvastatin.

Effect
HMG-CoA reductase inhibitor level may increase, raising the risk of adverse effects.

Nursing considerations
- Avoid giving atorvastatin with grapefruit juice.
- Fluvastatin and pravastatin are metabolized by other enzymes and may be less affected by grapefruit juice.
- Caution patient to take drug with a liquid other than grapefruit juice.
- Urge patient to report unexplained muscle pain, tenderness, or weakness to prescriber.

atorvastatin ▸◀ macrolide antibiotics
Lipitor   azithromycin, clarithromycin, erythromycin, telithromycin

Risk rating: 1
Severity: Major   **Onset: Delayed**   **Likelihood: Probable**

Cause
CYP3A4 metabolism of certain HMG-CoA reductase inhibitors, such as atorvastatin, may decrease.

Effect
HMG-CoA reductase inhibitor level may increase, raising the risk of severe myopathy or rhabdomyolysis.

Nursing considerations
- **⚠ ALERT** If atorvastatin is given with a macrolide antibiotic, watch for evidence of rhabdomyolysis, especially 5 to 21 days after macrolide starts. Evidence may include fatigue; muscle aches and weakness; joint pain; dark, red, or cola-colored urine; weight gain; seizures; and greatly increased serum CK level.
- Fluvastatin and pravastatin are metabolized by other enzymes and may be better choices when used with a macrolide antibiotic.

■ It may be safe to give atorvastatin with azithromycin.
■ Urge patient to report unexplained muscle pain, tenderness, or weakness to prescriber.

---

atorvastatin ◼▶◀◼ protease inhibitors

Lipitor   amprenavir, indinavir, lopinavir-ritonavir, nelfinavir, ritonavir, saquinavir

Risk rating: 2
Severity: Moderate   **Onset: Delayed**   **Likelihood: Suspected**

Cause
First-pass metabolism of atorvastatin by CYP3A4 in the GI tract may be inhibited.

Effect
Atorvastatin level may increase.

Nursing considerations
■ Monitor patient closely if a protease inhibitor is added to atorvastatin therapy.
◪ ALERT Watch for evidence of rhabdomyolysis, including dark or red urine, muscle weakness, and myalgia.
■ This interaction may be more likely when ritonavir and saquinavir are used together.
■ Tell patient to immediately report unexplained muscle weakness to prescriber.

---

atorvastatin ◼▶◀◼ rifamycins

Lipitor   rifabutin, rifampin, rifapentine

Risk rating: 2
Severity: Moderate   **Onset: Delayed**   **Likelihood: Suspected**

Cause
Rifamycins may induce CYP3A4 metabolism of HMG-CoA reductase inhibitors, such as atorvastatin, in the intestine and liver.

Effect
HMG-CoA reductase inhibitor effects may decrease.

Nursing considerations
■ Assess patient for expected response to therapy. If you suspect an interaction, consult prescriber or pharmacist; patient may need a different drug.

- Check serum cholesterol and lipid levels to monitor patient's response to therapy.
- Withhold HMG-CoA reductase inhibitor temporarily if something increases patient's risk of myopathy or rhabdomyolysis, such as sepsis, hypotension, major surgery, trauma, uncontrolled seizures, or a severe metabolic, endocrine, or electrolyte disorder.
- Pravastatin is less likely to interact with rifamycins and may be the best choice for combined use.

---

atorvastatin ◀▶ verapamil
Lipitor   Calan

Risk rating: 2
Severity: Moderate   **Onset: Delayed**   **Likelihood: Probable**

Cause
CYP3A4 metabolism of certain HMG-CoA reductase inhibitors, such as atorvastatin, may be decreased.

Effect
HMG-CoA reductase inhibitor level may increase, raising the risk of adverse effects.

Nursing considerations
- If possible, avoid giving atorvastatin with verapamil. If patient must take both drugs, consult prescriber; HMG-CoA reductase inhibitor dosage may be decreased.
- ⚡ ALERT Watch for evidence of rhabdomyolysis, including fatigue; muscle aches and weakness; joint pain; dark, red, or cola-colored urine; weight gain; seizures; and greatly increased serum CK level.
- Fluvastatin and pravastatin are metabolized by other enzymes and may be better choices for combined use.
- Urge patient to report unexplained muscle pain, tenderness, or weakness to prescriber.
- Obtain liver function test results at start of therapy and periodically thereafter. If ALT or AST level stays three times or more above the upper limit of normal, HMG-CoA reductase inhibitor will need to be stopped.

atracurium ▶◀ aminoglycosides
Tracrium

amikacin, gentamicin, kanamycin, neomycin, streptomycin, tobramycin

Risk rating: 1
Severity: Major   **Onset: Rapid**   **Likelihood: Probable**

Cause
These drugs may be synergistic.

Effect
Effects of nondepolarizing muscle relaxants, such as atracurium, may increase.

Nursing considerations
- Give these drugs together only when needed.
- The nondepolarizing muscle relaxant dose may need adjustment based on neuromuscular response.
- Monitor patient for prolonged respiratory depression.
- Provide ventilatory support as needed.

atracurium ▶◀ carbamazepine
Tracrium

Carbatrol, Epitol, Equetro, Tegretol

Risk rating: 2
Severity: Moderate   **Onset: Rapid**   **Likelihood: Probable**

Cause
The mechanism of this interaction is unknown.

Effect
The effect or duration of atracurium, a nondepolarizing muscle relaxant, may decrease.

Nursing considerations
- Monitor patient for decreased efficacy of the muscle relaxant.
- Dosage of the nondepolarizing muscle relaxant may need to be increased.
- Make sure patient is adequately sedated when receiving a nondepolarizing muscle relaxant.

atracurium ▶◀ clindamycin
Tracrium   Cleocin

Risk rating: 2
Severity: Moderate   **Onset: Rapid**   **Likelihood: Suspected**

Cause
Clindamycin may potentiate the action of nondepolarizing muscle relaxants, such as atracurium.

Effect
Action of the nondepolarizing muscle relaxant may increase.

Nursing considerations
■ If possible, avoid using clindamycin or other lincosamides with nondepolarizing muscle relaxants.
◪ **ALERT** Combined use may lead to profound, severe respiratory depression.
■ Monitor patient for respiratory distress.
■ Provide ventilatory support as needed.
■ Cholinesterase inhibitors or calcium may be useful in reversing drug effects.
■ Make sure patient is adequately sedated when receiving a nondepolarizing muscle relaxant.

atracurium ▶◀ magnesium sulfate
Tracrium

Risk rating: 2
Severity: Moderate   **Onset: Rapid**   **Likelihood: Suspected**

Cause
Magnesium probably potentiates the action of nondepolarizing muscle relaxants, such as atracurium.

Effect
The risk of profound, severe respiratory depression increases.

Nursing considerations
■ Use these drugs together cautiously.
■ The nondepolarizing muscle relaxant dosage may need adjustment.
■ Provide ventilatory support as needed.
■ Make sure patient is adequately sedated when receiving a nondepolarizing muscle relaxant.

atracurium ▰▰▰◖◗▰▰▰ polypeptide antibiotics
Tracrium
bacitracin, polymyxin B, vancomycin

Risk rating: 2
Severity: Moderate   **Onset: Rapid**   **Likelihood: Probable**

Cause
Polypeptide antibiotics may act synergistically with nondepolarizing muscle relaxants, such as atracurium.

Effect
Neuromuscular blockade may increase.

Nursing considerations
- If possible, avoid using polypeptide antibiotics with nondepolarizing muscle relaxants.
- Monitor neuromuscular function closely.
- Dosage of nondepolarizing muscle relaxant may need adjustment.
- Make sure patient is adequately sedated when receiving a nondepolarizing muscle relaxant.

atracurium ▰▰▰◖◗▰▰▰ quinine derivatives
Tracrium
quinidine, quinine

Risk rating: 2
Severity: Moderate   **Onset: Rapid**   **Likelihood: Suspected**

Cause
Quinine derivatives may act synergistically with nondepolarizing muscle relaxants, such as atracurium.

Effect
Effects of nondepolarizing muscle relaxants may increase.

Nursing considerations
⚡ **ALERT** This interaction may be life-threatening. Monitor neuromuscular function closely.
- The intensity and duration of neuromuscular blockade may be affected.
- The nondepolarizing muscle relaxant dosage may need adjustment.
- Make sure patient is adequately sedated when receiving a nondepolarizing muscle relaxant.

atracurium ▰▰▰ ▶◀ ▰▰▰ theophyllines
Tracrium   aminophylline, theophylline

Risk rating: 2
Severity: Moderate   **Onset: Rapid**   **Likelihood: Suspected**

Cause
These drugs may act antagonistically.

Effect
Neuromuscular blockade may be reversed.

Nursing considerations
- Monitor patient closely for lack of drug effect.
- Dosage of atracurium, a nondepolarizing muscle relaxant, may need adjustment.
- This interaction is dose dependent.
- Make sure patient is adequately sedated when receiving a nondepolarizing muscle relaxant.

atracurium ▰▰▰ ▶◀ ▰▰▰ verapamil
Tracrium   Calan

Risk rating: 2
Severity: Moderate   **Onset: Rapid**   **Likelihood: Suspected**

Cause
This interaction may stem from blockade of calcium channels in the skeletal muscle.

Effect
Effects of nondepolarizing muscle relaxants, such as atracurium, may increase.

Nursing considerations
- If possible, avoid using verapamil and nondepolarizing muscle relaxants together.
- If drugs are used together, monitor patient for prolonged respiratory depression.
- Nondepolarizing muscle relaxant dosage may need to be decreased.

atropine ►◄ phenothiazines
chlorpromazine,
fluphenazine, perphenazine,
prochlorperazine,
promethazine, thioridazine,
trifluoperazine

Risk rating: 2
Severity: Moderate   **Onset: Delayed**   **Likelihood: Suspected**

Cause
Anticholinergics, such as atropine, may antagonize phenothiazines.
Also, phenothiazine metabolism may increase.

Effect
Phenothiazine efficacy may decrease.

Nursing considerations
- Data regarding this interaction conflict.
- Monitor patient for decreased phenothiazine efficacy.
- Anticholinergic side effects may increase.
- Monitor patient for adynamic ileus, hyperpyrexia, hypoglycemia, and neurologic changes.

azithromycin ►◄ HMG-CoA reductase inhibitors
Zithromax

atorvastatin, lovastatin,
simvastatin

Risk rating: 1
Severity: Major   **Onset: Delayed**   **Likelihood: Probable**

Cause
CYP3A4 metabolism of certain HMG-CoA reductase inhibitors may
decrease.

Effect
HMG-CoA reductase inhibitor level may increase, raising the risk of
severe myopathy or rhabdomyolysis.

Nursing considerations
◪ **ALERT** If atorvastatin, lovastatin, or simvastatin is given with a
macrolide antibiotic, such as azithromycin, watch for evidence of
rhabdomyolysis, especially 5 to 21 days after macrolide therapy starts.
Evidence may include fatigue; muscle aches and weakness; joint pain;

dark, red, or cola-colored urine; weight gain; seizures; and greatly increased serum CK level.
■ Fluvastatin and pravastatin are metabolized by other enzymes and may be better choices when used with a macrolide antibiotic.
■ Urge patient to report unexplained muscle pain, tenderness, or weakness to prescriber.

azithromycin ▶◀ theophyllines

Zithromax   aminophylline, theophylline

Risk rating: 2
Severity: Moderate   Onset: Delayed   Likelihood: Established

Cause
Certain macrolides, such as azithromycin, inhibit metabolism of theophylline.

Effect
Serum theophylline level and risk of toxicity may increase.

Nursing considerations
■ When starting or stopping a macrolide, monitor serum theophylline level. Normal therapeutic range is 10 to 20 mcg/ml for adults and 5 to 15 mcg/ml for children.
■ Watch for evidence of toxicity, such as tachycardia, anorexia, nausea, vomiting, diarrhea, seizures, restlessness, irritability, and headache.
■ Describe adverse effects of theophylline and signs of toxicity, and tell patient to report them immediately to prescriber.

bacitracin ▶◀ nondepolarizing muscle relaxants

Baci-IM   atracurium, pancuronium, vecuronium

Risk rating: 2
Severity: Moderate   Onset: Rapid   Likelihood: Probable

Cause
Polypeptide antibiotics, such as bacitracin, may act synergistically with nondepolarizing muscle relaxants.

Effect
Neuromuscular blockade may increase.

Nursing considerations
■ If possible, avoid combining these drugs.

- Monitor neuromuscular function closely.
- Dosage of nondepolarizing muscle relaxant may need adjustment.
- Provide ventilatory support, as needed.
- Make sure patient is adequately sedated when receiving a nondepolarizing muscle relaxant.

belladonna ◄► phenothiazines
chlorpromazine, fluphenazine, perphenazine, prochlorperazine, promethazine, thioridazine, trifluoperazine

Risk rating: 2
Severity: **Moderate**   Onset: **Delayed**   Likelihood: **Suspected**

Cause
Anticholinergics, such as belladonna, may antagonize phenothiazines. Also, phenothiazine metabolism may increase.

Effect
Phenothiazine efficacy may decrease.

Nursing considerations
- Data regarding this interaction conflict.
- Monitor patient for decreased phenothiazine efficacy.
- Anticholinergic side effects may increase.
- Monitor patient for adynamic ileus, hyperpyrexia, hypoglycemia, and neurologic changes.

benazepril ◄► indomethacin
Lotensin   Indocin

Risk rating: 2
Severity: **Moderate**   Onset: **Rapid**   Likelihood: **Probable**

Cause
Indomethacin inhibits synthesis of prostaglandins, which benazepril and other ACE inhibitors need to lower blood pressure.

Effect
ACE inhibitor's hypotensive effect will be reduced.

Nursing considerations
⚑ ALERT Monitor blood pressure closely. Severe hypertension may persist until indomethacin is stopped.

■ If indomethacin can't be avoided, patient may need a different anti-hypertensive.
■ Other ACE inhibitors may interact with indomethacin. If you suspect an interaction, consult prescriber or pharmacist.
■ Remind patient that hypertension commonly causes no physical symptoms but sometimes may cause headache and dizziness.

---

benazepril ➤◀ potassium-sparing diuretics
Lotensin

amiloride, spironolactone, triamterene

Risk rating: 1
Severity: Major   Onset: Delayed   Likelihood: Probable

Cause
The mechanism of this interaction is unknown.

Effect
Serum potassium level may increase.

Nursing considerations
■ Use cautiously in patients at high risk for hyperkalemia, especially those with renal impairment.
■ Monitor BUN, creatinine, and serum potassium levels as needed.
■ ACE inhibitors other than benazepril may interact with potassium-sparing diuretics. If you suspect an interaction, consult prescriber or pharmacist.
■ Urge patient to immediately report an irregular heartbeat, a slow pulse, weakness, and other evidence of hyperkalemia.

---

benzphetamine ➤◀ MAO inhibitors
Didrex

phenelzine, tranylcypromine

Risk rating: 1
Severity: Major   Onset: Rapid   Likelihood: Suspected

Cause
This interaction probably stems from increased norepinephrine level at the synaptic cleft.

Effect
Anorexiant effects increase.

Nursing considerations
■ If possible, avoid giving these drugs together.

■ Headache and severe hypertension may occur rapidly if an amphetamine, such as benzphetamine, is given to patient who takes an MAO inhibitor.

◪ **ALERT** Death may result from hypertensive crisis and resulting cerebral hemorrhage.

■ Hypertensive reaction may occur for several weeks after stopping an MAO inhibitor.

benztropine ➤◀ phenothiazines

Cogentin

chlorpromazine, fluphenazine, perphenazine, prochlorperazine, promethazine, thioridazine, trifluoperazine

Risk rating: 2
Severity: Moderate   **Onset: Delayed**   **Likelihood: Suspected**

Cause
Anticholinergics, such as benztropine, may antagonize phenothiazines. Also, phenothiazine metabolism may increase.

Effect
Phenothiazine efficacy may decrease.

Nursing considerations
■ Data regarding this interaction conflict.
■ Monitor patient for decreased phenothiazine efficacy.
■ The phenothiazine dosage may need adjustment.
■ Anticholinergic side effects may increase.
■ Monitor patient for adynamic ileus, hyperpyrexia, hypoglycemia, and neurologic changes.

betamethasone ➤◀ cholinesterase inhibitors

Celestone

ambenonium, edrophonium, neostigmine, pyridostigmine

Risk rating: 1
Severity: Major   **Onset: Delayed**   **Likelihood: Probable**

Cause
In myasthenia gravis, betamethasone and other corticosteroids antagonize the effects of cholinesterase inhibitors by an unknown mechanism.

Effect
Patient may develop severe muscular depression refractory to cholinesterase inhibitor.

Nursing considerations
■ Corticosteroid therapy may have long-term benefits in myasthenia gravis.
■ Combined therapy may be attempted under strict supervision.
■ In myasthenia gravis, monitor patient for severe muscle deterioration.
◪ ALERT Be prepared to provide respiratory support and mechanical ventilation if needed.
■ Consult prescriber or pharmacist about safe corticosteroid delivery to maximize improvement in muscle strength.

betamethasone ▶◀ hydantoins
Celestone   ethotoin, fosphenytoin, phenytoin

Risk rating: 2
Severity: Moderate   Onset: Delayed   Likelihood: Established

Cause
Hydantoins induce liver enzymes, which stimulate metabolism of corticosteroids, such as betamethasone.

Effect
Corticosteroid effects may decrease.

Nursing considerations
■ Avoid giving hydantoins with corticosteroids if possible.
■ Monitor patient for decreased corticosteroid effects. Also monitor phenytoin level, and adjust dosage of either drug as needed.
■ Corticosteroid effects may decrease within days of starting phenytoin and may stay decreased 3 weeks after it stops.

betamethasone ▶◀ rifamycins
Celestone   rifabutin, rifampin, rifapentine

Risk rating: 1
Severity: Major   Onset: Delayed   Likelihood: Established

Cause
Rifamycins increase hepatic metabolism of corticosteroids, such as betamethasone.

Effect
Corticosteroid effects may decrease.

Nursing considerations
■ If possible, avoid giving rifamycins with corticosteroids.
■ Monitor patient for decreased corticosteroid effects, including loss of disease control.
■ Monitor patient closely for symptom control after increasing rifamycin dose. Drug may need to be stopped to regain control of disease.
■ Corticosteroid effects may decrease within days of starting rifampin and may stay decreased 2 to 3 weeks after it stops.

---

betamethasone ►◄ salicylates

Celestone

aspirin, bismuth subsalicylate, choline salicylate, magnesium salicylate, salsalate, sodium salicylate, sodium thiosalicylate

Risk rating: 2
Severity: Moderate   Onset: Delayed   Likelihood: Probable

Cause
Corticosteroids, such as betamethasone, stimulate hepatic metabolism of salicylates and may increase renal excretion.

Effect
Salicylate level and effects decrease.

Nursing considerations
■ If patient takes a salicylate and a corticosteroid, monitor salicylate efficacy.
■ Monitor salicylate level; dosage may need adjustment.
◧ ALERT Giving a salicylate while tapering a corticosteroid may result in salicylate toxicity.
■ Watch for evidence of salicylate toxicity, including diaphoresis, nausea, vomiting, tinnitus, hyperventilation, and CNS depression.
■ Patients with renal impairment may be at greater risk.

betaxolol 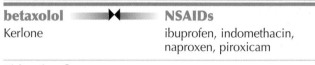 NSAIDs

Kerlone

ibuprofen, indomethacin,
naproxen, piroxicam

Risk rating: 2
Severity: Moderate   **Onset: Delayed**   **Likelihood: Probable**

Cause
NSAIDs may inhibit renal prostaglandin synthesis, allowing pressor
systems to be unopposed.

Effect
Beta blockers, such as betaxolol, may not be able to lower blood
pressure.

Nursing considerations
■ Avoid using these drugs together if possible.
■ Monitor blood pressure and other evidence of hypertension closely.
■ Talk with prescriber about ways to minimize interaction, such as ad-
justing beta blocker dosage or switching to sulindac as the NSAID.
■ Other NSAIDs may interact with beta blockers. If you suspect an
interaction, consult prescriber or pharmacist.

betaxolol   prazosin

Kerlone

Minipress

Risk rating: 2
Severity: Moderate   **Onset: Rapid**   **Likelihood: Probable**

Cause
The mechanism of this interaction is unknown.

Effect
Risk of orthostatic hypotension increases.

Nursing considerations
■ Assess patient's lying, sitting, and standing blood pressures closely,
especially when combined therapy starts.
■ To minimize effects of orthostatic hypotension, teach patient to
change positions slowly.
■ Interaction is confirmed only with propranolol but also may occur
with other beta blockers, such as betaxolol.

betaxolol ◄►◄ salicylates

Kerlone

aspirin, bismuth subsalicylate, choline salicylate, magnesium salicylate, salsalate, sodium salicylate, sodium thiosalicylate

Risk rating: 2
Severity: Moderate   **Onset: Rapid**   **Likelihood: Suspected**

Cause
Salicylates inhibit synthesis of prostaglandins, which beta blockers, such as betaxolol, need to reduce blood pressure. In patients with heart failure, the mechanism of this interaction is unknown.

Effect
Beta blocker effects decrease.

Nursing considerations
■ Watch closely for signs of heart failure and hypertension, and notify prescriber if they occur.
■ Talk with prescriber about switching patient to a different antihypertensive or antiplatelet drug.
■ Other beta blockers may interact with salicylates. If you suspect an interaction, consult prescriber or pharmacist.
■ Explain signs and symptoms of heart failure, and tell patient when to contact prescriber.

betaxolol ◄►◄ verapamil

Kerlone

Calan

Risk rating: 1
Severity: Major   **Onset: Rapid**   **Likelihood: Probable**

Cause
Verapamil may inhibit metabolism of beta blockers, such as betaxolol.

Effect
Effects of both drugs may increase.

Nursing considerations
■ Combining a beta blocker and verapamil is generally acceptable in patients with hypertension and unstable angina.
■ ALERT Risk of adverse effects increases, including heart failure, conduction disturbances, arrhythmias, and hypotension.

- Assess patient for adverse effects, including left ventricular dysfunction and AV conduction defects.
- Risk of interaction is greater when drugs are given I.V.
- Dosages of both drugs may need to be decreased.

biperiden ▸◂ phenothiazines

Akineton

chlorpromazine, fluphenazine, perphenazine, prochlorperazine, promethazine, thioridazine, trifluoperazine

Risk rating: 2
Severity: **Moderate**   Onset: **Delayed**   Likelihood: **Suspected**

Cause
Anticholinergics, such as biperiden, may antagonize phenothiazines. Also, phenothiazine metabolism may increase.

Effect
Phenothiazine efficacy may decrease.

Nursing considerations
- Data regarding this interaction conflict.
- Monitor patient for decreased phenothiazine efficacy.
- Phenothiazine dosage may need adjustment.
- Anticholinergic side effects may increase.
- Monitor patient for adynamic ileus, hyperpyrexia, hypoglycemia, and neurologic changes.

bisoprolol ▸◂ NSAIDs

Zebeta

ibuprofen, indomethacin, naproxen, piroxicam

Risk rating: 2
Severity: **Moderate**   Onset: **Delayed**   Likelihood: **Probable**

Cause
NSAIDs may inhibit renal prostaglandin synthesis, allowing pressor systems to be unopposed.

Effect
Beta blockers, such as bisoprolol, may not be able to lower blood pressure.

Nursing considerations
- Avoid using these drugs together if possible.

■ Monitor blood pressure and related signs and symptoms of hypertension closely.

■ Talk with prescriber about ways to minimize interaction, such as adjusting beta blocker dosage or switching to sulindac as the NSAID.

■ Other NSAIDs may interact with beta blockers. If you suspect an interaction, consult prescriber or pharmacist.

bisoprolol ▸◂ prazosin
Zebeta   Minipress

Risk rating: 2
Severity: Moderate   **Onset: Rapid**   **Likelihood: Probable**

Cause
The mechanism of this interaction is unknown.

Effect
Risk of orthostatic hypotension increases.

Nursing considerations
■ Assess patient's lying, sitting, and standing blood pressures closely, especially when combined therapy starts.

■ Adjust dosages of either drug as needed.

■ To minimize effects of orthostatic hypotension, teach patient to change positions slowly.

■ Interaction is confirmed only with propranolol but also may occur with other beta blockers, such as bisoprolol.

bisoprolol ▸◂ rifamycins
Zebeta   rifabutin, rifampin, rifapentine

Risk rating: 2
Severity: Moderate   **Onset: Delayed**   **Likelihood: Probable**

Cause
Rifamycins increase hepatic metabolism of beta blockers, such as bisoprolol.

Effect
Beta blocker effects decrease.

Nursing considerations
■ Monitor blood pressure and heart rate closely to assess beta blocker efficacy.

■ If beta blocker effects are decreased, consult prescriber; dosage may need to be increased.

■ Teach patient how to monitor blood pressure and heart rate and when to contact prescriber.

■ Other beta blockers may interact with rifamycins. If you suspect an interaction, consult prescriber or pharmacist.

---

bisoprolol ▶◀ salicylates

Zebeta

aspirin, bismuth subsalicylate, choline salicylate, magnesium salicylate, salsalate, sodium salicylate, sodium thiosalicylate

Risk rating: 2
Severity: Moderate   **Onset: Rapid**   **Likelihood: Suspected**

Cause
Salicylates inhibit synthesis of prostaglandins, which beta blockers, such as bisoprolol, need to lower blood pressure. In patients with heart failure, the mechanism of this interaction is unknown.

Effect
Beta blocker effects decrease.

Nursing considerations
■ Watch closely for signs of heart failure and hypertension, and notify prescriber if they occur.

■ Consult prescriber about switching patient to a different antihypertensive or antiplatelet drug.

■ Other beta blockers may interact with salicylates. If you suspect an interaction, consult prescriber or pharmacist.

■ Explain signs and symptoms of heart failure, and tell patient when to contact prescriber.

---

bisoprolol ▶◀ verapamil

Zebeta

Calan

Risk rating: 1
Severity: Major   **Onset: Rapid**   **Likelihood: Probable**

Cause
Verapamil may inhibit metabolism of beta blockers, such as bisoprolol.

Effect
Effects of both drugs may increase.

Nursing considerations
- Combining a beta blocker with verapamil is generally acceptable in patients with hypertension and unstable angina.
- **⚡ ALERT** Giving these drugs together increases risk of adverse effects, including heart failure, conduction disturbances, arrhythmias, and hypotension.
- Monitor patient for adverse effects, including left ventricular dysfunction and AV conduction defects.
- Risk of interaction is greater when drugs are given I.V.
- Dosages of both drugs may need to be decreased.

---

bosentan ━━━━▶◀━━━━ cyclosporine
Tracleer   Gengraf, Neoral, Sandimmune

Risk rating: 1
Severity: Major   **Onset: Delayed**   **Likelihood: Suspected**

Cause
Bosentan may increase cyclosporine metabolism. Cyclosporine may inhibit bosentan metabolism.

Effect
Bosentan level may increase. Cyclosporine level may decrease.

Nursing considerations
⚡ ALERT Use of bosentan with cyclosporine is contraindicated.
- Trough level of bosentan may increase 30 times above normal.
- Cyclosporine level may decrease by 50%.
- Watch for adverse effects from increased bosentan level, such as headache, nausea, vomiting, hypotension, and increased heart rate.

---

bumetanide ━━━━▶◀━━━━ aminoglycosides
Bumex   amikacin, gentamicin,
                                  kanamycin, neomycin,
                                  streptomycin, tobramycin

Risk rating: 1
Severity: Major   **Onset: Rapid**   **Likelihood: Suspected**

Cause
The mechanism of this interaction is unknown.

Effect
Interaction may cause synergistic ototoxicity and hearing loss of varying degrees, possibly permanent.

Nursing considerations
- Permanent hearing loss is more likely with this combination than when either drug is used alone.
- **ALERT** Renal insufficiency increases the risk of ototoxicity.
- Perform baseline and periodic hearing function tests.
- Other aminoglycosides may interact with loop diuretics, such as bumetanide. If you suspect an interaction, consult prescriber or pharmacist.
- Tell patient to immediately report ringing or roaring in the ears, muffled sounds, or any noticeable changes in hearing.
- Advise family members to stay alert for evidence of hearing loss.

bumetanide ━━━━◄ cisplatin
Bumex   Platinol

Risk rating: 2
Severity: **Moderate**   Onset: **Rapid**   Likelihood: **Suspected**

Cause
The mechanism of this interaction is unknown.

Effect
Interaction may cause additive ototoxicity.

Nursing considerations
- If possible, avoid giving a loop diuretic, such as bumetanide, and cisplatin together.
- Obtain hearing tests to detect early hearing loss.
- These drugs may cause ototoxicity much more severe than that caused by either drug alone.
- Ototoxicity may be permanent.
- Tell patient to report ringing in the ears, change in balance, or muffled sounds. Also, ask family members to watch for changes.

bumetanide ━━━━◄ thiazide diuretics
Bumex   chlorothiazide, hydrochloro-
                               thiazide, indapamide, methy-
                               clothiazide, metolazone, poly-
                               thiazide, trichlormethiazide

Risk rating: 2
Severity: **Moderate**   Onset: **Rapid**   Likelihood: **Probable**

Cause
The mechanism of this interaction is unclear.

Effect
Because these drugs work synergistically, they may cause profound diuresis and serious electrolyte abnormalities.

Nursing considerations
- This combination may be used for therapeutic benefit.
- Expect increased sodium, potassium, and chloride excretion and greater diuresis during combined therapy.
- Monitor patient for dehydration and electrolyte abnormalities.

---

bupropion ▶◀ ritonavir
Wellbutrin, Zyban   Norvir

Risk rating: 2
Severity: Moderate   Onset: Delayed   Likelihood: Suspected

Cause
Ritonavir may inhibit bupropion metabolism.

Effect
Large increases in serum bupropion level may occur.

Nursing considerations
⚠ **ALERT** Use together is contraindicated.
- If used together, risk of seizures from bupropion toxicity increases.
- To minimize the risk of interactions, urge patient to tell prescribers about all drugs and supplements he takes.

---

buspirone ▶◀ azole antifungals
BuSpar   fluconazole, itraconazole,
                             ketoconazole, miconazole

Risk rating: 2
Severity: Moderate   Onset: Delayed   Likelihood: Probable

Cause
Azole antifungal may inhibit the CYP3A4 isoenzyme responsible for buspirone metabolism.

Effect
Plasma buspirone level may increase.

Nursing considerations
- If patient is taking buspirone, monitor him closely when an azole antifungal is started or stopped or its dosage is changed.

- If patient is taking an azole antifungal, initial buspirone dose should be conservative.
- Monitor patient for signs of buspirone toxicity, including increased CNS effects (such as dizziness, drowsiness, and headache), vomiting, and diarrhea.
- Urge patient to tell prescriber about all drugs and supplements he takes and about any increase in adverse effects.

buspirone ⬛▶◀⬛ diltiazem
BuSpar   Cardizem

Risk rating: 2
Severity: Moderate   Onset: Delayed   Likelihood: Suspected

Cause
CYP3A4 metabolism of buspirone may decrease.

Effect
Buspirone level and adverse effects may increase.

Nursing considerations
- During buspirone therapy, monitor patient closely if diltiazem is started or stopped or its dosage is changed.
- Monitor patient for signs of buspirone toxicity, including increased CNS effects (such as dizziness, drowsiness, and headache), vomiting, and diarrhea.
- An antianxiety drug not metabolized by CYP3A4 (such as lorazepam) should be considered as alternative therapy if patient takes the calcium channel blocker diltiazem.
- Dihydropyridine calcium channel blockers (such as amlodipine and felodipine) that don't inhibit CYP3A4 metabolism probably wouldn't interfere with buspirone metabolism.
- Other calcium channel blockers may also have this interaction. If you suspect a drug interaction, consult prescriber or pharmacist.

buspirone ⬛▶◀⬛ grapefruit juice
BuSpar

Risk rating: 2
Severity: Moderate   Onset: Delayed   Likelihood: Probable

Cause
CYP3A4 metabolism of buspirone may be inhibited.

Effect
Buspirone level and adverse effects may increase.

Nursing considerations
■ If buspirone and grapefruit juice are taken together, buspirone adverse effects may increase, including dizziness, drowsiness, headache, vomiting, and diarrhea.
■ Advise patient to take buspirone with liquids other than grapefruit juice.
■ Urge patient to tell prescriber about all drugs and supplements he takes and about any increase in adverse effects.

---

buspirone ▶◀ **macrolide antibiotics**

BuSpar   clarithromycin, erythromycin,
                                    troleandomycin

Risk rating: 2
Severity: Moderate   **Onset: Delayed**   **Likelihood: Suspected**

Cause
CYP3A4 metabolism of buspirone may be inhibited by macrolide antibiotics.

Effect
Buspirone level and adverse effects may increase.

Nursing considerations
◤ ALERT Use of other macrolide antibiotics (such as azithromycin or dirithromycin) should be considered because they probably don't interact with buspirone. Consult prescriber or pharmacist.
■ During buspirone therapy, monitor patient closely if a macrolide antibiotic is started or stopped or its dosage is changed.
■ If patient takes a macrolide antibiotic, starting buspirone dose should be conservative.
■ Monitor patient for signs of buspirone toxicity, including increased CNS effects (such as dizziness, drowsiness, and headache), vomiting, and diarrhea.
■ Adjust buspirone dose as needed.

---

buspirone ▶◀ **rifamycins**

BuSpar   rifabutin, rifampin, rifapentine

Risk rating: 2
Severity: Moderate   **Onset: Delayed**   **Likelihood: Probable**

Cause
Buspirone metabolism may be increased via induction of CYP3A4 metabolism by rifamycins.

Effect
Buspirone effects may decrease.

Nursing considerations
■ Other rifamycins (such as rifaximin) may interact. If you suspect an interaction, consult prescriber or pharmacist.

■ Watch for expected buspirone effects when a rifamycin antibiotic is started or stopped or the dosage changes.

■ Advise patient to report increases or changes in anxiety if rifamycin antibiotic is started.

■ Urge patient to tell prescribers about all drugs and supplements he takes and about any increase in adverse effects.

---

buspirone ➤◀ verapamil
BuSpar   Calan

Risk rating: 2
Severity: Moderate   Onset: Delayed   Likelihood: Suspected

Cause
CYP3A4 metabolism of buspirone may decrease.

Effect
Buspirone level and adverse effects may increase.

Nursing considerations
■ Calcium channel blockers other than verapamil may interact with buspirone. If you suspect an interaction, consult prescriber or pharmacist.

■ During buspirone therapy, monitor patient closely if verapamil is started or stopped or the dosage changes.

■ Monitor patient for signs of buspirone toxicity, including increased CNS effects (such as dizziness, drowsiness, and headache), vomiting, and diarrhea.

■ An antianxiety drug not metabolized by CYP3A4 (such as lorazepam) should be considered as alternative therapy if patient takes verapamil.

■ Dihydropyridine calcium channel blockers (such as amlodipine and felodipine) that don't inhibit CYP3A4 metabolism probably wouldn't interfere with buspirone metabolism. Consult prescriber or pharmacist.

butabarbital 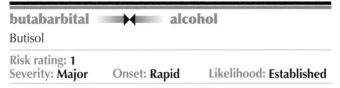 alcohol
Butisol

Risk rating: 1
Severity: **Major**   Onset: **Rapid**   Likelihood: **Established**

Cause
Acute alcohol intake inhibits hepatic metabolism of barbiturates, such as butabarbital. Chronic alcohol use increases barbiturate clearance, probably by inducing liver enzymes.

Effect
Acute alcohol intake with barbiturates can cause impaired hand-eye coordination, additive CNS effects, and death. Chronic alcohol use with barbiturates may cause drug tolerance, a need for increased barbiturate dosage, and an increased risk of adverse effects, including death.

Nursing considerations
◼ **ALERT** Because of the risk of serious adverse effects, including death, alcohol and barbiturates shouldn't be combined.
◼ Before barbiturate therapy starts, assess patient thoroughly for history or evidence of alcohol use.
◼ Other barbiturates interact with alcohol. If you suspect an interaction, consult prescriber or pharmacist.

butabarbital 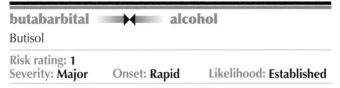 beta blockers
Butisol   metoprolol, propranolol

Risk rating: 2
Severity: **Moderate**   Onset: **Rapid**   Likelihood: **Probable**

Cause
Increased enzyme induction and first-pass hepatic metabolism of certain beta blockers reduce their availability.

Effect
Beta blocker efficacy may be reduced.

Nursing considerations
◼ Assess beta blocker efficacy by monitoring blood pressure, apical pulse, and presence of chest pain or headache, as appropriate.
◼ If patient has increased angina, rhythm problems, or blood pressure problems when starting a barbiturate, such as butabarbital, notify prescriber promptly. Beta blocker dosage may be increased.

■ Other beta blockers may interact with barbiturates. If you suspect an interaction, consult prescriber or pharmacist.
■ Explain the potential interaction between these drugs and the need to tell prescriber about any problems.

---

butabarbital ▶◀ corticosteroids

| Butisol | betamethasone, corticotropin, cortisone, cosyntropin, dexamethasone, fludrocortisone, hydrocortisone, methylprednisolone, prednisolone, prednisone, triamcinolone |

Risk rating: 2
Severity: Moderate   Onset: Delayed   Likelihood: Established

Cause
Butabarbital and other barbiturates induce liver enzymes, which stimulate corticosteroid metabolism.

Effect
Corticosteroid effects may be decreased.

Nursing considerations
■ Avoid giving barbiturates with corticosteroids, if possible.
■ If patient takes a corticosteroid, watch for worsening symptoms when a barbiturate is started or stopped.
■ During barbiturate treatment, corticosteroid dosage may need to be increased.

---

butabarbital ▶◀ methadone

| Butisol | Dolophine, Methadose |

Risk rating: 2
Severity: Moderate   Onset: Delayed   Likelihood: Suspected

Cause
The mechanism of this interaction is unknown, but barbiturates, such as butabarbital, probably increase hepatic metabolism of methadone.

Effect
Methadone effects may decrease, and patients on long-term therapy may notice opioid withdrawal symptoms.

Nursing considerations
■ If these drugs must be used together, monitor methadone efficacy.

- Check serum methadone level regularly.
- If methadone dosage is insufficient, it may be increased.
- Other barbiturates interact with methadone. If you suspect an interaction, consult prescriber or pharmacist.

butabarbital ▶◀ theophyllines
Butisol   aminophylline, theophylline

Risk rating: 2
Severity: Moderate   Onset: Delayed   Likelihood: Suspected

Cause
Butabarbital and other barbiturates may stimulate theophylline clearance by inducing the CYP pathway.

Effect
Theophylline level and efficacy may decrease.

Nursing considerations
- Monitor patient closely to determine theophylline efficacy.
- Monitor serum theophylline level regularly. Normal therapeutic range is 10 to 20 mcg/ml for adults and 5 to 15 mcg/ml for children.
- The theophylline dosage may need to be increased.
- Dyphylline undergoes renal elimination and may not be affected by this interaction.

calcium salts ▶◀ tetracyclines
calcium carbonate,   doxycycline, minocycline,
calcium citrate,   tetracycline
calcium gluconate,
calcium lactate,
tricalcium phosphate

Risk rating: 2
Severity: Moderate   Onset: Delayed   Likelihood: Probable

Cause
Calcium salts form an insoluble complex with tetracyclines that lowers tetracycline absorption.

Effect
Tetracycline level and efficacy decrease.

Nursing considerations
- Separate tetracyclines from calcium salts by at least 3 to 4 hours.

- Monitor efficacy of tetracycline in resolving infection. Notify prescriber if infection isn't responding to treatment.
- Doxycycline is somewhat less affected by this interaction.
- Advise against taking tetracycline with dairy products or calcium-fortified orange juice.
- Tell patient to separate tetracycline dose from calcium supplements by 3 to 4 hours.

---

candesartan ➤◄ potassium-sparing diuretics
Atacand

amiloride, spironolactone, triamterene

Risk rating: 1
Severity: Major   Onset: **Delayed**   Likelihood: **Suspected**

Cause
Both angiotensin II receptor antagonists, such as candesartan, and potassium-sparing diuretics may increase serum potassium level.

Effect
Risk of hyperkalemia may increase, especially among high-risk patients.

Nursing considerations
- High-risk patients include elderly people and those with renal impairment or type 2 diabetes; monitor these patients closely.
- Check serum potassium, BUN, and creatinine levels regularly. If they increase, notify prescriber.
- Advise patient to immediately report an irregular heartbeat, slow pulse, weakness, or other evidence of hyperkalemia.
- Give patient a list of foods high in potassium; stress the need to eat only moderate amounts.

---

captopril ➤◄ food
Capoten

Risk rating: 2
Severity: Moderate   Onset: **Rapid**   Likelihood: **Suspected**

Cause
Food decreases GI absorption of captopril.

Effect
Antihypertensive effectiveness may be reduced.

Nursing considerations
◪ ALERT Give captopril 1 hour before meals.
■ This interaction may occur with ACE inhibitors other than captopril. If you suspect a drug interaction, consult prescriber or pharmacist.
■ Food doesn't reduce absorption of enalapril or lisinopril.

---

captopril ━━━━▶◀━━━ indomethacin
Capoten   Indocin

Risk rating: 2
Severity: Moderate   **Onset: Rapid**   **Likelihood: Probable**

Cause
Indomethacin inhibits synthesis of prostaglandins, which captopril and other ACE inhibitors need to lower blood pressure.

Effect
ACE inhibitor's hypotensive effect will decrease.

Nursing considerations
◪ ALERT Monitor blood pressure closely. Severe hypertension may persist until indomethacin is stopped.
■ Patient taking indomethacin may need alternate antihypertensive.
■ Other ACE inhibitors may interact with indomethacin. If you suspect an interaction, consult prescriber or pharmacist.
■ Remind patient that hypertension commonly causes no physical symptoms but sometimes may cause headache and dizziness.

---

captopril ━━━━▶◀━━━ potassium-sparing diuretics
Capoten

amiloride, spironolactone, triamterene

Risk rating: 1
Severity: Major   **Onset: Delayed**   **Likelihood: Probable**

Cause
The mechanism of this interaction is unknown.

Effect
Serum potassium level may increase.

Nursing considerations
■ Use cautiously in patients at high risk for hyperkalemia, especially those with renal impairment.

- Monitor BUN, creatinine, and serum potassium level as needed.
- ACE inhibitors other than captopril may interact with potassium-sparing diuretics. If you suspect an interaction, consult prescriber or pharmacist.
- Urge patient to immediately report an irregular heartbeat, a slow pulse, weakness, and other evidence of hyperkalemia.

carbamazepine ➡◀ azole antifungals

Carbatrol, Epitol, Equetro, Tegretol

fluconazole, itraconazole, ketoconazole

Risk rating: 2
Severity: Moderate   Onset: Delayed   Likelihood: Suspected

Cause
Azole antifungals may inhibit CYP3A4 metabolism of carbamazepine.

Effect
Carbamazepine effects, including adverse effects, may increase.

Nursing considerations
- Monitor patient's response when an azole antifungal is started or stopped.
- Monitor carbamazepine level; therapeutic range is 4 to 12 mcg/ml.
- **ALERT** Watch for signs of anorexia or subtle appetite changes, which may indicate an excessive carbamazepine level.
- Monitor patient for signs of carbamazepine toxicity, including dizziness, ataxia, respiratory depression, tachycardia, arrhythmias, blood pressure changes, impaired consciousness, abnormal reflexes, nystagmus, seizures, nausea, vomiting, and urine retention.
- Other azole antifungals may interact with carbamazepine. If you suspect an interaction, consult prescriber or pharmacist.

carbamazepine ➡◀ bupropion

Carbatrol, Epitol, Equetro, Tegretol

Wellbutrin, Zyban

Risk rating: 2
Severity: Moderate   Onset: Delayed   Likelihood: Suspected

Cause
Carbamazepine increases hepatic metabolism of bupropion.

Effect
Bupropion level may decrease.

Nursing considerations
⚠ **ALERT** Bupropion is contraindicated in patients with a seizure disorder.
- Monitor patient's response to bupropion.
- Bupropion dosage may need adjustment.
- The risk of bupropion-related seizures may be reduced by keeping the daily dose below 450 mg (400 mg SR; 450 mg XL); giving the daily dose b.i.d. or t.i.d. (depending on preparation used) to avoid high peak levels; and increasing doses gradually.
- Urge patient to tell prescriber about all drugs and supplements he takes.

---

carbamazepine ▶◀ cimetidine
Carbatrol, Epitol,   Tagamet
Equetro, Tegretol

Risk rating: 2
Severity: Moderate   **Onset: Delayed**   **Likelihood: Suspected**

Cause
Cimetidine may inhibit hepatic metabolism of carbamazepine.

Effect
Carbamazepine plasma level and risk of toxicity may increase.

Nursing considerations
- Monitor patient's response when cimetidine starts (especially during the first 4 weeks of therapy) or stops.
- Monitor carbamazepine level; therapeutic range is 4 to 12 mcg/ml.
⚠ **ALERT** Watch for signs of anorexia or subtle appetite changes, which may indicate an excessive carbamazepine level.
- Monitor patient for signs of carbamazepine toxicity, including dizziness, ataxia, respiratory depression, tachycardia, arrhythmias, blood pressure changes, impaired consciousness, abnormal reflexes, nystagmus, seizures, nausea, vomiting, and urine retention.

---

carbamazepine ▶◀ cisatracurium
Carbatrol, Epitol,   Nimbex
Equetro, Tegretol

Risk rating: 2
Severity: Moderate   **Onset: Rapid**   **Likelihood: Probable**

Cause
The mechanism of this interaction is unknown.

Effect
The effect or duration of cisatracurium, a nondepolarizing muscle relaxant, may decrease.

Nursing considerations
- Monitor patient for decreased efficacy of muscle relaxant.
- Dosage of the nondepolarizing muscle relaxant may need to be increased.
- Make sure patient is adequately sedated when receiving a nondepolarizing muscle relaxant.

---

carbamazepine ➤◄ cyclosporine

Carbatrol, Epitol,   Gengraf, Neoral, Sandimmune
Equetro, Tegretol

Risk rating: 2
Severity: Moderate   **Onset: Delayed**   **Likelihood: Suspected**

Cause
Carbamazepine may induce hepatic metabolism of cyclosporine.

Effect
Cyclosporine level and effects may decrease.

Nursing considerations
- Monitor cyclosporine level; dosage may need adjustment.
- Watch for signs of rejection if carbamazepine therapy starts.
- Watch for signs of cyclosporine toxicity if carbamazepine therapy is stopped; signs of toxicity include hepatotoxicity, nephrotoxicity, nausea, vomiting, tremors, and seizures.

---

carbamazepine ➤◄ danazol

Carbatrol, Epitol,   Danocrine
Equetro, Tegretol

Risk rating: 2
Severity: Moderate   **Onset: Delayed**   **Likelihood: Suspected**

Cause
Danazol inhibits carbamazepine metabolism.

Effect
Carbamazepine level and toxicity may increase.

Nursing considerations
⚑ **ALERT** Avoid this combination if possible.

- Monitor carbamazepine level; therapeutic range is 4 to 12 mcg/ml.
- Carbamazepine dosage may need adjustment if danazol is started or stopped.

⚠ ALERT Watch for signs of anorexia or subtle appetite changes, which may indicate an excessive carbamazepine level.

- Monitor patient for evidence of carbamazepine toxicity, including dizziness, ataxia, respiratory depression, tachycardia, arrhythmias, blood pressure changes, impaired consciousness, abnormal reflexes, nystagmus, seizures, nausea, vomiting, and urine retention.

---

carbamazepine ▸◂ diltiazem

Carbatrol, Epitol,   Cardizem
Equetro, Tegretol

Risk rating: 2
Severity: Moderate   **Onset: Delayed**   **Likelihood: Suspected**

Cause
Diltiazem, a calcium channel blocker, may inhibit carbamazepine metabolism.

Effect
Carbamazepine level and risk of toxicity may increase.

Nursing considerations
- Monitor carbamazepine level; therapeutic range is 4 to 12 mcg/ml.
- If diltiazem therapy starts, watch for signs of carbamazepine toxicity, including dizziness, ataxia, respiratory depression, tachycardia, arrhythmias, blood pressure changes, impaired consciousness, abnormal reflexes, nystagmus, seizures, nausea, vomiting, and urine retention.
- If diltiazem therapy stops, watch for loss of carbamazepine effects (loss of seizure control). Carbamazepine dose may need to be increased.
- Urge patient to tell prescribers about all drugs and supplements he takes.
- Other calcium channel blockers may have this interaction. If you suspect an interaction, consult prescriber or pharmacist.

carbamazepine ▓▶◀▓ felbamate

Carbatrol, Epitol,   Felbatol
Equetro, Tegretol

Risk rating: 2
Severity: Moderate   **Onset: Delayed**   **Likelihood: Suspected**

Cause
The mechanism of this interaction is unknown. Carbamazepine metabolism may increase, or conversion of carbamazepine metabolites may decrease. Also, felbamate metabolism may increase.

Effect
Carbamazepine and felbamate levels and effects may decrease.

Nursing considerations
⚠ **ALERT** Monitor patient for loss of seizure control.
■ Monitor carbamazepine level; therapeutic range is 4 to 12 mcg/ml.
■ Dosage may need adjustment when felbamate starts.
■ Urge patient to tell prescribers about all drugs and supplements he takes.

carbamazepine ▓▶◀▓ felodipine

Carbatrol, Epitol,   Plendil
Equetro, Tegretol

Risk rating: 2
Severity: Moderate   **Onset: Delayed**   **Likelihood: Suspected**

Cause
The mechanism of this interaction is unknown. Carbamazepine may increase felodipine metabolism and decrease its availability.

Effect
Felodipine effects may decrease.

Nursing considerations
■ Felodipine dose may need to be increased.
■ If carbamazepine starts, watch for loss of blood pressure control, and urge patient to have blood pressure monitored.
■ If carbamazepine is stopped, watch for evidence of felodipine toxicity, such as peripheral vasodilation, hypotension, bradycardia, and palpitations.
■ Remind patient that hypertension commonly has no symptoms, although it may cause headache and dizziness.

carbamazepine ➤◄ fluoxetine

Carbatrol, Epitol,
Equetro, Tegretol

Prozac

Risk rating: 2
Severity: Moderate   **Onset: Delayed**   **Likelihood: Suspected**

Cause

The mechanism of this interaction is unknown. Fluoxetine may inhibit carbamazepine metabolism.

Effect

Carbamazepine level and risk of toxicity may increase.

Nursing considerations

■ Monitor carbamazepine level; therapeutic range is 4 to 12 mcg/ml.
■ **ALERT** Watch for signs of anorexia or subtle appetite changes, which may indicate excessive carbamazepine level.
■ Monitor patient for evidence of carbamazepine toxicity, including dizziness, ataxia, respiratory depression, tachycardia, arrhythmias, blood pressure changes, impaired consciousness, abnormal reflexes, nystagmus, seizures, nausea, vomiting, and urine retention.
■ Carbamazepine dosage may need adjustment if fluoxetine is started or stopped.
■ If fluoxetine starts during stabilized carbamazepine therapy, advise patient to report nausea, vomiting, dizziness, visual disturbances, difficulty balancing, tremors, or any new adverse effects.
■ SSRIs other than fluoxetine may interact with carbamazepine. If you suspect a drug interaction, consult prescriber or pharmacist.

carbamazepine ➤◄ grapefruit juice

Carbatrol, Epitol,
Equetro, Tegretol

Risk rating: 2
Severity: Moderate   **Onset: Delayed**   **Likelihood: Suspected**

Cause

CYP3A4 metabolism of carbamazepine may be inhibited.

Effect

Carbamazepine level and adverse effects may increase.

Nursing considerations

■ **ALERT** Avoid giving carbamazepine with grapefruit juice.
■ Carbamazepine adverse effects may be increased, including dizzi-

ness, ataxia, arrhythmias, impaired consciousness, worsening seizures, nausea, and vomiting.
- Therapeutic carbamazepine level is 4 to 12 mcg/ml.
- Advise patient to tell prescriber about all drugs and supplements he takes and any increase in adverse effects.

---

carbamazepine ▶◀ haloperidol
Carbatrol, Epitol,   Haldol
Equetro, Tegretol

Risk rating: 2
Severity: Moderate   Onset: Delayed   Likelihood: Suspected

Cause
Carbamazepine may increase haloperidol hepatic metabolism; haloperidol may inhibit carbamazepine metabolism.

Effect
Haloperidol effects may decrease; carbamazepine effects, including adverse effects, may increase.

Nursing considerations
- Monitor haloperidol level; therapeutic range is 5 to 20 ng/ml.
- Monitor carbamazepine level; therapeutic range is 4 to 12 mcg/ml.
- Watch for loss of haloperidol effects, including symptoms of psychomotor agitation, obsessive-compulsive rituals, withdrawn behavior, auditory hallucinations, delusions, and delirium.
- **⚡ ALERT** Watch for signs of anorexia or subtle appetite changes, which may indicate an excessive carbamazepine level.
- Watch for signs of carbamazepine toxicity, including dizziness, ataxia, respiratory depression, tachycardia, arrhythmias, blood pressure changes, impaired consciousness, abnormal reflexes, nystagmus, seizures, nausea, vomiting, and urine retention.

---

carbamazepine ▶◀ HMG-CoA reductase inhibitors
Carbatrol, Epitol,
Equetro, Tegretol   atorvastatin, lovastatin,
                            simvastatin

Risk rating: 2
Severity: Moderate   Onset: Delayed   Likelihood: Suspected

Cause
Carbamazepine may increase CYP3A4 metabolism of HMG-CoA reductase inhibitor.

Effect
HMG-CoA reductase inhibitor effects may be reduced.

Nursing considerations
- If possible, avoid use together.
- If use together can't be avoided, monitor serum cholesterol and lipid levels to assess patient's response to therapy.
- If hypercholesterolemia increases, notify prescriber.
- Pravastatin and rosuvastatin may be less likely to interact with carbamazepine and may be better choices than other HMG-CoA reductase inhibitors.

---

carbamazepine ➤◀ hormonal contraceptives
Carbatrol, Epitol, Ortho-Novum
Equetro, Tegretol

Risk rating: 2
Severity: Moderate   **Onset: Delayed**   **Likelihood: Suspected**

Cause
Hepatic metabolism of hormonal contraceptives may increase.

Effect
Contraceptive effectiveness may decrease.

Nursing considerations
- Other hormonal contraceptives may interact with carbamazepine. If you suspect a drug interaction, consult prescriber or pharmacist.
- Urge patient to use an alternative method of birth control to avoid unintended pregnancy.
- Larger hormonal contraceptive doses may be considered; consult prescriber about dosage to prevent breakthrough bleeding.

---

carbamazepine ➤◀ hydantoins
Carbatrol, Epitol, ethotoin, fosphenytoin,
Equetro, Tegretol phenytoin

Risk rating: 2
Severity: Moderate   **Onset: Delayed**   **Likelihood: Suspected**

Cause
Carbamazepine metabolism may increase. Carbamazepine also may decrease phenytoin availability.

Effect
Carbamazepine level and effects decrease. The effect of carbamazepine on phenytoin is variable.

Nursing considerations
■ Monitor serum levels of both drugs as appropriate, especially when starting or stopping either one.
■ Therapeutic carbamazepine level is 4 to 12 mcg/ml.
■ Therapeutic phenytoin level is 10 to 20 mcg/ml.
■ Dosage adjustments may be needed to maintain therapeutic effects and avoid toxicity.
■ Monitor patient for loss of drug effect (loss of seizure control).

---

carbamazepine ▶◀ isoniazid
Carbatrol, Epitol,
Equetro, Tegretol

Nydrazid

Risk rating: 2
Severity: Moderate   **Onset: Delayed**   **Likelihood: Suspected**

Cause
Isoniazid may inhibit carbamazepine metabolism. Carbamazepine may increase isoniazid hepatotoxicity.

Effect
Risk of carbamazepine toxicity and isoniazid hepatotoxicity increases.

Nursing considerations
■ Monitor carbamazepine level; therapeutic range is 4 to 12 mcg/ml.
■ Watch for signs of carbamazepine toxicity, including dizziness, ataxia, respiratory depression, tachycardia, arrhythmias, blood pressure changes, impaired consciousness, abnormal reflexes, nystagmus, seizures, nausea, vomiting, and urine retention.
■ Monitor liver function tests.
■ Advise patient to report signs of hepatotoxicity, including abdominal pain, loss of appetite, fatigue, yellow skin or eyes, and dark urine.

carbamazepine ◀▶ lamotrigine
Carbatrol, Epitol,   Lamictal
Equetro, Tegretol

Risk rating: 2
Severity: Moderate   Onset: Delayed   Likelihood: Suspected

Cause
Lamotrigine metabolism may increase. Lamotrigine may increase carbamazepine toxicity.

Effect
Lamotrigine effects may decrease. Carbamazepine metabolite level and risk of toxicity may increase.

Nursing considerations
■ Watch for expected lamotrigine effects when starting it in a patient who takes carbamazepine.
■ Lamotrigine dosage may need adjustment when starting or stopping carbamazepine or changing its dosage.
■ Monitor carbamazepine level when adding lamotrigine; therapeutic range is 4 to 12 mcg/ml.
■ Monitor patient for evidence of carbamazepine toxicity, including dizziness, ataxia, respiratory depression, tachycardia, arrhythmias, blood pressure changes, impaired consciousness, abnormal reflexes, nystagmus, seizures, nausea, vomiting, and urine retention.
■ Carbamazepine dosage may need reduction.

carbamazepine ◀▶ lithium
Carbatrol, Epitol,   Eskalith
Equetro, Tegretol

Risk rating: 2
Severity: Moderate   Onset: Delayed   Likelihood: Suspected

Cause
The mechanism of this interaction is unknown.

Effect
Risk of adverse CNS effects increases, including lethargy, muscle weakness, ataxia, tremor, and hyperreflexia.

Nursing considerations
■ Combination may be beneficial in treating bipolar depression and may be justified if benefits outweigh risks.
■ Some patients can tolerate combination without adverse effects.

carbamazepine ➤◄ macrolide antibiotics

Carbatrol, Epitol,
Equetro, Tegretol

clarithromycin, erythromycin,
troleandomycin

Risk rating: 1
Severity: Major   **Onset: Rapid**   **Likelihood: Established**

Cause
CYP3A4 metabolism of carbamazepine is inhibited, decreasing carbamazepine clearance.

Effect
Carbamazepine level and toxicity may increase.

Nursing considerations
⚡ ALERT If possible, avoid use together.
■ Consult prescriber or pharmacist about an alternative macrolide antibiotic (such as azithromycin) or an alternative anti-infective drug unlikely to interact with carbamazepine.
■ If using a macrolide antibiotic, monitor carbamazepine level; therapeutic range is 4 to 12 mcg/ml.
■ Monitor patient for evidence of carbamazepine toxicity, including dizziness, ataxia, respiratory depression, tachycardia, arrhythmias, blood pressure changes, impaired consciousness, abnormal reflexes, nystagmus, seizures, nausea, vomiting, and urine retention.
■ Carbamazepine dosage may need adjustment.

carbamazepine ➤◄ MAO inhibitors

Carbatrol, Epitol,
Equetro, Tegretol

isocarboxazid, phenelzine,
tranylcypromine

Risk rating: 1
Severity: Major   **Onset: Delayed**   **Likelihood: Suspected**

Cause
The mechanism of this interaction is unknown.

Effect
Risk of severe adverse effects, including hyperpyrexia, hyperexcitability, muscle rigidity, and seizures, may increase.

Nursing considerations
⚡ ALERT Use of carbamazepine with an MAO inhibitor is contraindicated.
⚡ ALERT Carbamazepine is structurally related to tricyclic antide-

pressants, which may cause hypertensive crisis, seizures, and death when given with MAO inhibitors.
■ MAO inhibitor should be stopped at least 14 days before carbamazepine starts.
■ Urge patient to tell prescriber about all drugs and supplements he takes and about any increase in adverse effects.

---

carbamazepine ▶◀ nefazodone
Carbatrol, Epitol,
Equetro, Tegretol

Risk rating: 1
Severity: Major   **Onset: Delayed**   **Likelihood: Suspected**

Cause
Nefazodone may inhibit CYP3A4 hepatic metabolism of carbamazepine. Carbamazepine may induce nefazodone metabolism.

Effect
Carbamazepine level and risk of adverse effects may increase. Nefazodone level and effects may decrease.

Nursing considerations
◤ ALERT Use of carbamazepine with nefazodone is contraindicated.
■ If drugs are combined for any reason, monitor carbamazepine serum level; therapeutic range is 4 to 12 mcg/ml.
■ Monitor patient for evidence of carbamazepine toxicity, including dizziness, ataxia, respiratory depression, tachycardia, arrhythmias, blood pressure changes, impaired consciousness, abnormal reflexes, nystagmus, seizures, nausea, vomiting, and urine retention.
■ Urge patient to tell prescriber about all drugs and supplements he takes and about any increase in adverse effects.

---

carbamazepine ▶◀ nondepolarizing muscle relaxants
Carbatrol, Epitol,
Equetro, Tegretol

atracurium, cisatracurium, mivacurium, pancuronium, rocuronium, vecuronium

Risk rating: 2
Severity: Moderate   **Onset: Rapid**   **Likelihood: Probable**

Cause
The mechanism of this interaction is unknown.

Effect
Effect or duration of nondepolarizing muscle relaxant may decrease.

Nursing considerations
- Monitor patient for decreased efficacy of muscle relaxant.
- Dosage of muscle relaxant may need to be increased.
- Make sure patient is adequately sedated when receiving a nondepolarizing muscle relaxant.

---

carbamazepine ➤◀ propoxyphene
Carbatrol, Epitol,   Darvon
Equetro, Tegretol

Risk rating: 2
Severity: Moderate   **Onset: Rapid**   **Likelihood: Suspected**

Cause
Hepatic metabolism of carbamazepine is inhibited, decreasing drug clearance.

Effect
Carbamazepine level and risk of toxicity may increase.

Nursing considerations
- **ALERT** Avoid combined use if possible.
- Monitor carbamazepine level; therapeutic range is 4 to 12 mcg/ml.
- Monitor patient for evidence of carbamazepine toxicity, including dizziness, ataxia, respiratory depression, tachycardia, arrhythmias, blood pressure changes, impaired consciousness, abnormal reflexes, nystagmus, seizures, nausea, vomiting, and urine retention.
- Consult prescriber or pharmacist about alternative analgesics to propoxyphene.

---

carbamazepine ➤◀ tricyclic antidepressants
Carbatrol, Epitol,   amitriptyline, desipramine,
Equetro, Tegretol   doxepin, imipramine,
                             nortriptyline

Risk rating: 2
Severity: Moderate   **Onset: Delayed**   **Likelihood: Probable**

Cause
Tricyclic antidepressants (TCAs) may compete with carbamazepine for hepatic metabolism. Carbamazepine may induce hepatic TCA metabolism.

Effect
Carbamazepine level and risk of toxicity may increase. TCA level and effects may decrease.

Nursing considerations
■ Other TCAs may interact with carbamazepine. If you suspect a drug interaction, consult prescriber or pharmacist.
■ Monitor carbamazepine level; therapeutic range is 4 to 12 mcg/ml.
■ Watch for evidence of carbamazepine toxicity, including dizziness, ataxia, respiratory depression, tachycardia, arrhythmias, blood pressure changes, impaired consciousness, abnormal reflexes, nystagmus, seizures, nausea, vomiting, and urine retention.

---

carbamazepine ◀▶ verapamil
Carbatrol, Epitol,   Calan
Equetro, Tegretol

Risk rating: 2
Severity: Moderate   Onset: Delayed   Likelihood: Suspected

Cause
Verapamil, a calcium channel blocker, may decrease hepatic metabolism of carbamazepine.

Effect
Carbamazepine level, effects, and toxic effects may increase.

Nursing considerations
■ Monitor carbamazepine level; therapeutic range is 4 to 12 mcg/ml.
■ Watch for evidence of carbamazepine toxicity, including dizziness, ataxia, respiratory depression, tachycardia, arrhythmias, blood pressure changes, impaired consciousness, abnormal reflexes, nystagmus, seizures, nausea, vomiting, and urine retention.
■ Carbamazepine dose may need to be reduced by 40% to 50%.
■ If verapamil is stopped, watch for loss of carbamazepine effect.
■ Other calcium channel blockers may interact with carbamazepine. If you suspect a drug interaction, consult prescriber or pharmacist.

carbamazepine 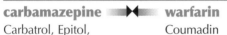 warfarin

Carbatrol, Epitol,   Coumadin
Equetro, Tegretol

Risk rating: 2
Severity: Moderate   Onset: Delayed   Likelihood: Suspected

Cause
Carbamazepine may increase hepatic metabolism of warfarin.

Effect
Anticoagulant effect of warfarin decreases.

Nursing considerations
■ If patient takes warfarin, monitor PT and INR when starting or
stopping carbamazepine or changing its dosage.
■ For an acute MI, atrial fibrillation, treatment of pulmonary embolism, prevention of systemic embolism, tissue heart valves, valvular
heart disease, or prophylaxis or treatment of venous thrombosis,
maintain INR at 2 to 3. For mechanical prosthetic valves or recurrent
systemic embolism, maintain INR at 3 to 4.5.

carbenicillin 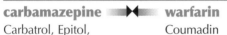 tetracyclines

Geocillin   demeclocycline, doxycycline,
                              minocycline, tetracycline

Risk rating: 1
Severity: Major   Onset: Delayed   Likelihood: Suspected

Cause
Tetracyclines may disrupt bactericidal activity of penicillins, such as
carbenicillin.

Effect
Penicillin efficacy may decrease.

Nursing considerations
■ If possible, avoid giving tetracyclines with penicillins.
■ Watch closely for lack of penicillin effect.

carbonic anhydrase ▶◀ salicylates
inhibitors

acetazolamide,
dichlorphenamide,
methazolamide

aspirin, choline salicylate,
magnesium salicylate,
salsalate, sodium salicylate,
sodium thiosalicylate

Risk rating: 2
Severity: Moderate   Onset: Delayed   Likelihood: Suspected

Cause
Carbonic anhydrase inhibitor is displaced from protein-binding sites,
and renal clearance is inhibited.

Effect
Carbonic anhydrase inhibitor level increases, causing acidosis and increased risk of salicylate penetration into the CNS.

Nursing considerations
■ Minimize or avoid combined use.
■ Monitor patient for evidence of salicylate toxicity, including lethar-
gy, confusion, fatigue, anorexia, urinary incontinence, tachypnea, and
hyperchloremic metabolic acidosis.
■ Chronic salicylate values higher than 15 mg/dl may produce toxicity.
Symptoms may appear in days to weeks.
■ Elderly patients and those with renal impairment are at greatest
risk of toxic effects.

carmustine ▶◀ cimetidine
BiCNU   Tagamet

Risk rating: 1
Severity: Major   Onset: Delayed   Likelihood: Suspected

Cause
The mechanism of interaction is unknown, but may involve additive
bone marrow suppression or decreased carmustine metabolism.

Effect
Carmustine myelosuppressive effects increase.

Nursing considerations
◱ ALERT Avoid combined use if possible.
■ Monitor CBC, WBC, and platelet counts if used together.
■ Be prepared to provide supportive measures, such as blood compo-
nents and granulocyte-colony stimulating factor, as ordered.

■ Consult prescriber or pharmacist for alternative drug to avoid severe myelosuppression.

■ H_2-receptor antagonists other than cimetidine may interact with carmustine. If you suspect an interaction, consult prescriber or pharmacist.

---

carteolol ◀▶ epinephrine
Cartrol

Risk rating: 1
Severity: Major   **Onset: Rapid**   **Likelihood: Established**

Cause
Alpha-receptor effects of epinephrine supersede the effects of non-selective beta blockers, such as caretolol, increasing vascular resistance.

Effect
Initial marked hypertensive effect is followed by reflex bradycardia.

Nursing considerations
⚡ ALERT Three days before planned use of epinephrine, stop the beta blocker. Or, if possible, don't use epinephrine.
■ Monitor blood pressure and pulse. If interaction occurs, give I.V. chlorpromazine, hydralazine, aminophylline, or atropine if needed.
■ Explain the risks of this interaction, and tell patient to carry medical identification at all times.
■ Other beta blockers may interact with epinephrine. If you suspect an interaction, consult prescriber or pharmacist.

---

carteolol ◀▶ ergot derivatives
Cartrol   dihydroergotamine, ergotamine

Risk rating: 2
Severity: Moderate   **Onset: Delayed**   **Likelihood: Suspected**

Cause
Carteolol- or other beta blocker–mediated blockade of peripheral $beta_2$ receptors allows unopposed ergot action.

Effect
Vasoconstrictive effects of ergot derivatives increase, causing peripheral ischemia, cold extremities, and possible gangrene.

Nursing considerations
■ Watch for evidence of peripheral ischemia.

- If needed, stop beta blocker and adjust ergot derivative.
- Other ergot derivatives may interact with beta blockers. If you suspect an interaction, consult prescriber or pharmacist

---

carteolol ━━━━◄►━━━━ NSAIDs

Cartrol

ibuprofen, indomethacin, naproxen, piroxicam

Risk rating: 2
Severity: Moderate   Onset: Delayed   Likelihood: Probable

Cause
NSAIDs may inhibit renal prostaglandin synthesis, allowing pressor systems to be unopposed.

Effect
Beta blockers, such as carteolol, may not be able to lower blood pressure.

Nursing considerations
- Avoid using these drugs together if possible.
- Monitor blood pressure and related signs and symptoms of hypertension closely.
- Consult prescriber about ways to avoid interaction, such as adjusting beta blocker dosage or switching to sulindac as the NSAID.
- Other NSAIDs may interact with beta blockers. If you suspect an interaction, consult prescriber or pharmacist.

---

carteolol ━━━━◄►━━━━ prazosin

Cartrol

Minipress

Risk rating: 2
Severity: Moderate   Onset: Rapid   Likelihood: Probable

Cause
The mechanism of this interaction is unknown.

Effect
Risk of orthostatic hypotension increases.

Nursing considerations
- Assess patient's lying, sitting, and standing blood pressures closely, especially when combined therapy starts.
- Adjust dosages of either drug based on patient effects.
- To minimize effects of orthostatic hypotension, teach patient to change positions slowly.

■ Interaction is confirmed only with propranolol, but also may occur with other beta blockers, such as carteolol.

---

carteolol ◄►► salicylates

Cartrol

aspirin, bismuth subsalicylate, choline salicylate, magnesium salicylate, salsalate, sodium salicylate, sodium thiosalicylate

Risk rating: 2
Severity: Moderate   Onset: Rapid   Likelihood: Suspected

Cause
Salicylates inhibit synthesis of prostaglandins, which carteolol and other beta blockers need to lower blood pressure. In patients with heart failure, the mechanism of this interaction is unknown.

Effect
Beta blocker effects decrease.

Nursing considerations
■ Watch closely for signs of heart failure and hypertension, and notify prescriber if they occur.
■ Consult prescriber about switching patient to a different antihypertensive or antiplatelet drug.
■ Other beta blockers may interact with salicylates. If you suspect an interaction, consult prescriber or pharmacist.
■ Explain signs and symptoms of heart failure, and tell patient when to contact prescriber.

---

carteolol ◄►► theophyllines

Cartrol

aminophylline, theophylline

Risk rating: 2
Severity: Moderate   Onset: Rapid   Likelihood: Probable

Cause
Theophylline clearance may be reduced up to 50%.

Effect
Theophylline efficacy may decrease.

Nursing considerations
■ When starting therapy with a nonselective beta blocker, such as carteolol, watch for decreased theophylline efficacy.

■ Monitor serum theophylline level closely, and notify prescriber about subtherapeutic level.
■ Normal therapeutic range for theophylline is 10 to 20 mcg/ml for adults and 5 to 15 mcg/ml for children.
■ Selective beta blockers may be preferred for patients who take theophylline, but the interaction remains with high doses of beta blocker.
■ Other beta blockers may interact with theophyllines. If you suspect an interaction, consult prescriber or pharmacist.

carteolol ▶◀ verapamil
Cartrol   Calan

Risk rating: 1
Severity: Major   **Onset: Rapid**   **Likelihood: Probable**

Cause
Verapamil may inhibit metabolism of beta blockers, such as carteolol.

Effect
Effects of both drugs may increase.

Nursing considerations
■ Combining a beta blocker and verapamil is generally acceptable in patients with hypertension and unstable angina.
▶ **ALERT** Risk of adverse effects increases, including heart failure, conduction disturbances, arrhythmias, and hypotension.
■ Assess patient for adverse effects, including left ventricular dysfunction and AV conduction defects.
■ Risk of interaction is greater when drugs are given I.V.
■ Dosages of both drugs may need to be decreased.

carvedilol ▶◀ cyclosporine
Coreg   Gengraf, Neoral, Sandimmune

Risk rating: 2
Severity: Moderate   **Onset: Delayed**   **Likelihood: Suspected**

Cause
Carvedilol may interfere with cyclosporine metabolism.

Effect
Cyclosporine level and risk of toxicity may increase.

Nursing considerations
■ Beta blockers other than carvedilol may interact with cyclosporine.

- Watch for evidence of cyclosporine toxicity, such as nephrotoxicity and neurotoxicity.
- Monitor serum creatinine level.
- Monitor cyclosporine level.

carvedilol ▶◀ salicylates

Coreg

aspirin, bismuth subsalicylate, choline salicylate, magnesium salicylate, salsalate, sodium salicylate, sodium thiosalicylate

Risk rating: 2
Severity: Moderate   Onset: Rapid   Likelihood: Suspected

Cause
Salicylates inhibit synthesis of prostaglandins, which carvedilol and other beta blockers need to lower blood pressure. In patients with heart failure, the mechanism of this interaction is unknown.

Effect
Beta blocker effects decrease.

Nursing considerations
- Watch closely for signs of heart failure and hypertension, and notify prescriber if they occur.
- Consult prescriber about switching patient to a different antihypertensive or antiplatelet drug.
- Other beta blockers may interact with salicylates. If you suspect an interaction, consult prescriber or pharmacist.
- Explain signs and symptoms of heart failure, and tell patient when to contact prescriber.

cephalosporins ▶◀ alcohol

cefoperazone, cefotetan, cefoxitin, ceftriaxone

Risk rating: 2
Severity: Moderate   Onset: Rapid   Likelihood: Probable

Cause
Certain cephalosporins may prevent complete alcohol metabolism.

Effect
Disulfiram-like reaction may occur if patient consumes alcohol after taking certain cephalosporins.

Nursing considerations
- If patient consumes alcohol, watch for disulfiram-like reaction that may include flushing, tachycardia, bronchospasm, sweating, nausea, and vomiting.
- Interaction may occur immediately or after several days.
- Cephalosporins with similar structure probably have similar effects. If you suspect an interaction, consult prescriber or pharmacist.

cephalosporins ◀▶ aminoglycosides

cefazolin, cefoperazone, cefotaxime, cefotetan, cefoxitin, ceftazidime, ceftizoxime, ceftriaxone, cefuroxime, cephradine

amikacin, gentamicin, kanamycin, neomycin, streptomycin, tobramycin

Risk rating: 2
Severity: **Moderate**   Onset: **Delayed**   Likelihood: **Suspected**

Cause
The mechanism of this interaction is unknown.

Effect
Bactericidal activity may increase against some organisms, but risk of nephrotoxicity also may increase.

Nursing considerations
- **ALERT** Check peak and trough aminoglycoside level after third dose. For peak level, draw blood 30 minutes after I.V. or 60 minutes after I.M. dose. For trough level, draw blood just before a dose.
- Assess BUN and creatinine levels.
- Monitor urine output, and check urine for increased protein, cell, or cast levels.
- If renal insufficiency develops, notify prescriber. Dosage may need to be reduced, or drug may need to be stopped.
- Other aminoglycosides may interact with cephalosporins. If you suspect an interaction, consult prescriber or pharmacist.

chloramphenicol ➡️◄ sulfonylureas

Chloromycetin

acetohexamide,
chlorpropamide,
glipizide, glyburide,
tolazamide, tolbutamide

Risk rating: 2
Severity: **Moderate**   Onset: **Delayed**   Likelihood: **Suspected**

Cause
Chloramphenicol reduces hepatic clearance of sulfonylureas.

Effect
Because sulfonylurea level is prolonged, hypoglycemia may occur.

Nursing considerations
■ Monitor patient for hypoglycemia.
■ Describe signs and symptoms of hypoglycemia, including diaphoresis, fatigue, headache, hunger, irritability, malaise, nervousness, rapid heart rate, tension, and trembling.
■ Instruct patient to eat a small carbohydrate snack or meal if hypoglycemia develops, preferably after checking blood glucose level.

chlordiazepoxide ➡️◄ alcohol

Librium

Risk rating: 2
Severity: **Moderate**   Onset: **Rapid**   Likelihood: **Established**

Cause
Alcohol inhibits hepatic enzymes, which decreases clearance and increases peak level of benzodiazepines, such as chlordiazepoxide.

Effect
Combining a benzodiazepine and alcohol may have additive or synergistic effects.

Nursing considerations
■ Advise against consuming alcohol while taking a benzodiazepine.
■ Before benzodiazepine therapy starts, assess patient thoroughly for history or evidence of alcohol use.
■ Watch for additive CNS effects, which may suggest benzodiazepine overdose.
■ Other benzodiazepines interact with alcohol. If you suspect an interaction, consult prescriber or pharmacist.

■ When a patient starts a benzodiazepine, stress the high risks of consuming alcohol.

---

chlordiazepoxide ➤◀ azole antifungals

Librium

fluconazole, itraconazole,
ketoconazole, miconazole

Risk rating: 2
Severity: Moderate   Onset: Rapid   Likelihood: Established

Cause
Azole antifungals decrease CYP3A4 metabolism of certain benzodiazepines, such as chlordiazepoxide.

Effect
Benzodiazepine effects are increased and prolonged, which may cause CNS depression and psychomotor impairment.

Nursing considerations
■ If patient takes fluconazole or miconazole, consult prescriber about giving a lower benzodiazepine dose or a drug not metabolized by CYP3A4, such as temazepam or lorazepam.
■ Caution that the effects of this interaction may last several days after stopping the azole antifungal.
■ Various benzodiazepine–azole antifungal combinations may interact. If you suspect an interaction, consult prescriber or pharmacist.

---

chlordiazepoxide ➤◀ protease inhibitors

Librium

amprenavir, atazanavir,
indinavir, lopinavir-ritonavir,
nelfinavir, ritonavir, saquinavir

Risk rating: 2
Severity: Moderate   Onset: Delayed   Likelihood: Suspected

Cause
Protease inhibitors may inhibit CYP3A4 metabolism of certain benzodiazepines, such as chlordiazepoxide.

Effect
Sedative effects of benzodiazepines may be increased and prolonged, leading to severe respiratory depression.

Nursing considerations
⚡ ALERT Don't combine chlordiazepoxide with protease inhibitors.

■ If patient takes any benzodiazepine–protease inhibitor combination, notify prescriber. Interaction could involve other drugs in the class.
■ Watch for evidence of oversedation and respiratory depression.
■ Teach patient and family about risks of using these drugs together.

chlordiazepoxide ▶◀ rifamycins

Librium

rifabutin, rifampin, rifapentine

Risk rating: 2
Severity: Moderate   Onset: Delayed   Likelihood: Suspected

Cause
Rifamycins may increase CYP3A4 metabolism of benzodiazepines, such as chlordiazepoxide.

Effect
Antianxiety, sedative, and sleep-inducing effects of benzodiazepines may decrease.

Nursing considerations
■ Watch for lack of benzodiazepine efficacy.
■ If benzodiazepine efficacy is reduced, notify prescriber; dosage may be changed.
■ Other benzodiazepines may interact with rifamycins. If you suspect an interaction, consult prescriber or pharmacist.
■ For insomnia, temazepam may be more effective because it doesn't undergo CYP3A4 metabolism.

chlorothiazide ▶◀ loop diuretics

Diuril

bumetanide, ethacrynic acid, furosemide, torsemide

Risk rating: 2
Severity: Moderate   Onset: Rapid   Likelihood: Probable

Cause
The mechanism of this interaction is unclear.

Effect
Because these drugs work synergistically, they may cause profound diuresis and serious electrolyte abnormalities.

Nursing considerations
■ This combination may be used for therapeutic benefit.
■ Expect increased sodium, potassium, and chloride excretion and greater diuresis.

■ Monitor patient for dehydration and electrolyte abnormalities.
■ Carefully adjust drugs using small or intermittent doses.

chlorothiazide ▶◀ sulfonylureas

Diuril

acetohexamide,
chlorpropamide,
glipizide, glyburide,
tolazamide, tolbutamide

Risk rating: 2
Severity: **Moderate**   Onset: **Delayed**   Likelihood: **Probable**

Cause
Chlorothiazide, a thiazide diuretic, may decrease insulin secretion
and tissue sensitivity to insulin, and it may increase sodium loss.

Effect
Risk of hyperglycemia and hyponatremia may increase.

Nursing considerations
■ Use these drugs together cautiously.
■ Monitor blood glucose and sodium levels regularly, and consult prescriber about dosage adjustments to maintain stable levels.
■ This interaction may occur several days to many months after dual
therapy starts but is readily reversible when the diuretic stops.
■ Describe signs and symptoms of hypoglycemia, including diaphoresis, fatigue, headache, hunger, irritability, malaise, nervousness, rapid
heart rate, tension, and trembling.
■ Instruct patient to eat a small carbohydrate snack or meal if hypoglycemia develops, preferably after checking blood glucose level.

chlorpromazine ▶◀ alcohol

Thorazine

Risk rating: 2
Severity: **Moderate**   Onset: **Rapid**   Likelihood: **Probable**

Cause
The mechanism of this interaction is unknown. It may be that these
substances produce CNS depression by working on different sites in
the brain. Also, alcohol may lower resistance to neurotoxic effects of
phenothiazines, such as chlorpromazine.

Effect
CNS depression may increase.

Nursing considerations
- Watch for extrapyramidal reactions, such as dystonic reactions and acute akathisia or restlessness.
- If patient takes a phenothiazine, warn that alcohol may worsen CNS depression and impair psychomotor skills.
- Discourage patient from drinking alcohol when taking a phenothiazine.

---

chlorpromazine ▬►◄▬ anticholinergics

Thorazine

atropine, belladonna, benztropine, biperiden, dicyclomine, hyoscyamine, oxybutynin, propantheline, scopolamine

Risk rating: 2
Severity: Moderate   Onset: Delayed   Likelihood: Suspected

Cause
Anticholinergics may antagonize phenothiazines, such as chlorpromazine. Also, phenothiazine metabolism may increase.

Effect
Phenothiazine efficacy may decrease.

Nursing considerations
- Data regarding this interaction conflict.
- Monitor patient for decreased phenothiazine efficacy.
- Phenothiazine dosage may need adjustment.
- Anticholinergic side effects may increase.
- Monitor patient for adynamic ileus, hyperpyrexia, hypoglycemia, and neurologic changes.

---

chlorpromazine ▬►◄▬ beta blockers

Thorazine

pindolol, propranolol

Risk rating: 1
Severity: Major   Onset: Delayed   Likelihood: Probable

Cause
Chlorpromazine may inhibit first-pass hepatic metabolism of propranolol.

Effect
Effects of both drugs and the risk of serious adverse reactions may increase.

Nursing considerations

■ If propranolol and chlorpromazine must be used together, monitor blood pressure and pulse rate regularly; propranolol dosage may need to be decreased.

■ Assess patient for adverse reactions to propranolol: fatigue, lethargy, dizziness, nausea, heart failure, and agranulocytosis.

■ Explain to patient and family the expected and adverse effects of these drugs and the risk of interaction.

■ Other beta blockers may interact with phenothiazines, such as chlorpromazine. If you suspect an interaction, consult prescriber or pharmacist.

chlorpromazine ➤◀ meperidine
Thorazine   Demerol

Risk rating: 2
Severity: Moderate   **Onset: Rapid**   **Likelihood: Probable**

Cause
Additive CNS depressant and cardiovascular effects may occur.

Effect
Excessive sedation and hypotension may occur.

Nursing considerations

■ Avoid using meperidine with phenothiazines, such as chlorpromazine.

■ These drugs have been used together to minimize opioid dosage and control nausea and vomiting, but risks may outweigh benefits.

■ Monitor patient for more severe and extended respiratory depression.

chlorpromazine ➤◀ quinolones
Thorazine   gatifloxacin, levofloxacin, moxifloxacin, sparfloxacin

Risk rating: 1
Severity: Major   **Onset: Delayed**   **Likelihood: Suspected**

Cause
The mechanism of this interaction is unknown.

Effect
Risk of life-threatening arrhythmias, including torsades de pointes, may increase.

Nursing considerations
⚠ ALERT Sparfloxacin is contraindicated in patients taking drugs that prolong the QTc interval, including phenothiazines, such as chlorpromazine.
■ Avoid giving levofloxacin.
■ Use gatifloxacin and moxifloxacin cautiously, with increased monitoring.
■ Quinolones that don't prolong the QTc interval or that aren't metabolized by CYP3A4 isoenzymes may be better alternatives.

chlorpropamide ➡◀ alcohol
Diabinese

Risk rating: 2
Severity: Moderate   Onset: Rapid   Likelihood: Established

Cause
Chronic alcohol use may interact with chlorpropamide by an unknown mechanism.

Effect
A disulfiram-like reaction may occur.

Nursing considerations
■ Alcohol also interacts with sulfonylureas other than chlorpropamide.
■ Naloxone may be used to antagonize a disulfiram-like reaction.
■ Tell patient who takes an oral antidiabetic to avoid ingesting more alcohol than an occasional single drink.
■ Urge patient to have regular follow-up blood tests to monitor diabetes and decrease episodes of hyperglycemia and hypoglycemia.
■ Describe the traits of a disulfiram-like reaction, including facial flushing and possible burning that spreads to the neck, headache, nausea, and tachycardia. Explain that it typically occurs within 20 minutes of alcohol intake and lasts for 1 to 2 hours.

chlorpropamide ➡◀ chloramphenicol
Diabinese   Chloromycetin

Risk rating: 2
Severity: Moderate   Onset: Delayed   Likelihood: Suspected

Cause
Chloramphenicol reduces hepatic clearance of sulfonylureas, such as chlorpropamide.

Effect

Because sulfonylurea level is prolonged, hypoglycemia may occur.

Nursing considerations

■ If patient takes a sulfonylurea, start chloramphenicol carefully, and monitor patient for hypoglycemia.

■ Describe signs and symptoms of hypoglycemia, including diaphoresis, fatigue, headache, hunger, irritability, malaise, nervousness, rapid heart rate, tension, and trembling.

■ Instruct patient to eat a small carbohydrate snack or meal if hypoglycemia develops, preferably after checking blood glucose level.

chlorpropamide ▬▶◀▬ diazoxide

Diabinese   Hyperstat, Proglycem

Risk rating: 2

Severity: Moderate   Onset: Delayed   Likelihood: Probable

Cause

Diazoxide may decrease insulin release or stimulate release of glucose and free fatty acids by various mechanisms.

Effect

The risk of hyperglycemia increases if a patient stabilized on a sulfonylurea, such as chlorpropamide, starts taking diazoxide.

Nursing considerations

■ Use these drugs together cautiously.

■ Monitor patient's blood glucose level regularly; consult prescriber about adjustments to either drug to maintain stable glucose level.

■ Teach patient to use a self-monitoring glucose meter and to report significant changes to prescriber.

■ Tell patient to stay alert for increased fatigue, thirst, eating, or urination and possible blurred vision or dry skin and mucous membranes as evidence of high blood glucose level.

chlorpropamide ▬▶◀▬ MAO inhibitors

Diabinese   isocarboxazid, phenelzine, tranylcypromine

Risk rating: 2

Severity: Moderate   Onset: Rapid   Likelihood: Suspected

Cause

The mechanism of this interaction is unknown.

Effect
MAO inhibitors increase the hypoglycemic effects of sulfonylureas, such as chlorpropamide.

Nursing considerations
■ If patient takes a sulfonylurea, start an MAO inhibitor carefully, monitoring patient for hypoglycemia.
■ Consult prescriber about adjustments to either drug to control glucose level and mental status.
■ Describe signs and symptoms of hypoglycemia, including diaphoresis, fatigue, headache, hunger, irritability, malaise, nervousness, rapid heart rate, tension, and trembling.
■ Instruct patient to eat a small carbohydrate snack or meal if hypoglycemia develops, preferably after checking blood glucose level.

---

chlorpropamide ◄► rifamycins
Diabinese   rifabutin, rifampin, rifapentine

Risk rating: 2
Severity: Moderate   **Onset: Delayed**   **Likelihood: Probable**

Cause
Rifamycins may increase hepatic metabolism of certain sulfonylureas, such as chlorpropamide.

Effect
The risk of hyperglycemia increases.

Nursing considerations
■ Use these drugs together cautiously.
■ Monitor patient's blood glucose level regularly; consult prescriber about adjustments to either drug to maintain stable glucose level.
■ Teach patient to use a self-monitoring glucose meter and to report significant changes to prescriber.
■ Tell patient to stay alert for increased fatigue, thirst, eating, or urination and possible blurred vision or dry skin and mucous membranes as evidence of high blood glucose level.

chlorpropamide ◢◤ salicylates

Diabinese

aspirin, choline salicylate, magnesium salicylate, salsalate, sodium salicylate, sodium thiosalicylate

Risk rating: 2
Severity: Moderate   **Onset: Delayed**   **Likelihood: Probable**

Cause
Salicylates reduce blood glucose level and prompt insulin secretion.

Effect
Hypoglycemic effects of chlorpropamide and other sulfonylureas increase.

Nursing considerations
- Monitor patient for hypoglycemia.
- Consult prescriber and patient about possibly replacing a salicylate with acetaminophen or an NSAID.
- Describe signs and symptoms of hypoglycemia, including diaphoresis, fatigue, headache, hunger, irritability, malaise, nervousness, rapid heart rate, tension, and trembling.
- Instruct patient to eat a small carbohydrate snack or meal if hypoglycemia develops, preferably after checking blood glucose level.

chlorpropamide ◢◤ sulfonamides

Diabinese

sulfasalazine, sulfisoxazole

Risk rating: 2
Severity: Moderate   **Onset: Delayed**   **Likelihood: Suspected**

Cause
Sulfonamides may hinder hepatic metabolism of sulfonylureas, such as chlorpropamide.

Effect
Prolonged sulfonylurea level increases risk of hypoglycemia.

Nursing considerations
- Monitor patient for hypoglycemia.
- Consult prescriber about adjustments to either drug to maintain stable glucose level.
- Glyburide doesn't interact and may be a good alternative to other sulfonylureas.

■ Describe signs and symptoms of hypoglycemia, including diaphoresis, fatigue, headache, hunger, irritability, malaise, nervousness, rapid heart rate, tension, and trembling.
■ Instruct patient to eat a small carbohydrate snack or meal if hypoglycemia develops, preferably after checking blood glucose level.

chlorpropamide ▶◀ thiazide diuretics

Diabinese

chlorothiazide, hydrochlorothiazide, indapamide, metolazone

Risk rating: 2
Severity: **Moderate**   Onset: **Delayed**   Likelihood: **Probable**

Cause
Thiazide diuretics may decrease insulin secretion and tissue sensitivity to insulin, and they may increase sodium loss.

Effect
The risk of hyperglycemia and hyponatremia may increase.

Nursing considerations
■ Use these drugs together cautiously.
■ Monitor patient's blood glucose and sodium levels regularly; consult prescriber about adjustments to either drug to maintain stable levels.
■ This interaction may occur several days to many months after dual therapy starts but is readily reversible when the diuretic stops.
■ Describe signs and symptoms of hypoglycemia, including diaphoresis, fatigue, headache, hunger, irritability, malaise, nervousness, rapid heart rate, tension, and trembling.
■ Instruct patient to eat a small carbohydrate snack or meal if hypoglycemia develops, preferably after checking blood glucose level.

chlorzoxazone ▶◀ disulfiram

Parafon Forte DSC

Antabuse

Risk rating: 2
Severity: **Moderate**   Onset: **Delayed**   Likelihood: **Probable**

Cause
Disulfiram inhibits hepatic metabolism of chlorzoxazone.

Effect
CNS depressant effects of chlorzoxazone may increase.

Nursing considerations
■ Monitor patient for increased CNS adverse effects including dizziness, drowsiness, headache, and light-headedness.
■ Signs of more severe toxicity include nausea, vomiting, diarrhea, loss of muscle tone, decreased or absent deep tendon reflexes, respiratory depression, and hypotension.
■ Advise patient to avoid hazardous activities that require alertness or physical coordination until CNS depressant effects are determined.
■ Chlorzoxazone dose may need to be reduced during combined therapy.

---

cholestyramine ▶◀ digoxin
LoCHOLEST, Prevalite, Questran

Lanoxin

Risk rating: 2
Severity: Moderate   **Onset: Delayed**   **Likelihood: Probable**

Cause
Cholestyramine may decrease digoxin absorption by binding to it. It also may interrupt digoxin metabolism in the liver.

Effect
Digoxin bioavailability and effects may be reduced.

Nursing considerations
■ Monitor digoxin level.
■ Monitor patient for decreased digoxin effects.
■ Adjust digoxin dose as needed.
■ Consider using digoxin capsules, because the interaction may be minimized.
■ Give cholestyramine 8 hours before or after digoxin to minimize the effects of the interaction.

---

cholestyramine ▶◀ furosemide
LoCHOLEST, Prevalite, Questran

Lasix

Risk rating: 2
Severity: Moderate   **Onset: Rapid**   **Likelihood: Suspected**

Cause
Cholestyramine may bind to furosemide, inhibiting furosemide absorption.

Effect
Furosemide effects may decrease.

Nursing considerations
- Cholestyramine should be taken at least 2 hours after furosemide.
- Monitor patient for expected furosemide effects, including reduction in peripheral edema, resolution of pulmonary edema, and decreased blood pressure in hypertensive patients.
- If furosemide is needed, consult prescriber or pharmacist about alternative cholesterol-lowering therapy.
- Bile acid sequestrants other than cholestyramine may interact with furosemide. If you suspect a drug interaction, consult prescriber or pharmacist.

---

cholestyramine ▶◀ **HMG-CoA reductase inhibitors**

LoCHOLEST, Prevalite, Questran

atorvastatin, fluvastatin, lovastatin, pravastatin, rosuvastatin, simvastatin

Risk rating: 2
Severity: **Moderate**   Onset: **Delayed**   Likelihood: **Suspected**

Cause
GI absorption of HMG-CoA reductase inhibitor may decrease.

Effect
HMG-CoA reductase inhibitor effects may decrease.

Nursing considerations
- **ALERT** Separate doses of HMG-CoA reductase inhibitor and cholestyramine, a bile acid sequestrant, by at least 4 hours.
- If possible, give cholestyramine before meals and HMG-CoA reductase inhibitor in the evening.
- Monitor serum cholesterol and lipid levels to assess patient's response to therapy.
- Help patient develop a daily plan to ensure proper intervals between drug doses.

cholestyramine ━━▶◀━━ hydrocortisone

LoCHOLEST, Prevalite, Questran

Cortef

Risk rating: 2
Severity: Moderate   **Onset: Delayed**   **Likelihood: Suspected**

Cause
Bile acid sequestrants, such as cholestyramine, interfere with GI absorption of hydrocortisone.

Effect
Hydrocortisone effects may decrease.

Nursing considerations
■ If patient needs hydrocortisone, consider a different cholesterol-lowering drug.
■ If drugs must be taken together, separate doses to help improve hydrocortisone absorption, even though doing so has no proven effect.
■ Check for expected hydrocortisone effects.
■ If needed, consult prescriber about increasing hydrocortisone dosage to achieve desired effect.
■ Help patient develop a daily plan to ensure proper intervals between drug doses.

cholestyramine ━━▶◀━━ thyroid hormones

LoCHOLEST, Prevalite, Questran

levothyroxine, liothyronine, liotrix, thyroid

Risk rating: 2
Severity: Moderate   **Onset: Delayed**   **Likelihood: Suspected**

Cause
Cholestyramine may prevent GI absorption of thyroid hormones.

Effect
Effects of exogenous thyroid hormone may be lost, and hypothyroidism may recur.

Nursing considerations
■ Separate doses by 6 hours.
■ Monitor patient for evidence of hypothyroidism, including weakness, fatigue, weight gain, coarse dry hair and skin, cold intolerance, muscle aches, constipation, depression, irritability, and memory loss.

■ Monitor thyroid function tests during combined therapy (TSH, 0.2 to 5.4 microunits/ml; T_3, 80 to 200 nanograms/dl; T_4, 5.4 to 11.5 mcg/dl).
■ Other thyroid hormones may interact with cholestyramine. If you suspect a drug interaction, consult prescriber or pharmacist.

cholestyramine ▬►◄▬ valproic acid

LoCHOLEST, Prevalite, Questran

divalproex sodium, valproate sodium, valproic acid

Risk rating: 2
Severity: Moderate   **Onset: Rapid**   **Likelihood: Suspected**

Cause
Cholestyramine may prevent GI absorption of valproic acid.

Effect
Valproic acid effects may decrease.

Nursing considerations
■ Give valproic acid at least 3 hours before or 3 hours after cholestyramine.
■ Watch for loss of seizure control.
■ Valproic acid dosage may need adjustment.

cilostazol ▬▬►◄▬▬ macrolide antibiotics

Pletal

clarithromycin, erythromycin, troleandomycin

Risk rating: 2
Severity: Moderate   **Onset: Delayed**   **Likelihood: Suspected**

Cause
Certain macrolide antibiotics inhibit CYP3A4 metabolism of cilostazol.

Effect
Cilostazol effects, including adverse effects, may increase.

Nursing considerations
■ Cilostazol dose may need to be decreased during combined therapy; consider cilostazol 50 mg b.i.d.
■ Watch for evidence of cilostazol toxicity, including severe headache, diarrhea, hypotension, hypotension, tachycardia, and arrhythmias.
■ Urge patient to tell prescriber about all drugs and supplements he takes and about any increase in adverse effects.

■ Other macrolide antibiotics may interact with cilostazol. If you suspect a drug interaction, consult prescriber or pharmacist.

---

cimetidine ━━━━▶◀━━━━ beta blockers
Tagamet   metoprolol, propranolol,
                                         timolol

Risk rating: 2
Severity: Moderate   **Onset: Rapid**   **Likelihood: Probable**

Cause
By inhibiting the CYP pathway, cimetidine reduces the first-pass metabolism of certain beta blockers.

Effect
Beta blocker clearance is decreased, increasing their action.

Nursing considerations
■ Monitor patient for severe bradycardia and hypotension.
■ If interaction occurs, notify prescriber; beta blocker dosage may be decreased.
■ Teach patient to monitor pulse rate. If it's significantly lower than usual, tell him to withhold beta blocker and to contact prescriber.
■ Instruct patient to change positions slowly to reduce effects of orthostatic hypotension.
■ Other beta blockers may interact with cimetidine. If you suspect an interaction, consult prescriber or pharmacist.

---

cimetidine ━━━━▶◀━━━━ carbamazepine
Tagamet   Carbatrol, Epitol, Equetro,
                                         Tegretol

Risk rating: 2
Severity: Moderate   **Onset: Delayed**   **Likelihood: Suspected**

Cause
Cimetidine may inhibit hepatic carbamazepine metabolism.

Effect
Carbamazepine level and risk of toxicity may increase.

Nursing considerations
■ Monitor patient's response when cimetidine is started (especially during the first 4 weeks) or stopped.
■ Monitor carbamazepine level; therapeutic range is 4 to 12 mcg/ml.

⚡ **ALERT** Watch for signs of anorexia or subtle appetite changes, which may indicate an excessive carbamazepine level.
■ Monitor patient for signs of carbamazepine toxicity, including dizziness, ataxia, respiratory depression, tachycardia, arrhythmias, blood pressure changes, impaired consciousness, abnormal reflexes, nystagmus, seizures, nausea, vomiting, and urine retention.
■ Carbamazepine dosage adjustment may be needed.

---

cimetidine ▸◂ carmustine
Tagamet   BiCNU

Risk rating: 1
Severity: Major   **Onset: Delayed**   **Likelihood: Suspected**

Cause
The mechanism of this interaction is unknown, but may involve additive bone marrow suppression or decreased carmustine metabolism by cimetidine.

Effect
Carmustine myelosuppressive effects increase.

Nursing considerations
⚡ **ALERT** Avoid combined use if possible.
■ Monitor CBC, WBC, and platelet counts.
■ Be prepared to provide supportive measures, such as blood components and granulocyte-colony stimulating factor.
■ H_2-receptor antagonists other than cimetidine interact with carmustine. If you suspect an interaction, consult prescriber or pharmacist.
■ Consult prescriber for alternative drug therapy to avoid severe myelosuppression.

---

cimetidine ▸◂ dofetilide
Tagamet   Tikosyn

Risk rating: 1
Severity: Major   **Onset: Delayed**   **Likelihood: Suspected**

Cause
Dofetilide renal elimination may be inhibited.

Effect
Dofetilide level and risk of ventricular arrhythmias, including torsades de pointes, may increase.

Nursing considerations

⚡ **ALERT** Use of dofetilide with cimetidine is contraindicated.

■ Monitor ECG for excessive prolongation of QTc interval and development of ventricular arrhythmias.

■ Omeprazole, ranitidine, and aluminum and magnesium antacids don't affect dofetilide elimination. Consult prescriber for alternative therapy.

■ Monitor renal function and QTc interval every 3 months during dofetilide therapy.

■ Urge patient to tell prescriber about all drugs and supplements he takes and about any increase in adverse effects.

---

cimetidine ━━━►◄━━━ lidocaine
Tagamet   Xylocaine

Risk rating: 2
Severity: Moderate   **Onset: Rapid**   **Likelihood: Established**

Cause
Hepatic lidocaine metabolism may decrease.

Effect
Risk of lidocaine toxicity increases.

Nursing considerations
■ Monitor patient for lidocaine toxicity: dizziness, somnolence, confusion, tremors, paresthesias, seizures, hypotension, arrhythmias, respiratory depression, and coma.

■ Adjust lidocaine dosage as ordered.

■ Consult prescriber or pharmacist for a safer H_2-receptor antagonist, such as ranitidine or famotidine, as an alternative to cimetidine. Monitor serum lidocaine level; therapeutic range is 1.5 to 6 mcg/ml.

■ Other H_2-receptor antagonists interact with lidocaine. If you suspect a drug interaction, consult prescriber or pharmacist.

---

cimetidine ━━━►◄━━━ metformin
Tagamet   Glucophage

Risk rating: 2
Severity: Moderate   **Onset: Rapid**   **Likelihood: Suspected**

Cause
Cimetidine reduces metformin clearance.

Effect

Metformin level and effects increase.

Nursing considerations

■ Monitor serum lactic acid level; reference range is 6 to 19 mg/dl.

⚠ ALERT Advise patient to report early symptoms of lactic acidosis, including malaise, myalgias, respiratory distress, increased somnolence, abdominal pain, nausea, and vomiting.

■ In addition to early symptoms of lactic acidosis, monitor patient for hypothermia, hypotension, and resistant bradyarrhythmias.

■ Monitor blood glucose level for possible hypoglycemia.

■ Metformin dosage may need adjustment when cimetidine is started or stopped.

■ Urge patient to tell prescriber about all drugs and supplements he takes and about any increase in adverse effects.

■ H_2-receptor antagonists other than cimetidine may interact with metformin. If you suspect an interaction, consult prescriber or pharmacist.

---

cimetidine ▶◀ moricizine

Tagamet   Ethmozine

Risk rating: 2
Severity: Moderate   **Onset: Delayed**   **Likelihood: Suspected**

Cause

Cimetidine inhibits hepatic metabolism of moricizine.

Effect

Moricizine effects, including adverse effects, may increase.

Nursing considerations

■ Monitor ECG when starting, changing, or stopping cimetidine.

■ Assess patient for evidence of increased moricizine toxicity, including arrhythmias, vomiting, lethargy, dizziness, syncope, hypotension, worsening heart failure, respiratory failure, and coma.

■ Consult prescriber or pharmacist for dosage adjustments of these drugs during combined therapy.

■ Urge patient to tell prescriber about all drugs and supplements he takes and about any increase in adverse effects.

■ H_2-receptor antagonists other than cimetidine may interact with moricizine. If you suspect a drug interaction, consult prescriber or pharmacist.

cimetidine 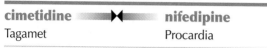 nifedipine
Tagamet   Procardia

Risk rating: 2
Severity: Moderate   **Onset: Delayed**   **Likelihood: Suspected**

Cause
The exact mechanism of this interaction is unknown; hepatic metabolism of nifedipine may be reduced.

Effect
Nifedipine effects, including adverse effects, may increase.

Nursing considerations
- Monitor patient for increased adverse effects, including hypotension, dizziness, light-headedness, syncope, peripheral edema, flushing, and nausea.
- Adjust the nifedipine dose as ordered.
- H_2-receptor antagonists other than cimetidine may interact with nifedipine. Calcium channel blockers other than nifedipine may interact with cimetidine. If you suspect an interaction, consult prescriber or pharmacist.

cimetidine ◄►► procainamide
Tagamet   Pronestyl

Risk rating: 2
Severity: Moderate   **Onset: Rapid**   **Likelihood: Established**

Cause
Cimetidine may reduce procainamide renal clearance.

Effect
Procainamide level and risk of toxicity may increase.

Nursing considerations
- **ALERT** Avoid combined use if possible.
- If drugs are used together, monitor procainamide level and its active metabolite NAPA. Therapeutic range for procainamide is 4 to 8 mcg/ml; therapeutic level of NAPA is 10 to 30 mcg/ml.
- Monitor patient for increased adverse effects, including severe hypotension, widening QRS complex, arrhythmias, seizures, oliguria, confusion, lethargy, nausea, and vomiting.
- Procainamide dosage may need adjustment.
- H_2-receptor antagonists other than cimetidine may interact with procainamide. If you suspect a drug interaction, consult prescriber or pharmacist.

cimetidine 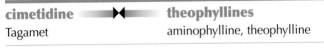 theophyllines
Tagamet   aminophylline, theophylline

Risk rating: 2
Severity: Moderate   Onset: Delayed   Likelihood: Established

Cause
Cimetidine inhibits hepatic metabolism of theophyllines.

Effect
Theophylline level and risk of toxicity may increase.

Nursing considerations
■ Monitor serum theophylline level closely. Normal therapeutic range is 10 to 20 mcg/ml for adults and 5 to 15 mcg/ml for children.
■ Watch for evidence of toxicity, such as tachycardia, anorexia, nausea, vomiting, diarrhea, seizures, restlessness, irritability, and headache.
■ The theophylline dosage may need to be decreased by 20% to 40%.
■ Describe adverse effects of theophylline and signs of toxicity, and tell patient to report them immediately to prescriber.
■ Giving ranitidine or famotidine instead of cimetidine for gastric hypersecretion may decrease risk of this interaction.

cimetidine 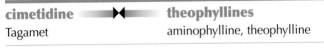 tricyclic antidepressants
Tagamet   amitriptyline, amoxapine, clomipramine, desipramine, doxepin, imipramine, nortriptyline, trimipramine

Risk rating: 2
Severity: Moderate   Onset: Rapid   Likelihood: Probable

Cause
Cimetidine may interfere with metabolism of tricyclic antidepressants (TCAs).

Effect
TCA level and bioavailability increase.

Nursing considerations
■ Monitor serum TCA level, and adjust dosage as prescribed.
■ If needed, consult prescriber about possible change from cimetidine to ranitidine.

■ Urge patient and family to watch for and report increased anticholinergic effects, dizziness, drowsiness, and psychosis.

---

ciprofloxacin ◄► didanosine
Cipro   Videx

Risk rating: 2
Severity: Moderate   **Onset: Rapid**   **Likelihood: Suspected**

Cause
Buffers in didanosine chewable tablets and pediatric powder for oral solution decrease GI absorption of ciprofloxacin.

Effect
Ciprofloxacin effects decrease.

Nursing considerations
■ Avoid use together. If it's unavoidable, give ciprofloxacin at least 2 hours before or 6 hours after didanosine.
■ The unbuffered form of didanosine doesn't affect ciprofloxacin absorption.
■ Help patient develop a daily plan to ensure proper intervals between drug doses.
■ To help avoid interactions, urge patient to tell prescribers about all drugs and supplements he takes.

---

ciprofloxacin ◄► iron salts
Cipro   ferrous fumarate, ferrous
                                         gluconate, ferrous sulfate

Risk rating: 2
Severity: Moderate   **Onset: Rapid**   **Likelihood: Probable**

Cause
Formation of an iron-quinolone complex decreases GI absorption of ciprofloxacin.

Effect
Effects of quinolone, such as ciprofloxacin, decrease.

Nursing considerations
■ Tell patient to separate ciprofloxacin from iron by at least 2 hours.
■ Help patient develop a daily plan to ensure proper intervals between drug doses.
■ Other quinolones may interact with iron.

ciprofloxacin ➤◄ milk
Cipro

Risk rating: 2
Severity: Moderate   **Onset: Rapid**   **Likelihood: Suspected**

Cause
GI absorption of some quinolones, such as ciprofloxacin, decreases.

Effect
Quinolone effects may decrease.

Nursing considerations
■ Advise patient not to take drug with milk, and to lengthen the time as much as possible between milk ingestion and the quinolone dose.
■ This interaction doesn't affect all quinolones.
■ Monitor patient for quinolone efficacy.

ciprofloxacin ➤◄ sucralfate
Cipro   Carafate

Risk rating: 2
Severity: Moderate   **Onset: Rapid**   **Likelihood: Probable**

Cause
Sucralfate decreases GI absorption of ciprofloxacin.

Effect
Ciprofloxacin effects decrease.

Nursing considerations
■ Avoid use together. If it's unavoidable, give sucralfate at least 6 hours after ciprofloxacin.
■ Monitor patient for resolving infection.
■ Help patient develop a daily plan to ensure proper intervals between drug doses.
■ To help avoid interactions, urge patient to tell prescribers about all drugs and supplements he takes.

cisapride ▶◀ antiarrhythmics

Propulsid

amiodarone, bretylium, disopyramide, flecainide, ibutilide, procainamide, propafenone, quinidine, sotalol

Risk rating: 1
Severity: Major   **Onset: Delayed**   **Likelihood: Suspected**

Cause
Cisapride causes added prolongation of the QT interval.

Effect
Risk of life-threatening arrhythmias may increase.

Nursing considerations
▷ **ALERT** Cisapride is contraindicated in patients taking class IA or class III antiarrhythmics, which prolong the QT interval.
■ Prolongation of the QT interval, torsades de pointes, other life-threatening arrhythmias, cardiac arrest, and sudden death may occur in patients taking cisapride.
■ Cisapride is available only on a restricted basis through a limited access program to patients who don't respond to all other standard treatments and who meet strict eligibility criteria.

cisapride ▶◀ aprepitant

Propulsid

Emend

Risk rating: 1
Severity: Major   **Onset: Delayed**   **Likelihood: Suspected**

Cause
Aprepitant may inhibit the CYP3A4 metabolism of cisapride.

Effect
Risk of life-threatening arrhythmias may increase.

Nursing considerations
▷ **ALERT** Use of aprepitant with cisapride is contraindicated.
■ Prolongation of the QT interval, torsades de pointes, other life-threatening arrhythmias, cardiac arrest, and sudden death may occur.
■ Cisapride is available only on a restricted basis through a limited access program to patients who don't respond to all other standard treatments and who meet strict eligibility criteria.

cisapride 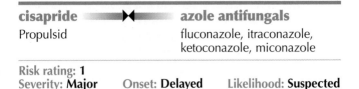 azole antifungals
Propulsid   fluconazole, itraconazole,
                             ketoconazole, miconazole

Risk rating: 1
Severity: Major   **Onset: Delayed**   **Likelihood: Suspected**

Cause
Azole antifungals may inhibit CYP3A4 hepatic metabolism of cisapride.

Effect
Cisapride level and risk of cardiotoxicity may increase.

Nursing considerations
◪ **ALERT** Use of azole antifungals with cisapride is contraindicated.
■ Prolongation of the QT interval, torsades de pointes, and other life-threatening arrhythmias may occur.
■ Cisapride is available only on a restricted basis through a limited access program to patients who don't respond to all other standard treatments and who meet strict eligibility criteria.

cisapride 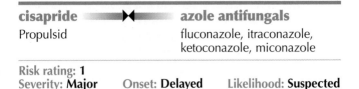 carbonic anhydrase inhibitors
Propulsid   acetazolamide, methazolamide

Risk rating: 1
Severity: Major   **Onset: Delayed**   **Likelihood: Suspected**

Cause
Electrolyte imbalance may increase the risk of additive QT interval prolongation.

Effect
Risk of life-threatening arrhythmias may increase.

Nursing considerations
◪ **ALERT** Use of carbonic anhydrase inhibitors with cisapride is contraindicated.
■ Prolongation of the QT interval, torsades de pointes, other life-threatening arrhythmias, cardiac arrest, and sudden death may occur.
■ Electrolyte disturbances increase the risk for arrhythmias; for example, hypokalemia may occur in patients with severe cirrhosis taking

carbonic anhydrase inhibitors or with inadequate oral electrolyte intake.

■ Cisapride is available only on a restricted basis through a limited access program to patients who don't respond to all other standard treatments and who meet strict eligibility criteria.

---

cisapride ▸◂ grapefruit juice
Propulsid

Risk rating: 1
Severity: Major   **Onset: Rapid**   **Likelihood: Suspected**

Cause
Grapefruit juice may inhibit CYP3A4 intestinal metabolism of cisapride.

Effect
Cisapride level and risk of life-threatening arrhythmias may increase.

Nursing considerations
◤ ALERT Don't give cisapride with grapefruit juice.
■ Prolongation of the QT interval, torsades de pointes, and other life-threatening arrhythmias may occur.
■ Cisapride is available only on a restricted basis through a limited access program to patients who don't respond to all other standard treatments and who meet strict eligibility criteria.
■ Advise patient not to take cisapride with any grapefruit product.

---

cisapride ▸◂ loop diuretics
Propulsid   bumetanide, ethacrynic acid,
                             furosemide, torsemide

Risk rating: 1
Severity: Major   **Onset: Delayed**   **Likelihood: Suspected**

Cause
Electrolyte imbalance may increase the risk of additive QT interval prolongation.

Effect
Risk of life-threatening arrhythmias may increase.

Nursing considerations
◤ ALERT Cisapride is contraindicated in patients taking loop diuretics because of possibly rapid potassium loss.

■ Prolongation of the QT interval, torsades de pointes, other life-threatening arrhythmias, cardiac arrest, and sudden death may occur.
■ Electrolyte disturbances increase the risk of arrhythmias.
■ Monitor serum electrolyte levels in patients taking cisapride.
■ Cisapride is available only on a restricted basis through a limited access program to patients who don't respond to all other standard treatments and who meet strict eligibility criteria.

cisapride ▶◀ macrolide antibiotics

Propulsid   clarithromycin, erythromycin, troleandomycin

Risk rating: 1
Severity: Major   **Onset: Delayed**   **Likelihood: Probable**

Cause
Certain macrolide antibiotics inhibit CYP3A4 hepatic metabolism of cisapride.

Effect
Cisapride level and risk of cardiotoxicity may increase.

Nursing considerations
⚠ **ALERT** Clarithromycin, erythromycin, and troleandomycin are contraindicated in patients taking cisapride.
■ Prolongation of the QT interval, torsades de pointes, and other life-threatening arrhythmias may occur.
■ Consult prescriber or pharmacist for alternative anti-infective therapy; azithromycin may be a safer alternative.
■ Cisapride is available only on a restricted basis through a limited access program to patients who don't respond to all other standard treatments and who meet strict eligibility criteria.

cisapride ▶◀ nefazodone

Propulsid

Risk rating: 1
Severity: Major   **Onset: Delayed**   **Likelihood: Suspected**

Cause
Nefazodone may inhibit CYP3A4 hepatic metabolism of cisapride.

Effect
Cisapride level and risk of cardiotoxicity may increase.

Nursing considerations

⚠ **ALERT** Use of nefazodone with cisapride is contraindicated.

■ Prolongation of the QT interval, torsades de pointes, and other life-threatening arrhythmias may occur.

■ Cisapride is available only on a restricted basis through a limited access program to patients who don't respond to all other standard treatments and who meet strict eligibility criteria.

■ Consult prescriber or pharmacist about alternative antidepressant therapy in patient taking cisapride.

---

cisapride ▶◀ nifedipine
Propulsid   Procardia

Risk rating: 2
Severity: Moderate   **Onset: Rapid**   **Likelihood: Suspected**

Cause
Enhanced GI motility caused by cisapride may increase the rate of nifedipine absorption.

Effect
Nifedipine level, effects, and adverse effects may increase.

Nursing considerations
■ Monitor blood pressure closely.

■ Monitor patient for adverse effects of nifedipine, such as dizziness, headache, light-headedness, flushing, and weakness.

■ Adjust the nifedipine dose as needed.

■ Because of the risk of serious arrhythmias and death, cisapride is available in the U.S. only through a limited access program.

---

cisapride ▶◀ nonnucleoside reverse transcriptase inhibitors
Propulsid   delavirdine, efavirenz

Risk rating: 1
Severity: Major   **Onset: Delayed**   **Likelihood: Suspected**

Cause
Metabolism of cisapride in the liver may be inhibited.

Effect
Cisapride level and risk of adverse effects, including life-threatening arrhythmias, may increase.

Nursing considerations

⚡ **ALERT** Use of cisapride with nonnucleoside reverse transcriptase inhibitors is contraindicated.

■ Elevated cisapride level may cause QT prolongation and serious cardiac arrhythmias.

■ Life-threatening arrhythmias, including torsades de pointes, QT prolongation, ventricular tachycardia, and ventricular fibrillation may occur.

■ Because of the risk of serious arrhythmias and death, cisapride is available in the U.S. only through a limited access program.

---

cisapride ▶◀	phenothiazines
Propulsid	chlorpromazine, fluphenazine, perphenazine, prochlor- perazine, promethazine, thioridazine, trifluoperazine

Risk rating: 1
Severity: Major　　**Onset: Delayed**　　**Likelihood: Suspected**

Cause
Phenothiazines may cause additive QT prolongation.

Effect
Risk of life-threatening arrhythmias, including torsades de pointes, may increase.

Nursing considerations

⚡ **ALERT** Use of phenothiazines with cisapride is contraindicated.

■ Prolonged QT interval, torsades de pointes, cardiac arrest, and sudden death may occur.

■ Because of the risk of serious arrhythmias and death, cisapride is available in the U.S. only through a limited access program.

---

cisapride ▶◀	protease inhibitors
Propulsid	amprenavir, atazanavir, indinavir, lopinavir-ritonavir, nelfinavir, ritonavir, saquinavir

Risk rating: 1
Severity: Major　　**Onset: Delayed**　　**Likelihood: Suspected**

Cause
Protease inhibitors may inhibit hepatic CYP3A4 metabolism of cisapride.

Effect
Cisapride level and risk of cardiotoxicity may increase.

Nursing considerations
◤ **ALERT** Use of cisapride with protease inhibitors is contraindicated.
■ Prolonged QT interval, torsades de pointes, cardiac arrest, and sudden death may occur.
■ Because of the risk of serious arrhythmias and death, cisapride is available in the U.S. only through a limited access program.

---

cisapride ▶◀	quinolones
Propulsid	gatifloxacin, levofloxacin, moxifloxacin, sparfloxacin

Risk rating: 1
Severity: Major   **Onset: Delayed**   **Likelihood: Suspected**

Cause
Cisapride may accelerate the rate of quinolone absorption.

Effect
Quinolone effects, including prolonged QTc interval, may increase.

Nursing considerations
◤ **ALERT** Use of cisapride with quinolones is contraindicated.
■ Prolonged QT interval, torsades de pointes, cardiac arrest, and sudden death may occur.
■ Because of the risk of serious arrhythmias and death, cisapride is available in the U.S. only through a limited access program.

---

cisapride ▶◀	telithromycin
Propulsid	Ketek

Risk rating: 1
Severity: Major   **Onset: Delayed**   **Likelihood: Suspected**

Cause
Telithromycin may inhibit hepatic CYP3A4 metabolism of cisapride.

Effect
Cisapride level and risk of cardiotoxicity may increase.

Nursing considerations
◤ **ALERT** Use of cisapride with telithromycin is contraindicated.
■ Prolonged QT interval, torsades de pointes, cardiac arrest, and sudden death may occur.

■ Because of the risk of serious arrhythmias and death, cisapride is available in the U.S. only through a limited access program.

---

cisapride ▶◀ tetracyclic antidepressants

Propulsid

maprotiline

Risk rating: 1
Severity: Major   **Onset: Delayed**   **Likelihood: Suspected**

Cause
Tetracyclic antidepressants may cause additive prolongation of the QT interval.

Effect
Risk of life-threatening arrhythmias, including torsades de pointes, may increase.

Nursing considerations
◪ ALERT Use of tetracyclic antidepressants with cisapride is contra-indicated.
■ Prolonged QT interval, torsades de pointes, cardiac arrest, and sudden death may occur.
■ Because of the risk of serious arrhythmias and death, cisapride is available in the U.S. only through a limited access program.

---

cisapride ▶◀ thiazide diuretics

Propulsid

chlorothiazide, hydrochlorothiazide, indapamide, methyclothiazide, metolazone, polythiazide, trichlormethiazide

Risk rating: 1
Severity: Major   **Onset: Delayed**   **Likelihood: Suspected**

Cause
Added QT interval prolongation may occur because of electrolyte loss from thiazide diuretics.

Effect
Risk of life-threatening arrhythmias, including torsades de pointes, may increase.

Nursing considerations
◪ ALERT Use of thiazide diuretics with cisapride is contraindicated.

■ Prolonged QT interval, torsades de pointes, cardiac arrest, and sudden death may occur.
■ Because of the risk of serious arrhythmias and death, cisapride is available in the U.S. only through a limited access program.

cisapride ▬▬▬►◄▬▬▬ tricyclic antidepressants
Propulsid

amitriptyline, amoxapine, clomipramine, desipramine, doxepin, imipramine, nortriptyline, protriptyline, trimipramine

Risk rating: 1
Severity: Major   **Onset: Delayed**   **Likelihood: Suspected**

Cause
Tricyclic antidepressants (TCAs) may cause additive prolongation of the QT interval.

Effect
Risk of life-threatening arrhythmias, including torsades de pointes, may increase.

Nursing considerations
◪ ALERT Use of TCAs with cisapride is contraindicated.
■ Prolonged QT interval, torsades de pointes, cardiac arrest, and sudden death may occur.
■ Because of the risk of serious arrhythmias and death, cisapride is available in the U.S. only through a limited access program.

cisapride ▬▬▬►◄▬▬▬ voriconazole
Propulsid   Vfend

Risk rating: 1
Severity: Major   **Onset: Delayed**   **Likelihood: Suspected**

Cause
Voriconazole may inhibit CYP3A4 hepatic metabolism of cisapride.

Effect
Risk of life-threatening arrhythmias, including torsades de pointes, may increase.

Nursing considerations
◪ ALERT Use of cisapride with voriconazole is contraindicated.

■ Prolonged QT interval, torsades de pointes, cardiac arrest, and sudden death may occur.
■ Because of the risk of serious arrhythmias and death, cisapride is available in the U.S. only through a limited access program.

cisatracurium ▶◀ carbamazepine

Nimbex

Carbatrol, Epitol, Equetro, Tegretol

Risk rating: 2
Severity: Moderate   **Onset: Rapid**   **Likelihood: Probable**

Cause
The mechanism of this interaction is unknown.

Effect
Effect or duration of cisatracurium, a nondepolarizing muscle relaxant, may decrease.

Nursing considerations
■ Monitor patient for decreased efficacy of muscle relaxant.
■ Cisatracurium dosage may need to be increased.
■ Make sure patient is adequately sedated when receiving a nondepolarizing muscle relaxant.

cisatracurium ▶◀ magnesium sulfate

Nimbex

Risk rating: 2
Severity: Moderate   **Onset: Rapid**   **Likelihood: Suspected**

Cause
Magnesium probably potentiates the action of nondepolarizing muscle relaxants, such as cisatracurium.

Effect
Risk of profound, severe respiratory depression increases.

Nursing considerations
■ Use these drugs together cautiously.
■ Cisatracurium dosage may need to be adjusted.
■ Monitor patient for respiratory distress.
■ Make sure patient is adequately sedated when receiving a nondepolarizing muscle relaxant.

cisatracurium ◄► phenytoin

Nimbex   Dilantin

Risk rating: 2
Severity: Moderate   **Onset: Rapid**   **Likelihood: Probable**

Cause
Phenytoin has effects at prejunctional sites similar to those of nondepolarizing muscle relaxants, such as cisatracurium.

Effect
Nondepolarizing muscle relaxant effect or duration may decrease.

Nursing considerations
■ Monitor patient for decreased efficacy of the muscle relaxant.
■ Cisatracurium dosage may need to be increased.
■ Atracurium may be a suitable alternative because this interaction
may not occur in all patients.
■ Make sure patient is adequately sedated when receiving a nonde-
polarizing muscle relaxant.

cisplatin ◄► loop diuretics

Platinol   bumetanide, ethacrynic acid,
                                      furosemide

Risk rating: 2
Severity: Moderate   **Onset: Rapid**   **Likelihood: Suspected**

Cause
The mechanism of this interaction is unknown.

Effect
Interaction may cause additive ototoxicity.

Nursing considerations
■ If possible, avoid giving loop diuretics and cisplatin together.
■ If drugs are given together, obtain hearing tests to detect early hear-
ing loss.
■ Combined therapy may cause ototoxicity much more severe than
therapy with either drug alone.
■ Ototoxicity caused by combined therapy may be permanent.
■ Tell patient to report ringing in the ears, a change in balance, or
muffled sounds. Also, ask family members to watch for changes.

citalopram ━━━▶◀━━━ MAO inhibitors
Celexa   isocarboxazid, phenelzine,
                                selegiline, tranylcypromine

Risk rating: 1
Severity: Major   **Onset: Rapid**   **Likelihood: Probable**

Cause
Serotonin may accumulate rapidly in the CNS.

Effect
The risk of serotonin syndrome increases.

Nursing considerations
⚡ **ALERT** Don't use these drugs together.
■ Allow 2 weeks after stopping citalopram before giving an MAO inhibitor.
■ Allow 2 weeks after stopping an MAO inhibitor before giving an SSRI, such as citalopram.
■ Describe the traits of serotonin syndrome, including confusion, restlessness, incoordination, muscle tremors and rigidity, fever, and sweating.
■ Explain that serotonin-induced symptoms can be fatal if not treated immediately.

citalopram ━━━▶◀━━━ selective 5-HT$_1$ receptor agonists
Celexa   almotriptan, eletriptan,
                                frovatriptan, naratriptan,
                                rizatriptan, sumatriptan,
                                zolmitriptan

Risk rating: 1
Severity: Major   **Onset: Rapid**   **Likelihood: Suspected**

Cause
Serotonin may accumulate rapidly in the CNS.

Effect
The risk of serotonin syndrome increases.

Nursing considerations
⚡ **ALERT** If possible, avoid combined use of these drugs.
■ If combined use can't be avoided, start with lowest dosages possible, and assess patient closely.
■ Stop the selective 5-HT$_1$ receptor agonist at first sign of interaction.

■ In some patients, migraine frequency may increase and antimigraine drug efficacy may decrease when an SSRI, such as citalopram, is started.

■ Describe the traits of serotonin syndrome, including confusion, restlessness, incoordination, muscle tremors and rigidity, fever, and sweating.

■ Explain that serotonin-induced symptoms can be fatal if not treated immediately.

---

citalopram　━━▶◀━━　St. John's wort
Celexa

Risk rating: 2
Severity: Moderate　　**Onset: Rapid**　　**Likelihood: Suspected**

Cause
St. John's wort may cause additive inhibition of serotonin reuptake.

Effect
The sedative-hypnotic effects of citalopram may increase.

Nursing considerations
◪ ALERT Discourage use of St. John's wort with an SSRI, such as citalopram.

■ In addition to oversedation, mild serotonin-like symptoms may occur, including confusion, diaphoresis, tremor, and muscle twitching.

■ Inform the patient about the dangers of this combination.

■ Urge patient to consult prescriber before taking any herb.

---

clarithromycin　━━▶◀━━　benzodiazepines
Biaxin　　　　　　　　　　alprazolam, diazepam,
　　　　　　　　　　　　　midazolam, triazolam

Risk rating: 2
Severity: Moderate　　**Onset: Rapid**　　**Likelihood: Suspected**

Cause
Macrolide antibiotics, such as clarithromycin, may decrease metabolism of certain benzodiazepines.

Effect
Sedative effects of benzodiazepines may be increased or prolonged.

Nursing considerations
■ Consult prescriber about decreasing benzodiazepine dosage during antibiotic therapy.

- Lorazepam, oxazepam, and temazepam probably don't interact with macrolide antibiotics; substitution may be possible.
- Urge patient to promptly report oversedation.

clarithromycin ➤◀ ergot derivatives
Biaxin   dihydroergotamine, ergotamine

Risk rating: 1
Severity: Major   **Onset: Rapid**   **Likelihood: Probable**

Cause
Macrolide antibiotics, such as clarithromycin, interfere with hepatic metabolism of ergotamine, although exact mechanism of this interaction is unknown.

Effect
Patient may develop symptoms of acute ergotism.

Nursing considerations
- Monitor patient for evidence of peripheral ischemia, including pain in limb muscles while exercising and later at rest; numbness and tingling of fingers and toes; cool, pale, or cyanotic limbs; red or violet blisters on hands or feet; and gangrene.
- Dosage of ergot drug may need to be decreased, or both drugs may need to be stopped.
- Consult prescriber about a different anti-infective drug that's less likely to interact with ergot derivatives.
- ◖ ALERT Sodium nitroprusside may be used to treat macrolide–ergot-induced vasospasm.
- Explain evidence of ergot-induced peripheral ischemia. Urge patient to report it promptly to prescriber.

clarithromycin ➤◀ HMG-CoA reductase inhibitors
Biaxin   atorvastatin, lovastatin, simvastatin

Risk rating: 1
Severity: Major   **Onset: Delayed**   **Likelihood: Probable**

Cause
CYP3A4 metabolism of certain HMG-CoA reductase inhibitors may decrease.

Effect
HMG-CoA reductase inhibitor level may increase, raising the risk of severe myopathy or rhabdomyolysis.

Nursing considerations
⚠ ALERT If atorvastatin, lovastatin, or simvastatin is given with a macrolide antibiotic, such as clarithromycin, watch for evidence of rhabdomyolysis, especially 5 to 21 days after macrolide starts. Evidence may include fatigue; muscle aches and weakness; joint pain; dark, red, or cola-colored urine; weight gain; seizures; and greatly increased serum CK level.

■ Fluvastatin and pravastatin are metabolized by other enzymes and may be better choices when used with a macrolide antibiotic.

■ Urge patient to report unexplained muscle pain, tenderness, or weakness to prescriber.

---

clarithromycin ▶◀ methylprednisolone
Biaxin   Medrol

Risk rating: 2
Severity: Moderate   **Onset: Delayed**   **Likelihood: Established**

Cause
The mechanism of this interaction is unclear.

Effect
Methylprednisolone effects, including toxic effects, may increase.

Nursing considerations
■ This interaction may be used for therapeutic benefit because it may be possible to reduce methylprednisolone dosage.
■ Methylprednisolone dosage may need adjustment.
■ Monitor patient for adverse or toxic effects, such as euphoria, insomnia, peptic ulceration, and cushingoid effects.

---

clarithromycin ▶◀ repaglinide
Biaxin   Prandin

Risk rating: 2
Severity: Moderate   **Onset: Delayed**   **Likelihood: Suspected**

Cause
Certain macrolide antibiotics, such as clarithromycin, may inhibit metabolism of repaglinide.

Effect

Repaglinide level and effects, including adverse effects, may increase.

Nursing considerations

- Monitor blood glucose level closely.
- Repaglinide dose should be adjusted as needed.
- Monitor patient for evidence of hypoglycemia, including hunger, dizziness, shakiness, sweating, confusion, and light-headedness.
- Advise patient to carry glucose tablets or another simple sugar in case of hypoglycemia.
- Make sure patient and family know what to do if hypoglycemia occurs.

---

clarithromycin ▶◀ rifamycins

Biaxin   rifabutin, rifampin, rifapentine

Risk rating: 2
Severity: Moderate   **Onset: Delayed**   **Likelihood: Suspected**

Cause

Metabolism of rifamycin may be inhibited. Metabolism of macrolide antibiotic, such as clarithromycin, may be increased.

Effect

Adverse effects of rifamycin may increase. Antimicrobial effects of macrolide antibiotic may decrease.

Nursing considerations

- Monitor patient for increased rifamycin adverse effects, such as abdominal pain, anorexia, nausea, vomiting, diarrhea, and rash.
- Monitor patient for decreased response to clarithromycin.
- Rifabutin and clarithromycin usually cause nausea, vomiting, or diarrhea. This interaction doesn't occur with azithromycin or dirithromycin; these drugs may be better choices.
- Giving clarithromycin with rifabutin may increase the risk of neutropenia.

clarithromycin ▬▶◀▬ theophyllines
Biaxin   aminophylline, theophylline

Risk rating: **2**
Severity: **Moderate**   Onset: **Delayed**   Likelihood: **Established**

Cause
Certain macrolides, such as clarithromycin, inhibit metabolism of
theophylline.

Effect
Theophylline level and risk of toxicity may increase.

Nursing considerations
- When starting or stopping a macrolide, monitor theophylline level.
Normal therapeutic range is 10 to 20 mcg/ml for adults and 5 to
15 mcg/ml for children.
- Consult prescriber about possibility of using another antibiotic.
- Watch for evidence of theophylline toxicity, such as tachycardia,
anorexia, nausea, vomiting, diarrhea, seizures, restlessness, irritability,
and headache.
- Describe adverse effects of theophylline and signs of toxicity, and
tell patient to report them immediately to prescriber.

clindamycin ▬▶◀▬ nondepolarizing muscle relaxants
Cleocin

atracurium, mivacurium,
pancuronium, rocuronium,
vecuronium

Risk rating: **2**
Severity: **Moderate**   Onset: **Rapid**   Likelihood: **Suspected**

Cause
Clindamycin may potentiate the actions of nondepolarizing muscle
relaxants.

Effect
Nondepolarizing muscle relaxant effects may increase.

Nursing considerations
- If possible, avoid using clindamycin and other lincosamides with
nondepolarizing muscle relaxants.
- Monitor patient for respiratory depression.

■ Provide ventilatory support as needed.
■ Cholinesterase inhibitors or calcium may be useful in reversing drug effects.
■ Make sure patient is adequately sedated when receiving a nondepolarizing muscle relaxant.

---

clomipramine ▶◀ fluoxetine
Anafranil   Prozac, Sarafem

Risk rating: 2
Severity: Moderate   Onset: Delayed   Likelihood: Probable

Cause
Fluoxetine may inhibit hepatic metabolism of tricyclic antidepressants (TCAs), such as clomipramine.

Effect
Serum TCA level and toxicity may increase.

Nursing considerations
■ Monitor serum TCA level and watch closely for evidence of toxicity, such as increased anticholinergic effects, delirium, dizziness, drowsiness, and psychosis.
■ Report evidence of increased TCA level or toxicity; dosage may need to be decreased.
■ If TCA starts when patient already takes fluoxetine, TCA dosage may need to be decreased by up to 75% to avoid interaction.
■ Other TCAs may interact with fluoxetine. If you suspect an interaction, consult prescriber or pharmacist.

---

clomipramine ▶◀ fluvoxamine
Anafranil   Luvox

Risk rating: 2
Severity: Moderate   Onset: Delayed   Likelihood: Probable

Cause
Fluvoxamine may inhibit oxidative metabolism of tricyclic antidepressants (TCAs), such as clomipramine, by CYP2D6 pathway.

Effect
TCA level and risk of toxicity increase.

Nursing considerations
■ If combined use can't be avoided, TCA dosage may need to be decreased.

- Monitor TCA level.
- Report evidence of toxicity or increased TCA level.
- Inhibitory effects of fluvoxamine may take up to 2 weeks to dissipate after drug is stopped.
- Using the TCA desipramine may avoid this interaction.
- Urge patient and family to watch for and report increased anticholinergic effects, dizziness, drowsiness, and psychosis.

clomipramine ◄►◄ MAO inhibitors
Anafranil   isocarboxazid, phenelzine, tranylcypromine

Risk rating: 1
Severity: Major   **Onset: Rapid**   **Likelihood: Suspected**

Cause
The mechanism of this interaction is unknown.

Effect
Risk of hyperpyretic crisis, seizures, and death increases.

Nursing considerations
⚡ ALERT Don't give a tricyclic antidepressant (TCA), such as clomipramine, with or within 2 weeks of an MAO inhibitor.
- Clomipramine and imipramine may be more likely than other TCAs to interact with MAO inhibitors.
- Watch for adverse effects, including confusion, hyperexcitability, rigidity, seizures, increased temperature, increased pulse, increased respiration, sweating, mydriasis, flushing, headache, coma, and DIC.

clomipramine ◄►◄ quinolones
Anafranil   gatifloxacin, levofloxacin, moxifloxacin, sparfloxacin

Risk rating: 1
Severity: Major   **Onset: Delayed**   **Likelihood: Suspected**

Cause
The mechanism of this interaction is unknown.

Effect
Life-threatening arrhythmias, including torsades de pointes, may increase.

Nursing considerations
⚡ **ALERT** Sparfloxacin is contraindicated in patients taking a tricyclic antidepressant (TCA), such as clomipramine, because QTc interval may be prolonged.

⚡ **ALERT** Avoid giving levofloxacin with a TCA.

■ Use gatifloxacin and moxifloxacin cautiously with a TCA.

■ If possible, use other quinolone antibiotics that don't prolong the QTc interval or aren't metabolized by the CYP3A4 isoenzyme.

---

clomipramine ➤◀ rifamycins
Anafranil   rifabutin, rifampin

Risk rating: 2
Severity: Moderate   **Onset: Delayed**   **Likelihood: Suspected**

Cause
Metabolism of tricyclic antidepressants (TCAs), such as clomipramine, in the liver may increase.

Effect
TCA level and efficacy may decrease.

Nursing considerations
■ Monitor serum TCA level to maintain therapeutic range.

■ Urge patient and family to watch for adverse reactions, including increased drowsiness and dizziness, for several weeks after rifamycin stops. Tell them to notify prescriber promptly.

■ Other TCAs may interact with rifamycins. If you suspect an interaction, consult prescriber or pharmacist.

---

clomipramine ➤◀ sertraline
Anafranil   Zoloft

Risk rating: 2
Severity: Moderate   **Onset: Delayed**   **Likelihood: Suspected**

Cause
Hepatic metabolism of clomipramine, a tricyclic antidepressant (TCA), by CYP2D6 may be inhibited.

Effect
Therapeutic and toxic effects of certain TCAs may increase.

Nursing considerations
■ If possible, avoid this drug combination.

■ Watch for evidence of TCA toxicity and serotonin syndrome.

■ Signs of serotonin syndrome include confusion, myoclonus, and hyperreflexia.
■ Monitor serum TCA levels when starting or stopping sertraline.
■ If abnormalities occur, decrease TCA dosage or stop drug.

---

clomipramine ◄►► sympathomimetics
Anafranil

direct: dobutamine, epinephrine, norepinephrine, phenylephrine
mixed: dopamine, ephedrine

Risk rating: 2
Severity: Moderate   **Onset: Rapid**   **Likelihood: Established**

Cause
Tricyclic antidepressants (TCAs), such as clomipramine, increase the effects of direct-acting sympathomimetics and decrease the effects of indirect-acting sympathomimetics.

Effect
When sympathomimetic effects increase, the risk of hypertension and arrhythmias increases. When sympathomimetic effects decrease, blood pressure control decreases.

Nursing considerations
■ If possible, avoid using these drugs together.
■ Watch patient closely for hypertension and heart rhythm changes; they may warrant reduction of sympathomimetic dosage.
■ If patient takes a mixed-acting sympathomimetic, watch for negative effects; dosage may need to be altered.
■ Other TCAs and sympathomimetics may interact. If you suspect an interaction, consult prescriber or pharmacist.

---

clomipramine ◄►► valproic acid
Anafranil

divalproex sodium, valproate sodium, valproic acid

Risk rating: 2
Severity: Moderate   **Onset: Delayed**   **Likelihood: Suspected**

Cause
Valproic acid may inhibit hepatic metabolism of tricyclic antidepressants (TCAs), such as clomipramine.

Effect
TCA level and adverse effects may increase.

Nursing considerations
■ Use these drugs together cautiously.
■ If patient is stable on valproic acid, start TCA at reduced dosage and adjust upward slowly to address symptoms and serum level.
■ If patient is stable on a TCA, monitor serum level and patient status closely when starting or stopping valproic acid.
■ Explain signs and symptoms to watch for when these drugs are combined.
■ Other TCAs may interact with valproic acid. If you suspect an interaction, consult prescriber or pharmacist.

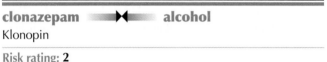

clonazepam ➤◀ alcohol
Klonopin

Risk rating: 2
Severity: Moderate   Onset: Rapid   Likelihood: Established

Cause
Alcohol inhibits hepatic enzymes, which decreases clearance and increases peak level of benzodiazepines, such as clonazepam.

Effect
Combining a benzodiazepine and alcohol may have additive or synergistic effects.

Nursing considerations
■ Advise against consuming alcohol while taking a benzodiazepine.
■ Before benzodiazepine therapy starts, assess patient thoroughly for history or evidence of alcohol use.
■ Watch for additive CNS effects, which may suggest benzodiazepine overdose.
■ Other benzodiazepines interact with alcohol. If you suspect an interaction, consult prescriber or pharmacist.

---

clonazepam ➤◀ azole antifungals
Klonopin   fluconazole, itraconazole,
                        ketoconazole, miconazole

Risk rating: 2
Severity: Moderate   Onset: Rapid   Likelihood: Established

Cause
Azole antifungals decrease CYP3A4 metabolism of certain benzodiazepines, such as clonazepam.

Effect
Benzodiazepine effects are increased and prolonged, which may cause CNS depression and psychomotor impairment.

Nursing considerations
■ If patient takes fluconazole or miconazole, consult prescriber about giving a lower benzodiazepine dose or a drug not metabolized by CYP3A4, such as temazepam or lorazepam.
■ Caution that the effects of this interaction may last several days after stopping the azole antifungal.
■ Explain that taking these drugs together may increase sedative effects; tell patient to report such effects promptly.
■ Various benzodiazepine–azole antifungal combinations may interact. If you suspect an interaction, consult prescriber or pharmacist.

---

clonazepam ━━━━►◄━━━━ protease inhibitors
Klonopin

amprenavir, atazanavir, indinavir, lopinavir-ritonavir, nelfinavir, ritonavir, saquinavir

Risk rating: 2
Severity: Moderate　　Onset: **Delayed**　　Likelihood: **Suspected**

Cause
Protease inhibitors may inhibit CYP3A4 metabolism of certain benzodiazepines, such as clonazepam.

Effect
Sedative effects of benzodiazepines may be increased and prolonged, leading to severe respiratory depression.

Nursing considerations
■ If patient takes any benzodiazepine–protease inhibitor combination, notify prescriber. Interaction could involve other drugs in the class.
■ Watch for evidence of oversedation and respiratory depression.
■ Explain the risks of using these drugs together.

---

clonazepam ━━━━►◄━━━━ rifamycins
Klonopin

rifabutin, rifampin, rifapentine

Risk rating: 2
Severity: Moderate　　Onset: **Delayed**　　Likelihood: **Suspected**

Cause
Rifamycins may increase CYP3A4 metabolism of benzodiazepines, such as clonazepam.

Effect
Antianxiety, sedative, and sleep-inducing effects of benzodiazepines may decrease.

Nursing considerations
■ Watch for lack of benzodiazepine efficacy, and notify prescriber; dosage may be changed.
■ Other benzodiazepines may interact with rifamycins. If you suspect an interaction, consult prescriber or pharmacist.
■ For insomnia, temazepam may be more effective because it doesn't undergo CYP3A4 metabolism.

clonidine ━━━▶◀━━	beta blockers
Catapres	acebutolol, atenolol, betaxolol, carteolol, esmolol, metoprolol, nadolol, penbutolol, pindolol, propranolol, timolol

Risk rating: 1
Severity: Major   **Onset: Delayed**   **Likelihood: Suspected**

Cause
The mechanism of this interaction is unclear.

Effect
Potentially life-threatening hypertension may occur.

Nursing considerations
■ Life-threatening hypertension may occur after simultaneously stopping clonidine and a beta blocker.
■ It's unknown whether hypertension is caused by an interaction or withdrawal syndrome linked to each drug.
■ Closely monitor blood pressure after starting or stopping the beta blocker or clonidine.
■ When stopping combined therapy, gradually withdraw the beta blocker first to minimize adverse reactions.

clonidine ━━━◀▶━━━ tricyclic antidepressants

Catapres

amitriptyline, amoxapine, clomipramine, desipramine, doxepin, imipramine, nortriptyline, protriptyline, trimipramine

Risk rating: 1
Severity: Major   **Onset: Rapid**   **Likelihood: Probable**

Cause
Tricyclic antidepressants (TCAs) inhibit alpha$_2$-adrenergic receptors, which clonidine stimulates for blood pressure control.

Effect
Clonidine efficacy in reducing blood pressure decreases.

Nursing considerations
- Life-threatening increases in blood pressure may occur.
- The intensity of this effect depends on the dosage of both drugs.
- **◤ ALERT** Tell prescriber that patient takes a TCA.
- Tell patient to keep an up-to-date list of all drugs he takes, so prescriber can avoid possible interactions.
- Other types of antidepressants can be used as an alternative treatment without this potential interaction.

clorazepate ━━━◀▶━━━ alcohol

Tranxene

Risk rating: 2
Severity: Moderate   **Onset: Rapid**   **Likelihood: Established**

Cause
Alcohol inhibits hepatic enzymes, which decreases clearance and increases peak level of benzodiazepines, such as clorazepate.

Effect
Combining a benzodiazepine and alcohol may have additive or synergistic effects.

Nursing considerations
- Advise against consuming alcohol while taking a benzodiazepine.
- Before benzodiazepine therapy starts, assess patient thoroughly for history or evidence of alcohol use.
- Watch for additive CNS effects, which may suggest benzodiazepine overdose.

clorazepate ━━━▶◀━━━ azole antifungals

Tranxene   fluconazole, itraconazole,
                            ketoconazole, miconazole

Risk rating: 2
Severity: Moderate   **Onset: Rapid**   **Likelihood: Established**

Cause
Azole antifungals decrease CYP3A4 metabolism of certain benzodiazepines, such as clorazepate.

Effect
Benzodiazepine effects are increased and prolonged, which may cause CNS depression and psychomotor impairment.

Nursing considerations
■ If patient takes fluconazole or miconazole, consult prescriber about giving a lower benzodiazepine dose or a drug not metabolized by CYP3A4, such as temazepam or lorazepam.
■ Caution that the effects of this interaction may last several days after stopping the azole antifungal.
■ Explain that taking these drugs together may increase sedative effects; tell patient to report such effects promptly.
■ Explain alternative methods of inducing sleep or relieving anxiety during antifungal therapy.
■ Various benzodiazepine–azole antifungal combinations may interact. If you suspect an interaction, consult prescriber or pharmacist.

clorazepate ━━━▶◀━━━ protease inhibitors

Tranxene   amprenavir, atazanavir,
                            indinavir, lopinavir-ritonavir,
                            nelfinavir, ritonavir, saquinavir

Risk rating: 2
Severity: Moderate   **Onset: Delayed**   **Likelihood: Suspected**

Cause
Protease inhibitors may inhibit CYP3A4 metabolism of certain benzodiazepines, such as clorazepate.

Effect
Sedative effects of benzodiazepines may be increased and prolonged, leading to severe respiratory depression.

Nursing considerations
◼ ALERT Don't combine clorazepate with a protease inhibitor.

- If patient takes any benzodiazepine–protease inhibitor combination, notify prescriber. Interaction could involve other drugs in the class.
- Watch for evidence of oversedation and respiratory depression.
- Teach patient and family about the risks of using these drugs together.

---

clorazepate ▶◀ rifamycins
Tranxene   rifabutin, rifampin, rifapentine

Risk rating: 2
Severity: **Moderate**   Onset: **Delayed**   Likelihood: **Suspected**

Cause
Rifamycins may increase CYP3A4 metabolism of benzodiazepines, such as clorazepate.

Effect
Antianxiety, sedative, and sleep-inducing effects of benzodiazepines may be decreased.

Nursing considerations
- Watch for lack of benzodiazepine efficacy, and notify prescriber; dosage may be changed.
- Other benzodiazepines may interact with rifamycins. If you suspect an interaction, consult prescriber or pharmacist.
- For insomnia, temazepam may be more effective because it doesn't undergo CYP3A4 metabolism.

---

clozapine ▶◀ ritonavir
Clozaril   Norvir

Risk rating: 1
Severity: **Major**   Onset: **Delayed**   Likelihood: **Suspected**

Cause
Ritonavir may inhibit clozapine metabolism.

Effect
Clozapine level and risk of toxicity may increase.

Nursing considerations
- **⚡ ALERT** Use of clozapine with ritonavir is contraindicated.
- Increased clozapine dose may increase risk of seizures.
- Watch for evidence of clozapine toxicity, including agranulocytosis, ECG changes, and seizures.

■ Monitor ECG. Clozapine-induced ECG changes should normalize after drug is stopped.

---

clozapine ▶◀ **serotonin reuptake inhibitors**

Clozaril

citalopram, fluoxetine, fluvoxamine, sertraline

Risk rating: 2
Severity: **Moderate**   Onset: **Delayed**   Likelihood: **Established**

Cause
Serotonin reuptake inhibitors inhibit hepatic metabolism of clozapine.

Effect
Clozapine level and risk of toxicity increase.

Nursing considerations
■ Not all serotonin reuptake inhibitors share this interaction. If you suspect an interaction, consult prescriber or pharmacist.
■ Monitor serum clozapine level.
■ Assess patient for increased adverse effects or toxicity, including agranulocytosis, ECG changes, and seizures.
■ Adjust clozapine dose as needed when adding or withdrawing a serotonin reuptake inhibitor.

---

colchicine ▶◀ **cyclosporine**

Gengraf, Neoral, Sandimmune

Risk rating: 2
Severity: **Moderate**   Onset: **Delayed**   Likelihood: **Suspected**

Cause
The mechanism of this interaction is unknown.

Effect
Severe adverse effects, including toxicity, may occur.

Nursing considerations
■ Watch for GI, hepatic, renal, and neuromuscular adverse effects.
■ Check cyclosporine level.
■ Monitor LDH, liver enzyme, bilirubin, and creatinine levels.
■ If an interaction is suspected and both drugs must be used, adjust cyclosporine dose as needed.
■ Adverse effects should quickly subside once either drug is stopped.

colestipol ▶◀ digoxin
Colestid   Lanoxin

Risk rating: 2
Severity: Moderate   **Onset: Rapid**   **Likelihood: Suspected**

Cause
Colestipol may bind with digoxin and decrease its GI absorption. Colestipol also may interfere with normal recycling of digoxin between the liver and intestines.

Effect
Digoxin effects may decrease.

Nursing considerations
- Colestipol may be useful in treating digoxin toxicity.
- If patient is taking colestipol routinely, monitor serum digoxin level. Therapeutic range is 0.8 to 2 nanograms/ml.
- Assess patient for expected digoxin effects, including decreased heart rate, arrhythmia conversion, maintenance of converted rhythm, and improvement of heart failure symptoms.
- Bile acid sequestrants other than colestipol (such as cholestyramine) may also have this interaction. If you suspect a drug interaction, consult prescriber or pharmacist.

colestipol ▶◀ furosemide
Colestid   Lasix

Risk rating: 2
Severity: Moderate   **Onset: Rapid**   **Likelihood: Suspected**

Cause
Colestipol may bind to furosemide, inhibiting furosemide absorption.

Effect
Furosemide effects may decrease.

Nursing considerations
- Separate doses; colestipol should be taken at least 2 hours after furosemide.
- Monitor patient for expected furosemide effects, including reduction in peripheral edema, resolution of pulmonary edema, and decreased blood pressure in hypertensive patients.
- Monitor urine output and blood pressure to assess diuretic effect.
- If furosemide must be used, consult prescriber or pharmacist about alternative cholesterol-lowering therapy.

■ Help patient develop a daily plan to ensure proper intervals between drug doses.

■ Bile acid sequestrants other than colestipol may interact with furosemide. If you suspect an interaction, consult prescriber or pharmacist.

---

colestipol ▶◀ HMG-CoA reductase inhibitors
Colestid

atorvastatin, fluvastatin, lovastatin, pravastatin, rosuvastatin, simvastatin

Risk rating: 2
Severity: Moderate   Onset: Delayed   Likelihood: Suspected

Cause
GI absorption of HMG-CoA reductase inhibitor may decrease.

Effect
HMG-CoA reductase inhibitor effects may decrease.

Nursing considerations
◨ ALERT Separate doses of HMG-CoA reductase inhibitor and bile acid sequestrant, such as colestipol, by at least 4 hours.

■ If possible, give bile acid sequestrant before meals and HMG-CoA reductase inhibitor in the evening.

■ Monitor serum cholesterol and lipid levels to assess patient's response to therapy.

■ Help patient develop a daily plan to ensure proper intervals between drug doses.

---

colestipol ▶◀ hydrocortisone
Colestid   Cortef

Risk rating: 2
Severity: Moderate   Onset: Delayed   Likelihood: Suspected

Cause
Bile acid sequestrants, such as colestipol, interfere with GI absorption of hydrocortisone.

Effect
Hydrocortisone effects may decrease.

Nursing considerations
■ If patient needs hydrocortisone, consider a different cholesterol-lowering drug as an alternative to colestipol.
■ Check for expected hydrocortisone effects.
■ Help patient develop a daily plan to ensure proper intervals between drug doses.

corticotropin ━━━▶◀━━━ barbiturates
amobarbital, butabarbital, pentobarbital, phenobarbital, primidone, secobarbital

Risk rating: 2
Severity: Moderate   Onset: Delayed   Likelihood: Established

Cause
Barbiturates induce liver enzymes, which stimulate metabolism of corticosteroids, such as corticotropin.

Effect
Corticosteroid effects may decrease.

Nursing considerations
■ Avoid giving barbiturates with corticosteroids, if possible.
■ If patient takes a corticosteroid, watch for worsening symptoms when barbiturate is started or stopped.
■ During barbiturate treatment, corticosteroid dosage may need to be increased.

corticotropin ━━━▶◀━━━ cholinesterase inhibitors
ambenonium, edrophonium, neostigmine, pyridostigmine

Risk rating: 1
Severity: Major   Onset: Delayed   Likelihood: Probable

Cause
In myasthenia gravis, corticotropin and other corticosteroids antagonize the effects of cholinesterase inhibitors by an unknown mechanism.

Effect
Patient may develop severe muscular depression refractory to cholinesterase inhibitor.

Nursing considerations
- Corticosteroid therapy may have long-term benefits in myasthenia gravis.
- Combined therapy may be attempted under strict supervision.
- Monitor patient with myasthenia gravis for severe muscle deterioration.

⚠ **ALERT** Be prepared to provide respiratory support and mechanical ventilation if needed.

- Consult prescriber or pharmacist about safe corticosteroid delivery to maximize improvement in muscle strength.

---

corticotropin ▬▶◀▬ hydantoins
ethotoin, fosphenytoin, phenytoin

Risk rating: 2
Severity: Moderate   Onset: Delayed   Likelihood: Established

Cause
Hydantoins induce liver enzymes, which stimulate metabolism of corticosteroids, such as corticotropin.

Effect
Corticosteroid effects may be decreased.

Nursing considerations
- Avoid giving hydantoins with corticosteroids if possible.
- If drugs must be given together, monitor patient for decreased corticosteroid effects. Also monitor phenytoin level, and adjust dosage of either drug as needed.
- Corticosteroid effects may decrease within days of starting phenytoin and may stay decreased 3 weeks after it stops.
- Dosage of either or both drugs may need to be increased.

cortisone ▬▬►◄▬▬ barbiturates

amobarbital, butabarbital, pentobarbital, phenobarbital, primidone, secobarbital

Risk rating: 2
Severity: **Moderate**   Onset: **Delayed**   Likelihood: **Established**

Cause
Barbiturates induce liver enzymes, which stimulate metabolism of corticosteroids, such as cortisone.

Effect
Corticosteroid effects may be decreased.

Nursing considerations
■ Avoid giving barbiturates with corticosteroids, if possible.
■ If patient takes a corticosteroid, watch for worsening symptoms when a barbiturate is started or stopped.
■ During barbiturate treatment, corticosteroid dosage may need to be increased.

cortisone ▬▬►◄▬▬ cholinesterase inhibitors

ambenonium, edrophonium, neostigmine, pyridostigmine

Risk rating: 1
Severity: **Major**   Onset: **Delayed**   Likelihood: **Probable**

Cause
In myasthenia gravis, cortisone and other corticosteroids antagonize the effects of cholinesterase inhibitors by an unknown mechanism.

Effect
Patient may develop severe muscular depression refractory to cholinesterase inhibitor.

Nursing considerations
■ Corticosteroid therapy may have long-term benefits in myasthenia gravis.
■ Combined therapy may be attempted under strict supervision.
■ If patient has myasthenia gravis, watch for severe muscle deterioration.
🔔 ALERT Be prepared to provide respiratory support and mechanical ventilation if needed.

■ Consult prescriber or pharmacist about safe corticosteroid delivery to maximize improvement in muscle strength.

---

cortisone ━━━━►◄━━━━ **hydantoins**

ethotoin, fosphenytoin, phenytoin

Risk rating: 2
Severity: Moderate   Onset: Delayed   Likelihood: Established

Cause
Hydantoins induce liver enzymes, which stimulate metabolism of corticosteroids, such as cortisone.

Effect
Corticosteroid effects may be decreased.

Nursing considerations
■ Avoid giving hydantoins with corticosteroids if possible.
■ If drugs must be given together, monitor patient for decreased corticosteroid effects. Also monitor phenytoin level, and adjust dosage of either drug as needed.
■ Corticosteroid effects may decrease within days of starting phenytoin and may stay decreased 3 weeks after it stops.
■ Dosage of either or both drugs may need to be increased.

---

cortisone ━━━━►◄━━━━ **rifamycins**

rifabutin, rifampin, rifapentine

Risk rating: 1
Severity: Major   Onset: Delayed   Likelihood: Established

Cause
Rifamycins increase hepatic metabolism of corticosteroids, such as cortisone.

Effect
Corticosteroid effects may be decreased.

Nursing considerations
■ If possible, avoid giving rifamycins with corticosteroids.
■ Monitor patient for decreased corticosteroid effects, including loss of disease control.
■ Monitor patient closely for symptom control after increasing rifamycin dose. Drug may need to be stopped to regain control of disease.

■ Corticosteroid effects may decrease within days of starting rifampin and may stay decreased 2 to 3 weeks after it stops.
■ Corticosteroid dose may need to be doubled after adding rifampin.

---

cortisone ▶◀ salicylates

aspirin, bismuth subsalicylate, choline salicylate, magnesium salicylate, salsalate, sodium salicylate, sodium thiosalicylate

Risk rating: 2
Severity: Moderate   Onset: Delayed   Likelihood: Probable

Cause
Cortisone and other corticosteroids stimulate hepatic metabolism of salicylates and may increase renal excretion.

Effect
Salicylate level and effects decrease.

Nursing considerations
■ Monitor salicylate efficacy and level; dosage may need adjustment.
⚠ **ALERT** Giving a salicylate while tapering a corticosteroid may result in salicylate toxicity.
■ Watch for evidence of salicylate toxicity, including diaphoresis, nausea, vomiting, tinnitus, hyperventilation, and CNS depression.
■ Patients with renal impairment may be at greater risk.

---

cosyntropin ▶◀ barbiturates

Cortrosyn

amobarbital, butabarbital, pentobarbital, phenobarbital, primidone, secobarbital

Risk rating: 2
Severity: Moderate   Onset: Delayed   Likelihood: Established

Cause
Barbiturates induce liver enzymes, which stimulate metabolism of corticosteroids, such as cosyntropin.

Effect
Corticosteroid effects may decrease.

Nursing considerations
■ Avoid giving barbiturates with corticosteroids, if possible.

■ If patient takes a corticosteroid, watch for worsening symptoms when a barbiturate is started or stopped.
■ During barbiturate treatment, corticosteroid dosage may need to be increased.

---

cosyntropin ▶◀ cholinesterase inhibitors

Cortrosyn   ambenonium, edrophonium, neostigmine, pyridostigmine

---

Risk rating: 1
Severity: **Major**   Onset: **Delayed**   Likelihood: **Probable**

Cause
In myasthenia gravis, cosyntropin and other corticosteroids antagonize the effects of cholinesterase inhibitors by an unknown mechanism.

Effect
Patient may develop severe muscular depression refractory to cholinesterase inhibitor.

Nursing considerations
■ Corticosteroids may have long-term benefits in myasthenia gravis.
■ Combined therapy may be attempted under strict supervision.
■ If patient has myasthenia gravis, watch for severe muscle deterioration.
⚡ ALERT Be prepared to provide respiratory support and mechanical ventilation if needed.
■ Consult prescriber or pharmacist about safe corticosteroid delivery to maximize improvement in muscle strength.

---

cosyntropin ▶◀ hydantoins

Cortrosyn   ethotoin, fosphenytoin, phenytoin

Risk rating: 2
Severity: **Moderate**   Onset: **Delayed**   Likelihood: **Established**

Cause
Hydantoins induce liver enzymes, which stimulate metabolism of corticosteroids, such as cosyntropin.

Effect
Corticosteroid effects may be decreased.

Nursing considerations
■ Avoid giving hydantoins with corticosteroids if possible.
■ Monitor patient for decreased corticosteroid effects. Also monitor phenytoin level, and adjust dosage of either drug as needed.
■ Corticosteroid effects may decrease within days of starting phenytoin and may stay decreased 3 weeks after it stops.
■ Dosage of either or both drugs may need to be increased.

cyclophosphamide ▶◀ succinylcholine
Cytoxan   Anectine

Risk rating: 2
Severity: Moderate   **Onset: Rapid**   **Likelihood: Probable**

Cause
Cyclophosphamide decreases succinylcholine metabolism by inhibiting cholinesterase activity.

Effect
Prolonged neuromuscular blockade caused by succinylcholine may occur.

Nursing considerations
■ Avoid using succinylcholine in a patient who has been receiving cyclophosphamide, if possible.
■ Effect of cyclophosphamide on plasma cholinesterase level is dose dependent.
■ If succinylcholine is given, measure plasma cholinesterase level.
■ If cholinesterase level declines, succinylcholine dosage may need to be reduced.
■ Monitor patient for prolonged neuromuscular blockade.

cyclosporine ▶◀ amiodarone
Gengraf, Neoral,   Cordarone, Pacerone
Sandimmune

Risk rating: 2
Severity: Moderate   **Onset: Delayed**   **Likelihood: Suspected**

Cause
Amiodarone may inhibit cyclosporine metabolism.

Effect
Cyclosporine level and risk of nephrotoxicity may increase.

Nursing considerations
- Closely monitor cyclosporine level when amiodarone is started or stopped or its dosage is changed.
- Because of amiodarone's long half-life, monitor cyclosporine level for several weeks after any dose alterations.
- Cyclosporine dosage may need reduction (up to 50% in some cases) to keep cyclosporine level in the desired range.
- Monitor patient for signs of nephrotoxicity.
- Monitor BUN and creatinine levels and urine output.
- Check urine for increased proteins, cells, or casts.
- If renal insufficiency develops, notify prescriber.

---

cyclosporine ◗◖ azole antifungals

Gengraf, Neoral, Sandimmune

fluconazole, itraconazole, ketoconazole, voriconazole

Risk rating: 2
Severity: Moderate   Onset: Delayed   Likelihood: Established

Cause
Azole antifungals decrease cyclosporine metabolism.

Effect
Cyclosporine level and toxicity may increase.

Nursing considerations
- Cyclosporine level may increase 1 to 3 days after starting an azole antifungal and persist for more than 1 week after stopping it.
- Monitor cyclosporine level.
- Adjust cyclosporine dosage to maintain therapeutic level.
- Cyclosporine dose may need to be decreased by 68% to 97%.
- Monitor patient for hepatotoxicity and nephrotoxicity.

---

cyclosporine ◗◖ bosentan

Gengraf, Neoral, Sandimmune

Tracleer

Risk rating: 1
Severity: Major   Onset: Delayed   Likelihood: Suspected

Cause
Bosentan may increase cyclosporine metabolism. Cyclosporine may inhibit bosentan metabolism.

Effect
Bosentan level may increase. Cyclosporine level may decrease.

Nursing considerations
⚠ **ALERT** Use of bosentan with cyclosporine is contraindicated.
■ Trough level of bosentan may increase 30 times over normal.
■ Cyclosporine level may decrease by 50%.
■ Watch for adverse effects from increased bosentan level, such as headache, nausea, vomiting, hypotension, and increased heart rate.

---

cyclosporine ◄►	carbamazepine
Gengraf, Neoral, Sandimmune	Carbatrol, Epitol, Equetro, Tegretol

Risk rating: 2
Severity: **Moderate**   Onset: **Delayed**   Likelihood: **Suspected**

Cause
Carbamazepine may induce hepatic metabolism of cyclosporine.

Effect
Cyclosporine level and effects may decrease.

Nursing considerations
■ Monitor cyclosporine level.
■ If carbamazepine therapy is started, observe patient for signs of rejection or decreased clinical effect.
■ If carbamazepine therapy is stopped, observe patient for signs of cyclosporine toxicity, such as hepatotoxicity, nephrotoxicity, nausea, vomiting, tremors, and seizures.
■ Cyclosporine dosage may need adjustment.
■ Advise patient to report signs of organ rejection; for example, decreased urine output in kidney transplant patients or shortness of breath and decreased stamina in heart transplant patients.

---

cyclosporine ◄►	carvedilol
Gengraf, Neoral, Sandimmune	Coreg

Risk rating: 2
Severity: **Moderate**   Onset: **Delayed**   Likelihood: **Suspected**

Cause
Carvedilol, a beta blocker, may disrupt cyclosporine metabolism.

Effect
Cyclosporine level and risk of toxicity may increase.

Nursing considerations
- Monitor patient for signs and symptoms of cyclosporine toxicity, such as nephrotoxicity and neurotoxicity.
- Monitor serum creatinine level.
- Monitor cyclosporine level.
- Adjust cyclosporine dosage to maintain therapeutic level.
- Other beta blockers may interact with cyclosporine.

---

cyclosporine ▶◀ colchicine
Gengraf, Neoral,
Sandimmune

Risk rating: 2
Severity: Moderate   **Onset: Delayed**   **Likelihood: Suspected**

Cause
The mechanism for this interaction is unknown.

Effect
Severe adverse effects, including toxicity, may occur.

Nursing considerations
- Watch for GI, hepatic, renal, and neuromuscular adverse effects.
- Monitor cyclosporine level.
- Monitor LDH, liver enzyme, bilirubin, and creatinine levels.
- If an interaction is suspected and both drugs must be used, adjust cyclosporine dose as needed.
- Adverse reactions should quickly subside once either drug stops.

---

cyclosporine ▶◀ diltiazem
Gengraf, Neoral,   Cardizem
Sandimmune

Risk rating: 2
Severity: Moderate   **Onset: Delayed**   **Likelihood: Established**

Cause
Diltiazem may inhibit cyclosporine metabolism in the liver.

Effect
Cyclosporine level and risk of toxicity may increase.

Nursing considerations
- Monitor cyclosporine level when adding or stopping diltiazem.
- Adjust cyclosporine dosage as needed. It may need to be reduced by 20% to 50%.

- Monitor patient for arthralgia and encephalopathy, which may occur when cyclosporine and diltiazem are given together.
- Adverse reactions should subside when diltiazem is stopped.

⚠ ALERT Rejection episodes may increase when diltiazem stops because cyclosporine level may be reduced. Monitor patient closely.

cyclosporine ▶◀ etoposide

Gengraf, Neoral, Sandimmune

VePesid

Risk rating: **2**
Severity: **Moderate**   Onset: **Delayed**   Likelihood: **Established**

Cause
Cyclosporine may decrease etoposide clearance and inhibit its metabolism.

Effect
Etoposide level and risk of toxicity may increase.

Nursing considerations
- Monitor patient for evidence of etoposide toxicity, including myelosuppression, nausea, vomiting, and diarrhea.
- Monitor CBC for evidence of leukopenia and thrombocytopenia.
- Adjust etoposide dosage as needed.

cyclosporine ▶◀ foscarnet

Gengraf, Neoral, Sandimmune

Foscavir

Risk rating: **1**
Severity: **Major**   Onset: **Delayed**   Likelihood: **Suspected**

Cause
Foscarnet and cyclosporine may work synergistically to cause nephrotoxicity.

Effect
Risk of renal failure may be increased.

Nursing considerations
- Individualize foscarnet dosage based on renal function.
- Monitor renal function carefully.
- If nephrotoxicity occurs, consider stopping foscarnet.
- Nephrotoxicity should resolve when foscarnet is stopped.

cyclosporine ▶◀ grapefruit juice, high-fat food
Gengraf, Neoral, Sandimmune

Risk rating: 2
Severity: Moderate **Onset: Rapid** **Likelihood: Probable**

Cause
Some foods may inhibit the intestinal enzyme responsible for cyclosporine metabolism.

Effect
Cyclosporine level may increase.

Nursing considerations
- Despite dosage reduction, cyclosporine level may be increased when taken with grapefruit juice.
- Monitor cyclosporine level.
- Advise patient to avoid taking cyclosporine with grapefruit juice.
- If patient drinks grapefruit juice, watch for cyclosporine toxicity, including hepatotoxicity, nephrotoxicity, nausea, vomiting, tremors, and seizures.
- Advise patient that high-fat meals may increase cyclosporine level.

cyclosporine ▶◀ HMG-CoA reductase inhibitors
Neoral

atorvastatin, lovastatin, pravastatin, rosuvastatin, simvastatin

Risk rating: 1
Severity: Major **Onset: Delayed** **Likelihood: Probable**

Cause
Metabolism of some HMG-CoA reductase inhibitors may decrease.

Effect
HMG-CoA reductase inhibitor level and adverse effects may increase.

Nursing considerations
- If possible, avoid use together.
- HMG-CoA reductase inhibitor dosage may need to be decreased.
- Monitor serum cholesterol and lipid levels to assess patient's response to therapy.

◪ **ALERT** Assess patient for evidence of rhabdomyolysis: fatigue; muscle aches and weakness; joint pain; dark, red, or cola-colored urine; weight gain; seizures; and greatly increased serum CK level.
■ Urge patient to report unexplained muscle pain, tenderness, or weakness to prescriber.

---

cyclosporine ▶◀ hydantoins

Gengraf, Neoral,   ethotoin, fosphenytoin,
Sandimmune   phenytoin

Risk rating: 1
Severity: Major   **Onset: Delayed**   **Likelihood: Probable**

Cause
Cyclosporine absorption may decrease or metabolism may increase.

Effect
Cyclosporine level may decrease.

Nursing considerations
■ Patients may be at risk for transplant rejection when cyclosporine is given with phenytoin.
■ Cyclosporine level decreases within 48 hours of phenytoin treatment and returns to normal within 1 week of stopping phenytoin.
■ Monitor cyclosporine level closely.
■ Adjust cyclosporine dose as needed.

---

cyclosporine ▶◀ imipenem and cilastatin

Gengraf, Neoral,   Primaxin
Sandimmune

Risk rating: 2
Severity: Moderate   **Onset: Rapid**   **Likelihood: Suspected**

Cause
Additive or synergistic toxicity may occur.

Effect
Adverse CNS effects of both drugs may increase.

Nursing considerations
■ Monitor patient for adverse CNS effects, including confusion, agitation, and tremors.
■ Decreasing cyclosporine dose may decrease risk of adverse effects.

■ Consider giving an alternative antibiotic if an interaction is suspected.
■ Adverse effects should improve after stopping imipenem and cilastatin.

---

cyclosporine ▸◂ metoclopramide
Gengraf, Neoral,   Reglan
Sandimmune

Risk rating: 2
Severity: **Moderate**   Onset: **Delayed**   Likelihood: **Suspected**

Cause
Metoclopramide increases gastric emptying time, which may increase cyclosporine absorption.

Effect
Cyclosporine level and risk of toxicity may increase.

Nursing considerations
■ Monitor cyclosporine level closely.
■ Watch for cyclosporine toxicity, including hepatotoxicity, nephrotoxicity, nausea, vomiting, tremors, and seizures.
■ Consider decreasing cyclosporine dose as needed.
■ It isn't known whether altering dosage or schedule of metoclopramide would decrease risk or severity of interaction.

---

cyclosporine ▸◂ nefazodone
Gengraf, Neoral,
Sandimmune

Risk rating: 2
Severity: **Moderate**   Onset: **Delayed**   Likelihood: **Probable**

Cause
Nefazodone, an antidepressant, may inhibit cyclosporine metabolism.

Effect
Cyclosporine level and risk of toxicity may increase.

Nursing considerations
■ For a patient taking cyclosporine, consider another antidepressant.
■ Monitor cyclosporine level closely.
■ Signs and symptoms of toxicity may include shakiness, headaches, tremor, hypertension, and fatigue.
■ Decrease cyclosporine dose as needed.

cyclosporine ▶◀ nicardipine

Gengraf, Neoral,
Sandimmune

Cardene

Risk rating: 2
Severity: Moderate   **Onset: Delayed**   **Likelihood: Suspected**

Cause
Nicardipine may inhibit cyclosporine metabolism in the liver.

Effect
Cyclosporine level and risk of renal toxicity may increase.

Nursing considerations
- Monitor cyclosporine level. Trough level may be elevated.
- Assess renal function.
- Monitor patient for signs and symptoms of toxicity.
- Adjust cyclosporine dose as needed.
- If nicardipine is stopped, consider increasing the cyclosporine dose to prevent rejection.

cyclosporine ▶◀ orlistat

Gengraf, Neoral,
Sandimmune

Xenical

Risk rating: 1
Severity: Major   **Onset: Delayed**   **Likelihood: Probable**

Cause
Orlistat may decrease cyclosporine absorption.

Effect
Cyclosporine level may be decreased.

Nursing considerations
- Avoid orlistat in patients being treated with cyclosporine.
- Monitor cyclosporine level.
- Increasing the cyclosporine dose may not result in an elevated drug level.

cyclosporine ▶◀ quinolones

Gengraf, Neoral, Sandimmune

ciprofloxacin, norfloxacin

Risk rating: 2
Severity: Moderate   Onset: Delayed   Likelihood: Suspected

Cause
Norfloxacin may inhibit cyclosporine metabolism.

Effect
Cyclosporine level may be elevated and cyclosporine-induced nephrotoxicity may occur.

Nursing considerations
- Monitor cyclosporine level.
- Monitor renal function.
- Consult prescriber or pharmacist if you suspect an interaction.
- Consider an alternative antibiotic to the quinolone if renal toxicity occurs or cyclosporine level increases.
- Not all quinolones share this interaction. Ofloxacin and levofloxacin don't appear to interact with cyclosporine.

cyclosporine ▶◀ rifamycins

Gengraf, Neoral, Sandimmune

rifabutin, rifampin, rifapentine

Risk rating: 2
Severity: Moderate   Onset: Delayed   Likelihood: Suspected

Cause
Rifamycins inhibit cyclosporine metabolism.

Effect
Immunosuppressive effects of cyclosporine may decrease.

Nursing considerations
- Avoid using rifamycins during cyclosporine treatment if possible.
- Cyclosporine effects may decrease within 2 days after starting a rifamycin and may continue 1 to 3 weeks after it's stopped.
- Monitor cyclosporine level often during and after rifamycin treatment.
- Adjust cyclosporine dose as needed.
- Cyclosporine level may remain decreased despite dosage increases.
- Assess patient for signs and symptoms of rejection.
- Monitor creatinine level during and after rifamycin treatment.

cyclosporine ■■■■►◄■■■■ serotonin reuptake inhibitors

Gengraf, Neoral, Sandimmune

fluoxetine, fluvoxamine, paroxetine, sertraline

Risk rating: 2
Severity: Moderate   **Onset: Delayed**   **Likelihood: Suspected**

Cause
Serotonin reuptake inhibitors inhibit cyclosporine metabolism.

Effect
Cyclosporine level and risk of toxicity may increase.

Nursing considerations
■ Consider use of citalopram as an alternative to these serotonin reuptake inhibitors because this interaction probably won't occur.
■ Monitor cyclosporine level when adding or stopping a serotonin reuptake inhibitor.
■ Adjust cyclosporine dose as needed.

cyclosporine ■■■■►◄■■■■ sirolimus

Gengraf, Neoral, Sandimmune

Rapamune

Risk rating: 2
Severity: Moderate   **Onset: Delayed**   **Likelihood: Probable**

Cause
The mechanism of this interaction is unknown.

Effect
Sirolimus level and risk of toxicity may increase.

Nursing considerations
■ Give sirolimus 4 hours after cyclosporine.
■ Monitor patient for evidence of sirolimus toxicity, such as anxiety, headache, hypertension, and thrombocytopenia.
■ Sirolimus level may decrease when cyclosporine is stopped.
■ Anticipate need for increased sirolimus dosage if cyclosporine is stopped.

cyclosporine 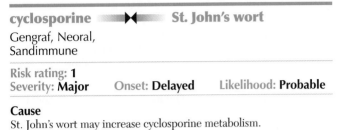 St. John's wort

Gengraf, Neoral,
Sandimmune

Risk rating: 1
Severity: Major   Onset: **Delayed**   Likelihood: **Probable**

Cause
St. John's wort may increase cyclosporine metabolism.

Effect
Cyclosporine level and efficacy may decrease.

Nursing considerations
- Discourage use of St. John's wort with cyclosporine.
- Monitor patient for signs and symptoms of rejection.
- Warn patient to consult prescriber before taking OTC or herbal products.

cyclosporine ▶◀ terbinafine

Gengraf, Neoral,   Lamisil
Sandimmune

Risk rating: 2
Severity: Moderate   Onset: **Delayed**   Likelihood: **Suspected**

Cause
Terbinafine may increase cyclosporine metabolism.

Effect
Cyclosporine level may decrease.

Nursing considerations
- Monitor cyclosporine level.
- Adjust cyclosporine dose as needed.
- Closely monitor patient for signs and symptoms of rejection when terbinafine is started or stopped.

danazol ▶◀ carbamazepine

Danocrine

Carbatrol, Epitol, Equetro, Tegretol

Risk rating: 2
Severity: Moderate   **Onset: Delayed**   **Likelihood: Suspected**

Cause
Danazol inhibits carbamazepine metabolism.

Effect
Carbamazepine level and toxicity may increase.

Nursing considerations
■ **ALERT** Avoid this combination if possible.
■ Monitor carbamazepine level; therapeutic range is 4 to 12 mcg/ml.
■ If danazol is started or stopped, carbamazepine dosage may need adjustment.
■ **ALERT** Watch for signs of anorexia or subtle appetite changes, which may indicate excessive carbamazepine level.
■ Watch for carbamazepine toxicity: dizziness, ataxia, respiratory depression, tachycardia, arrhythmias, blood pressure changes, impaired consciousness, abnormal reflexes, nystagmus, seizures, nausea, vomiting, and urine retention.

delavirdine ▶◀ amprenavir

Rescriptor

Agenerase

Risk rating: 2
Severity: Moderate   **Onset: Delayed**   **Likelihood: Suspected**

Cause
Amprenavir may induce CYP3A4 metabolism of delavirdine. Delavirdine may inhibit CYP3A4 metabolism of amprenavir.

Effect
Amprenavir level may increase. Delavirdine level may decrease.

Nursing considerations
■ If amprenavir starts, watch for decreased delavirdine effects.
■ Review common adverse reactions caused by this interaction: headache, fatigue, rash, and GI complaints.
■ Caution patient to report bothersome effects but not to alter regimen without consulting prescriber.

delavirdine ►◄ benzodiazepines

Rescriptor

alprazolam, midazolam,
triazolam

Risk rating: 2
Severity: Moderate   Onset: Delayed   Likelihood: Suspected

Cause
Nonnucleoside reverse-transcriptase inhibitors, such as delavirdine,
may inhibit CYP3A4 metabolism of some benzodiazepines.

Effect
Sedative effects of benzodiazepines may be increased or prolonged,
leading to respiratory depression.

Nursing considerations
 ⚡ **ALERT** Don't combine alprazolam, midazolam, or triazolam with
delavirdine.
 ■ Other benzodiazepines and nonnucleoside reverse-transcriptase in-
hibitors may interact. If you suspect an interaction, consult prescriber
or pharmacist.
 ■ Explain the risk of oversedation and respiratory depression.
 ■ Urge patient to promptly report any suspected interaction.

delavirdine ►◄ ergot derivatives

Rescriptor

dihydroergotamine, ergotamine

Risk rating: 1
Severity: Major   Onset: Delayed   Likelihood: Suspected

Cause
Nonnucleoside reverse-transcriptase inhibitors, such as delavirdine,
may decrease CYP3A4 metabolism of ergot derivatives.

Effect
Risk of ergot-induced peripheral vasospasm and ischemia may increase.

Nursing considerations
 ⚡ **ALERT** Use of ergot derivatives with delavirdine is contraindicated.
 ■ Watch for evidence of peripheral ischemia: pain in limb muscles
while exercising and later at rest; numbness and tingling of fingers
and toes; cool, pale, or cyanotic limbs; red or violet blisters on hands
or feet; and gangrene.
 ■ Ergot toxicity may cause nausea, vomiting, lassitude, impaired mental function, delirium, severe dyspnea, hypotension, hypertension, rapid or weak pulse, unconsciousness, limb spasms, seizures, and shock.

- Give vasodilators for vasospasm and diazepam for seizures.
- Other nonnucleoside reverse-transcriptase inhibitors, such as nevirapine, may interact with ergot derivatives. If you suspect an interaction, consult prescriber or pharmacist.

demeclocycline ▰▰◀◀ iron salts

Declomycin

ferrous fumarate, ferrous gluconate, ferrous sulfate, iron polysaccharide

Risk rating: 2
Severity: Moderate   Onset: Delayed   Likelihood: Probable

Cause
Demeclocycline and other tetracyclines form insoluble chelates with iron salts, which may reduce absorption of both substances.

Effect
Tetracycline and iron salt levels and effects may decrease.

Nursing considerations
⚠ **ALERT** If possible, avoid giving these drugs together.
- Separate doses by 3 to 4 hours.
- If you suspect an interaction, consult prescriber or pharmacist; an enteric-coated or sustained-release iron salt may reduce interaction.
- Watch for expected therapeutic response to tetracycline.
- Assess patient for evidence of iron deficiency: fatigue, dyspnea, tachycardia, palpitations, dizziness, and orthostatic hypotension.

demeclocycline ▰▰◀◀ penicillins

Declomycin

amoxicillin, ampicillin, carbenicillin, cloxacillin, dicloxacillin, nafcillin, oxacillin, penicillin G, penicillin V, piperacillin, ticarcillin

Risk rating: 1
Severity: Major   Onset: Delayed   Likelihood: Suspected

Cause
Demeclocycline and other tetracyclines may disrupt penicillin's bactericidal activity.

Effect
Penicillin efficacy may be reduced.

Nursing considerations
■ If possible, avoid giving tetracyclines with penicillins.
■ Monitor patient closely for lack of penicillin effect.

desipramine ━━━▶◀━━━ cimetidine
Norpramin   Tagamet

Risk rating: 2
Severity: Moderate   Onset: Rapid   Likelihood: Probable

Cause
Cimetidine may interfere with metabolism of tricyclic antidepressants (TCAs), such as desipramine.

Effect
TCA level and bioavailability increase.

Nursing considerations
■ When starting or stopping cimetidine, monitor serum TCA level and adjust dosage as needed.
■ Tell prescriber if TCA level or effect increases; dosage may need to be decreased.
■ If needed, consult prescriber about possible change from cimetidine to ranitidine.
■ Urge patient and family to watch for and report increased anticholinergic effects, dizziness, drowsiness, and psychosis.

desipramine ━━━▶◀━━━ fluoxetine
Norpramin   Prozac, Sarafem

Risk rating: 2
Severity: Moderate   Onset: Delayed   Likelihood: Probable

Cause
Fluoxetine may inhibit hepatic metabolism of tricyclic antidepressants (TCAs), such as desipramine.

Effect
Serum TCA level and toxicity may increase.

Nursing considerations
■ Monitor serum TCA level and watch closely for evidence of toxicity, such as increased anticholinergic effects, delirium, dizziness, drowsiness, and psychosis.
■ Report evidence of increased TCA level or toxicity; dosage may need to be decreased.

■ If TCA starts when patient already takes fluoxetine, TCA dosage may need to be decreased by up to 75% to avoid interaction.
■ Other TCAs may interact with fluoxetine. If you suspect an interaction, consult prescriber or pharmacist.

desipramine ━━▶◀━━ MAO inhibitors

Norpramin

isocarboxazid, phenelzine, tranylcypromine

Risk rating: 1
Severity: Major   **Onset: Rapid**   **Likelihood: Suspected**

Cause
The mechanism of this interaction is unknown.

Effect
The risk of hyperpyretic crisis, seizures, and death increases.

Nursing considerations
⚡ ALERT Don't give a tricyclic antidepressant, such as desipramine, with or within 2 weeks of an MAO inhibitor.
■ Watch for adverse effects, including confusion, hyperexcitability, rigidity, seizures, increased temperature, increased pulse, increased respiration, sweating, mydriasis, flushing, headache, coma, and DIC.

desipramine ━━▶◀━━ paroxetine

Norpramin

Paxil

Risk rating: 2
Severity: Moderate   **Onset: Delayed**   **Likelihood: Suspected**

Cause
Paroxetine may decrease desipramine metabolism in some people and increase it in others.

Effect
Therapeutic and toxic effects of certain tricyclic antidepressants (TCAs), such as desipramine, may increase.

Nursing considerations
■ When starting or stopping paroxetine, monitor TCA level and adjust dosage as needed.
■ Watch for adverse reactions, such as increased drowsiness, dizziness, confusion, heart rate or rhythm changes, and urine retention.

■ Watch closely for evidence of serotonin syndrome, such as delirium, bizarre movements, and tachycardia. Alert prescriber if they occur; TCA may need to be stopped.

■ Symptoms of serotonin syndrome may resolve within 24 hours of stopping a TCA and starting a short course of cyproheptadine.

◤ ALERT TCAs other than desipramine may have this interaction.

desipramine ▶◀ quinolones

Norpramin

gatifloxacin, levofloxacin, moxifloxacin, sparfloxacin

Risk rating: 1
Severity: Major   Onset: Delayed   Likelihood: Suspected

Cause
The mechanism of this interaction if unknown.

Effect
Life-threatening arrhythmias, including torsades de pointes, may increase when certain tricyclic antidepressants (TCAs), such as desipramine, and quinolones are used together.

Nursing considerations
◤ ALERT Sparfloxacin is contraindicated in patients taking a TCA because the QTc interval may be prolonged.

◤ ALERT Avoid giving levofloxacin with a TCA.

■ Use gatifloxacin and moxifloxacin cautiously with TCAs.

■ If possible, use other quinolones that don't prolong the QTc interval or aren't metabolized by the CYP3A4 isoenzyme.

desipramine ▶◀ rifamycins

Norpramin

rifabutin, rifampin

Risk rating: 2
Severity: Moderate   Onset: Delayed   Likelihood: Suspected

Cause
Hepatic metabolism of tricyclic antidepressants (TCAs), such as desipramine, may increase.

Effect
TCA level and efficacy may decrease.

Nursing considerations
■ When starting, stopping, or changing the dosage of a rifamycin, monitor serum TCA level to maintain therapeutic range.

■ Watch for resolution of depression as TCA dosage is adjusted to therapeutic level during rifamycin therapy.
■ Urge patient and family to watch for adverse reactions, including increased drowsiness and dizziness, for several weeks after rifamycin stops. Tell them to notify prescriber promptly.
■ Other TCAs may interact with rifamycins. If you suspect an interaction, consult prescriber or pharmacist.

desipramine ■■■▶◀■■ sertraline
Norpramin   Zoloft

Risk rating: 2
Severity: Moderate   Onset: Delayed   Likelihood: Suspected

Cause
Hepatic metabolism of a tricyclic antidepressant (TCA), such as desipramine, by CYP2D6 may be inhibited.

Effect
Therapeutic and toxic effects of certain TCAs may increase.

Nursing considerations
■ If possible, avoid this drug combination.
■ Watch for evidence of TCA toxicity and serotonin syndrome.
■ Signs of serotonin syndrome include delirium, bizarre movements, and tachycardia.
■ Monitor serum TCA levels when starting or stopping sertraline.
■ If abnormalities occur, decrease TCA dosage or stop drug.

desipramine ■■■▶◀■■ sympathomimetics
Norpramin   *direct:* dobutamine,
                                   epinephrine, norepinephrine,
                                   phenylephrine
                                   mixed: dopamine, ephedrine,
                                   metaraminol

Risk rating: 2
Severity: Moderate   Onset: Rapid   Likelihood: Established

Cause
Tricyclic antidepressants (TCAs), such as desipramine, increase the effects of direct-acting sympathomimetics and decrease the effects of indirect-acting sympathomimetics.

Effect
When sympathomimetic effects increase, the risk of hypertension and arrhythmias increases. When sympathomimetic effects decrease, blood pressure control decreases.

Nursing considerations
- If possible, avoid using these drugs together.
- Watch closely for hypertension and heart rhythm changes; they may warrant reduction of sympathomimetic dosage.
- If patient takes a mixed-acting sympathomimetic, watch for negative effects; dosage may need to be altered.
- Other TCAs and sympathomimetics may interact. If you suspect an interaction, consult prescriber or pharmacist.

---

desipramine ▶◀ terbinafine

Norpramin   Lamisil

Risk rating: **2**
Severity: **Moderate**   Onset: **Delayed**   Likelihood: **Suspected**

Cause
Hepatic metabolism of tricyclic antidepressants (TCAs), such as desipramine, may be inhibited.

Effect
Therapeutic and toxic effects of certain TCAs may increase.

Nursing considerations
- Check for abnormal TCA levels; report them to prescriber.
- TCA dosage may be decreased while patient takes terbinafine.
- Interaction may cause vertigo, fatigue, loss of appetite, ataxia, muscle twitching, and trouble swallowing.
- Terbinafine's inhibitory effects may take several weeks to dissipate after drug is stopped.
- Describe signs and symptoms of interaction.

---

desipramine ▶◀ valproic acid

Norpramin   divalproex sodium, valproate
                          sodium, valproic acid

Risk rating: **2**
Severity: **Moderate**   Onset: **Delayed**   Likelihood: **Suspected**

Cause
Valproic acid may inhibit hepatic metabolism of tricyclic antidepressants (TCAs), such as desipramine.

Effect
TCA level and adverse effects may increase.

Nursing considerations
■ Use these drugs together cautiously.
■ If patient is stable on valproic acid, start TCA at reduced dosage and adjust upward slowly to address symptoms and serum levels.
■ If patient is stable on a TCA, monitor serum level and patient status closely when starting or stopping valproic acid.
■ Explain signs and symptoms of interaction.
■ Other TCAs may interact with valproic acid. If you suspect an interaction, consult prescriber or pharmacist.

---

dexamethasone ▶◀ aprepitant
Decadron   Emend

Risk rating: 2
Severity: Moderate   **Onset: Delayed**   **Likelihood: Suspected**

Cause
Aprepitant may inhibit first-pass metabolism of certain corticosteroids, such as dexamethasone.

Effect
Corticosteroid level may be increased and half-life prolonged.

Nursing considerations
■ Corticosteroid dosage may need to be decreased.
■ When starting or stopping aprepitant, adjust corticosteroid dosage as needed.
■ Watch closely for evidence of increased corticosteroid level, such as insomnia, euphoria, increased appetite, mood changes, and increased blood glucose level.
■ Tell patient to report symptoms of increased blood glucose level, including increased thirst or hunger and frequent urination.

dexamethasone ▰▶◀▰ barbiturates

Decadron

amobarbital, butabarbital, pentobarbital, phenobarbital, primidone, secobarbital

Risk rating: 2
Severity: Moderate   Onset: Delayed   Likelihood: Established

Cause
Barbiturates induce liver enzymes, which stimulate metabolism of corticosteroids, such as dexamethasone.

Effect
Corticosteroid effects may be decreased.

Nursing considerations
■ Avoid giving barbiturates with corticosteroids.
■ If patient takes a corticosteroid, watch for worsening symptoms when a barbiturate is started or stopped.
■ During barbiturate treatment, corticosteroid dosage may need to be increased.

dexamethasone ▰▶◀▰ cholinesterase inhibitors

Decadron

ambenonium, edrophonium, neostigmine, pyridostigmine

Risk rating: 1
Severity: Major   Onset: Delayed   Likelihood: Probable

Cause
In myasthenia gravis, dexamethasone and other corticosteroids antagonize the effects of cholinesterase inhibitors.

Effect
Severe muscular depression may develop that's refractory to the cholinesterase inhibitor.

Nursing considerations
■ Corticosteroids may have long-term benefits in myasthenia gravis.
■ Combined therapy may be attempted under strict supervision.
■ Monitor patient for severe muscle deterioration.
■ **ALERT** Be prepared to provide respiratory support and mechanical ventilation if needed.
■ Consult prescriber or pharmacist about safe corticosteroid delivery to maximize improvement in muscle strength.

dexamethasone ▶◀ hydantoins
Decadron

ethotoin, fosphenytoin, phenytoin

Risk rating: 2
Severity: **Moderate**   Onset: **Delayed**   Likelihood: **Established**

Cause
Hydantoins induce liver enzymes, which stimulate metabolism of corticosteroids, such as dexamethasone. Dexamethasone may enhance hepatic clearance of phenytoin.

Effect
Corticosteroid effects may decrease.

Nursing considerations
■ Avoid giving hydantoins with corticosteroids if possible.
■ Watch for decreased corticosteroid effects, monitor phenytoin level, and adjust dosage of either drug as needed.
■ Dosage of either or both drugs may need to be increased.
■ Corticosteroid effects may decrease within days of starting phenytoin and may stay decreased 3 weeks after it stops.

dexamethasone ▶◀ rifamycins
Decadron

rifabutin, rifampin, rifapentine

Risk rating: 1
Severity: **Major**   Onset: **Delayed**   Likelihood: **Established**

Cause
Rifamycins increase hepatic metabolism of corticosteroids, such as dexamethasone.

Effect
Corticosteroid effects may decrease.

Nursing considerations
■ If possible, avoid giving rifamycins with corticosteroids.
■ Watch for decreased corticosteroid effects, including loss of disease control.
■ Watch closely for symptom control after increasing rifamycin dose. Drug may need to be stopped to regain control of disease.
■ Corticosteroid effects may decrease within days of starting rifampin and may stay decreased 2 to 3 weeks after it stops.
■ Corticosteroid dose may need to be doubled after adding rifampin.

dexamethasone ➤◄ salicylates

Decadron

aspirin, bismuth subsalicylate, choline salicylate, magnesium salicylate, salsalate, sodium salicylate, sodium thiosalicylate

Risk rating: 2
Severity: Moderate   Onset: Delayed   Likelihood: Probable

Cause
Dexamethasone and other corticosteroids stimulate hepatic metabolism of salicylates and may increase their renal excretion.

Effect
Salicylate level and effects decrease.

Nursing considerations
■ Monitor salicylate level and efficacy; dosage may need adjustment.
❦ ALERT Giving a salicylate while tapering a corticosteroid may result in salicylate toxicity.
■ Watch for evidence of salicylate toxicity, including diaphoresis, nausea, vomiting, tinnitus, hyperventilation, and CNS depression.
■ Patients with renal impairment may be at greater risk.

dexmethylphenidate ➤◄ MAO inhibitors

Focalin

isocarboxazid, phenelzine, tranylcypromine

Risk rating: 1
Severity: Major   Onset: Delayed   Likelihood: Suspected

Cause
The mechanism of this interaction is unknown.

Effect
The risk of hypertensive crisis increases.

Nursing considerations
❦ ALERT Use of dexmethylphenidate with MAO inhibitors is contraindicated.
■ Don't use dexmethylphenidate within 14 days after stopping an MAO inhibitor.
■ Monitor blood pressure closely if methylphenidate is given with an MAO inhibitor.
■ Teach patient and parent to monitor and record blood pressure.

dextroamphetamine ►◄ MAO inhibitors

Dexedrine   phenelzine, tranylcypromine

Risk rating: 1
Severity: Major   **Onset: Rapid**   **Likelihood: Suspected**

Cause
This interaction probably stems from increased norepinephrine levels at the synaptic cleft.

Effect
Anorexiant effects increase.

Nursing considerations
■ If possible, avoid giving these drugs together.
■ Headache and severe hypertension may occur rapidly if an amphetamine, such as dextroamphetamine, is given to patient who takes an MAO inhibitor.
■ **ALERT** Death may result from hypertensive crisis and resulting cerebral hemorrhage.
■ Monitor patient for hypotension, hyperpyrexia, and seizures.
■ Hypertensive reaction may occur for several weeks after stopping an MAO inhibitor.

dextroamphetamine ►◄ SSRIs

Dexedrine   fluoxetine, fluvoxamine,
                                   paroxetine, sertraline

Risk rating: 1
Severity: Major   **Onset: Rapid**   **Likelihood: Suspected**

Cause
The mechanism of this interaction is unknown.

Effect
Sympathomimetic effects and risk of serotonin syndrome increase.

Nursing considerations
■ If these drugs must be used together, watch closely for increased CNS effects, such as anxiety, jitteriness, agitation, and restlessness.
■ Mild serotonin-like symptoms may develop, including anxiety, dizziness, restlessness, nausea, and vomiting.
■ Explain the risk of interaction and the need to avoid amphetamines, such as dextroamphetamine.
■ Describe the traits of serotonin syndrome, including CNS irritability, motor weakness, shivering, myoclonus, and altered consciousness.

dextroamphetamine ▶◀ urine alkalinizers

Dexedrine   potassium citrate, sodium
                             acetate, sodium bicarbonate,
                             sodium citrate, sodium lactate,
                             tromethamine

Risk rating: 2
Severity: Moderate   Onset: Rapid   Likelihood: Established

Cause
When urine is alkaline, amphetamine clearance is prolonged.

Effect
In amphetamine overdose, the toxic period will be extended, increasing the risk of injury.

Nursing considerations
◣ ALERT Avoid drugs that may alkalinize the urine, particularly during overdose with an amphetamine, such as dextroamphetamine.
■ Watch for evidence of amphetamine toxicity, such as dermatoses, marked insomnia, irritability, hyperactivity, and personality changes.
■ If patient takes an anorexiant, advise against excessive use of sodium bicarbonate as an antacid.

dextromethorphan ▶◀ MAO inhibitors

Robitussin DM   isocarboxazid, phenelzine,
                             tranylcypromine

Risk rating: 1
Severity: Major   Onset: Rapid   Likelihood: Suspected

Cause
MAO inhibitor may decrease serotonin metabolism. Dextromethorphan may decrease synaptic reuptake of serotonin.

Effect
Risk of serotonin syndrome increases.

Nursing considerations
■ If possible, avoid giving these drugs together.
◣ ALERT Combined use may cause hyperpyrexia, abnormal muscle movement, hypotension, coma, and death.
■ If patient takes an MAO inhibitor, caution against taking OTC cough and cold medicines that contain dextromethorphan.

diazepam ▸◂ alcohol
Valium

Risk rating: 2
Severity: Moderate   **Onset: Rapid**   **Likelihood: Established**

Cause
Alcohol inhibits hepatic enzymes, which decreases clearance and increases peak levels of benzodiazepines, such as diazepam.

Effect
Effects may be additive or synergistic.

Nursing considerations
■ Advise against consuming alcohol while taking a benzodiazepine.
■ Before benzodiazepine therapy starts, assess patient thoroughly for history or evidence of alcohol use.
■ Watch for additive CNS effects, which may suggest benzodiazepine overdose.
■ Other benzodiazepines interact with alcohol. If you suspect an interaction, consult prescriber or pharmacist.

diazepam ▸◂ azole antifungals
Valium   fluconazole, itraconazole,
                          ketoconazole, miconazole

Risk rating: 2
Severity: Moderate   **Onset: Rapid**   **Likelihood: Established**

Cause
Azole antifungals decrease CYP3A4 metabolism of certain benzodiazepines, such as diazepam.

Effect
Benzodiazepine effects are increased and prolonged, which may cause CNS depression and psychomotor impairment.

Nursing considerations
■ If patient takes fluconazole or miconazole, consult prescriber about giving a lower benzodiazepine dose or a drug not metabolized by CYP3A4, such as temazepam or lorazepam.
■ Caution that the effects of this interaction may last several days after stopping the azole antifungal.
■ Explain that taking these drugs together may increase sedative effects; tell patient to report such effects promptly.

■ Explain alternative methods of inducing sleep or relieving anxiety during antifungal therapy.
■ Various benzodiazepine–azole antifungal combinations may interact. If you suspect an interaction, consult prescriber or pharmacist.

---

diazepam ━━━▶◀━━━ macrolide antibiotics
Valium   clarithromycin, erythromycin

Risk rating: 2
Severity: Moderate   **Onset: Rapid**   **Likelihood: Suspected**

Cause
Macrolide antibiotics may decrease the metabolism of certain benzodiazepines, such as diazepam.

Effect
Sedative effects of benzodiazepines may be increased or prolonged.

Nursing considerations
■ Consult prescriber about decreasing benzodiazepine dosage.
■ Lorazepam, oxazepam, and temazepam probably don't interact with macrolide antibiotics; substitution may be possible.
■ Urge patient to promptly report oversedation.

---

diazepam ━━━▶◀━━━ protease inhibitors
Valium   amprenavir, atazanavir,
                                         indinavir, lopinavir-ritonavir,
                                         nelfinavir, ritonavir, saquinavir

Risk rating: 2
Severity: Moderate   **Onset: Delayed**   **Likelihood: Suspected**

Cause
Protease inhibitors may inhibit CYP3A4 metabolism of certain benzodiazepines, such as diazepam.

Effect
Sedative effects of benzodiazepines may be increased and prolonged, leading to severe respiratory depression.

Nursing considerations
◤ ALERT Don't combine alprazolam with protease inhibitors.
■ If patient takes any benzodiazepine–protease inhibitor combination, notify prescriber. Interaction could involve other drugs in the class.
■ Watch for evidence of oversedation and respiratory depression.
■ Teach patient and family about the risks of combined use.

diazepam ━━━◄►━━━ rifamycins
Valium   rifabutin, rifampin, rifapentine

Risk rating: 2
Severity: Moderate   Onset: Delayed   Likelihood: Suspected

Cause
Rifamycins may increase CYP3A4 metabolism of benzodiazepines, such as diazepam.

Effect
Antianxiety, sedative, and sleep-inducing effects of benzodiazepines may be decreased.

Nursing considerations
- Watch for expected benzodiazepine effects and lack of efficacy.
- If benzodiazepine efficacy is reduced, dosage may be changed.
- Other benzodiazepines may interact with rifamycins. If you suspect an interaction, consult prescriber or pharmacist.
- For insomnia, temazepam may be more effective because it doesn't undergo CYP3A4 metabolism.

diazoxide ━━━◄►━━━ sulfonylureas
Hyperstat, Proglycem   acetohexamide,
                               chlorpropamide, glipizide,
                               glyburide, tolazamide,
                               tolbutamide

Risk rating: 2
Severity: Moderate   Onset: Delayed   Likelihood: Probable

Cause
Diazoxide may decrease insulin release or stimulate release of glucose and free fatty acids by various mechanisms.

Effect
Risk of hyperglycemia increases if a patient stabilized on a sulfonylurea starts diazoxide.

Nursing considerations
- Use these drugs together cautiously.
- Monitor patient's blood glucose level regularly, and consult prescriber about adjustments to either drug to maintain stable level.
- Teach patient to monitor the blood glucose level.
- Tell patient to stay alert for evidence of high blood glucose level, such as increased fatigue, thirst, eating, or urination and possible blurred vision or dry skin and mucous membranes.

diclofenac ⧓ aminoglycosides

Cataflam | amikacin, gentamicin, kanamycin, netilmicin, streptomycin, tobramycin

Risk rating: **2**
Severity: **Moderate** Onset: **Delayed** Likelihood: **Suspected**

Cause
Diclofenac and other NSAIDs may reduce glomerular filtration rate (GFR), causing aminoglycosides to accumulate.

Effect
Aminoglycoside level in premature infants may increase.

Nursing considerations
- Before NSAID starts, aminoglycoside dose should be reduced.

ALERT Check peak and trough levels after the third dose. For peak level, draw blood 30 minutes after an I.V. or 60 minutes after an I.M. dose. For trough level, draw blood just before a dose.

- Monitor patient's renal function.
- Although only indomethacin is known to interact with aminoglycosides, other NSAIDs probably do as well. If you suspect an interaction, consult prescriber or pharmacist.
- Other drugs cleared by GFR may have a similar interaction.

dicloxacillin ⧓ food

Risk rating: **2**
Severity: **Moderate** Onset: **Delayed** Likelihood: **Suspected**

Cause
Food may delay or reduce GI absorption of penicillins, such as dicloxacillin.

Effect
Penicillin efficacy may decrease.

Nursing considerations
- Food may affect penicillin absorption and peak level.
- Penicillin V and amoxicillin don't have this interaction and may be given without regard to meals.
- If patient takes a penicillin with food, watch for lack of drug efficacy.
- Tell patient to take penicillin 1 hour before or 2 hours after a meal.

dicloxacillin ━━►◄━━ tetracyclines

demeclocycline, doxycycline, minocycline, tetracycline

Risk rating: 1
Severity: Major   **Onset: Delayed**   **Likelihood: Suspected**

Cause
Tetracyclines may adversely affect the bactericidal activity of penicillins, such as dicloxacillin.

Effect
Penicillin efficacy may be reduced.

Nursing considerations
- If possible, avoid giving tetracyclines with penicillins.
- Monitor patient closely for lack of penicillin effect.

dicyclomine ━━►◄━━ phenothiazines

chlorpromazine, fluphenazine, mesoridazine, perphenazine, prochlorperazine, promethazine, thioridazine, trifluoperazine

Risk rating: 2
Severity: Moderate   **Onset: Delayed**   **Likelihood: Suspected**

Cause
Dicyclomine and other anticholinergics may antagonize phenothiazines. Also, phenothiazine metabolism may increase.

Effect
Phenothiazine efficacy may decrease.

Nursing considerations
- Data regarding this interaction conflict.
- Monitor patient for decreased phenothiazine efficacy.
- Phenothiazine dosage may need adjustment.
- Adverse anticholinergic effects may increase.
- Monitor patient for adynamic ileus, hyperpyrexia, hypoglycemia, and neurologic changes.

didanosine ▬▶◀▬ azole antifungals
Videx   itraconazole, ketoconazole

Risk rating: 2
Severity: Moderate   **Onset: Rapid**   **Likelihood: Suspected**

Cause
Inert ingredients in chewable didanosine tablets decrease absorption of azole antifungals.

Effect
Efficacy of azole antifungals may decrease.

Nursing considerations
■ To minimize interaction, instruct patient to take antifungal 2 hours before didanosine.
■ Monitor patient for lack of response to antifungal drug.
■ Help patient develop a plan to ensure proper dosage intervals.
■ Other azole antifungals may interact with didanosine. If you suspect an interaction, consult prescriber or pharmacist.

didanosine ▬▶◀▬ quinolones
Videx   ciprofloxacin, lomefloxacin,
                               norfloxacin, ofloxacin

Risk rating: 2
Severity: Moderate   **Onset: Rapid**   **Likelihood: Suspected**

Cause
Buffers in didanosine chewable tablets and pediatric powder for oral solution decrease GI absorption of quinolones.

Effect
Quinolone effects decrease.

Nursing considerations
■ Avoid use together. If it's unavoidable, give the quinolone at least 2 hours before or 6 hours after didanosine.
■ Monitor patient for improvement in infection.
■ Unbuffered didanosine doesn't affect quinolone absorption.
■ Help patient develop a plan to ensure proper dosage intervals.

digoxin ━━━━▶◀━━━━ amiodarone
Lanoxin   Cordarone

Risk rating: 1
Severity: Major   **Onset: Delayed**   **Likelihood: Probable**

Cause
The mechanism for this interaction is unknown.

Effect
Digoxin level and risk of toxicity may increase.

Nursing considerations
■ Watch for evidence of digoxin toxicity, such as arrhythmias, nausea, vomiting, and agitation.
■ Monitor digoxin level; digoxin dosage may need to be reduced during amiodarone treatment.
■ Higher amiodarone doses cause greatest increase in digoxin level.
■ Because amiodarone has a long half-life, effects of interaction may persist after amiodarone is stopped.

digoxin ━━━━▶◀━━━━ cholestyramine
Lanoxin   LoCHOLEST, Prevalite,
                                 Questran

Risk rating: 2
Severity: Moderate   **Onset: Delayed**   **Likelihood: Probable**

Cause
Cholestyramine may decrease digoxin absorption by binding to it. Cholestyramine also may interrupt digoxin metabolism in the liver.

Effect
Digoxin bioavailability and effects may decrease.

Nursing considerations
■ Monitor digoxin level.
■ Watch for decreased digoxin effects; dosage may need adjustment.
■ Digoxin capsules may minimize the interaction.
■ Give cholestyramine 8 hours before or after digoxin.
■ Cholestyramine may be useful in treating digoxin toxicity.

digoxin ◄►◄ colestipol
Lanoxin   Colestid

Risk rating: 2
Severity: Moderate   Onset: Rapid   Likelihood: Suspected

Cause
Colestipol may bind with digoxin and decrease its GI absorption. Colestipol also may interfere with normal recycling of digoxin between liver and intestine.

Effect
Digoxin effects may decrease.

Nursing considerations
- Colestipol may be useful in treating digoxin toxicity.
- If you suspect an interaction, consult prescriber or pharmacist.
- If patient takes colestipol routinely, monitor digoxin level. Therapeutic range for digoxin is 0.8 to 2 nanograms/ml.
- Monitor patient for expected digoxin effects, including decreased heart rate, arrhythmia conversion, maintenance of converted rhythm, and improvement of heart failure symptoms.
- If digoxin level or effects decrease, dosage may need adjustment.

digoxin ◄►◄ indomethacin
Lanoxin   Indocin

Risk rating: 2
Severity: Moderate   Onset: Delayed   Likelihood: Suspected

Cause
Indomethacin may reduce renal digoxin elimination.

Effect
Digoxin level and risk of toxicity may increase.

Nursing considerations
- This interaction may not occur in patients with normal renal function.
- ⚡ ALERT Use cautiously in preterm infants with decreased renal function; digoxin dose may need to be reduced by half when indomethacin starts.
- Monitor digoxin level. Therapeutic range is 0.8 to 2 nanograms/ml.
- Check renal function tests and urine output.
- Watch for evidence of digoxin toxicity: arrhythmias (bradycardia and AV blocks, more common in children; ventricular ectopy, more common in adults), lethargy, drowsiness, confusion, hallucinations, head-

aches, syncope, visual disturbances, nausea, vomiting, diarrhea, anorexia, and failure to thrive.

digoxin ▶◀ itraconazole
Lanoxin   Sporanox

Risk rating: 2
Severity: Moderate   **Onset: Delayed**   **Likelihood: Established**

Cause
Renal digoxin clearance may decrease and absorption increase.

Effect
Digoxin level and risk of toxicity may increase.

Nursing considerations
■ Monitor digoxin level. Therapeutic range is 0.8 to 2 nanograms/ml.
■ Watch for evidence of digoxin toxicity: arrhythmias (bradycardia, AV block, and ventricular ectopy), lethargy, drowsiness, confusion, hallucinations, headaches, syncope, visual disturbances, nausea, anorexia, vomiting, and diarrhea.
■ Digoxin dosage may need reduction.
■ Azole antifungals other than itraconazole may interact with digoxin. If you suspect an interaction, consult prescriber or pharmacist.

digoxin ▶◀ macrolide antibiotics
Lanoxin   clarithromycin, erythromycin

Risk rating: 1
Severity: Major   **Onset: Delayed**   **Likelihood: Established**

Cause
Macrolide antibiotics may alter GI flora and increase digoxin absorption. Clarithromycin may inhibit renal clearance of digoxin.

Effect
Digoxin level and risk of toxicity may increase.

Nursing considerations
■ Monitor digoxin level. Therapeutic range is 0.8 to 2 nanograms/ml.
■ Watch for evidence of digoxin toxicity: arrhythmias (bradycardia, AV blocks, and ventricular ectopy), lethargy, drowsiness, confusion, hallucinations, headaches, syncope, visual disturbances, nausea, anorexia, vomiting, and diarrhea.
■ Digoxin dosage may need reduction.

⚡ ALERT Neither clarithromycin nor erythromycin affects the serum level of digoxin given I.V. Capsule form of digoxin may increase digoxin availability and decrease risk of interaction.
■ Other macrolide antibiotics may interact with digoxin. If you suspect an interaction, consult prescriber or pharmacist.

---

digoxin ▶◀ metoclopramide
Lanoxin   Reglan

Risk rating: 2
Severity: Moderate   **Onset: Delayed**   **Likelihood: Probable**

Cause
Increased GI motility may decrease digoxin absorption.

Effect
Digoxin level and effects may decrease.

Nursing considerations
■ Monitor patient for decreased digoxin level; therapeutic range is 0.8 to 2 nanograms/ml.
■ Watch for expected digoxin effects: decreased heart rate, arrhythmia conversion, maintenance of converted rhythm, and improvement of heart failure symptoms.
■ If digoxin level or effects decrease, dosage may need adjustment.
⚡ ALERT This interaction may not occur with high bioavailability digoxin forms, including capsules, elixir, and tablets with a high dissolution rate.
■ Urge patient to tell prescriber about increased adverse effects.

---

digoxin ▶◀ propafenone
Lanoxin   Rythmol

Risk rating: 1
Severity: Major   **Onset: Delayed**   **Likelihood: Established**

Cause
Digoxin distribution and renal and nonrenal digoxin clearance may decrease.

Effect
Digoxin level and risk of toxicity may increase.

Nursing considerations
■ Monitor digoxin level. Therapeutic range is 0.8 to 2 nanograms/ml.

■ Check ECG for digoxin toxicity: arrhythmias, such as bradycardia and AV blocks, ventricular ectopy, and shortened QTc interval.
■ Watch for other evidence of digoxin toxicity: lethargy, drowsiness, confusion, hallucinations, headaches, syncope, visual disturbances, nausea, anorexia, failure to thrive, vomiting, and diarrhea.
■ If propafenone starts or stops during digoxin therapy, digoxin dosage may need adjustment.

digoxin ━━━━▶◀━━━━ quinidine
Lanoxin

Risk rating: 1
Severity: **Major**   Onset: **Delayed**   Likelihood: **Established**

Cause
Total renal and biliary digoxin clearance decreases.

Effect
Digoxin level and risk of toxicity may increase.

Nursing considerations
■ Monitor digoxin level. Therapeutic range is 0.8 to 2 nanograms/ml.
■ Some patients may have toxicity even with serum digoxin level in therapeutic range.
■ Watch for signs of digoxin toxicity: arrhythmias (bradycardia, AV blocks, and ventricular ectopy), lethargy, drowsiness, confusion, hallucinations, headaches, syncope, visual disturbances, nausea, anorexia, vomiting, and diarrhea.
■ If quinidine starts, digoxin dosage may need reduction of up to 50%.

digoxin ━━━━▶◀━━━━ spironolactone
Lanoxin   Aldactone

Risk rating: 2
Severity: **Moderate**   Onset: **Rapid**   Likelihood: **Suspected**

Cause
Spironolactone may lessen digoxin's ability to strengthen myocardial contraction. It also may decrease renal clearance of digoxin.

Effect
Digoxin level may increase; positive inotropic effect may decrease.

Nursing considerations
■ Watch for expected digoxin effects, especially in heart failure.
■ Monitor digoxin level. Therapeutic range is 0.8 to 2 nanograms/ml.

⚠ **ALERT** Spironolactone may interfere with determination of serum digoxin level, causing falsely elevated level.
■ During spironolactone therapy, digoxin dosage may need adjustment; however, remember that spironolactone may cause falsely elevated digoxin level.

---

digoxin ━━━►◄━━━ St. John's wort
Lanoxin

Risk rating: 2
Severity: Moderate   **Onset: Delayed**   **Likelihood: Suspected**

Cause
St. John's wort may decrease absorption and availability of digoxin.

Effect
Digoxin level and effects may decrease.

Nursing considerations
■ Watch for decreased digoxin level. Therapeutic range is 0.8 to 2 nanograms/ml.
■ Monitor patient for expected digoxin effects: decreased heart rate, arrhythmia conversion, maintenance of converted rhythm, and improvement of heart failure symptoms.
■ Advise patient to avoid taking St. John's wort with digoxin.
■ If patient stabilized on combined use stops taking St. John's wort, monitor digoxin level and adjust dosage as needed.

---

digoxin ━━━►◄━━━ tetracyclines
Lanoxin   demeclocycline, doxycycline, minocycline, tetracycline

Risk rating: 1
Severity: Major   **Onset: Delayed**   **Likelihood: Suspected**

Cause
Tetracyclines may alter GI flora and increase digoxin absorption.

Effect
Digoxin level and risk of toxicity may increase.

Nursing considerations
⚠ **ALERT** Effects of tetracyclines on digoxin may persist for several months after antibiotic is stopped.
■ Monitor digoxin level. Therapeutic range is 0.8 to 2 nanograms/ml.

■ Watch for signs of digoxin toxicity: arrhythmias (bradycardia, AV block, and ventricular ectopy), lethargy, drowsiness, confusion, hallucinations, headaches, syncope, visual disturbances, nausea, anorexia, vomiting, and diarrhea.
■ Digoxin dosage may need reduction.
■ Capsule form may increase digoxin availability and decrease the risk of interaction.

---

digoxin ▶◀ thiazide diuretics
Lanoxin

chlorothiazide, hydrochlorothiazide, indapamide, methyclothiazide, metolazone, polythiazide, trichlormethiazide

Risk rating: 1
Severity: Major   **Onset: Delayed**   **Likelihood: Probable**

Cause
Thiazide diuretics increase urinary excretion of potassium and magnesium, which are needed for proper cardiac muscle function.

Effect
Electrolyte imbalances may contribute to digoxin-induced arrhythmias.

Nursing considerations
■ Monitor serum potassium and magnesium levels.
■ Give potassium or magnesium supplements as ordered.
■ Consult prescriber about dietary sodium restriction or potassium-sparing diuretics to prevent further losses.
■ Monitor ECG for arrhythmias.
■ Urge patient to eat potassium-rich foods: fruits (such as avocados, bananas, and cantaloupes), broccoli, potatoes, and spinach.

---

digoxin ▶◀ thioamines
Lanoxin

methimazole, propylthiouracil

Risk rating: 2
Severity: Moderate   **Onset: Delayed**   **Likelihood: Established**

Cause
Digoxin level may increase in hypothyroidism or when a hyperthyroid patient becomes euthyroid.

Effect
Digoxin effects and risk of toxicity increase.

Nursing considerations
- Monitor digoxin level. Therapeutic range is 0.8 to 2 nanograms/ml.
- Watch for digoxin toxicity: arrhythmias (bradycardia, AV block, and ventricular ectopy), lethargy, drowsiness, confusion, hallucinations, headaches, syncope, visual disturbances, nausea, anorexia, vomiting, and diarrhea.
- Monitor thyroid function tests (TSH, 0.2 to 5.4 microunits/ml; T_3, 80 to 200 nanograms/dl; and T_4, 5.4 to 11.5 mcg/dl).
- If hyperthyroid patient becomes euthyroid, digoxin dosage may need reduction.
- If patient is euthyroid and taking a thioamine when digoxin starts, no special precautions are needed.

---

digoxin ▸◂ thyroid hormones
Lanoxin   levothyroxine, liothyronine, liotrix, thyroid

Risk rating: 2
Severity: Moderate   Onset: Delayed   Likelihood: Established

Cause
Digoxin level may decrease in hyperthyroidism or when a hypothyroid patient becomes euthyroid.

Effect
Digoxin effects may decrease.

Nursing considerations
- Monitor digoxin level. Therapeutic range is 0.8 to 2 nanograms/ml.
- Watch for expected digoxin effects: decreased heart rate, arrhythmia conversion, maintenance of converted rhythm, and improvement of heart failure symptoms.
- Monitor thyroid function tests (TSH, 0.2 to 5.4 microunits/ml; T_3, 80 to 200 nanograms/dl; and T_4, 5.4 to 11.5 mcg/dl).
- If hypothyroid patient becomes euthyroid, digoxin dosage may need to be increased.
- If patient is euthyroid and taking a thyroid hormone when digoxin starts, no special precautions are needed.

digoxin 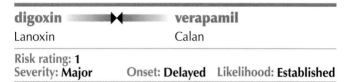 verapamil
Lanoxin   Calan

Risk rating: 1
Severity: Major   **Onset: Delayed**   **Likelihood: Established**

Cause
Verapamil decreases digoxin elimination. Verapamil and digoxin have additive effects that decrease AV conduction.

Effect
Digoxin level, effects, and risk of toxicity may increase.

Nursing considerations
■ Monitor digoxin level. Therapeutic range is 0.8 to 2 nanograms/ml.
■ Watch for signs of digoxin toxicity: arrhythmias (bradycardia, AV block, and ventricular ectopy), lethargy, drowsiness, confusion, hallucinations, headaches, syncope, visual disturbances, nausea, anorexia, vomiting, and diarrhea.
■ Digoxin dosage may need reduction.
■ Urge patient to report adverse reactions that may suggest toxicity: nausea, vomiting, diarrhea, appetite loss, and visual disturbances.

dihydroergotamine ▶◀ beta blockers
D.H.E. 45   carteolol, nadolol, penbutolol,
                                  pindolol, propranolol, timolol

Risk rating: 2
Severity: Moderate   **Onset: Delayed**   **Likelihood: Suspected**

Cause
Vasoconstriction and blockade of peripheral beta$_2$ receptors allow unopposed ergot action.

Effect
Vasoconstrictive effects of ergot derivatives, such as dihydroergotamine, increase.

Nursing considerations
■ Watch for evidence of peripheral ischemia, cold extremities, and possible gangrene.
■ If needed, stop beta blocker and adjust ergot derivative.
■ Other ergot derivatives may interact with beta blockers. If you suspect an interaction, consult prescriber or pharmacist.

dihydroergotamine ➤◄ itraconazole
D.H.E. 45   Sporanox

Risk rating: 1
Severity: Major   **Onset: Delayed**   **Likelihood: Suspected**

Cause
Itraconazole may inhibit CYP3A4 metabolism of ergot derivatives, such as dihydroergotamine.

Effect
Risk of ergot toxicity may increase.

Nursing considerations
❯ ALERT Use of these drugs together is contraindicated.
- Signs of ergot toxicity include peripheral vasospasm and ischemia.

dihydroergotamine ➤◄ macrolide antibiotics
D.H.E. 45   clarithromycin, erythromycin,
                                       troleandomycin

Risk rating: 1
Severity: Major   **Onset: Rapid**   **Likelihood: Probable**

Cause
Macrolide antibiotics interfere with hepatic metabolism of ergotamine, although exact mechanism is unknown.

Effect
Patient may develop symptoms of acute ergotism, mainly peripheral ischemia.

Nursing considerations
- Watch for evidence of peripheral ischemia: pain in limb muscles while exercising and later at rest; numbness and tingling of fingers and toes; cool, pale, or cyanotic limbs; red or violet blisters on hands or feet; and gangrene.
- Dosage of ergot derivative, such as dihydroergotamine, may need to be decreased, or both drugs may need to be stopped.
- Consider a different anti-infective drug that's less likely to interact with an ergot derivative.
❯ ALERT Sodium nitroprusside may be given for macrolide-ergot–induced vasospasm.
- Explain evidence of ergot-induced peripheral ischemia. Urge patient to report it promptly.

dihydroergotamine ▶◀ nitrates

D.H.E. 45

amyl nitrite, isosorbide
dinitrate, nitroglycerin

Risk rating: 2
Severity: Moderate   Onset: Rapid   Likelihood: Suspected

Cause
Dihydroergotamine metabolism decreases, increasing its availability
and antagonizing nitrate-induced coronary vasodilation.

Effect
Increased dihydroergotamine availability may increase systolic blood
pressure and decrease antianginal effects.

Nursing considerations
■ Use these drugs together cautiously in patients with angina.
■ Monitor patient for evidence of ergotism: peripheral ischemia,
paresthesia, headache, nausea, and vomiting.
■ Urge patient to immediately report possible peripheral ischemia:
numbness or tingling in fingers and toes, red blisters on hands or feet.
Dihydroergotamine dosage may need to be decreased.

dihydroergotamine ▶◀ nonnucleoside reverse-
transcriptase inhibitors

D.H.E. 45

delavirdine, efavirenz

Risk rating: 1
Severity: Major   Onset: Delayed   Likelihood: Suspected

Cause
Nonnucleoside reverse-transcriptase inhibitors may decrease CYP3A4
metabolism of ergot derivatives, such as dihydroergotamine.

Effect
Risk of ergot-induced peripheral vasospasm and ischemia may increase.

Nursing considerations
◪ ALERT Use of ergot derivatives with delavirdine or efavirenz is contraindicated.
■ Watch for evidence of peripheral ischemia: pain in limb muscles
while exercising and later at rest; numbness and tingling of fingers
and toes; cool, pale, or cyanotic limbs; red or violet blisters on hands
or feet; and gangrene.

- Ergot toxicity also may cause nausea, vomiting, lassitude, impaired mental function, delirium, severe dyspnea, hypotension, hypertension, rapid or weak pulse, unconsciousness, limb spasms, seizures, and shock.
- Give vasodilator for vasospasm and diazepam for seizures as needed.
- Other nonnucleoside reverse-transcriptase inhibitors, such as nevirapine, may interact with ergot derivatives. If you suspect an interaction, consult prescriber or pharmacist.

dihydroergotamine ⋈ protease inhibitors

D.H.E. 45

amprenavir, atazanavir, indinavir, lopinavir-ritonavir, nelfinavir, ritonavir, saquinavir

Risk rating: 1
Severity: Major   Onset: **Delayed**   Likelihood: **Probable**

Cause
Protease inhibitors may interfere with CYP3A4 metabolism of ergot derivatives, such as dihydroergotamine.

Effect
Risk of ergot-induced peripheral vasospasm and ischemia may increase.

Nursing considerations
⚑ ALERT Use of ergot derivatives with protease inhibitors is contraindicated.
- Watch for evidence of peripheral ischemia: pain in limb muscles while exercising and later at rest; numbness and tingling of fingers and toes; cool, pale, or cyanotic limbs; red or violet blisters on hands or feet; and gangrene.
⚑ ALERT Sodium nitroprusside may be given for ergot-induced vasospasm.
- If patient takes a protease inhibitor, consult prescriber and pharmacist about alternative treatments for migraine pain.
⚑ ALERT Urge patient to tell prescriber about increased adverse effects.

dihydroergotamine ➤◀ selective 5-HT$_1$ receptor agonists

D.H.E. 45

frovatriptan, naratriptan, rizatriptan, sumatriptan, zolmitriptan

Risk rating: 1
Severity: Major   **Onset: Rapid**   **Likelihood: Suspected**

Cause
Combined use may have additive effects.

Effect
Risk of vasospastic effects increases.

Nursing considerations
⚠ **ALERT** Use of these drugs or any two selective 5-HT$_1$ receptor agonists within 24 hours of each other is contraindicated.

■ Combined use may cause severe vasospastic effects, including sustained coronary artery vasospasm that triggers MI.

■ Warn patient not to mix migraine drugs within 24 hours of each other; advise calling prescriber if a drug isn't effective.

diltiazem ➤◀ benzodiazepines

Cardizem

diazepam, midazolam, triazolam

Risk rating: 2
Severity: Moderate   **Onset: Rapid**   **Likelihood: Probable**

Cause
Diltiazem may decrease metabolism of some benzodiazepines.

Effect
Benzodiazepine effects may increase.

Nursing considerations
■ Watch for signs of increased CNS depression: sedation, dizziness, confusion, asthenia, ataxia, altered level of consciousness, hypoactive reflexes, hypotension, bradycardia, and respiratory depression.

■ Lower benzodiazepine dose may be needed.

■ Explain the risk of increased and prolonged CNS effects.

■ Warn patient to avoid hazardous activities until effects of this combination are clear.

■ Other benzodiazepines may interact with diltiazem. If you suspect an interaction, consult prescriber or pharmacist.

diltiazem ━━━▶◀━━━ buspirone
Cardizem   BuSpar

Risk rating: 2
Severity: Moderate   Onset: Delayed   Likelihood: Suspected

Cause
CYP3A4 metabolism of buspirone may decrease.

Effect
Buspirone level and adverse effects may increase.

Nursing considerations
■ If patient takes buspirone, watch closely when the calcium channel blocker diltiazem starts or stops or when its dosage changes.
■ Watch for signs of buspirone toxicity: increased CNS effects (dizziness, drowsiness, and headache), vomiting, and diarrhea.
■ Adjust buspirone dose as needed.
■ If patient takes diltiazem, prescriber may consider an antianxiety drug not metabolized by CYP3A4, such as lorazepam.
■ Dihydropyridine calcium channel blockers that don't inhibit CYP3A4 metabolism, such as amlodipine and felodipine, probably won't disrupt buspirone metabolism.
■ Other calcium channel blockers may have this interaction. If you suspect an interaction, consult prescriber or pharmacist.

diltiazem ━━━▶◀━━━ carbamazepine
Cardizem   Carbatrol, Epitol, Equetro,
                                  Tegretol

Risk rating: 2
Severity: Moderate   Onset: Delayed   Likelihood: Suspected

Cause
Diltiazem may inhibit carbamazepine metabolism.

Effect
Carbamazepine level and risk of toxicity may increase.

Nursing considerations
■ Monitor carbamazepine level; therapeutic range is 4 to 12 mcg/ml.
■ If diltiazem therapy starts, watch for signs of carbamazepine toxicity: dizziness, ataxia, respiratory depression, tachycardia, arrhythmias, blood pressure changes, impaired consciousness, abnormal reflexes, nystagmus, seizures, nausea, vomiting, and urine retention.

■ If diltiazem therapy stops, watch for loss of carbamazepine effects (loss of seizure control). Dosage may need to be increased.

■ Calcium channel blockers other than diltiazem may have this interaction. If you suspect an interaction, consult prescriber or pharmacist.

---

diltiazem ◄►◄ cyclosporine

Cardizem   Gengraf, Neoral, Sandimmune

Risk rating: 2
Severity: **Moderate**   Onset: **Delayed**   Likelihood: **Established**

Cause
Diltiazem may inhibit cyclosporine metabolism in the liver.

Effect
Cyclosporine level and risk of toxicity may increase.

Nursing considerations
■ When starting or stopping diltiazem, monitor cyclosporine level.
■ Cyclosporine dosage may need to be reduced by 20% to 50%.
■ Watch for arthralgia and encephalopathy.
■ Adverse reactions typically subside when diltiazem stops.
🗈 **ALERT** Rejection episodes may increase when diltiazem is stopped because cyclosporine level may be reduced.

---

diltiazem ◄►◄ HMG-CoA reductase inhibitors

Cardizem
atorvastatin, lovastatin, simvastatin

Risk rating: 2
Severity: **Moderate**   Onset: **Delayed**   Likelihood: **Probable**

Cause
CYP3A4 metabolism of certain HMG-CoA reductase inhibitors may be inhibited.

Effect
HMG-CoA reductase inhibitor level may increase, raising the risk of toxicity, including myositis and rhabdomyolysis.

Nursing considerations
■ If possible, avoid use together.
■ Assess patient for evidence of rhabdomyolysis: fatigue; muscle aches and weakness; joint pain; dark, red, or cola-colored urine; weight gain; seizures; and greatly increased serum CK level.

⚡ **ALERT** If patient may have rhabdomyolysis, notify prescriber and obtain renal function tests and serum potassium, sodium, calcium, lactic acid, and myoglobin levels.

■ Pravastatin is less likely to interact with diltiazem than other HMG-CoA reductase inhibitors and may be best choice for combined use.

■ Urge patient to report unexplained muscle pain, tenderness, or weakness to prescriber.

diltiazem ▶◀ methylprednisolone
Cardizem   Medrol

Risk rating: 2
Severity: Moderate   **Onset: Delayed**   **Likelihood: Suspected**

Cause
Methylprednisolone CYP3A4 metabolism may be inhibited.

Effect
Methylprednisolone effects and risk of toxicity may increase.

Nursing considerations
■ Monitor patient for appropriate response to methylprednisolone.
■ Watch for signs of methylprednisolone toxicity: nervousness, sleepiness, depression, psychoses, weakness, decreased hearing, lower leg edema, skin disorders, hypertension, muscle weakness, and seizures.
■ Methylprednisolone dosage may need adjustment.
■ Advise patient to report increased adverse effects.
■ Corticosteroids other than methylprednisolone may interact with diltiazem. If you suspect an interaction, consult prescriber or pharmacist.

diltiazem ▶◀ moricizine
Cardizem   Ethmozine

Risk rating: 2
Severity: Moderate   **Onset: Delayed**   **Likelihood: Suspected**

Cause
Moricizine metabolism may decrease; diltiazem metabolism may increase.

Effect
Moricizine effects (including adverse effects) may increase; diltiazem effects may decrease.

Nursing considerations
- Watch for expected effects of diltiazem.
- Urge patient to report increased angina or symptoms of hypertension, including headache, dizziness, and blurred vision.
- Watch for increased adverse moricizine effects, particularly headache, dizziness, and paresthesia.
- Caution patient to avoid hazardous activities if adverse CNS reactions or blurred vision occurs. These adverse effects may be more common with increased moricizine level.
- Dosage adjustment may be needed when either drug starts, stops, or changes dosage. Consult prescriber or pharmacist.

diltiazem ➤◀ quinidine
Cardizem

Risk rating: 2
Severity: Moderate   **Onset: Delayed**   **Likelihood: Suspected**

Cause
Hepatic metabolism of quinidine may be inhibited.

Effect
Quinidine effects and risk of toxicity may increase.

Nursing considerations
- Monitor quinidine level. Therapeutic range is 2 to 6 mcg/ml.
- Watch ECG for widened QRS complexes, prolonged QT and PR intervals, and ventricular arrhythmias, including torsades de pointes.
- Monitor patient for signs of quinidine toxicity: hypotension, seizures, ataxia, anuria, respiratory distress, irritability, and hallucinations.
- Explain that adverse GI effects, especially diarrhea, may signal quinidine toxicity. Tell patient to alert prescriber.
- Adjust quinidine dosage if needed.

diltiazem ➤◀ tacrolimus
Cardizem   Prograf

Risk rating: 2
Severity: Moderate   **Onset: Delayed**   **Likelihood: Suspected**

Cause
Hepatic metabolism of tacrolimus by CYP3A4 may be inhibited.

Effect
Tacrolimus level and risk of toxicity may increase.

Nursing considerations
- Diltiazem may have similar effects on cyclosporine and sirolimus.
- Monitor tacrolimus level. Therapeutic range for liver transplants is 5 to 20 nanograms/ml and for kidney transplants is 7 to 20 nanograms/ml for the first 3 months, 5 to 15 nanograms/ml through 1 year.
- Monitor patient for tacrolimus toxicity: delirium, confusion, agitation, tremor, adverse GI effects, and abnormal renal function tests.
- Tacrolimus dosage may need adjustment when diltiazem starts, stops, or changes dosage.

diltiazem ▶◀ theophyllines
Cardizem   aminophylline, theophylline

Risk rating: 2
Severity: **Moderate**   Onset: **Delayed**   Likelihood: **Suspected**

Cause
Theophylline metabolism may be inhibited.

Effect
Theophylline level and risk of toxicity may increase.

Nursing considerations
- Watch for evidence of toxicity, such as tachycardia, anorexia, nausea, vomiting, diarrhea, seizures, restlessness, irritability, and headache.
- Monitor serum theophylline level closely. Normal therapeutic range is 10 to 20 mcg/ml for adults and 5 to 15 mcg/ml for children.
- Describe adverse effects of theophylline and signs of toxicity, and tell patient to report them immediately to prescriber.

disopyramide ▶◀ quinolones
Norpace   gatifloxacin, levofloxacin, moxifloxacin, sparfloxacin

Risk rating: 1
Severity: **Major**   Onset: **Delayed**   Likelihood: **Suspected**

Cause
The mechanism of this interaction is unknown.

Effect
Risk of life-threatening arrhythmias, including torsades de pointes, increases.

Nursing considerations

◤ **ALERT** Use of sparfloxacin with an antiarrhythmic, such as disopyramide, is contraindicated.

■ Avoid giving a class IA or class III antiarrhythmics with gatifloxacin, levofloxacin, or moxifloxacin.

■ Quinolones that aren't metabolized by CYP3A4 isoenzymes or that don't prolong the QT interval may be given with antiarrhythmics.

■ Monitor ECG for prolonged QTc interval.

■ Tell patient to report a rapid heartbeat, shortness of breath, dizziness, fainting, and chest pain.

---

disopyramide ▸◀ vardenafil
Norpace   Levitra

Risk rating: 1
Severity: Major   **Onset: Rapid**   **Likelihood: Suspected**

Cause
The mechanism of this interaction is unknown.

Effect
QTc interval may be prolonged, particularly in patients with previous QT-interval prolongation and those taking certain antiarrhythmics, such as disopyramide. This increases the risk of such life-threatening arrhythmias as torsades de pointes.

Nursing considerations

◤ **ALERT** Use of vardenafil with a class IA or class III antiarrhythmic is contraindicated.

■ Monitor ECG before and periodically after patient starts vardenafil.

■ Urge patient to report light-headedness, faintness, palpitations, and chest pain or pressure while taking vardenafil.

■ To reduce risk of adverse effects, patients age 65 and older should start with 5 mg vardenafil, half the usual starting dose.

---

disulfiram ▸◀ alcohol
Antabuse

Risk rating: 1
Severity: Major   **Onset: Rapid**   **Likelihood: Established**

Cause
Disulfiram inhibits alcohol metabolism, which causes acetaldehyde—a toxic metabolite—to accumulate.

Effect
A disulfiram reaction occurs.

Nursing considerations
⚠ ALERT Patients taking disulfiram shouldn't be exposed to or consume any products containing alcohol, including back rub preparations, cough syrups, liniments, and shaving lotion.

⚠ ALERT Disulfiram should be taken only if patient has abstained from alcohol for at least 12 hours. Make sure patient understands the consequences of disulfiram use and consents to its use.

■ Disulfiram reaction may cause flushing, throbbing headache, dyspnea, nausea, copious vomiting, diaphoresis, thirst, chest pain, palpitations, hyperventilation, hypotension, syncope, anxiety, weakness, blurred vision, confusion, and arthropathy. More severe reactions may include respiratory depression, cardiovascular collapse, arrhythmias, MI, acute heart failure, seizures, unconsciousness, or death.

■ Mild reactions may occur in sensitive patient at a blood alcohol level of 5 to 10 mg/dl; symptoms are fully developed at 50 mg/dl; unconsciousness typically occurs at 125 to 150 mg/dl level. Reaction may last 30 minutes to several hours or as long as alcohol stays in the blood.

■ Caution family not to give disulfiram to patient without his knowledge; severe reaction or death could result if patient drinks alcohol.

---

disulfiram ━━━▶◀━━━ chlorzoxazone
Antabuse   Parafon Forte DSC

Risk rating: 2
Severity: Moderate   **Onset: Delayed**   **Likelihood: Probable**

Cause
Disulfiram inhibits hepatic metabolism of chlorzoxazone.

Effect
CNS depressant effects of chlorzoxazone may increase.

Nursing considerations
■ Watch for increased adverse CNS effects including dizziness, drowsiness, headache, and light-headedness.

■ Signs of more severe toxicity include nausea, vomiting, diarrhea, loss of muscle tone, decreased or absent deep tendon reflexes, respiratory depression, and hypotension.

■ Advise patient to avoid hazardous activities until CNS depressant effects are known.

■ Chlorzoxazone dose may need to be reduced.

■ Urge patient to tell prescriber about increased adverse effects.

disulfiram ▬▶◀▬ metronidazole
Antabuse   Flagyl

Risk rating: 2
Severity: Moderate   **Onset: Delayed**   **Likelihood: Suspected**

Cause
Interaction may stem from excess dopaminergic activity.

Effect
Risk of acute psychosis or confusion increases.

Nursing considerations
■ **ALERT** Avoid use together.
■ Disulfiram given alone may cause acute encephalopathy, paranoid ideas, disorientation, impaired memory, ataxia, and confusion.
■ Monitor patient for acute psychosis and confusion.
■ If adverse effects occur, consult prescriber; one or both drugs may need to be stopped.
■ Urge patient to tell prescriber about increased adverse effects.

disulfiram ▬▶◀▬ phenytoin
Antabuse   Dilantin

Risk rating: 2
Severity: Moderate   **Onset: Rapid**   **Likelihood: Established**

Cause
Disulfiram inhibits hepatic metabolism of phenytoin and may interfere with elimination.

Effect
Phenytoin level, effects, and risk of toxicity may increase.

Nursing considerations
■ Monitor phenytoin level; therapeutic range is 10 to 20 mcg/ml.
■ Watch for evidence of phenytoin toxicity: drowsiness, nausea, vomiting, nystagmus, ataxia, dysarthria, tremor, slurred speech, hypotension, arrhythmias, respiratory depression, and coma.
■ If disulfiram is stopped, assess patient for loss of phenytoin effects (loss of seizure control).
■ Adjust phenytoin dose as ordered.
■ Hydantoins other than phenytoin may interact with disulfiram. If you suspect an interaction, consult prescriber or pharmacist.

disulfiram ►◄ theophyllines
Antabuse   aminophylline, theophylline

Risk rating: 2
Severity: **Moderate**   Onset: **Delayed**   Likelihood: **Suspected**

Cause
Disulfiram inhibits theophylline metabolism.

Effect
Theophylline effects, including toxic effects, increase.

Nursing considerations
■ Watch for evidence of toxicity, such as tachycardia, anorexia, nausea, vomiting, diarrhea, seizures, restlessness, irritability, and headache.
■ Monitor serum theophylline level closely. Normal therapeutic range is 10 to 20 mcg/ml for adults and 5 to 15 mcg/ml for children.
■ Because disulfiram exerts dose-dependent inhibition of theophylline, theophylline dosage may need adjustment.
■ Describe adverse effects of theophylline and signs of toxicity, and tell patient to report them immediately to prescriber.

divalproex sodium ►◄ tricyclic antidepressants
Depakote   amitriptyline, amoxapine, clomipramine, desipramine, doxepin, imipramine, nortriptyline, trimipramine

Risk rating: 2
Severity: **Moderate**   Onset: **Delayed**   Likelihood: **Suspected**

Cause
Valproic acid, such as divalproex sodium, may inhibit hepatic metabolism of tricyclic antidepressants (TCAs).

Effect
Levels and adverse effects of TCAs may increase.

Nursing considerations
■ Use these drugs together cautiously.
■ If patient is stable on valproic acid, start TCA at reduced dosage and adjust upward slowly to address symptoms and serum level.
■ If patient is stable on a TCA, monitor serum level and patient status closely when starting or stopping valproic acid.
■ Explain signs and symptoms to watch for.

■ Other TCAs may interact with valproic acid. If you suspect an interaction, consult prescriber or pharmacist.

---

dobutamine ▶◀ methyldopa
Dobutrex   Aldomet

Risk rating: 2
Severity: Moderate   **Onset: Rapid**   **Likelihood: Suspected**

Cause
The mechanism of this interaction is unknown.

Effect
Pressor response of sympathomimetics, such as dobutamine, may increase, resulting in hypertension.

Nursing considerations
■ Monitor patient's blood pressure closely.
■ If patient takes methyldopa, explain that many OTC products contain drugs that can raise blood pressure. Urge patient to read labels carefully or check with prescriber before using a new product.
■ Teach patient to monitor blood pressure at home.

---

dobutamine ▶◀ tricyclic antidepressants
Dobutrex   amitriptyline, amoxapine,
                                  clomipramine, desipramine,
                                  doxepin, imipramine,
                                  nortriptyline, trimipramine

Risk rating: 2
Severity: Moderate   **Onset: Rapid**   **Likelihood: Established**

Cause
Tricyclic antidepressants (TCAs) increase the effects of direct-acting sympathomimetics, such as dobutamine, and decrease the effects of indirect-acting sympathomimetics.

Effect
When sympathomimetic effects increase, the risk of hypertension and arrhythmias increases. When sympathomimetic effects decrease, blood pressure control decreases.

Nursing considerations
■ If possible, avoid using these drugs together.
■ Watch closely for hypertension and heart rhythm changes; they may warrant reduction of dobutamine dosage.

- If patient takes a mixed-acting sympathomimetic, watch for negative effects; dosage may need to be altered.
- Other TCAs and sympathomimetics may interact. If you suspect an interaction, consult prescriber or pharmacist.

---

dofetilide ━━━▶◀━━━ azole antifungals
Tikosyn   itraconazole, ketoconazole

Risk rating: 1
Severity: Major   **Onset: Delayed**   **Likelihood: Suspected**

Cause
Dofetilide renal elimination may be inhibited.

Effect
Dofetilide level and risk of ventricular arrhythmias, including torsades de pointes, may increase.

Nursing considerations
◪ ALERT Use of dofetilide with itraconazole or ketoconazole is contraindicated.
- Monitor ECG for excessive prolongation of QTc interval or development of ventricular arrhythmias.
- Consult prescriber about alternative anti-infective therapy.
- Urge patient to tell prescriber about increased adverse effects.
- Other azole antifungals may interact with dofetilide. If you suspect an interaction, consult prescriber or pharmacist.

---

dofetilide ━━━▶◀━━━ cimetidine
Tikosyn   Tagamet

Risk rating: 1
Severity: Major   **Onset: Delayed**   **Likelihood: Suspected**

Cause
Dofetilide renal elimination may be inhibited.

Effect
Dofetilide level and risk of ventricular arrhythmias, including torsades de pointes, may increase.

Nursing considerations
◪ ALERT Use of dofetilide with cimetidine is contraindicated.
- Monitor ECG for excessive prolongation of QTc interval and development of ventricular arrhythmias.

■ Omeprazole, ranitidine, and aluminum and magnesium antacids don't affect dofetilide elimination. Consult prescriber or pharmacist about them as alternatives to cimetidine.

■ During dofetilide therapy, monitor renal function and QTc interval every 3 months.

---

dofetilide ◄►◄ megestrol
Tikosyn   Megace

Risk rating: 1
Severity: Major   **Onset: Delayed**   **Likelihood: Suspected**

Cause
Dofetilide renal elimination may be inhibited.

Effect
Dofetilide level and the risk of ventricular arrhythmias, including torsades de pointes, increase.

Nursing considerations
◪ ALERT Use of dofetilide with megestrol is contraindicated.

■ Monitor ECG for excessive prolongation of QTc interval and development of ventricular arrhythmias.

■ During dofetilide therapy, monitor renal function and QTc interval every 3 months.

■ Watch for prolonged diarrhea, sweating, and vomiting, and alert prescriber. Electrolyte imbalance may increase risk of arrhythmias.

■ Urge patient to tell prescriber about increased adverse effects.

---

dofetilide ◄►◄ prochlorperazine
Tikosyn   Compazine

Risk rating: 1
Severity: Major   **Onset: Delayed**   **Likelihood: Suspected**

Cause
Dofetilide renal elimination may be inhibited.

Effect
Dofetilide level and risk of ventricular arrhythmias, including torsades de pointes, increase.

Nursing considerations
◪ ALERT Use of dofetilide with prochlorperazine is contraindicated.

■ Monitor ECG for excessive prolongation of QTc interval and development of ventricular arrhythmias.

■ During dofetilide therapy, monitor renal function and QTc interval every 3 months.
■ Consult prescriber or pharmacist for alternative to prochlorperazine to control nausea and vomiting or symptoms of psychosis.

---

dofetilide ▶◀ thiazide diuretics

Tikosyn

chlorothiazide, hydrochloro-thiazide, indapamide, methy-clothiazide, metolazone, poly-thiazide, trichlormethiazide

Risk rating: 1
Severity: Major   **Onset: Delayed**   **Likelihood: Suspected**

Cause
Use of a thiazide diuretic increases potassium excretion.

Effect
Hypokalemia increases risk of ventricular arrhythmias, including torsades de pointes.

Nursing considerations
🔌 ALERT Use of dofetilide with a thiazide diuretic is contraindicated.
■ Monitor ECG for excessive prolongation of the QTc interval and development of ventricular arrhythmias.
■ A similar interaction is likely with loop diuretics.
■ Dofetilide clearance is decreased when used with a thiazide diuretic.

---

dofetilide ▶◀ trimethoprim, trimethoprim-sulfamethoxazole

Tikosyn

Proloprim, Septra

Risk rating: 1
Severity: Major   **Onset: Delayed**   **Likelihood: Suspected**

Cause
Dofetilide renal elimination may be inhibited.

Effect
Dofetilide level and risk of ventricular arrhythmias, including torsades de pointes, increase.

Nursing considerations
🔌 ALERT Use of dofetilide with trimethoprim or trimethoprim-sulfamethoxazole is contraindicated.

- Monitor ECG for excessive prolongation of QTc interval and development of ventricular arrhythmias.
- During dofetilide therapy, monitor renal function and QTc interval every 3 months.
- Watch for prolonged diarrhea, sweating, and vomiting, and alert prescriber. Electrolyte imbalance may increase risk of arrhythmias.
- Consult prescriber or pharmacist about alternative anti-infective.

dofetilide ▶◀ verapamil
Tikosyn   Calan

Risk rating: 1
Severity: Major   **Onset: Delayed**   **Likelihood: Suspected**

Cause
Verapamil may increase dofetilide absorption.

Effect
Dofetilide level and risk of ventricular arrhythmias, including torsades de pointes, increase.

Nursing considerations
⚠ ALERT Use of dofetilide with verapamil is contraindicated.
- Monitor ECG for excessive prolongation of QTc interval and development of ventricular arrhythmias.
- During dofetilide therapy, monitor renal function and QTc interval every 3 months.

dofetilide ▶◀ ziprasidone
Tikosyn   Geodon

Risk rating: 1
Severity: Major   **Onset: Delayed**   **Likelihood: Suspected**

Cause
Each of these drugs may lengthen the QTc interval; joint use may have additive effects.

Effect
Risk of ventricular arrhythmias, including torsades de pointes, increases.

Nursing considerations
⚠ ALERT Use of dofetilide with ziprasidone is contraindicated.
- Monitor ECG for excessive prolongation of QTc interval and development of ventricular arrhythmias.

■ During dofetilide therapy, monitor renal function and QTc interval every 3 months.
■ If patient takes dofetilide, consult prescriber or pharmacist about antipsychotic other than ziprasidone.
■ Urge patient to tell prescriber about increased adverse effects.

---

dopamine ▶◀ MAO inhibitors

Intropin   isocarboxazid, phenelzine, tranylcypromine

Risk rating: 1
Severity: Major   **Onset: Rapid**   **Likelihood: Established**

Cause
Norepinephrine accumulates with MAO inhibition and is released by indirect and mixed-acting sympathomimetics, such as dopamine.

Effect
Pressor response at receptor sites increases, increasing the risk of severe headache, hypertension, high fever, and hypertensive crisis.

Nursing considerations
■ Avoid giving dopamine with an MAO inhibitor.
■ Direct-acting sympathomimetics interact minimally.
◪ **ALERT** Warn patient that OTC medicines, such as decongestants, may cause this interaction.
■ Phentolamine can be administered to block epinephrine- and norepinephrine-induced vasoconstriction and reduce blood pressure.

---

dopamine ▶◀ methyldopa

Intropin   Aldomet

Risk rating: 2
Severity: Moderate   **Onset: Rapid**   **Likelihood: Suspected**

Cause
The mechanism of this interaction is unknown.

Effect
Pressor response of sympathomimetics, such as dopamine, may be increased, resulting in hypertension.

Nursing considerations
■ Monitor patient's blood pressure closely.
■ If patient takes methyldopa, explain that many OTC products con-

tain drugs that can raise blood pressure. Urge patient to read labels carefully or check with prescriber before using a new product.
■ Teach patient to monitor blood pressure at home.

---

dopamine ━━━►◄━━━ tricyclic antidepressants

Intropin

amitriptyline, amoxapine, clomipramine, desipramine, doxepin, imipramine, nortriptyline, trimipramine

Risk rating: 2
Severity: **Moderate**   Onset: **Rapid**   Likelihood: **Established**

Cause
Tricyclic antidepressants (TCAs) increase effects of direct-acting sympathomimetics and decrease effects of indirect-acting sympathomimetics.

Effect
When sympathomimetic effects increase, the risk of hypertension and arrhythmias increases. When sympathomimetic effects decrease, blood pressure control decreases.

Nursing considerations
■ If possible, avoid using these drugs together.
■ Watch patient closely for hypertension and heart rhythm changes; dopamine dosage may need reduction.
■ If patient takes a mixed-acting sympathomimetic, such as dopamine, watch for negative effects; dosage may need to be altered.
■ Other TCAs and sympathomimetics may interact. If you suspect an interaction, consult prescriber or pharmacist.

---

doxepin ━━━►◄━━━ cimetidine

Sinequan

Tagamet

Risk rating: 2
Severity: **Moderate**   Onset: **Rapid**   Likelihood: **Probable**

Cause
Cimetidine may interfere with metabolism of tricyclic antidepressants (TCAs), such as doxepin.

Effect
TCA level and bioavailability increase.

Nursing considerations
■ When starting or stopping cimetidine, monitor TCA level and adjust dosage as needed.
■ If needed, consult prescriber about possible change from cimetidine to ranitidine.
■ Urge patient and family to watch for and report increased anticholinergic effects, dizziness, drowsiness, and psychosis.

---

doxepin ▶◀ **MAO inhibitors**

Sinequan   isocarboxazid, phenelzine,
                             tranylcypromine

Risk rating: 1
Severity: Major   **Onset: Rapid**   **Likelihood: Suspected**

Cause
The mechanism of this interaction is unknown.

Effect
Risk of hyperpyretic crisis, seizures, and death increases.

Nursing considerations
⚡ ALERT Don't give a tricyclic antidepressant, such as doxepin, with or within 2 weeks of an MAO inhibitor.
■ Watch for adverse effects, including confusion, hyperexcitability, rigidity, seizures, increased temperature, increased pulse, increased respiration, sweating, mydriasis, flushing, headache, coma, and DIC.

---

doxepin ▶◀ **quinolones**

Sinequan   gatifloxacin, levofloxacin,
                             moxifloxacin, sparfloxacin

Risk rating: 1
Severity: Major   **Onset: Delayed**   **Likelihood: Suspected**

Cause
The mechanism of this interaction is unknown.

Effect
Risk of life-threatening arrhythmias, including torsades de pointes, may increase when certain of these drugs are used together.

Nursing considerations
⚡ ALERT Sparfloxacin is contraindicated in patients taking a tricyclic antidepressant (TCA), such as doxepin, because QTc interval may be prolonged.

▶ **ALERT** Avoid giving levofloxacin with a TCA.
■ Use gatifloxacin and moxifloxacin cautiously with a TCA.
■ If possible, use a quinolone that doesn't prolong the QTc interval or isn't metabolized by CYP3A4.

---

doxepin ◀▶ rifamycins
Sinequan   rifabutin, rifampin

Risk rating: 2
Severity: Moderate   Onset: Delayed   Likelihood: Suspected

Cause
Metabolism of tricyclic antidepressants (TCAs), such as doxepin, in the liver may increase.

Effect
TCA level and efficacy may decrease.

Nursing considerations
■ When starting, stopping, or changing dosage of a rifamycin, monitor serum TCA level to maintain therapeutic range.
■ Watch for resolution of depression as TCA dosage is adjusted to therapeutic level during rifamycin therapy.
■ Urge patient and family to watch for adverse reactions, including increased drowsiness and dizziness, for several weeks after rifamycin stops. Tell them to notify prescriber promptly.
■ Other TCAs may interact with rifamycins. If you suspect an interaction, consult prescriber or pharmacist.

---

doxepin ◀▶ sertraline
Sinequan   Zoloft

Risk rating: 2
Severity: Moderate   Onset: Delayed   Likelihood: Suspected

Cause
Hepatic metabolism of tricyclic antidepressants (TCAs), such as doxepin, by CYP2D6 may be inhibited.

Effect
Therapeutic and toxic effects of certain TCAs may increase.

Nursing considerations
■ If possible, avoid this drug combination.
■ Watch for evidence of TCA toxicity and serotonin syndrome.

- Signs of serotonin syndrome include delirium, bizarre movements, and tachycardia.
- Monitor serum TCA level when starting or stopping sertraline.
- If abnormalities occur, decrease TCA dosage or stop drug.

---

doxepin ▶◀ sympathomimetics

Sinequan

direct: dobutamine, epinephrine, norepinephrine, phenylephrine
mixed: dopamine, ephedrine, metaraminol

Risk rating: 2
Severity: Moderate   **Onset: Rapid**   **Likelihood: Established**

Cause
Tricyclic antidepressants (TCAs), such as doxepin, increase the effects of direct-acting sympathomimetics and decrease the effects of indirect-acting sympathomimetics.

Effect
When sympathomimetic effects increase, the risk of hypertension and arrhythmias increases. When sympathomimetic effects decrease, blood pressure control decreases.

Nursing considerations
- If possible, avoid using these drugs together.
- Watch patient closely for hypertension and heart rhythm changes; they may warrant reduction of sympathomimetic dosage.
- If patient takes a mixed-acting sympathomimetic, watch for negative effects; dosage may need to be altered.
- Other TCAs and sympathomimetics may interact. If you suspect an interaction, consult prescriber or pharmacist.

---

doxepin ▶◀ valproic acid

Sinequan

divalproex sodium, valproate sodium, valproic acid

Risk rating: 2
Severity: Moderate   **Onset: Delayed**   **Likelihood: Suspected**

Cause
Valproic acid may inhibit hepatic metabolism of tricyclic antidepressants (TCAs), such as doxepin.

Effect
TCA level and adverse effects may increase.

Nursing considerations
- Use these drugs together cautiously.
- If patient is stable on valproic acid, start TCA at reduced dosage and adjust upward slowly.
- If patient is stable on a TCA, monitor serum level and patient status closely when starting or stopping valproic acid.
- Explain signs and symptoms of interaction.
- Other TCAs may interact with valproic acid. If you suspect an interaction, consult prescriber or pharmacist.

---

doxycycline ▶◀ aluminum salts
Vibramycin

aluminum carbonate,
aluminum hydroxide,
magaldrate

Risk rating: 2
Severity: Moderate   Onset: Delayed   Likelihood: Probable

Cause
Formation of an insoluble chelate with aluminum may decrease absorption of tetracyclines, such as doxycycline.

Effect
Tetracycline levels may decline more than 50%, reducing efficacy.

Nursing considerations
- Separate doses by at least 3 hours.
- If patient must take these drugs together, notify prescriber. Doxycycline dosage may need adjustment.
- Monitor patient for reduced anti-infective response, including infection flare-up, fever, and malaise.
- Other tetracyclines may interact with aluminum salts. If you suspect an interaction, consult prescriber or pharmacist.
- Help patient develop a plan to ensure proper dosage intervals.

doxycycline ▶◀ barbiturates

Vibramycin

amobarbital, butabarbital, pentobarbital, phenobarbital, primidone, secobarbital

Risk rating: 2
Severity: Moderate   Onset: Delayed   Likelihood: Suspected

Cause
Barbiturates may increase hepatic metabolism of doxycycline, a tetracycline.

Effect
Doxycycline level and effects may decrease.

Nursing considerations
■ Monitor patient for expected doxycycline effects.
■ Doxycycline dose may need to be increased.
■ Effects of barbiturates on doxycycline may persist for weeks after barbiturate is stopped.
■ Consult prescriber or pharmacist about using a tetracycline that doesn't interact with barbiturates, such as demeclocycline, oxytetracycline, or tetracycline.
■ Urge patient to tell prescriber if he isn't improving with doxycycline.

doxycycline ▶◀ calcium salts

Vibramycin

calcium carbonate, calcium citrate, calcium gluconate, calcium lactate, tricalcium phosphate

Risk rating: 2
Severity: Moderate   Onset: Delayed   Likelihood: Probable

Cause
Calcium salts form an insoluble complex with tetracyclines, such as doxycycline, that lowers tetracycline absorption.

Effect
Decreased tetracycline level decreases anti-infective efficacy.

Nursing considerations
■ Separate tetracyclines from calcium salts by at least 3 to 4 hours.
■ Monitor tetracycline efficacy. Notify prescriber if infection isn't responding.
■ Doxycycline is somewhat less affected by this interaction.

■ Advise against taking tetracycline with dairy products or calcium-fortified orange juice.

doxycycline ▬▬►◄▬▬ iron salts
Vibramycin

ferrous fumarate, ferrous gluconate, ferrous sulfate, iron polysaccharide

Risk rating: 2
Severity: **Moderate**   Onset: **Delayed**   Likelihood: **Probable**

Cause
Doxycycline and other tetracyclines form insoluble chelates with iron salts, which may reduce absorption of both substances.

Effect
Tetracycline and iron salt levels and effects may decrease.

Nursing considerations
◆ ALERT If possible, avoid giving tetracyclines with iron salts.
■ If they must be given together, separate doses by 3 to 4 hours.
■ If you suspect an interaction, consult prescriber or pharmacist; an enteric-coated or sustained-release iron salt may reduce interaction.
■ Monitor patient for expected response to tetracycline.
■ Assess for evidence of iron deficiency, including fatigue, dyspnea, tachycardia, palpitations, dizziness, and orthostatic hypotension.

doxycycline ▬▬►◄▬▬ magnesium salts, oral
Vibramycin

magaldrate, magnesium carbonate, magnesium citrate, magnesium gluconate, magnesium hydroxide, magnesium oxide, magnesium sulfate, magnesium trisilicate

Risk rating: 2
Severity: **Moderate**   Onset: **Delayed**   Likelihood: **Probable**

Cause
Magnesium salts form an insoluble complex with tetracyclines, such as doxycycline, that lowers tetracycline absorption.

Effect
Decreased tetracycline level decreases anti-infective efficacy.

Nursing considerations
- Separate tetracyclines from magnesium salts by at least 3 to 4 hours.
- Monitor efficacy of tetracycline in resolving infection. Notify prescriber if infection isn't responding.
- Tell patient to separate tetracycline dose from magnesium-based antacids, laxatives, and supplements by 3 to 4 hours.

---

doxycycline ▶◀ penicillins
Vibramycin

amoxicillin, ampicillin, carbenicillin, cloxacillin, dicloxacillin, nafcillin, oxacillin, penicillin G, penicillin V, piperacillin, ticarcillin

Risk rating: 1
Severity: Major   **Onset: Delayed**   **Likelihood: Suspected**

Cause
Tetracyclines, such as doxycycline, may adversely affect bactericidal activity of penicillins.

Effect
Penicillin efficacy may be reduced.

Nursing considerations
- If possible, avoid giving tetracyclines with penicillins.
- Monitor patient closely for lack of penicillin effect.

---

doxycycline ▶◀ phenytoin
Vibramycin

Dilantin

Risk rating: 2
Severity: Moderate   **Onset: Delayed**   **Likelihood: Probable**

Cause
Phenytoin induces doxycycline metabolism, and doxycycline may be displaced from plasma proteins.

Effect
Doxycycline elimination may increase, and effects may decrease.

Nursing considerations
- Hydantoins other than phenytoin may interact with doxycycline. If you suspect an interaction, consult prescriber or pharmacist.
- If patient takes phenytoin, watch for expected doxycycline effects.

- Doxycycline dose may need to be doubled to maintain therapeutic level; consult prescriber for dosage increase.
- Consult prescriber or pharmacist about using a tetracycline that doesn't interact with phenytoin.
- Urge patient to tell prescriber if he isn't improving.

---

edrophonium ▶◀ corticosteroids

Tensilon

betamethasone, corticotropin, cortisone, cosyntropin, dexamethasone, fludrocortisone, hydrocortisone, methylprednisolone, prednisolone, prednisone, triamcinolone

Risk rating: 1
Severity: Major   Onset: Delayed   Likelihood: Probable

Cause

In myasthenia gravis, corticosteroids antagonize cholinesterase inhibitors, such as edrophonium, by an unknown mechanism.

Effect

Patient may develop severe muscular depression refractory to cholinesterase inhibitor.

Nursing considerations

- Corticosteroids may have long-term benefits in myasthenia gravis.
- Combined therapy may be attempted under strict supervision.
- Monitor patient for severe muscle deterioration.
- ⚑ ALERT Provide respiratory support and mechanical ventilation if needed.
- Consult prescriber or pharmacist about safe corticosteroid delivery to maximize improvement in muscle strength.

---

efavirenz ▶◀ benzodiazepines

Sustiva

alprazolam, midazolam, triazolam

Risk rating: 2
Severity: Moderate   Onset: Delayed   Likelihood: Suspected

Cause

Nonnucleoside reverse-transcriptase inhibitors, such as efavirenz, may inhibit CYP3A4 metabolism of certain benzodiazepines.

Effect
Sedative effects of benzodiazepines may be increased or prolonged.

Nursing considerations
ALERT Don't combine listed benzodiazepines with efavirenz.
- Explain the risk of oversedation and respiratory depression.
- Urge patient to promptly report any suspected interaction.
- Other benzodiazepines and nonnucleoside reverse-transcriptase inhibitors may interact. If you suspect an interaction, consult prescriber or pharmacist.

---

efavirenz ▶◀ **ergot derivatives**

Sustiva   dihydroergotamine, ergotamine

Risk rating: 1
Severity: Major   Onset: **Delayed**   Likelihood: **Suspected**

Cause
Nonnucleoside reverse-transcriptase inhibitors, such as efavirenz, may decrease CYP3A4 metabolism of ergot derivatives.

Effect
Risk of ergot-induced peripheral vasospasm and ischemia increases.

Nursing considerations
ALERT Use of ergot derivatives with efavirenz is contraindicated.
- Monitor patient for peripheral ischemia: pain in limb muscles while exercising and later at rest; numbness and tingling of fingers and toes; cool, pale, or cyanotic limbs; red or violet blisters on hands or feet; and gangrene.
- Ergot toxicity also may cause nausea, vomiting, lassitude, impaired mental function, delirium, severe dyspnea, hypotension, hypertension, rapid or weak pulse, unconsciousness, limb spasms, seizures, and shock.
- Give vasodilator for vasospasm and diazepam for seizures as needed.
- Other nonnucleoside reverse-transcriptase inhibitors, such as nevirapine, may interact with ergot derivatives. If you suspect an interaction, consult prescriber or pharmacist.

eletriptan ▶◀ azole antifungals

Relpax

itraconazole, ketoconazole

Risk rating: 2
Severity: Moderate   **Onset: Delayed**   **Likelihood: Suspected**

Cause
Azole antifungals inhibit CYP3A4 metabolism of certain 5-HT_1 receptor agonists, such as eletriptan.

Effect
Selective 5-HT_1 receptor agonist level and adverse effects increase.

Nursing considerations
◼ **ALERT** Don't give eletriptan within 72 hours or almotriptan within 7 days of itraconazole or ketoconazole.
◼ Adverse effects of selective 5-HT_1 receptor agonists include coronary artery vasospasm, dizziness, nausea, paresthesia, and somnolence.

eletriptan ▶◀ serotonin reuptake inhibitors

Relpax

citalopram, fluoxetine, fluvoxamine, nefazodone, paroxetine, sertraline, venlafaxine

Risk rating: 1
Severity: Major   **Onset: Rapid**   **Likelihood: Suspected**

Cause
Serotonin may accumulate rapidly in the CNS.

Effect
Risk of serotonin syndrome increases.

Nursing considerations
◼ **ALERT** If possible, avoid combined use of these drugs.
◼ Start with lowest dosages possible, and assess patient closely.
◼ Stop eletriptan, a selective 5-HT_1 receptor agonist, at the first sign of interaction, and start an antiserotonergic.
◼ In some patients, migraine frequency may increase and antimigraine drug efficacy may decrease when a serotonin reuptake inhibitor is started.
◼ Describe the traits of serotonin syndrome: CNS irritability, motor weakness, shivering, muscle twitching, and altered consciousness.

■ Explain that serotonin syndrome can be fatal if not treated immediately.

---

enalapril ▶◀ indomethacin
Vasotec   Indocin

Risk rating: 2
Severity: Moderate   **Onset: Rapid**   **Likelihood: Probable**

Cause
Indomethacin inhibits synthesis of prostaglandins, which eletriptan, an ACE inhibitor, needs to lower blood pressure.

Effect
ACE inhibitor's hypotensive effect decreases.

Nursing considerations
◪ **ALERT** Monitor blood pressure closely. Severe hypertension may persist until indomethacin is stopped.
■ If indomethacin can't be avoided, patient may need a different antihypertensive.
■ Remind patient that hypertension commonly causes no physical symptoms but sometimes may cause headache and dizziness.
■ Other ACE inhibitors may interact with indomethacin. If you suspect an interaction, consult prescriber or pharmacist.

---

enalapril ▶◀ potassium-sparing diuretics
Vasotec

amiloride, spironolactone, triamterene

Risk rating: 1
Severity: Major   **Onset: Delayed**   **Likelihood: Probable**

Cause
The mechanism of this interaction is unknown.

Effect
Serum potassium level may increase.

Nursing considerations
■ Use cautiously in patients at high risk for hyperkalemia, especially those with renal impairment.
■ Monitor BUN, creatinine, and serum potassium levels as needed.

■ ACE inhibitors other than enalapril may interact with potassium-sparing diuretics. If you suspect an interaction, consult prescriber or pharmacist.

■ Urge patient to immediately report an irregular heartbeat, a slow pulse, weakness, and other evidence of hyperkalemia.

enalapril ▶◀ salicylates

Vasotec

aspirin, bismuth subsalicylate, choline salicylate, magnesium salicylate, salsalate, sodium salicylate

Risk rating: 2
Severity: Moderate   Onset: Rapid   Likelihood: Suspected

Cause
Salicylates inhibit synthesis of prostaglandins, which enalapril, an ACE inhibitor, needs to lower blood pressure.

Effect
ACE inhibitor's hypotensive effect decreases.

Nursing considerations
■ This interaction is more likely in people with hypertension, coronary artery disease, and possibly heart failure.

ephedrine ▶◀ MAO inhibitors

isocarboxazid, phenelzine, tranylcypromine

Risk rating: 1
Severity: Major   Onset: Rapid   Likelihood: Established

Cause
Norepinephrine accumulates with MAO inhibition and is released by indirect and mixed-acting sympathomimetics, such as ephedrine.

Effect
Pressor response at receptor sites increases, increasing the risk of severe headache, hypertension, high fever, and hypertensive crisis.

Nursing considerations
■ Avoid giving indirect or mixed-acting sympathomimetics with an MAO inhibitor.

■ If drugs are given together, phentolamine can block epinephrine- and norepinephrine-induced vasoconstriction and reduce blood pressure.

■ Direct-acting sympathomimetics interact minimally.
■ **ALERT** Warn patient that OTC medicines, such as decongestants, may cause this interaction.

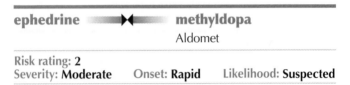

ephedrine ━━━━▶◀━━━━ methyldopa
Aldomet

Risk rating: 2
Severity: Moderate   **Onset: Rapid**   **Likelihood: Suspected**

Cause
The mechanism of this interaction is unknown.

Effect
Pressor response of sympathomimetics, such as ephedrine, may increase, resulting in hypertension.

Nursing considerations
■ Monitor patient's blood pressure closely.
■ If patient takes methyldopa, explain that many OTC products contain drugs that can raise blood pressure. Urge patient to read labels carefully or check with prescriber before using a new product.
■ Teach patient to monitor blood pressure at home.

ephedrine ━━━━▶◀━━━━ tricyclic antidepressants
amitriptyline, amoxapine, clomipramine, desipramine, doxepin, imipramine, nortriptyline, trimipramine

Risk rating: 2
Severity: Moderate   **Onset: Rapid**   **Likelihood: Established**

Cause
Tricyclic antidepressants (TCAs) increase effects of direct-acting and decrease effects of indirect-acting sympathomimetics.

Effect
When sympathomimetic effects increase, the risk of hypertension and arrhythmias increases. When sympathomimetic effects decrease, blood pressure control decreases.

Nursing considerations
■ If possible, avoid using these drugs together.
■ If patient takes a mixed-acting sympathomimetic, such as ephedrine, watch for negative effects; dosage may need to be altered.

■ Watch patient closely for hypertension and heart rhythm changes; they may warrant reduction of sympathomimetic dosage.
■ Other TCAs and sympathomimetics may interact. If you suspect an interaction, consult prescriber or pharmacist.

epinephrine ▶◀ beta blockers

Adrenalin

carteolol, nadolol, penbutolol, pindolol, propranolol, timolol

Risk rating: 1
Severity: **Major**   Onset: **Rapid**   Likelihood: **Established**

Cause
Alpha-receptor effects of epinephrine supersede the effects of non-selective beta blockers, increasing vascular resistance.

Effect
Marked hypertensive effects are followed by reflex bradycardia.

Nursing considerations
⚡ ALERT Three days before planned use of epinephrine, stop the beta blocker. Or, if possible, don't use epinephrine.
■ If drugs must be used together, monitor blood pressure and pulse closely. If interaction occurs, give I.V. chlorpromazine, hydralazine, aminophylline, or atropine if needed.
■ Explain the risks of interaction, and tell patient to carry medical identification at all times.
■ Other beta blockers may interact with epinephrine. If you suspect an interaction, consult prescriber or pharmacist.

epinephrine ▶◀ methyldopa

Adrenalin

Aldomet

Risk rating: 2
Severity: **Moderate**   Onset: **Rapid**   Likelihood: **Suspected**

Cause
The mechanism of this interaction is unknown.

Effect
Pressor response of sympathomimetics, such as epinephrine, may increase, resulting in hypertension.

Nursing considerations
■ Monitor patient's blood pressure closely.

■ If patient takes methyldopa, explain that many OTC products contain drugs that can raise blood pressure. Urge patient to read labels carefully or check with prescriber before using a new product.
■ Teach patient to monitor blood pressure at home.

---

epinephrine ▶◀ tricyclic antidepressants

Adrenalin

amitriptyline, amoxapine, clomipramine, desipramine, doxepin, imipramine, nortriptyline, trimipramine

Risk rating: 2
Severity: **Moderate**   Onset: **Rapid**   Likelihood: **Established**

Cause
Tricyclic antidepressants (TCAs) increase the effects of direct-acting sympathomimetics, such as epinpehrine.

Effect
When sympathomimetic effects increase, the risk of hypertension and arrhythmias increases.

Nursing considerations
■ If possible, avoid using these drugs together.
■ Watch patient closely for hypertension and heart rhythm changes; they may warrant reduction of sympathomimetic dosage.
■ Other TCAs and sympathomimetics may interact. If you suspect an interaction, consult prescriber or pharmacist.

---

eplerenone ▶◀ protease inhibitors

Inspra

nelfinavir, ritonavir

Risk rating: 1
Severity: **Major**   Onset: **Delayed**   Likelihood: **Suspected**

Cause
Protease inhibitors inhibit eplerenone metabolism.

Effect
Eplerenone level rises, causing hyperkalemia and increasing the risk of life-threatening arrhythmias.

Nursing considerations
◼ ALERT Use of nelfinavir or ritonavir with eplerenone is contraindicated.

■ Potent CYP3A4 inhibitors increase the eplerenone level and the risk of hyperkalemia-induced arrhythmias—some fatal.
■ Monitor patient's serum potassium level.
■ Tell patient to report nausea, irregular heartbeat, or slowed pulse to prescriber.

---

eprosartan ▸◂ potassium-sparing diuretics
Teveten

amiloride, spironolactone, triamterene

Risk rating: 1
Severity: Major   **Onset: Delayed**   **Likelihood: Suspected**

Cause
Angiotensin II receptor antagonists, such as eprosartan, and potassium-sparing diuretics may increase serum potassium level.

Effect
Risk of hyperkalemia may increase, especially among high-risk patients.

Nursing considerations
■ High-risk patients include elderly people and those with renal impairment, type 2 diabetes, or decreased renal perfusion; monitor these patients closely.
■ Check serum potassium, BUN, and creatinine levels regularly. If they increase, notify prescriber.
■ Advise patient to immediately report an irregular heart beat, slow pulse, weakness, or other evidence of hyperkalemia.
■ Give patient a list of foods high in potassium; stress the need to eat only moderate amounts

---

ergonovine ▸◂ protease inhibitors
Ergotrate

amprenavir, atazanavir, indinavir, lopinavir-ritonavir, nelfinavir, ritonavir, saquinavir

Risk rating: 1
Severity: Major   **Onset: Delayed**   **Likelihood: Probable**

Cause
Protease inhibitors may interfere with CYP3A4 metabolism of ergot derivatives, such as ergonovine.

Effect
Risk of ergot-induced peripheral vasospasm and ischemia may increase.

Nursing considerations
⚠ ALERT Use of ergot derivatives with protease inhibitors is contraindicated.

- Monitor patient for evidence of peripheral ischemia, including pain in limb muscles while exercising and later at rest; numbness and tingling of fingers and toes; cool, pale, or cyanotic limbs; red or violet blisters on hands or feet; and gangrene.
- Sodium nitroprusside may be given for ergot-induced vasospasm.
- If patient takes a protease inhibitor, consult prescriber or pharmacist about alternative treatments for migraine pain.
- Urge patient to tell prescriber about increased adverse effects.

---

ergotamine ■■■▶◀■■■ beta blockers

Ergomar

carteolol, nadolol, penbutolol, pindolol, propranolol, timolol

Risk rating: 2
Severity: Moderate   Onset: Delayed   Likelihood: Suspected

Cause
Vasoconstriction and blockade of peripheral beta$_2$ receptors allow unopposed ergot action.

Effect
Vasoconstrictive effects of ergot derivatives, such as ergotamine, increase.

Nursing considerations
- Watch for peripheral ischemia, cold limbs, and possible gangrene.
- If needed, stop beta blocker and adjust ergot derivative.
- Other ergot derivatives may interact with beta blockers. If you suspect an interaction, consult prescriber or pharmacist.

ergotamine ━━━━▶◀━━━━ itraconazole

Ergomar   Sporanox

Risk rating: 1
Severity: Major   **Onset: Delayed**   **Likelihood: Suspected**

Cause
Itraconazole inhibits CYP3A4 metabolism of ergot derivatives, such as ergotamine.

Effect
Risk of ergot toxicity may increase.

Nursing considerations
◤ ALERT Use of these drugs together is contraindicated.
■ Signs of ergot toxicity include peripheral vasospasm and ischemia.
■ Caution against use of ergot derivatives (for migraine, for example) while taking itraconazole; consult prescriber about alternatives.

ergotamine ━━━━▶◀━━━━ macrolide antibiotics

Ergomar   clarithromycin, erythromycin,
                                       troleandomycin

Risk rating: 1
Severity: Major   **Onset: Rapid**   **Likelihood: Probable**

Cause
Macrolide antibiotics interfere with hepatic metabolism of ergot derivatives, such as ergotamine.

Effect
Symptoms of acute ergotism, mainly peripheral ischemia, may develop.

Nursing considerations
■ Monitor patient for evidence of peripheral ischemia, including pain in limb muscles while exercising and later at rest; numbness and tingling of fingers and toes; cool, pale, or cyanotic limbs; red or violet blisters on hands or feet; and gangrene.
■ Dosage of ergot derivative may need to be decreased, or both drugs may need to be stopped.
■ Consider a different anti-infective drug that's less likely to interact with ergot derivative.
◤ ALERT Sodium nitroprusside may be given for macrolide-ergot–induced vasospasm.

■ Explain evidence of ergot-induced peripheral ischemia. Urge patient to report it promptly to prescriber.

ergotamine ━━━▶◀━━━ nonnucleoside reverse-transcriptase inhibitors
Ergomar

delavirdine, efavirenz

Risk rating: 1
Severity: Major   **Onset: Delayed**   **Likelihood: Suspected**

Cause
Nonnucleoside reverse-transcriptase inhibitors may decrease CYP3A4 metabolism of ergot derivatives, such as ergotamine.

Effect
Risk of ergot-induced peripheral vasospasm and ischemia may increase.

Nursing considerations
⚠ ALERT Use of ergot derivatives with delavirdine or efavirenz is contraindicated.
■ Monitor patient for evidence of peripheral ischemia: pain in limb muscles while exercising and later at rest; numbness and tingling of fingers and toes; cool, pale, or cyanotic limbs; red or violet blisters on hands or feet; and gangrene.
■ Ergot toxicity also may cause nausea, vomiting, lassitude, impaired mental function, delirium, severe dyspnea, hypotension, hypertension, rapid or weak pulse, unconsciousness, limb spasm, seizures, and shock.
■ Give vasodilator for vasospasm and diazepam for seizures as needed.
■ Other nonnucleoside reverse-transcriptase inhibitors, such as nevirapine, may interact with ergot derivatives. If you suspect an interaction, consult prescriber or pharmacist.

ergotamine ━━━▶◀━━━ protease inhibitors
Ergomar

amprenavir, atazanavir, indinavir, lopinavir-ritonavir, nelfinavir, ritonavir, saquinavir

Risk rating: 1
Severity: Major   **Onset: Delayed**   **Likelihood: Probable**

Cause
Protease inhibitors may interfere with CYP3A4 metabolism of ergot derivatives, such as ergotamine.

Effect
Risk of ergot-induced peripheral vasospasm and ischemia may increase.

Nursing considerations
⚠ **ALERT** Use of ergotamine with protease inhibitors is contraindicated.
■ Watch for evidence of peripheral ischemia: pain in limb muscles while exercising and later at rest; numbness and tingling of fingers and toes; cool, pale, or cyanotic limbs; red or violet blisters on hands or feet; and gangrene.
■ Sodium nitroprusside may be given for ergot-induced vasospasm.
■ If patient takes a protease inhibitor, consult prescriber or pharmacist about alternative treatments for migraine pain.
■ Urge patient to tell prescriber about increased adverse effects.

---

ergotamine ▶◀ **selective 5-HT$_1$ receptor agonists**
Ergomar

frovatriptan, naratriptan, rizatriptan, sumatriptan, zolmitriptan

Risk rating: **1**		
Severity: **Major**	Onset: **Rapid**	Likelihood: **Suspected**

Cause
Combined use may have additive effects.

Effect
Risk of vasospastic effects increases.

Nursing considerations
⚠ **ALERT** Use of these drugs or any two selective 5-HT$_1$ receptor agonists within 24 hours of each other is contraindicated.
■ Combined use may cause severe vasospastic effects, including sustained coronary artery vasospasm that triggers MI.
■ Warn patient not to mix migraine headache drugs within 24 hours of each other, but to call prescriber if a drug isn't effective.

ergotamine ▶◀ sibutramine
Ergomar   Meridia

Risk rating: 1
Severity: Major   **Onset: Rapid**   **Likelihood: Suspected**

Cause
Drugs may cause additive serotonergic effects.

Effect
Risk of serotonin syndrome may increase.

Nursing considerations
⚠ **ALERT** If possible, avoid giving sibutramine with an ergot derivative, such as ergotamine.
■ Watch for evidence of serotonin syndrome: excitement, hypomania, restlessness, loss of consciousness, confusion, disorientation, anxiety, agitation, motor weakness, myoclonus, tremor, hemiballismus, hyperreflexia, ataxia, dysarthria, incoordination, hyperthermia, shivering, papillary dilation, diaphoresis, emesis, hypertension, and tachycardia.
■ If serotonin syndrome occurs, stop these drugs and provide supportive care as needed.
■ Other ergot derivatives may interact with sibutramine. If you suspect an interaction, consult prescriber or pharmacist.
■ Urge patient to tell prescriber about increased adverse effects.

erythromycin ▶◀ benzodiazepines
E-mycin, Eryc   alprazolam, diazepam,
                               midazolam, triazolam

Risk rating: 2
Severity: Moderate   **Onset: Rapid**   **Likelihood: Suspected**

Cause
Macrolide antibiotics, such as erythromycin, may decrease metabolism of certain benzodiazepines.

Effect
Sedative effects of benzodiazepines may be increased or prolonged.

Nursing considerations
■ Talk with prescriber about decreasing benzodiazepine dosage during antibiotic therapy.
■ Lorazepam, oxazepam, and temazepam probably don't interact with macrolide antibiotics; substitution may be possible.
■ Urge patient to promptly report oversedation.

erythromycin ▶◀ ergot derivatives

E-mycin, Eryc   dihydroergotamine, ergotamine

Risk rating: 1
Severity: Major   **Onset: Rapid**   **Likelihood: Probable**

Cause
Macrolide antibiotics, such as erythromycin, interfere with hepatic metabolism of ergotamine.

Effect
Symptoms of acute ergotism, primarily peripheral ischemia, may develop.

Nursing considerations
■ Watch for evidence of peripheral ischemia: pain in limb muscles while exercising and later at rest; numbness and tingling of fingers and toes; cool, pale, or cyanotic limbs; red or violet blisters on hands or feet; and gangrene.
■ Dosage of ergot derivative may need to be decreased, or both drugs may need to be stopped.
■ Consider a different anti-infective that's less likely to interact with ergot derivative.
■ Sodium nitroprusside may be given for macrolide-ergot–induced vasospasm.
■ Explain evidence of ergot-induced peripheral ischemia. Urge patient to report it promptly to prescriber.

erythromycin ▶◀ food, grapefruit juice

E-mycin, Eryc

Risk rating: 2
Severity: Moderate   **Onset: Delayed**   **Likelihood: Suspected**

Cause
Food may decrease GI absorption of erythromycin stearate and certain erythromycin base forms. Grapefruit may inhibit metabolism of erythromycin and other macrolide antibiotics.

Effect
With food, efficacy of certain macrolide antibiotics may decrease. With grapefruit, macrolide level and adverse effects may increase.

Nursing considerations
■ Give erythromycin stearate and non–enteric-coated erythromycin base tablets 2 hours before or after a meal.

■ Enteric-coated tablets aren't affected by food and may be taken without regard to meals.
■ Give erythromycin estolate, erythromycin ethylsuccinate, and enteric-coated tablets of erythromycin base with food to decrease GI adverse effects.
■ Advise patient to take a macrolide antibiotic with liquid other than grapefruit juice.

---

erythromycin ➤◀ HMG-CoA reductase inhibitors

E-mycin, Eryc

atorvastatin, lovastatin, simvastatin

Risk rating: 1
Severity: Major   Onset: Delayed   Likelihood: Probable

Cause
CYP3A4 metabolism of certain HMG-CoA reductase inhibitors may be decreased.

Effect
HMG-CoA reductase inhibitor level and risk of severe myopathy or rhabdomyolysis may increase.

Nursing considerations
⚡ **ALERT** If these drugs are given with a macrolide antibiotic, such as erythromycin, watch for evidence of rhabdomyolysis, especially 5 to 21 days after macrolide starts. Evidence may include fatigue; muscle aches and weakness; joint pain; dark, red, or cola-colored urine; weight gain; seizures; and greatly increased serum CK level.
■ Fluvastatin and pravastatin are metabolized by other enzymes and may be better choices when used with a macrolide antibiotic.
■ Urge patient to report muscle pain, tenderness, or weakness.

---

erythromycin ➤◀ methylprednisolone

E-mycin, Eryc

Medrol

Risk rating: 2
Severity: Moderate   Onset: Delayed   Likelihood: Established

Cause
The mechanism of this interaction is unclear.

Effect
Methylprednisolone effects, including toxic effects, may increase.

Nursing considerations
■ This interaction may be used for therapeutic benefit because it may be possible to reduce methylprednisolone dosage.
■ Monitor patient for adverse or toxic effects, such as euphoria, insomnia, peptic ulceration, and cushingoid effects.

---

erythromycin ▶◀ quinolones
E-mycin, Eryc

gatifloxacin, levofloxacin, moxifloxacin, sparfloxacin

Risk rating: 1
Severity: Major   **Onset: Delayed**   **Likelihood: Suspected**

Cause
The mechanism of this interaction is unknown.

Effect
Risk of life-threatening arrhythmias, including torsades de pointes, increases.

Nursing considerations
◆ ALERT Use of sparfloxacin with erythromycin is contraindicated.
■ Avoid use of levofloxacin with erythromycin because doing so may prolong the QT interval.
■ Use cautiously with gatifloxacin and moxifloxacin.
■ Monitor ECG for prolonged QTc interval and arrhythmias.
■ Tell patient to report palpitations, dizziness, shortness of breath, and chest pain.
■ Macrolides other than erythromycin may interact with quinolones. If you suspect an interaction, consult prescriber or pharmacist.
■ Monitor serum electrolyte levels; electrolyte disturbances increase the risk of ventricular arrhythmias.

---

erythromycin ▶◀ repaglinide
E-mycin, Eryc

Prandin

Risk rating: 2
Severity: Moderate   **Onset: Delayed**   **Likelihood: Suspected**

Cause
Certain macrolide antibiotics, such as erythromycin, may inhibit metabolism of repaglinide.

Effect
Repaglinide level, effects, and adverse effects may increase.

Nursing considerations
■ Monitor blood glucose level closely when starting or stopping a macrolide antibiotic.
■ Adjust repaglinide dosage as needed.
■ Monitor patient for evidence of hypoglycemia: hunger, dizziness, shakiness, sweating, confusion, and light-headedness.
■ Advise patient to carry glucose tablets or another simple sugar in case of hypoglycemia.
■ Make sure patient and family know what to do about hypoglycemia.

---

erythromycin ▶◀ rifamycins
E-mycin, Eryc   rifabutin, rifampin, rifapentine

Risk rating: 2
Severity: Moderate   **Onset: Delayed**   **Likelihood: Suspected**

Cause
Metabolism of rifamycin may decrease. Metabolism of macrolide antibiotic, such as erythromycin, may increase.

Effect
Adverse effects of rifamycins may increase. Antimicrobial effects of macrolide antibiotics may decrease.

Nursing considerations
■ Monitor patient for increased rifamycin adverse effects: abdominal pain, anorexia, nausea, vomiting, diarrhea, and rash.
■ Monitor patient for decreased response to macrolide antibiotic.

---

erythromycin ▶◀ theophyllines
E-mycin, Eryc   aminophylline, theophylline

Risk rating: 2
Severity: Moderate   **Onset: Delayed**   **Likelihood: Established**

Cause
Certain macrolides, such as erythromycin, inhibit theophylline metabolism. Theophylline increases renal clearance and decreases availability of oral erythromycin.

Effect
Theophylline level and risk of toxicity may increase. Erythromycin level may decrease.

Nursing considerations

■ When starting or stopping a macrolide, monitor theophylline level. Therapeutic range is 10 to 20 mcg/ml for adults and 5 to 15 mcg/ml for children.

■ If patient takes theophylline, watch for decreased erythromycin efficacy; tell prescriber promptly.

■ Consult prescriber about possibility of using another antibiotic.

■ Watch for evidence of toxicity: tachycardia, anorexia, nausea, vomiting, diarrhea, seizures, restlessness, irritability, and headache.

■ Describe adverse effects of theophylline and signs of toxicity, and tell patient to report them immediately to prescriber.

---

escitalopram ▶◀ MAO inhibitors

Lexapro

isocarboxazid, phenelzine, selegiline, tranylcypromine

Risk rating: 1
Severity: Major   **Onset: Rapid**   **Likelihood: Probable**

Cause

Serotonin may accumulate rapidly in the CNS.

Effect

Risk of serotonin syndrome increases.

Nursing considerations

◪ ALERT Don't use these drugs together.

■ Allow 2 weeks after stopping escitalopram before giving an MAO inhibitor. Allow 2 weeks after stopping an MAO inhibitor before giving an SSRI.

■ The selective MAO type-B inhibitor selegiline has been given with fluoxetine, paroxetine, or sertraline to patients with Parkinson's disease without negative effects.

■ Describe the traits of serotonin syndrome: CNS irritability, motor weakness, shivering, myoclonus, and altered consciousness.

■ Urge patient to promptly report adverse effects to prescriber.

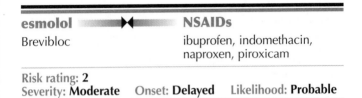

esmolol ▶◀ NSAIDs

Brevibloc

ibuprofen, indomethacin,
naproxen, piroxicam

Risk rating: 2
Severity: Moderate   **Onset: Delayed**   **Likelihood: Probable**

Cause
NSAIDs may inhibit renal prostaglandin synthesis, allowing pressor systems to be unopposed.

Effect
Esmolol, a beta blocker, may not be able to lower blood pressure.

Nursing considerations
- Avoid using these drugs together if possible
- Monitor blood pressure and other evidence of hypertension closely.
- Talk with prescriber about ways to minimize interaction, such as adjusting beta blocker dosage or switching to sulindac as the NSAID.
- Explain risks of using these drugs together, and teach patient how to monitor his own blood pressure.
- Other NSAIDs may interact with beta blockers. If you suspect an interaction, consult prescriber or pharmacist.

esmolol ▶◀ prazosin

Brevibloc

Minipress

Risk rating: 2
Severity: Moderate   **Onset: Rapid**   **Likelihood: Probable**

Cause
The mechanism of this interaction is unknown.

Effect
Effect of these drugs on orthostatic hypotension increases.

Nursing considerations
- Assess patient's lying, sitting, and standing blood pressures closely, especially when combined therapy starts.
- Adjust dosages of either drug based on patient effects.
- To minimize effects of orthostatic hypotension, teach patient to change positions slowly.
- Interaction is confirmed only with propranolol but also may occur with other beta blockers, such as esmolol.

esmolol 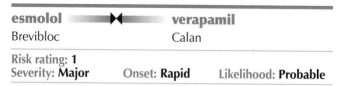 verapamil
Brevibloc   Calan

Risk rating: 1
Severity: Major   **Onset: Rapid**   **Likelihood: Probable**

Cause
Verapamil may inhibit metabolism of esmolol, a beta blocker.

Effect
Effects of both drugs may be increased.

Nursing considerations
▪ Combination therapy is common in patients with hypertension and unstable angina.
◪ **ALERT** Combined use increases risk of adverse effects, including heart failure, conduction disturbances, arrhythmias, and hypotension.
▪ Monitor patient for adverse effects, including left ventricular dysfunction and AV conduction defects.
▪ Risk of interaction is greater when drugs are given I.V.
▪ Dosages of both drugs may need to be decreased.

esomeprazole 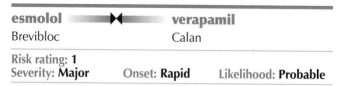 azole antifungals
Nexium   itraconazole, ketoconazole

Risk rating: 2
Severity: Moderate   **Onset: Rapid**   **Likelihood: Suspected**

Cause
Esomeprazole, a proton pump inhibitor, increases gastric pH, which may impair dissolution of azole antifungals.

Effect
Efficacy of azole antifungals may decrease.

Nursing considerations
▪ Tell prescriber about combined use; an alternative may be available.
▪ If no alternative is possible, suggest taking the azole antifungal with an acidic beverage, such as cola.
▪ Monitor patient for lack of response to antifungal.
▪ If patient can't tolerate acidic beverages and antifungal therapy appears to be ineffective, antifungal dosage may need to be increased.
▪ Other drugs that increase gastric pH may interact with azole antifungals. If you suspect an interaction, consult prescriber or pharmacist.

estazolam ▶◀ alcohol
ProSom

Risk rating: 2
Severity: Moderate   **Onset: Rapid**   **Likelihood: Established**

Cause
Alcohol inhibits hepatic enzymes, which decreases clearance and increases peak levels of benzodiazepines, such as estazolam.

Effect
Additive or synergistic effects may develop.

Nursing considerations
■ Before benzodiazepine therapy starts, assess patient thoroughly for history or evidence of alcohol use.
■ Watch for additive CNS effects, which may suggest benzodiazepine overdose.
■ Other benzodiazepines interact with alcohol. If you suspect an interaction, consult prescriber or pharmacist.
■ When patient starts a benzodiazepine, stress the high risks of consuming alcohol.

estazolam ▶◀ azole antifungals
ProSom   fluconazole, itraconazole, ketoconazole, miconazole

Risk rating: 2
Severity: Moderate   **Onset: Rapid**   **Likelihood: Established**

Cause
Azole antifungals decrease CYP3A4 metabolism of certain benzodiazepines, such as estazolam.

Effect
Benzodiazepine effects are increased and prolonged, which may cause CNS depression and psychomotor impairment.

Nursing considerations
■ If patient takes fluconazole or miconazole, consult prescriber about a lower benzodiazepine dose or a drug not metabolized by CYP3A4, such as temazepam or lorazepam.
■ Caution that the effects of this interaction may last several days after stopping the azole antifungal.
■ Explain that taking these drugs together may increase sedative effects; tell patient to report such effects promptly.

■ Explain alternative methods of inducing sleep or relieving anxiety.
■ Various benzodiazepine–azole antifungal combinations may interact. If you suspect an interaction, consult prescriber or pharmacist.

estazolam ━━━►◄ protease inhibitors
ProSom   amprenavir, atazanavir,
                      indinavir, lopinavir-ritonavir,
                      nelfinavir, ritonavir, saquinavir

Risk rating: 2
Severity: Moderate   **Onset: Delayed**   **Likelihood: Suspected**

Cause
Protease inhibitors may inhibit CYP3A4 metabolism of certain benzodiazepines, such as estazolam.

Effect
Sedative effects may be increased and prolonged.

Nursing considerations
◆ **ALERT** Don't combine estazolam with protease inhibitors.
■ If patient takes any benzodiazepine–protease inhibitor combination, notify prescriber. Interaction could involve others in the class.
■ Watch for evidence of oversedation and respiratory depression.
■ Teach patient and family about the risks of combining these drugs.

estazolam ━━━►◄ rifamycins
ProSom   rifabutin, rifampin, rifapentine

Risk rating: 2
Severity: Moderate   **Onset: Delayed**   **Likelihood: Suspected**

Cause
Rifamycins may increase CYP3A4 metabolism of benzodiazepines, such as estazolam.

Effect
Antianxiety, sedative, and sleep-inducing effects may decrease.

Nursing considerations
■ Watch for expected benzodiazepine effects and lack of efficacy.
■ If benzodiazepine efficacy is reduced, notify prescriber; dosage may be changed.
■ Other benzodiazepines may interact with rifamycins. If you suspect an interaction, consult prescriber or pharmacist.

■ For insomnia, temazepam may be more effective because it doesn't undergo CYP3A4 metabolism.

estrogens ━━━◄► corticosteroids

conjugated estrogens, esterified estrogens, estradiol, estrone, estropipate, ethinyl estradiol

hydrocortisone, prednisolone, prednisone

Risk rating: 2
Severity: Moderate   Onset: Delayed   Likelihood: Suspected

Cause
Estrogens may inhibit hepatic metabolism of corticosteroids.

Effect
Therapeutic and toxic corticosteroid effects may increase.

Nursing considerations
■ Assess effect of corticosteroid when given with estrogens.
■ Watch for evidence of corticosteroid toxicity: nervousness, sleepiness, depression, psychosis, weakness, decreased hearing, lower leg edema, skin disorders, hypertension, muscle weakness, and seizures.
■ Corticosteroid dosage may need adjustment.
■ Estrogen may continue to affect corticosteroid therapy for an unknown length of time after estrogen is stopped.
■ Other corticosteroids may interact with estrogens. If you suspect an interaction, consult prescriber or pharmacist.
■ Tell patient to report increased adverse effects.

estrogens ━━━◄► phenytoin

conjugated estrogens, esterified estrogens, estradiol, estrone, estropipate, ethinyl estradiol

Dilantin

Risk rating: 2
Severity: Moderate   Onset: Delayed   Likelihood: Suspected

Cause
Phenytoin may induce hepatic metabolism of estrogens. Estrogens may increase water retention, worsen seizures, and alter phenytoin protein-binding.

Effect
Risk of spotting, breakthrough bleeding, and pregnancy increases.
Seizure control may decrease.

Nursing considerations
⚡ ALERT Advise patient that breakthrough bleeding, spotting, and
amenorrhea are signs of contraceptive failure.
- Estrogen dose may need to be altered to obtain cycle control.
- Seizures may worsen in patients who take hormonal contraceptives.
- Watch for increased seizure activity when estrogen therapy starts.
- Hydantoins other than phenytoin may interact with estrogens. If
you suspect an interaction, consult prescriber or pharmacist.
- If patient takes phenytoin, suggest a nonhormonal contraceptive.

---

estrogens ◄►◄ rifamycins

conjugated estrogens,
esterified estrogens,
estradiol, estrone,
estropipate, ethinyl
estradiol

rifabutin, rifampin, rifapentine

Risk rating: 2
Severity: Moderate   Onset: Delayed   Likelihood: Suspected

Cause
Rifamycins induce hepatic metabolism of estrogens.

Effect
Estrogen level and efficacy may be reduced.

Nursing considerations
- Watch for menstrual disturbances, such as spotting, intermenstrual
bleeding, or amenorrhea.
- Explain that contraception may fail during combined therapy.
- Estrogen dose may need to be increased; consult prescriber.
- If patient takes a rifamycin, suggest a nonhormonal contraceptive.
- Urge patient to take the full course of rifamycin exactly as pre-
scribed to minimize risk of continued infection.

estrogens ━━━━▶◀━━━ **thyroid hormones**

conjugated estrogens,
esterified estrogens,
estradiol, estrone,
estropipate, ethinyl
estradiol

levothyroxine, liotrix

Risk rating: 2
Severity: Moderate   Onset: Delayed   Likelihood: Probable

Cause
Estrogen increases thyroxine-binding globulin level. Because thyroid
hormone binds to it, T_3 and T_4 levels decrease, and TSH is secreted.

Effect
Efficacy of thyroid hormone replacement decreases in hypothyroid
women.

Nursing considerations
■ Check serum TSH, T_3, and T_4 levels about 12 weeks after hypothy-
roid patient starts estrogen therapy.
■ Therapeutic range for TSH is 0.2 to 5.4 microunits/ml; for T_3, 80 to
200 nanogram/dl; and for T_4, 5.4 to 11.5 mcg/dl.
■ Watch for evidence of hypothyroidism, including weakness, fatigue,
weight gain, coarse dry hair, rough skin, cold intolerance, muscle
aches, constipation, depression, irritability, and memory loss.
■ Adjust thyroid hormone dose as ordered.
■ Explain that thyroid hormone dose may need to be altered.
■ Tell patient to report evidence of hypothyroidism, such as fatigue,
weight gain, cold intolerance, and constipation.

estrogens ━━━━▶◀━━━ **topiramate**

conjugated estrogens,
esterified estrogens,
estradiol, estrone,
estropipate, ethinyl
estradiol

Topamax

Risk rating: 2
Severity: Moderate   Onset: Delayed   Likelihood: Suspected

Cause
Topiramate may increase estrogen metabolism.

Effect
Estrogen efficacy may decrease.

Nursing considerations
■ Watch for worsening vasomotor symptoms: hot flashes, diaphoresis, headache, nausea, palpitations, dizziness, and a skin-crawling feeling.
■ Estrogen replacement or hormonal contraceptive dosage may need to be increased; consult prescriber or pharmacist.
■ Tell patient that topiramate may decrease estrogen efficacy.
■ Urge patient to report loss of effect—such as spotting, break-through bleeding, and amenorrhea—or increased adverse effects.
■ If patient takes topiramate, suggest a nonhormonal contraceptive.

ethacrynic acid ➤◄ aminoglycosides
Edecrin

amikacin, gentamicin, kanamycin, neomycin, netilmicin, streptomycin, tobramycin

Risk rating: 1
Severity: Major   Onset: **Rapid**   Likelihood: **Suspected**

Cause
The mechanism of the interaction is unknown.

Effect
Synergistic ototoxicity increases risk of hearing loss, possibly permanent.

Nursing considerations
◤ **ALERT** Patients with renal insufficiency are at increased risk for ototoxicity.
■ Perform baseline and periodic hearing function tests.
■ Other aminoglycosides may interact with loop diuretics, such as ethacrynic acid. If you suspect an interaction, consult prescriber or pharmacist.
■ Tell patient to immediately report ringing or roaring in the ears, muffled sounds, or any noticeable changes in hearing.
■ Advise family members to stay alert for evidence of hearing loss.

ethacrynic acid ➤◄ cisplatin
Edecrin

Platinol

Risk rating: 2
Severity: Moderate   Onset: **Rapid**   Likelihood: **Suspected**

Cause
The mechanism of this interaction is unknown.

Effect
Interaction may cause additive ototoxicity.

Nursing considerations
- Avoid giving a loop diuretic, such as ethacrynic acid, with cisplatin.
- Obtain hearing tests to detect early hearing loss.
- Combined, these drugs may cause ototoxicity much more severe than that of either drug alone and possibly permanent.
- Tell patient to report ringing in the ears, change in balance, or muffled sounds. Also, ask family members to watch for changes.

---

ethacrynic acid ▶◀ thiazide diuretics

Edecrin

chlorothiazide, hydrochloro-thiazide, indapamide, methy-clothiazide, metolazone, poly-thiazide, trichlormethiazide

Risk rating: 2
Severity: **Moderate**   Onset: **Rapid**   Likelihood: **Probable**

Cause
The mechanism of this interaction is unclear.

Effect
Because these drugs work synergistically, they may cause profound diuresis and serious electrolyte abnormalities.

Nursing considerations
- This combination may be used together for therapeutic benefit.
- Expect increased sodium, potassium, and chloride excretion and greater diuresis during combined therapy.
- Monitor patient for dehydration and electrolyte abnormalities.
- Carefully adjust drugs using small or intermittent doses.

---

etodolac ▶◀ aminoglycosides

Lodine

amikacin, gentamicin, kanamycin, netilmicin, streptomycin, tobramycin

Risk rating: 2
Severity: **Moderate**   Onset: **Delayed**   Likelihood: **Suspected**

Cause
Etodolac, an NSAID, may reduce glomerular filtration rate (GFR), causing aminoglycosides to accumulate.

Effect
Aminoglycoside level in premature infants may increase.

Nursing considerations
■ Before NSAID starts, aminoglycoside dose should be reduced.
◪ **ALERT** Check peak and trough aminoglycoside levels after third dose. For peak level, draw blood 30 minutes after I.V. or 60 minutes after I.M. dose. For trough level, draw blood just before a dose.
■ Monitor patient's renal function.
■ Although only indomethacin is known to interact with aminoglycosides, other NSAIDs probably do as well. If you suspect an interaction, consult prescriber or pharmacist.
■ Other drugs cleared by GFR may have a similar interaction.

---

etoposide ▶◀ cyclosporine
VePesid   Gengraf, Neoral, Sandimmune

Risk rating: 2
Severity: Moderate   Onset: Delayed   Likelihood: Established

Cause
Etoposide clearance may be decreased and metabolism inhibited by cyclosporine.

Effect
Etoposide level and risk of toxicity may increase.

Nursing considerations
■ Monitor patient for evidence of etoposide toxicity, including myelosuppression, nausea, vomiting and diarrhea.
■ Monitor CBC for evidence of leukopenia and thrombocytopenia.
■ Adjust etoposide dosage as needed.

---

felbamate ▶◀ carbamazepine
Felbatol   Carbatrol, Epitol, Equetro,
                                 Tegretol

Risk rating: 2
Severity: Moderate   Onset: Delayed   Likelihood: Suspected

Cause
The exact mechanism is unknown. Carbamazepine metabolism may increase, or conversion of carbamazepine metabolites may decrease. Carbamazepine also may increase felbamate metabolism.

Effect
Carbamazepine and felbamate levels and effects may decrease.

Nursing considerations
⚠ **ALERT** Monitor patient for loss of seizure control.
■ The active epoxide metabolite of carbamazepine may compensate for decreased carbamazepine level.
■ Monitor carbamazepine level; therapeutic range is 4 to 12 mcg/ml.
■ Dosage adjustments may be needed when felbamate starts.

---

felodipine ▶◀ barbiturates
Plendil   amobarbital, butabarbital,
                                 pentobarbital, phenobarbital,
                                 primidone, secobarbital

Risk rating: 2
Severity: Moderate   Onset: Delayed   Likelihood: Suspected

Cause
Felodipine metabolism may increase and availability decrease.

Effect
Felodipine effects may decrease.

Nursing considerations
■ Felodipine dose may need to be increased during combined use.
■ Watch for loss of blood pressure control if barbiturate starts.
■ Watch for evidence of felodipine toxicity (peripheral vasodilation, hypotension, bradycardia, and palpitations) if barbiturate is stopped.
■ Other barbiturates may interact with felodipine. If you suspect an interaction, consult prescriber or pharmacist.
■ Urge patient to have blood pressure monitored if barbiturate starts. Remind patient that hypertension may cause no physical symptoms.

---

felodipine ▶◀ carbamazepine
Plendil   Carbatrol, Epitol, Equetro,
                                 Tegretol

Risk rating: 2
Severity: Moderate   Onset: Delayed   Likelihood: Suspected

Cause
Felodipine metabolism may increase and availability decrease.

Effect
Felodipine effects may decrease.

Nursing considerations
■ Watch for loss of blood pressure control if carbamazepine starts.
■ Felodipine dose may need to be increased.
■ Watch for evidence of felodipine toxicity (peripheral vasodilation, hypotension, bradycardia, and palpitations) if carbamazepine stops.
■ Advise patient to tell prescriber about all drugs and supplements he takes and about any increase in adverse effects.
■ Urge patient to have blood pressure monitored if carbamazepine starts. Remind patient that hypertension may cause no symptoms.

---

felodipine ➤◀ grapefruit juice
Plendil

Risk rating: 2
Severity: Moderate   **Onset: Rapid**   **Likelihood: Probable**

Cause
Felodipine metabolism may be decreased by grapefruit juice.

Effect
Felodipine level, effects, and risk of adverse effects may increase.

Nursing considerations
◗ **ALERT** Avoid giving felodipine with grapefruit juice.
■ Watch for increased felodipine effects: prolonged hypotension, bradycardia, palpitations, flushing, headache, dizziness, and edema.
■ Urge patient to take felodipine with liquids other than grapefruit juice.
■ Urge patient to tell prescriber about increased adverse effects.

---

felodipine ➤◀ hydantoins
Plendil   ethotoin, fosphenytoin, phenytoin

Risk rating: 2
Severity: Moderate   **Onset: Delayed**   **Likelihood: Suspected**

Cause
Hydantoins may increase felodipine metabolism and decrease its availability.

Effect
Felodipine effects may decrease.

Nursing considerations
■ Felodipine dose may need to be increased.

■ Watch for loss of blood pressure control if patient who takes felodipine starts a hydantoin.
■ Watch for evidence of felodipine toxicity (peripheral vasodilation, hypotension, bradycardia, and palpitations) if a hydantoin is stopped.
■ Urge patient to have blood pressure monitored if hydantoin therapy starts. Remind patient that hypertension may cause no symptoms.
■ Urge patient to tell prescriber about increased adverse effects.

felodipine ━━━◀▶━━━ itraconazole
Plendil   Sporanox

Risk rating: 2
Severity: **Moderate**   Onset: **Delayed**   Likelihood: **Probable**

Cause
Itraconazole may inhibit felodipine CYP3A4 metabolism.

Effect
Felodipine level and adverse effects may increase.

Nursing considerations
■ Felodipine dose may need to be adjusted.
■ Closely monitor patients age 65 and older and patients with liver impairment; they're at increased risk for elevated felodipine level.
■ Monitor patient for adverse felodipine effects, including increased peripheral edema, hypotension, and tachycardia.
■ Azole antifungals other than itraconazole may interact with felodipine. If you suspect an interaction, consult prescriber or pharmacist.
■ Urge patient to tell prescriber about increased adverse effects.

fenoprofen ━━━◀▶━━━ aminoglycosides
                          amikacin, gentamicin,
                          kanamycin, netilmicin,
                          streptomycin, tobramycin

Risk rating: 2
Severity: **Moderate**   Onset: **Delayed**   Likelihood: **Suspected**

Cause
Fenoprofen, an NSAID, may reduce glomerular filtration rate (GFR), causing aminoglycosides to accumulate.

Effect
Aminoglycoside level in premature infants may increase.

Nursing considerations
■ Before NSAID starts, aminoglycoside dose should be reduced.
■ ALERT Check peak and trough aminoglycoside levels after third dose. For peak level, draw blood 30 minutes after I.V. or 60 minutes after I.M. dose. For trough level, draw blood just before a dose.
■ Monitor patient's renal function.
■ Although only indomethacin is known to interact with aminoglycosides, other NSAIDs probably do as well. If you suspect an interaction, consult prescriber or pharmacist.
■ Other drugs cleared by GFR may have a similar interaction.

---

fentanyl ━━━━▸◂━━━━ **amiodarone**
Sublimaze   Cordarone, Pacerone

Risk rating: 1
Severity: Major   **Onset: Rapid**   **Likelihood: Suspected**

Cause
The mechanism of this interaction is unknown.

Effect
Risk of profound bradycardia, sinus arrest, and hypotension increases.

Nursing considerations
■ It isn't known if these effects are related to fentanyl anesthesia or anesthesia in general; use cautiously together.
■ Monitor hemodynamic function.
■ Keep inotropic, chronotropic, and pressor support available.
■ ALERT Bradycardia caused by this interaction usually doesn't respond to atropine.

---

fentanyl ━━━━▸◂━━━━ **protease inhibitors**
Sublimaze   amprenavir, indinavir,
                                             nelfinavir, ritonavir, saquinavir

Risk rating: 1
Severity: Major   **Onset: Delayed**   **Likelihood: Suspected**

Cause
Metabolism of fentanyl in the GI tract and liver may be inhibited.

Effect
Fentanyl level may increase and half-life lengthen.

Nursing considerations
⚠ **ALERT** If patient takes a protease inhibitor, watch closely for respiratory depression if fentanyl is added.
- Because fentanyl half-life is prolonged, monitoring period should be extended, even after fentanyl is stopped.
- Keep naloxone available to treat respiratory depression.
- If fentanyl is continuously infused, dosage should be decreased.

---

fexofenadine ━━▶◀━━ fruit juices
Allegra   apple, grapefruit, orange

Risk rating: 2
Severity: Moderate   Onset: Rapid   Likelihood: Suspected

Cause
Fruit juices may decrease fexofenadine absorption.

Effect
Fexofenadine level and effects may decline.

Nursing considerations
- Advise against taking fexofenadine with these fruit juices.
- Watch for expected clinical effects, including relief of seasonal allergic rhinitis or relief of chronic urticaria.
- In patients with impaired renal function, maximum daily dosage recommendations are 60 mg for adults and 30 mg for children.

---

flecainide ━━▶◀━━ ritonavir
Tambocor   Norvir

Risk rating: 1
Severity: Major   Onset: Delayed   Likelihood: Suspected

Cause
Ritonavir may inhibit CYP2D6 metabolism of flecainide.

Effect
Flecainide level and risk of toxicity may increase.

Nursing considerations
⚠ **ALERT** Ritonavir is contraindicated in patients taking flecainide.
- Monitor serum flecainide level; therapeutic range is 0.2 to 1 mcg/ml.
- Watch for flecainide toxicity: slowed or irregular pulse, palpitations, shortness of breath, hypotension, and new or worsened heart failure.
- Monitor ECG for conduction disturbances (prolonged PR, QRS, and QT intervals), new or worsened arrhythmias, ventricular tachy-

cardia, ventricular fibrillation, tachycardia, bradycardia, second- or third-degree AV block, and sinus arrest.

fluconazole ━━━━▶◀━━━━ benzodiazepines
Diflucan

alprazolam, chlordiazepoxide, clonazepam, clorazepate, diazepam, estazolam, flurazepam, midazolam, quazepam, triazolam

Risk rating: 2
Severity: Moderate   **Onset: Rapid**   **Likelihood: Established**

Cause
Azole antifungals, such as fluconazole, decrease CYP3A4 metabolism of certain benzodiazepines.

Effect
Benzodiazepine effects are increased and prolonged, which may cause CNS depression and psychomotor impairment.

Nursing considerations
■ If patient takes fluconazole, talk with prescriber about giving a lower benzodiazepine dose or a drug not metabolized by CYP3A4, such as temazepam or lorazepam.
■ Caution that the effects of this interaction may last several days after stopping the azole antifungal.
■ Explain the risk of sedation; tell patient to report it promptly.
■ Explain alternative methods of inducing sleep or relieving anxiety during antifungal therapy.
■ Various azole antifungal–benzodiazepine combinations may interact. If you suspect an interaction, consult prescriber or pharmacist.

fluconazole ━━━━▶◀━━━━ HMG-CoA reductase inhibitors
Diflucan

atorvastatin, fluvastatin, lovastatin, pravastatin, rosuvastatin, simvastatin

Risk rating: 2
Severity: Moderate   **Onset: Rapid**   **Likelihood: Probable**

Cause
Azole antifungals, such as fluconazole, may inhibit hepatic metabolism of HMG-CoA reductase inhibitors.

Effect
HMG-CoA reductase inhibitor level and adverse effects may increase.

Nursing considerations
■ If possible, avoid use together.
■ HMG-CoA reductase inhibitor dosage may need to be decreased.
■ Monitor serum cholesterol and lipid levels.
⚡ ALERT Assess patient for evidence of rhabdomyolysis: fatigue; muscle aches and weakness; joint pain; dark, red, or cola-colored urine; weight gain; seizures; and greatly increased serum CK level.
■ Pravastatin is least affected by this interaction and may be preferable for use with an azole antifungal, if needed.

---

fluconazole ▶◀ nisoldipine
Diflucan   Sular

Risk rating: 2
Severity: Moderate   Onset: Delayed   Likelihood: Suspected

Cause
Azole antifungals, such as fluconazole, inhibit CYP3A4, which is needed for nisoldipine metabolism.

Effect
Nisoldipine level, effects, and risk of adverse effects may increase.

Nursing considerations
■ Tell prescriber about combined use; an alternative may be available.
■ If drugs must be taken together, watch for orthostatic hypotension, which stems from increased nisoldipine effect.
■ Tell patient to report adverse nisoldipine effects, including chest pain, dizziness, headache, weight gain, nausea, palpitations, and peripheral edema.

---

fluconazole ▶◀ protease inhibitors
Diflucan   amprenavir, atazanavir,
                           indinavir, lopinavir-ritonavir,
                           nelfinavir, ritonavir, saquinavir

Risk rating: 2
Severity: Moderate   Onset: Delayed   Likelihood: Suspected

Cause
Azole antifungals, such as fluconazole, may inhibit metabolism of protease inhibitors.

Effect

Protease inhibitor level may increase.

Nursing considerations

- Protease inhibitor dosage may need to be decreased.
- Watch for increased protease inhibitor effects: hyperglycemia, onset of diabetes, rash, GI complaints, and altered liver function tests.
- Advise patient to report increased hunger or thirst, frequent urination, fatigue, and dry, itchy skin.
- Tell patient not to change dosage or stop either drug without consulting prescriber.

---

fluconazole ◄►◄ rifamycins

Diflucan   rifabutin, rifampin, rifapentine

Risk rating: 2
Severity: Moderate   Onset: Delayed   Likelihood: Suspected

Cause

Rifamycins may decrease level of azole antifungals, such as fluconazole.

Effect

Infection may recur.

Nursing considerations

- Tell prescriber about combined use; an alternative may be available.
- If drugs must be taken together and the antifungal appears ineffective, antifungal dosage may need to be increased.
- Teach patient to recognize evidence of infection and to contact prescriber promptly if it recurs.

---

fluconazole ◄►◄ sirolimus

Diflucan   Rapamune

Risk rating: 2
Severity: Moderate   Onset: Delayed   Likelihood: Suspected

Cause

Azole antifungals, such as fluconazole, inhibit CYP3A4, which is needed for sirolimus metabolism.

Effect

Sirolimus level, effects, and risk of adverse effects and toxicity may increase.

Nursing considerations

■ Monitor trough level of sirolimus in whole blood when starting or stopping an azole antifungal. Therapeutic levels vary with other drugs patient receives—cyclosporine, for example.

■ Watch for signs of sirolimus toxicity, such as anemia, leukopenia, thrombocytopenia, hypokalemia, hyperlipemia, fever, interstitial lung disease, and diarrhea.

■ Other CYP3A4 inhibitors may interact with sirolimus. If you suspect an interaction, consult prescriber or pharmacist.

■ Urge patient to promptly report new onset of fever higher than 100° F (38° C), fatigue, shortness of breath, easy bruising, gum bleeding, muscle twitches, palpitations, or chest discomfort or pain.

---

fluconazole ➡◀ tolterodine
Diflucan   Detrol

Risk rating: 2
Severity: Moderate   Onset: Delayed   Likelihood: Suspected

Cause
Azole antifungals, such as fluconazole, inhibit CYP3A4, which is needed for tolterodine metabolism.

Effect
Tolterodine level, effects, and risk of adverse effects may increase.

Nursing considerations
■ Tell prescriber about combined use; an alternative may be available.
■ Watch for evidence of tolterodine overdose, such as dry mouth, urine retention, constipation, dizziness, and headache.
■ Explain adverse tolterodine effects and need to report them.
■ Other CYP3A4 inhibitors may interact with tolterodine. If you suspect an interaction, consult prescriber or pharmacist.

---

fluconazole ➡◀ tricyclic antidepressants
Diflucan   amitriptyline, imipramine, nortriptyline

Risk rating: 2
Severity: Moderate   Onset: Delayed   Likelihood: Suspected

Cause
Azole antifungals, such as fluconazole, may inhibit metabolism of tricyclic antidepressants (TCAs) by CYP pathways.

Effect
TCA level and risk of toxicity may increase.

Nursing considerations
■ When starting or stopping an azole antifungal, monitor serum TCA level and adjust dosage as needed.
■ After starting an azole antifungal, check sitting and standing blood pressure for changes.
■ Watch for adverse reactions, such as increased drowsiness, dizziness, confusion, heart rate or rhythm changes, and urine retention.

---

fluconazole ▶◀ vinca alkaloids
Diflucan   vinblastine, vincristine

Risk rating: 1
Severity: Major   **Onset: Delayed**   **Likelihood: Probable**

Cause
Azole antifungals, such as fluconazole, inhibit CYP3A4, which is needed for vinca alkaloid metabolism.

Effect
Risk of vinca alkaloid toxicity increases.

Nursing considerations
■ If possible, avoid giving these drugs together.
■ Watch for evidence of toxicity, such as constipation, myalgia, hypertension, hyponatremia, and neutropenia.
■ Explain adverse vinca alkaloid effects and need to report them.
■ Stop azole antifungal as soon as possible.

---

fludrocortisone ▶◀ barbiturates
Florinef   amobarbital, butabarbital,
                          pentobarbital, phenobarbital,
                          primidone, secobarbital

Risk rating: 2
Severity: Moderate   **Onset: Delayed**   **Likelihood: Established**

Cause
Barbiturates induce liver enzymes, which stimulate metabolism of corticosteroids, such as fludrocortisone.

Effect
Corticosteroid effects may be decreased.

Nursing considerations
- Avoid giving barbiturates with corticosteroids, if possible.
- If patient takes a corticosteroid, watch for worsening symptoms when a barbiturate is started or stopped.
- Corticosteroid dosage may need to be increased.

---

fludrocortisone ◢◣ cholinesterase inhibitors
Florinef   ambenonium, edrophonium, neostigmine, pyridostigmine

Risk rating: 1
Severity: Major   **Onset: Delayed**   **Likelihood: Probable**

Cause
In myasthenia gravis, fludrocortisone and other corticosteroids antagonize the effects of cholinesterase inhibitors.

Effect
Patient may develop severe muscular depression refractory to cholinesterase inhibitor.

Nursing considerations
- Corticosteroids may have long-term benefits in myasthenia gravis.
- Combined therapy may be attempted under strict supervision.
- In myasthenia gravis, watch for severe muscle deterioration.
- **⚡ ALERT** Be prepared to provide respiratory support and mechanical ventilation if needed.
- Consult prescriber or pharmacist about safe corticosteroid delivery to maximize improvement in muscle strength.

---

fludrocortisone ◢◣ hydantoins
Florinef   ethotoin, fosphenytoin, phenytoin

Risk rating: 2
Severity: Moderate   **Onset: Delayed**   **Likelihood: Established**

Cause
Hydantoins induce liver enzymes, which stimulate metabolism of corticosteroids, such as fludrocortisone.

Effect
Corticosteroid effects may decrease.

Nursing considerations
- Avoid giving hydantoins with corticosteroids if possible.

- Monitor patient for decreased corticosteroid effects. Also monitor phenytoin level, and adjust dosage of either drug as needed.
- Corticosteroid effects may decrease within days of starting phenytoin and may stay decreased 3 weeks after it stops.
- Dosage of either or both drugs may need to be increased.

fludrocortisone ◀▶ rifamycins

Florinef   rifabutin, rifampin, rifapentine

Risk rating: 1
Severity: Major   **Onset: Delayed**   **Likelihood: Established**

Cause
Rifamycins increase hepatic metabolism of corticosteroids, such as fludrocortisone.

Effect
Corticosteroid effects may be decreased.

Nursing considerations
- If possible, avoid giving rifamycins with corticosteroids.
- Monitor patient for decreased corticosteroid effects, including loss of disease control.
- Watch closely for symptom control after increasing rifamycin dose. Drug may need to be stopped to regain control of disease.
- Corticosteroid effects may decrease within days of starting rifampin and may stay decreased 2 to 3 weeks after it stops.
- Corticosteroid dose may need to be doubled after adding rifampin.

fludrocortisone ◀▶ salicylates

Florinef   aspirin, bismuth subsalicylate, choline salicylate, magnesium salicylate, salsalate, sodium salicylate, sodium thiosalicylate

Risk rating: 2
Severity: Moderate   **Onset: Delayed**   **Likelihood: Probable**

Cause
Corticosteroids, such as fludrocortisone, stimulate hepatic metabolism of salicylates and may increase renal excretion.

Effect
Salicylate level and effects decrease.

Nursing considerations
- Monitor salicylate level and efficacy; dosage may need adjustment.
- **⚠ ALERT** Giving a salicylate while tapering a corticosteroid may result in salicylate toxicity.
- Watch for evidence of salicylate toxicity, including diaphoresis, nausea, vomiting, tinnitus, hyperventilation, and CNS depression.
- Patients with renal impairment may be at greater risk.

---

fluoxetine ▶◀ carbamazepine
Prozac, Sarafem

Carbatrol, Epitol, Equetro, Tegretol

Risk rating: 2
Severity: Moderate   **Onset: Delayed**   **Likelihood: Suspected**

Cause
Fluoxetine may inhibit carbamazepine metabolism.

Effect
Carbamazepine level and risk of toxicity may increase.

Nursing considerations
- Monitor carbamazepine level; therapeutic range is 4 to 12 mcg/ml.
- Carbamazepine dosage may need adjustment if fluoxetine starts or stops.
- **⚠ ALERT** Watch for signs of anorexia or subtle appetite changes, which may indicate excessive carbamazepine level.
- Watch for evidence of carbamazepine toxicity: dizziness, ataxia, respiratory depression, tachycardia, arrhythmias, blood pressure changes, impaired consciousness, abnormal reflexes, nystagmus, seizures, nausea, vomiting, and urine retention.
- When fluoxetine starts during stabilized carbamazepine therapy, urge patient to report nausea, vomiting, dizziness, visual disturbances, difficulty balancing, tremors, and any new adverse effects.
- SSRIs other than fluoxetine may interact with carbamazepine. If you suspect an interaction, consult prescriber or pharmacist.

fluoxetine ◄►◄ hydantoins

Prozac, Sarafem

ethotoin, fosphenytoin, phenytoin

Risk rating: 2
Severity: Moderate   **Onset: Delayed**   **Likelihood: Suspected**

Cause
Fluoxetine may inhibit hydantoin metabolism.

Effect
Serum hydantoin level, effects, and risk of toxicity may increase.

Nursing considerations
- Monitor serum hydantoin level. Therapeutic range for phenytoin is 10 to 20 mcg/ml.
- Hydantoin dosage may need adjustment.
- Watch for evidence of hydantoin toxicity: drowsiness, nausea, vomiting, nystagmus, ataxia, dysarthria, tremor, slurred speech, hypotension, arrhythmias, respiratory depression, and coma.
- For patients taking fosphenytoin, the metabolites formate and phosphate may contribute to signs of toxicity. Symptoms of formate toxicity are similar to methanol toxicity. An elevated phosphate level may cause hypocalcemia with paresthesia, muscle spasms, and seizures.
- Urge patient to tell prescriber about increased adverse effects.

fluoxetine ◄► MAO inhibitors

Prozac, Sarafem

isocarboxazid, phenelzine, selegiline, tranylcypromine

Risk rating: 1
Severity: Major   **Onset: Rapid**   **Likelihood: Probable**

Cause
Serotonin may accumulate rapidly in the CNS.

Effect
Risk of serotonin syndrome increases.

Nursing considerations
◼ ALERT Don't use these drugs together.
- Allow 5 weeks after stopping fluoxetine before giving an MAO inhibitor. Allow 2 weeks after stopping an MAO inhibitor before giving an SSRI, such as fluoxetine.
- The selective MAO type-B inhibitor selegiline has been given with fluoxetine, paroxetine, or sertraline to patients with Parkinson's disease without negative effects.

- Describe the traits of serotonin syndrome, including CNS irritability, motor weakness, shivering, myoclonus, and altered consciousness.
- Urge patient to promptly report these and other adverse effects to prescriber.

---

fluoxetine ▶◀ propafenone

Prozac, Sarafem   Rythmol

Risk rating: 2
Severity: Moderate   Onset: Delayed   Likelihood: Suspected

Cause
Certain serotonin reuptake inhibitors, such as fluoxetine, may inhibit CYP2D6 metabolism of propafenone.

Effect
Propafenone level and risk of adverse effects may increase.

Nursing considerations
- Monitor cardiac function closely.
- Tell patient to promptly report dizziness, drowsiness, ataxia, tremor, palpitations, chest pain, edema, dyspnea, and other new symptoms.
- Citalopram doesn't inhibit CYP2D6 and may be a safer choice.

---

fluoxetine ▶◀ selective 5-HT$_1$ receptor agonists

Prozac, Sarafem

almotriptan, eletriptan, frovatriptan, naratriptan, rizatriptan, sumatriptan, zolmitriptan

Risk rating: 1
Severity: Major   Onset: Rapid   Likelihood: Suspected

Cause
Serotonin may accumulate rapidly in the CNS.

Effect
Risk of serotonin syndrome increases.

Nursing considerations
- **⚠ ALERT** If possible, avoid combined use of these drugs.
- Start with lowest dosages possible, and assess patient closely.
- Stop selective 5-HT$_1$ receptor agonist at the first sign of interaction, and start an antiserotonergic.

■ In some patients, migraine frequency may increase and antimigraine drug efficacy may decrease when an SSRI, such as fluoxetine, is started.

■ Describe traits of serotonin syndrome: CNS irritability, motor weakness, shivering, muscle twitching, and altered consciousness.

■ Explain that serotonin syndrome can be fatal if not treated immediately.

---

fluoxetine ◄►◄ sibutramine

Prozac, Sarafem   Meridia

Risk rating: 1
Severity: Major   **Onset: Rapid**   **Likelihood: Suspected**

Cause
Serotonin may accumulate rapidly in the CNS.

Effect
Risk of serotonin syndrome increases.

Nursing considerations
◼ **ALERT** If possible, don't give these drugs together.

■ Watch carefully for adverse effects; they need immediate attention.

■ Describe traits of serotonin syndrome: CNS irritability, motor weakness, shivering, muscle twitching, and altered consciousness.

■ Explain that serotonin syndrome can be fatal if not treated immediately.

---

fluoxetine ◄►◄ St. John's wort

Prozac, Sarafem

Risk rating: 2
Severity: Moderate   **Onset: Rapid**   **Likelihood: Suspected**

Cause
St. John's wort may cause additive inhibition of serotonin reuptake.

Effect
The sedative-hypnotic effects of SSRIs, such as fluoxetine, may increase.

Nursing considerations
◼ **ALERT** Discourage use of St. John's wort with an SSRI.

■ In addition to oversedation, mild serotonin-like symptoms may occur, including anxiety, dizziness, nausea, restlessness, and vomiting.

■ Inform the patient about the dangers of this combination.
■ Urge patient to consult prescriber before taking any herb.

---

fluoxetine ━━━▶◀━━━ sympathomimetics

Prozac, Sarafem

amphetamine,
dextroamphetamine,
methamphetamine,
phentermine

Risk rating: 1
Severity: Major   **Onset: Rapid**   **Likelihood: Suspected**

Cause
The mechanism of this interaction is unknown.

Effect
Sympathomimetic effects and risk of serotonin syndrome increase.

Nursing considerations
■ Watch closely for increased CNS effects, such as anxiety, jitteriness, agitation, and restlessness.
■ Mild serotonin-like symptoms may develop, including anxiety, dizziness, restlessness, nausea, and vomiting.
■ Explain risk of interaction and need to avoid sympathomimetics.
■ Describe traits of serotonin syndrome: CNS irritability, motor weakness, shivering, myoclonus, and altered consciousness.

---

fluoxetine ━━━▶◀━━━ tricyclic antidepressants

Prozac, Sarafem

amitriptyline, amoxapine,
clomipramine, desipramine,
doxepin, imipramine,
nortriptyline, trimipramine

Risk rating: 2
Severity: Moderate   **Onset: Delayed**   **Likelihood: Probable**

Cause
Fluoxetine may inhibit hepatic metabolism of tricyclic antidepressants (TCAs).

Effect
Serum TCA level and toxicity may increase.

Nursing considerations
■ Monitor serum TCA level and watch closely for evidence of toxicity,

such as increased anticholinergic effects, delirium, dizziness, drowsiness, and psychosis.

■ Report evidence of increased TCA level or toxicity; dosage may need to be decreased.

■ If TCA starts when patient already takes fluoxetine, TCA dosage may need to be decreased by up to 75% to avoid interaction.

■ Inhibitory effects of fluoxetine may take several weeks to dissipate after drug is stopped.

■ Other TCAs may interact with fluoxetine. If you suspect an interaction, consult prescriber or pharmacist.

fluphenazine ➤◄ alcohol
Prolixin

Risk rating: 2
Severity: Moderate   **Onset: Rapid**   **Likelihood: Probable**

Cause
These substances may produce CNS depression by working on different sites in the brain. Also, alcohol may lower resistance to neurotoxic effects of phenothiazines, such as fluphenazine.

Effect
CNS depression may increase.

Nursing considerations
■ Watch for extrapyramidal reactions, such as dystonic reactions and acute akathisia or restlessness.

■ If patient takes a phenothiazine, warn that alcohol may worsen CNS depression and impair psychomotor skills.

■ Discourage alcohol consumption during phenothiazine therapy.

fluphenazine ➤◄ anticholinergics
Prolixin   atropine, belladonna,
                        benztropine, biperiden,
                        dicyclomine, hyoscyamine,
                        oxybutynin, propantheline,
                        scopolamine

Risk rating: 2
Severity: Moderate   **Onset: Delayed**   **Likelihood: Suspected**

Cause
Anticholinergics may antagonize phenothiazines, such as fluphenazine. Also, phenothiazine metabolism may increase.

Effect
Phenothiazine efficacy may decrease.

Nursing considerations
- Data regarding this interaction conflict.
- Monitor patient for decreased phenothiazine efficacy.
- Phenothiazine dosage may need adjustment.
- Anticholinergic side effects may increase.
- Monitor patient for adynamic ileus, hyperpyrexia, hypoglycemia, and neurologic changes.

---

fluphenazine ➤◀ quinolones
Prolixin   gatifloxacin, levofloxacin,
                                 moxifloxacin, sparfloxacin

Risk rating: 1
Severity: Major   **Onset: Delayed**   **Likelihood: Suspected**

Cause
The mechanism of this interaction is unknown.

Effect
Risk of life-threatening arrhythmias, including torsades de pointes, may increase.

Nursing considerations
⚠ ALERT Sparfloxacin is contraindicated with drugs that prolong the QTc interval, including phenothiazines, such as fluphenazine.
- Avoid giving levofloxacin with fluphenazine.
- Use gatifloxacin and moxifloxacin cautiously with fluphenazine and with increased monitoring.
- Quinolones that don't prolong the QTc interval or that aren't metabolized by CYP3A4 isoenzymes may be better alternatives.

---

flurazepam ➤◀ alcohol
Dalmane

Risk rating: 2
Severity: Moderate   **Onset: Rapid**   **Likelihood: Established**

Cause
Alcohol inhibits hepatic enzymes, which decreases clearance and increases peak levels of benzodiazepines, such as flurazepam.

Effect
Additive or synergistic effects may develop.

Nursing considerations
■ Before benzodiazepine therapy starts, assess patient thoroughly for history or evidence of alcohol use.
■ Watch for additive CNS effects, which may suggest benzodiazepine overdose.

---

flurazepam ━━━►◄━━━ **azole antifungals**
Dalmane   fluconazole, itraconazole,
                             ketoconazole, miconazole

Risk rating: 2
Severity: Moderate   Onset: Rapid   Likelihood: Established

Cause
Azole antifungals decrease CYP3A4 metabolism of certain benzodiazepines, such as flurazepam.

Effect
Benzodiazepine effects are increased and prolonged, which may cause CNS depression and psychomotor impairment.

Nursing considerations
■ If patient takes fluconazole, consult prescriber about a lower benzodiazepine dose or a drug not metabolized by CYP3A4, such as temazepam or lorazepam.
■ Various benzodiazepine–azole antifungal combinations may interact. If you suspect an interaction, consult prescriber or pharmacist.
■ Caution that the effects of this interaction may last several days after stopping the azole antifungal.
■ Explain that sedative effects may increase and should be reported.

---

flurazepam ━━━►◄━━━ **protease inhibitors**
Dalmane   amprenavir, atazanavir,
                             indinavir, lopinavir-ritonavir,
                             nelfinavir, ritonavir, saquinavir

Risk rating: 2
Severity: Moderate   Onset: Delayed   Likelihood: Suspected

Cause
Protease inhibitors may inhibit CYP3A4 metabolism of certain benzodiazepines, such as flurazepam.

Effect
Sedative effects may be increased and prolonged.

Nursing considerations
■ **ALERT** Don't combine flurazepam with protease inhibitors.
■ If patient takes any benzodiazepine–protease inhibitor combination, notify prescriber. Interaction could involve related drugs.
■ Watch for oversedation and respiratory depression.
■ Teach patient and family about risks of taking these drugs together.

---

flurazepam ▶◀ rifamycins
Dalmane   rifabutin, rifampin, rifapentine

Risk rating: 2
Severity: Moderate   **Onset: Delayed**   **Likelihood: Suspected**

Cause
Rifamycins may increase CYP3A4 metabolism of benzodiazepines, such as flurazepam.

Effect
Antianxiety, sedative, and sleep-inducing effects may decrease.

Nursing considerations
■ Watch for expected benzodiazepine effects and lack of efficacy.
■ If benzodiazepine efficacy is reduced, notify prescriber; dosage may be changed.
■ Other benzodiazepines may interact with rifamycins. If you suspect an interaction, consult prescriber or pharmacist.
■ For insomnia, temazepam may be more effective because it doesn't undergo CYP3A4 metabolism.

---

flurbiprofen ▶◀ aminoglycosides
Ansaid   amikacin, gentamicin,
                                  kanamycin, netilmicin,
                                  streptomycin, tobramycin

Risk rating: 2
Severity: Moderate   **Onset: Delayed**   **Likelihood: Suspected**

Cause
Flurbiprofen and other NSAIDs may reduce glomerular filtration rate (GFR), causing aminoglycosides to accumulate.

Effect
Aminoglycoside level in premature infants may increase.

Nursing considerations
■ Before NSAID starts, aminoglycoside dose should be reduced.

▶ ALERT Check peak and trough aminoglycoside levels after third dose. For peak level, draw blood 30 minutes after I.V. or 60 minutes after I.M. dose. For trough level, draw blood just before a dose.
- Monitor patient's renal function.
- Although only indomethacin is known to interact with aminoglycosides, other NSAIDs probably do as well. If you suspect an interaction, consult prescriber or pharmacist.
- Other drugs cleared by GFR may have a similar interaction.

fluvastatin ▶◀	azole antifungals
Lescol	fluconazole, itraconazole, ketoconazole, voriconazole

Risk rating: 2
Severity: Moderate   **Onset: Rapid**   **Likelihood: Probable**

Cause
Azole antifungals may inhibit hepatic metabolism of HMG-CoA reductase inhibitors, such as fluvastatin.

Effect
Fluvastatin level and adverse effects may increase.

Nursing considerations
- If possible, avoid use together.
- Fluvastatin dosage may need to be decreased.
- Monitor serum cholesterol and lipid levels.

▶ ALERT Assess patient for evidence of rhabdomyolysis: fatigue; muscle aches and weakness; joint pain; dark, red, or cola-colored urine; weight gain; seizures; and greatly increased CK level.
- Pravastatin is the HMG-CoA reductase inhibitor least affected by this interaction and may be preferable to use with an azole antifungal.

fluvastatin ▶◀	bile acid sequestrants
Lescol	cholestyramine, colestipol

Risk rating: 2
Severity: Moderate   **Onset: Delayed**   **Likelihood: Suspected**

Cause
GI absorption of HMG-CoA reductase inhibitors, such as fluvastatin, may decrease.

Effect
Fluvastatin effects may decrease.

Nursing considerations
- Separate doses of these drugs by at least 4 hours.
- If possible, give bile acid sequestrant before meals and fluvastatin in the evening.
- Monitor serum cholesterol and lipid levels.
- Obtain liver function test results at start of therapy and periodically thereafter. If ALT or AST level stays three times or more above upper limit of normal, fluvastatin will need to be stopped.
- Help patient develop a plan to ensure proper dosage intervals.

---

fluvastatin ◄►◄ gemfibrozil
Lescol   Lopid

Risk rating: 1
Severity: **Major**   Onset: **Delayed**   Likelihood: **Suspected**

Cause
The mechanism of this interaction is unknown.

Effect
Severe myopathy or rhabdomyolysis may occur.

Nursing considerations
- Avoid use together.
- If patient has severe hyperlipidemia, combined therapy may be an option, but only with careful monitoring.
- **⚡ ALERT** Assess patient for evidence of rhabdomyolysis: fatigue; muscle aches and weakness; joint pain; dark, red, or cola-colored urine; weight gain; seizures; and greatly increased CK level.
- Watch for evidence of acute renal failure: decreased urine output, elevated BUN and creatinine levels, edema, dyspnea, tachycardia, distended neck veins, nausea, vomiting, poor appetite, weakness, fatigue, confusion, and agitation.
- Urge patient to report muscle pain, tenderness, or weakness.

---

fluvastatin ◄►◄ rifamycins
Lescol   rifabutin, rifampin, rifapentine

Risk rating: 2
Severity: **Moderate**   Onset: **Delayed**   Likelihood: **Suspected**

Cause
Rifamycins may induce CYP3A4 metabolism of HMG-CoA reductase inhibitors, such as fluvastatin, in the intestine and liver.

Effect
Fluvastatin effects may decrease.

Nursing considerations
■ Assess response to therapy. If you suspect an interaction, consult prescriber or pharmacist; patient may need a different drug.
■ Check serum cholesterol and lipid levels.
■ Obtain liver function test results at start of therapy and periodically thereafter. If ALT or AST level stays three times or more above upper limit of normal, fluvastatin will need to be stopped.
◼ ALERT Withhold fluvastatin temporarily if patient's risk of myopathy or rhabdomyolysis increases, for example, if he has sepsis, hypotension, major surgery, trauma, uncontrolled seizures, or a severe metabolic, endocrine, or electrolyte disorder.
■ Pravastatin is an HMG-CoA reductase inhibitor less likely to interact with rifamycins; it may be the best choice for combined use.

---

fluvoxamine ▸◀ hydantoins
Luvox

ethotoin, fosphenytoin, phenytoin

Risk rating: 2
Severity: Moderate   **Onset: Delayed**   **Likelihood: Suspected**

Cause
Fluvoxamine may inhibit CYP2C9 and CYP2C19 metabolism of hydantoins.

Effect
Hydantoin level and risk of toxic effects may increase.

Nursing considerations
■ Monitor serum hydantoin level. Therapeutic range for phenytoin is 10 to 20 mcg/ml.
■ Hydantoin dosage may need adjustment.
■ When fluvoxamine starts, watch for hydantoin toxicity: drowsiness, nausea, vomiting, nystagmus, ataxia, dysarthria, tremor, slurred speech, hypotension, arrhythmias, respiratory depression, and coma.
■ If patient takes fosphenytoin, the metabolites formate and phosphate may add to signs of toxicity. Formate toxicity is similar to methanol toxicity. An increased phosphate level may cause hypocalcemia with paresthesia, muscle spasms, and seizures.
■ When fluvoxamine stops, watch for loss of anticonvulsant effect and increased seizure activity.

fluvoxamine ➤◀ MAO inhibitors

Luvox

isocarboxazid, phenelzine, selegiline, tranylcypromine

Risk rating: 1
Severity: Major   **Onset: Rapid**   **Likelihood: Probable**

Cause
Serotonin may accumulate rapidly in the CNS.

Effect
Risk of serotonin syndrome increases.

Nursing considerations
◪ ALERT Don't use these drugs together.
■ Allow 2 weeks after stopping fluvoxamine before giving an MAO inhibitor. Allow 2 weeks after stopping an MAO inhibitor before giving an SSRI, such as fluvoxamine.
■ The selective MAO type-B inhibitor selegiline has been given with fluoxetine, paroxetine, or sertraline to patients with Parkinson's disease without negative effects.
■ Describe the traits of serotonin syndrome, including CNS irritability, motor weakness, shivering, myoclonus, and altered consciousness.
■ Urge patient to promptly report adverse effects.

fluvoxamine ➤◀ selective 5-HT$_1$ receptor agonists

Luvox

almotriptan, eletriptan, frovatriptan, naratriptan, rizatriptan, sumatriptan, zolmitriptan

Risk rating: 1
Severity: Major   **Onset: Rapid**   **Likelihood: Suspected**

Cause
Serotonin may accumulate rapidly in the CNS.

Effect
Risk of serotonin syndrome increases.

Nursing considerations
◪ ALERT If possible, avoid combined use of these drugs.
■ Start with lowest dosages possible, and assess patient closely.
■ Stop the selective 5-HT$_1$ receptor agonist at first sign of interaction.

- In some patients, migraine frequency may increase and antimigraine drug efficacy may decrease when an SSRI, such as fluvoxamine, is started.
- Describe traits of serotonin syndrome: CNS irritability, motor weakness, shivering, muscle twitching, and altered consciousness.
- Explain that serotonin syndrome can be fatal if not treated immediately.

fluvoxamine ━━▶◀━━ sibutramine
Luvox   Meridia

Risk rating: 1
Severity: Major   **Onset: Rapid**   **Likelihood: Suspected**

Cause
Serotonin may accumulate rapidly in the CNS.

Effect
Risk of serotonin syndrome increases.

Nursing considerations
⚡ ALERT If possible, don't give these drugs together.
- Watch carefully for adverse effects; they need immediate attention.
- Describe traits of serotonin syndrome: CNS irritability, motor weakness, shivering, muscle twitching, and altered consciousness.
- Explain that serotonin syndrome can be fatal if not treated immediately.

fluvoxamine ━━▶◀━━ St. John's wort
Luvox

Risk rating: 2
Severity: Moderate   **Onset: Rapid**   **Likelihood: Suspected**

Cause
St. John's wort may cause additive inhibition of serotonin reuptake.

Effect
Sedative-hypnotic effects of SSRIs, such as fluvoxamine, may increase.

Nursing considerations
⚡ ALERT Discourage use of St. John's wort with an SSRI.
- Explain the dangers of this combination.
- In addition to oversedation, mild serotonin-like symptoms may occur, including anxiety, dizziness, nausea, restlessness, and vomiting.
- Urge patient to consult prescriber before taking any herb.

fluvoxamine ▶◀ sympathomimetics

Luvox

amphetamine,
dextroamphetamine,
methamphetamine,
phentermine

Risk rating: 1
Severity: Major   **Onset: Rapid**   **Likelihood: Suspected**

Cause
The mechanism of this interaction is unknown.

Effect
Sympathomimetic effects and risk of serotonin syndrome increase.

Nursing considerations
■ Watch closely for increased CNS effects, such as anxiety, jitteriness, agitation, and restlessness.
■ Mild serotonin-like symptoms may develop, including anxiety, dizziness, restlessness, nausea, and vomiting.
■ Inform patient of the risk of interaction and the need to avoid sympathomimetics.
■ Describe the traits of serotonin syndrome, including CNS irritability, motor weakness, shivering, myoclonus, and altered consciousness.

fluvoxamine ▶◀ tacrine

Luvox

Cognex

Risk rating: 2
Severity: Moderate   **Onset: Delayed**   **Likelihood: Suspected**

Cause
Fluvoxamine may inhibit CYP1A2 metabolism of tacrine.

Effect
Tacrine level, effects, and adverse effects may increase.

Nursing considerations
■ Avoid use together if possible.
■ If combined use can't be avoided, watch for tacrine toxicity: nausea, vomiting, salivation, sweating, bradycardia, hypotension, and seizures.
◪ **ALERT** Watch for progressive muscle weakness (a symptom of tacrine toxicity), which can be fatal if respiratory muscles are involved.
■ Monitor liver function tests. Urge patient to report signs of hepatotoxicity: abdominal pain, loss of appetite, fatigue, yellow skin or eye discoloration, and dark urine.

■ Consult prescriber or pharmacist ; SSRIs that aren't metabolized by CYP1A2 metabolism, such as fluoxetine, may be safer alternatives.

fluvoxamine ▶◀ theophyllines
Luvox   aminophylline, theophylline

Risk rating: 2
Severity: Moderate   Onset: Delayed   Likelihood: Suspected

Cause
Fluvoxamine inhibits hepatic CYP1A2 metabolism of theophylline.

Effect
Theophylline level and risk of toxicity may increase.

Nursing considerations
■ When adding fluvoxamine to regimen, monitor theophylline level closely. Therapeutic range is 10 to 20 mcg/ml for adults and 5 to 15 mcg/ml for children.
■ If patient who takes fluvoxamine starts theophylline, theophylline dosage may be reduced by 33%.
■ Watch for evidence of toxicity: tachycardia, anorexia, nausea, vomiting, diarrhea, seizures, restlessness, irritability, and headache.
■ Describe adverse effects of theophylline and signs of toxicity, and tell patient to report them immediately.

fluvoxamine ▶◀ tricyclic antidepressants
Luvox   amitriptyline, clomipramine,
                         imipramine, trimipramine

Risk rating: 2
Severity: Moderate   Onset: Delayed   Likelihood: Probable

Cause
Fluvoxamine may inhibit oxidative metabolism of tricyclic antidepressants (TCAs) via CYP2D6 pathway.

Effect
TCA level and risk of toxicity increase.

Nursing considerations
■ If combined use can't be avoided, TCA dosage may be decreased.
■ When starting or stopping fluvoxamine, monitor serum TCA level.
■ Report evidence of toxicity or increased TCA level.
■ Inhibitory effects of fluvoxamine may take up to 2 weeks to dissipate after drug is stopped.

■ Using the TCA desipramine may avoid this interaction.
■ Urge patient and family to watch for and report increased anticholinergic effects, dizziness, drowsiness, and psychosis.

---

folic acid ◄► hydantoins
Folvite   ethotoin, fosphenytoin,
                                     phenytoin

Risk rating: 2
Severity: Moderate   Onset: Delayed   Likelihood: Suspected

Cause
The mechanism of this interaction is unknown but probably involves altered metabolic process.

Effect
Hydantoin level and effects may decrease.

Nursing considerations
■ Monitor hydantoin level. Therapeutic range for phenytoin is 10 to 20 mcg/ml.
■ Hydantoin dosage may need adjustment.
■ If folic acid is started during hydantoin therapy, watch for loss of anticonvulsant effect and increased seizure activity.
■ If folic acid is stopped during hydantoin therapy, watch for evidence of hydantoin toxicity: drowsiness, nausea, vomiting, nystagmus, ataxia, dysarthria, tremor, slurred speech, hypotension, arrhythmias, respiratory depression, and coma.
■ Urge patient to tell prescriber about increased adverse effects.

---

foscarnet ◄► cyclosporine
Foscavir   Gengraf, Neoral, Sandimmune

Risk rating: 1
Severity: Major   Onset: Delayed   Likelihood: Suspected

Cause
Synergistic drug effects may cause nephrotoxicity.

Effect
Risk of renal failure may be increased.

Nursing considerations
■ Base foscarnet dosage on patient's renal function.
■ Expect cyclosporine level to stay within normal limits.

- Monitor renal function carefully.
- If nephrotoxicity occurs, foscarnet may need to be stopped.
- Nephrotoxicity should resolve once foscarnet is stopped.

fosinopril ▶◀ indomethacin
Monopril   Indocin

Risk rating: 2
Severity: Moderate   **Onset: Rapid**   **Likelihood: Probable**

Cause
Indomethacin inhibits synthesis of prostaglandins, which fosinopril and other ACE inhibitors need to lower blood pressure.

Effect
ACE inhibitor's hypotensive effect decreases.

Nursing considerations
⚡ **ALERT** Monitor blood pressure closely. Severe hypertension may persist until indomethacin is stopped.
- If indomethacin can't be avoided, patient may need a different antihypertensive.
- Other ACE inhibitors may interact with indomethacin. If you suspect an interaction, consult prescriber or pharmacist.
- Remind patient that hypertension commonly causes no physical symptoms but sometimes may cause headache and dizziness.

fosinopril ▶◀ potassium-sparing diuretics
Monopril

amiloride, spironolactone, triamterene

Risk rating: 1
Severity: Major   **Onset: Delayed**   **Likelihood: Probable**

Cause
The mechanism of this interaction is unknown.

Effect
Potassium level may increase.

Nursing considerations
- Use cautiously in patients at high risk for hyperkalemia, especially those with renal impairment.
- Monitor BUN, creatinine, and serum potassium levels as needed.

■ ACE inhibitors other than fosinopril may interact with potassium-sparing diuretics. If you suspect an interaction, consult prescriber or pharmacist.

■ Urge patient to immediately report an irregular heartbeat, a slow pulse, weakness, and other evidence of hyperkalemia.

---

fosinopril 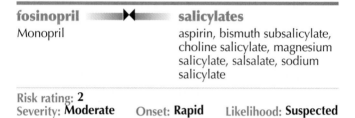 salicylates

Monopril

aspirin, bismuth subsalicylate, choline salicylate, magnesium salicylate, salsalate, sodium salicylate

Risk rating: 2
Severity: Moderate   **Onset: Rapid**   **Likelihood: Suspected**

Cause
Salicylates inhibit synthesis of prostaglandins, which fosinopril and other ACE inhibitors need to lower blood pressure.

Effect
ACE inhibitor's hypotensive effect will decrease.

Nursing considerations
■ This interaction is more likely in people with hypertension, coronary artery disease, or possibly heart failure.

---

fosphenytoin 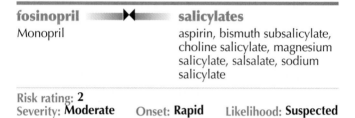 corticosteroids

Cerebyx

betamethasone, corticotropin, cortisone, cosyntropin, dexamethasone, fludrocortisone, hydrocortisone, methylprednisolone, prednisolone, prednisone, triamcinolone

Risk rating: 2
Severity: Moderate   **Onset: Delayed**   **Likelihood: Established**

Cause
Fosphenytoin and other hydantoins induce liver enzymes, which stimulate corticosteroid metabolism. Dexamethasone may enhance hepatic clearance of phenytoin.

Effect
Corticosteroid effects may be decreased.

Nursing considerations
- Avoid giving hydantoins with corticosteroids if possible.
- Watch for decreased corticosteroid effects, and monitor phenytoin level.
- Corticosteroid effects may decrease within days of starting hydantoin and may stay decreased 3 weeks after it stops.
- Dosage of one or both drugs may need to be increased.

fosphenytoin ▶◀ fluvoxamine
Cerebyx   Luvox

Risk rating: 2
Severity: Moderate   **Onset: Delayed**   **Likelihood: Suspected**

Cause
Fluvoxamine may inhibit CYP2C9 and CYP2C19 metabolism of hydantoins, such as fosphenytoin.

Effect
Serum hydantoin level and risk of toxic effects may increase.

Nursing considerations
- Monitor hydantoin level. Therapeutic range for phenytoin is 10 to 20 mcg/ml.
- Hydantoin dosage may need adjustment.
- When fluvoxamine starts, watch for hydantoin toxicity: drowsiness, nausea, vomiting, nystagmus, ataxia, dysarthria, tremor, slurred speech, hypotension, arrhythmias, respiratory depression, and coma.
- With fosphenytoin, the metabolites formate and phosphate may add to signs of toxicity. Formate toxicity is similar to methanol toxicity. An increased phosphate level may cause hypocalcemia with paresthesia, muscle spasms, and seizures.
- When fluvoxamine stops, watch for loss of anticonvulsant effect and increased seizure activity.

fosphenytoin ▶◀ folic acid
Cerebyx   Folvite

Risk rating: 2
Severity: Moderate   **Onset: Delayed**   **Likelihood: Suspected**

Cause
The mechanism of this interaction is unknown but probably involves altered metabolic process.

Effect
Level and effects of hydantoin, such as fosphenytoin, may decrease.

Nursing considerations
- Monitor hydantoin level. Therapeutic range for phenytoin is 10 to 20 mcg/ml.
- Hydantoin dosage may need adjustment.
- If folic acid is started during hydantoin therapy, watch for loss of anticonvulsant effect and increased seizure activity.
- If folic acid is stopped during hydantoin therapy, watch for signs of hydantoin toxicity: drowsiness, nausea, vomiting, nystagmus, ataxia, dysarthria, tremor, slurred speech, hypotension, arrhythmias, respiratory depression, and coma.
- Urge patient to tell prescriber about increased adverse effects.

---

fosphenytoin ➤◄ methadone
Cerebyx   Dolophine, Methadose

Risk rating: 2
Severity: Moderate   Onset: Delayed   Likelihood: Suspected

Cause
The mechanism of this interaction is unknown but probably involves altered metabolic process.

Effect
Level and effects of hydantoin, such as fosphenytoin, may decrease.

Nursing considerations
- Monitor hydantoin level. Therapeutic range for phenytoin is 10 to 20 mcg/ml.
- Hydantoin dosage may need adjustment.
- If methadone is started during hydantoin therapy, watch for loss of anticonvulsant effect and increased seizure activity.
- If methadone is stopped during hydantoin therapy, watch for evidence of hydantoin toxicity: drowsiness, nausea, vomiting, nystagmus, ataxia, dysarthria, tremor, slurred speech, hypotension, arrhythmias, respiratory depression, and coma.
- Urge patient to tell prescriber about increased adverse effects.

fosphenytoin ◄►◄ mirtazapine
Cerebyx   Remeron

Risk rating: 2
Severity: Moderate   **Onset: Delayed**   **Likelihood: Suspected**

Cause
Fosphenytoin and other hydantoins may increase CYP3A3 and CYP3A4 metabolism of mirtazapine.

Effect
Mirtazapine level and effects may decrease.

Nursing considerations
■ Assess patient for expected mirtazapine effects, including improvement of depression and stabilization of mood.
■ Record mood changes, and monitor patient for suicidal tendencies.
■ If a hydantoin starts, mirtazapine dosage may need to be increased.
■ If a hydantoin stops, watch for mirtazapine toxicity: disorientation, drowsiness, impaired memory, tachycardia, severe hypotension, heart failure, seizures, CNS depression, and coma.
■ Urge patient to tell prescriber about increased adverse effects.

fosphenytoin ◄►◄ sertraline
Cerebyx   Zoloft

Risk rating: 2
Severity: Moderate   **Onset: Delayed**   **Likelihood: Suspected**

Cause
Sertraline may inhibit metabolism of hydantoin, such as fosphenytoin.

Effect
Hydantoin level, effects, and risk of toxicity may increase.

Nursing considerations
■ Monitor hydantoin level. Therapeutic range for phenytoin is 10 to 20 mcg/ml.
■ Hydantoin dosage may need adjustment.
■ If sertraline starts during hydantoin therapy, watch for evidence of hydantoin toxicity: drowsiness, nausea, vomiting, nystagmus, ataxia, dysarthria, tremor, slurred speech, hypotension, arrhythmias, respiratory depression, and coma.
■ If sertraline stops during hydantoin therapy, watch for decreased anticonvulsant effect and increased seizure activity.
■ Urge patient to tell prescriber about increased adverse effects.

fosphenytoin 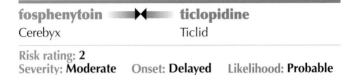 ticlopidine
Cerebyx   Ticlid

Risk rating: 2
Severity: Moderate   Onset: Delayed   Likelihood: Probable

Cause
Ticlopidine may inhibit hepatic metabolism of hydantoins, such as fosphenytoin.

Effect
Hydantoin level and risk of adverse effects may increase.

Nursing considerations
■ Monitor hydantoin level. Therapeutic range for phenytoin is 10 to 20 mcg/ml.
■ Hydantoin level may increase gradually over a month.
■ Hydantoin dosage may need adjustment.
■ If ticlopidine starts during hydantoin therapy, watch for adverse CNS effects of hydantoins, including vertigo, ataxia, and somnolence.
■ If ticlopidine stops during hydantoin therapy, watch for decreased anticonvulsant effect and increased seizure activity.

frovatriptan ◄►► ergot derivatives
Frova   dihydroergotamine, ergotamine

Risk rating: 1
Severity: Major   Onset: Rapid   Likelihood: Suspected

Cause
Combined use may have additive effects.

Effect
Risk of vasospastic effects increases.

Nursing considerations
◤ **ALERT** Use of these drugs or any two selective 5-HT$_1$ receptor agonists within 24 hours of each other is contraindicated.
■ Combined use may cause severe vasospastic effects, including sustained coronary artery vasospasm that triggers MI.
■ Warn patient not to mix migraine headache drugs within 24 hours of each other, but to call prescriber if a drug isn't effective.

frovatriptan ▬▶◀▬ serotonin reuptake inhibitors

Frova

citalopram, fluoxetine, fluvoxamine, nefazodone, paroxetine, sertraline, venlafaxine

Risk rating: 1
Severity: Major   **Onset: Rapid**   **Likelihood: Suspected**

Cause
Serotonin may accumulate rapidly in the CNS.

Effect
Risk of serotonin syndrome increases.

Nursing considerations
◖ ALERT If possible, avoid combined use of these drugs.
■ Start with lowest dosages possible, and assess patient closely.
■ Stop frovatriptan, a selective 5-HT$_1$ receptor agonist, at the first sign of interaction, and start an antiserotonergic.
■ In some patients, migraine frequency may increase and antimigraine drug efficacy may decrease when a serotonin reuptake inhibitor is started.
■ Describe traits of serotonin syndrome: CNS irritability, motor weakness, shivering, muscle twitching, and altered consciousness.
■ Explain that serotonin syndrome can be fatal if not treated immediately.

furosemide ▬▶◀▬ aminoglycosides

Lasix

amikacin, gentamicin, kanamycin, neomycin, netilmicin, streptomycin, tobramycin

Risk rating: 1
Severity: Major   **Onset: Rapid**   **Likelihood: Suspected**

Cause
The mechanism of this interaction is unknown.

Effect
Synergistic ototoxicity may cause hearing loss of varying degrees, possibly permanent.

Nursing considerations
⚠ ALERT Patients with renal insufficiency are at increased risk for ototoxicity.

■ Perform baseline and periodic hearing function tests.

■ Other aminoglycosides may interact with loop diuretics, such as furosemide. If you suspect an interaction, consult prescriber or pharmacist.

■ Tell patient to immediately report ringing or roaring in the ears, muffled sounds, or any noticeable changes in hearing.

■ Advise family members to stay alert for evidence of hearing loss.

---

furosemide ━━━▶◀━━━ bile acid sequestrants

Lasix   cholestyramine, colestipol

Risk rating: 2
Severity: Moderate   **Onset: Rapid**   **Likelihood: Suspected**

Cause
Bile acid sequestrant may inhibit furosemide absorption.

Effect
Furosemide effects may decrease.

Nursing considerations
■ Separate doses; bile acid sequestrant should be taken at least 2 hours after furosemide.

■ If you suspect an interaction, consult prescriber or pharmacist.

■ Monitor patient for expected furosemide effects: reduction in peripheral edema, resolution of pulmonary edema, or decreased blood pressure in hypertensive patients.

■ If patient needs furosemide, consult prescriber or pharmacist about a different cholesterol-lowering drug.

■ Help patient develop a plan to ensure proper dosage intervals.

---

furosemide ━━━▶◀━━━ cisplatin

Lasix   Platinol

Risk rating: 2
Severity: Moderate   **Onset: Rapid**   **Likelihood: Suspected**

Cause
The mechanism of this interaction is unknown.

Effect
Additive ototoxicity may be much more severe than that of either drug used alone, causing permanent hearing loss.

Nursing considerations
■ If possible, avoid giving loop diuretics, such as furosemide, with cisplatin.
■ Obtain hearing tests to detect early hearing loss.
■ Tell patient to report ringing in the ears, change in balance, or muffled sounds. Also, ask family members to watch for changes.

---

furosemide ■━━►◄━━ thiazide diuretics
Lasix

chlorothiazide, hydrochlorothiazide, indapamide, methyclothiazide, metolazone, polythiazide, trichlormethiazide

Risk rating: 2
Severity: **Moderate**   Onset: **Rapid**   Likelihood: **Probable**

Cause
The mechanism of this interaction is unclear.

Effect
Synergistic effects may cause profound diuresis and serious electrolyte abnormalities.

Nursing considerations
■ These drugs may be used together for therapeutic benefit.
■ Expect increased sodium, potassium, and chloride excretion and greater diuresis during combined therapy.
■ Monitor patient for dehydration and electrolyte abnormalities.
■ Adjust drugs carefully, using small or intermittent doses.

---

gatifloxacin ■━━►◄━━ antiarrhythmics
Tequin

amiodarone, bretylium, disopyramide, procainamide, quinidine, sotalol

Risk rating: 1
Severity: **Major**   Onset: **Delayed**   Likelihood: **Suspected**

Cause
The mechanism of this interaction is unknown.

Effect
Risk of life-threatening arrhythmias, including torsades de pointes, increases when certain quinolones, such as gatifloxacin, are combined with antiarrhythmics.

Nursing considerations
■ Avoid giving class IA or class III antiarrhythmics with gatifloxacin.
■ Quinolones that aren't metabolized by CYP3A4 isoenzymes or that don't prolong the QT interval may be given with antiarrhythmics.
■ Monitor ECG for prolonged QTc interval.
■ Tell patient to report a rapid heartbeat, shortness of breath, dizziness, fainting, and chest pain.

---

gatifloxacin ▶◀ erythromycin
Tequin   E-mycin, Eryc

Risk rating: 1
Severity: Major   **Onset: Delayed**   **Likelihood: Suspected**

Cause
The mechanism of this interaction is unknown.

Effect
Risk of life-threatening arrhythmias, including torsades de pointes, increases when certain quinolones, such as gatifloxacin, are combined with erythromycin.

Nursing considerations
■ Use gatifloxacin cautiously with erythromycin.
■ Monitor QTc interval closely.
■ Tell patient to report palpitations, dizziness, shortness of breath, and chest pain.

---

gatifloxacin ▶◀ phenothiazines
Tequin   chlorpromazine, fluphenazine,
                                    mesoridazine, perphenazine,
                                    prochlorperazine,
                                    promethazine, thioridazine

Risk rating: 1
Severity: Major   **Onset: Delayed**   **Likelihood: Suspected**

Cause
The mechanism of this interaction is unknown.

Effect
Risk of life-threatening arrhythmias, including torsades de pointes, may increase when certain quinolones, such as gatifloxacin, are combined with phenothiazines.

Nursing considerations
▪ Use gatifloxacin cautiously, with increased monitoring.
▪ Quinolones that don't prolong the QTc interval or that aren't metabolized by CYP3A4 isoenzymes may be better alternatives.

---

gatifloxacin ➤◀ tricyclic antidepressants

Tequin

amitriptyline, amoxapine, clomipramine, desipramine, doxepin, imipramine, nortriptyline, trimipramine

Risk rating: 1
Severity: Major   **Onset: Delayed**   **Likelihood: Suspected**

Cause
The mechanism of this interaction is unknown.

Effect
Life-threatening arrhythmias, including torsades de pointes, may increase when certain quinolones, such as gatifloxacin, are combined with tricyclic antidepressants (TCAs).

Nursing considerations
▪ Use gatifloxacin cautiously with TCAs.
▪ If possible, use other quinolone antibiotics that don't prolong the QTc interval or aren't metabolized by the CYP3A4 isoenzyme.

---

gemfibrozil ➤◀ HMG-CoA reductase inhibitors

Lopid

atorvastatin, fluvastatin, lovastatin, pravastatin, rosuvastatin, simvastatin

Risk rating: 1
Severity: Major   **Onset: Delayed**   **Likelihood: Suspected**

Cause
The mechanism of this interaction is unknown.

Effect
Severe myopathy or rhabdomyolysis may occur.

Nursing considerations
⚠ **ALERT** Avoid use together.
▪ If patient has severe hyperlipidemia, combined therapy may be an option, but only with careful monitoring.

■ Assess patient for evidence of rhabdomyolysis: fatigue; muscle aches and weakness; joint pain; dark, red, or cola-colored urine; weight gain; seizures; and greatly increased CK level.

■ Watch for evidence of acute renal failure: decreased urine output, elevated BUN and creatinine levels, edema, dyspnea, tachycardia, distended neck veins, nausea, vomiting, poor appetite, weakness, fatigue, confusion, and agitation.

■ Urge patient to report muscle pain, tenderness, or weakness.

---

gentamicin ━━━▸◂━━━ cephalosporins

Garamycin | cefazolin, cefoperazone, cefotaxime, cefotetan, cefoxitin, ceftazidime, ceftizoxime, ceftriaxone, cefuroxime, cephradine

Risk rating: 2
Severity: **Moderate**   Onset: **Delayed**   Likelihood: **Suspected**

Cause
The mechanism of this interaction is unknown.

Effect
Bactericidal activity may increase against some organisms, but the risk of nephrotoxicity also may increase.

Nursing considerations
◙ ALERT Check peak and trough gentamicin levels after third dose. For peak level, draw blood 30 minutes after an I.V. or 60 minutes after an I.M. dose. For trough level, draw blood just before a dose.

■ Assess BUN and creatinine levels.

■ Monitor urine output, and check urine for increased protein, cell, or cast levels.

■ If renal insufficiency develops, notify prescriber. Dosage may need to be reduced, or drug may need to be stopped.

■ Aminoglycosides other than gentamicin may interact with cephalosporins. If you suspect an interaction, consult prescriber or pharmacist.

gentamicin ▸◂ loop diuretics

Garamycin

bumetanide, ethacrynic acid, furosemide, torsemide

Risk rating: 1
Severity: Major   **Onset: Rapid**   **Likelihood: Suspected**

Cause
The mechanism of this interaction is unknown.

Effect
Synergistic ototoxicity may cause hearing loss of varying degrees, possibly permanent.

Nursing considerations
⚠ **ALERT** Patients with renal insufficiency are at increased risk for ototoxicity.
■ Perform baseline and periodic hearing function tests.
■ Aminoglycosides other than gentamicin may interact with loop diuretics. If you suspect an interaction, consult prescriber or pharmacist.
■ Tell patient to immediately report ringing or roaring in the ears, muffled sounds, or any noticeable changes in hearing.
■ Advise family members to stay alert for evidence of hearing loss.

gentamicin ▸◂ nondepolarizing muscle relaxants

Garamycin

atracurium, mivacurium, pancuronium, rocuronium, vecuronium

Risk rating: 1
Severity: Major   **Onset: Rapid**   **Likelihood: Probable**

Cause
These drugs may be synergistic.

Effect
Effects of nondepolarizing muscle relaxants may increase.

Nursing considerations
■ Give these drugs together only when needed.
■ The nondepolarizing muscle relaxant dose may need adjustment based on neuromuscular response.
■ Monitor patient for prolonged respiratory depression.
■ Provide ventilatory support as needed.

gentamicin ━━━━▶◀━━━━ NSAIDs

Garamycin

diclofenac, etodolac,
fenoprofen, flurbiprofen,
ibuprofen, indomethacin,
ketoprofen, ketorolac,
meclofenamate, nabumetone,
naproxen, oxaprozin,
piroxicam, sulindac, tolmetin

Risk rating: 2
Severity: Moderate   Onset: Delayed   Likelihood: Suspected

Cause
NSAIDs may reduce glomerular filtration rate (GFR), causing aminoglycosides, such as gentamicin, to accumulate.

Effect
Aminoglycoside level in premature infants may increase.

Nursing considerations
■ Before NSAID therapy starts, aminoglycoside dose should be reduced.
◤ ALERT Check aminoglycoside peak and trough levels after third dose. For peak level, draw blood 30 minutes after I.V. or 60 minutes after I.M. dose. For trough level, draw blood just before a dose.
■ Monitor patient's renal function.
■ Although only indomethacin is known to interact with aminoglycosides, other NSAIDs probably do as well. If you suspect an interaction, consult prescriber or pharmacist.
■ Other drugs cleared by GFR may have a similar interaction.

gentamicin ━━━━▶◀━━━━ penicillins

Garamycin

ampicillin, nafcillin, oxacillin,
penicillin G, piperacillin,
ticarcillin

Risk rating: 2
Severity: Moderate   Onset: Delayed   Likelihood: Probable

Cause
The mechanism of this interaction is unknown.

Effect
Penicillins may inactivate certain aminoglycosides, such as gentamicin, decreasing their therapeutic effects.

Nursing considerations

⚠ ALERT Check peak and trough aminoglycoside levels after third dose. For peak level, draw blood 30 minutes after I.V. or 60 minutes after I.M. dose. For trough level, draw blood just before a dose.

■ Penicillin affects gentamicin more than amikacin and netilmicin.

■ Monitor patient's renal function.

■ Other aminoglycosides may interact with penicillins. If you suspect an interaction, consult prescriber or pharmacist.

---

gentamicin ▬▬▬►◄▬▬ succinylcholine

Garamycin   Anectine, Quelicin

Risk rating: 2
Severity: Moderate   Onset: Rapid   Likelihood: Probable

Cause

Gentamicin and other aminoglycosides may stabilize the postjunctional membrane and disrupt prejunctional calcium influx and acetylcholine output, causing a synergistic interaction with succinylcholine.

Effect

Neuromuscular effects of succinylcholine are potentiated.

Nursing considerations

■ After succinylcholine use, delay aminoglycoside delivery as long as possible after adequate respirations return.

■ If drugs must be given together, use extreme caution, and monitor respiratory status closely.

⚠ ALERT Patients with renal impairment and those receiving aminoglycosides by peritoneal instillation have an increased risk of prolonged neuromuscular blockade.

■ If respiratory depression occurs, patient may need mechanical ventilation. Give I.V. calcium or a cholinesterase inhibitor if needed.

---

glimepiride ▬▬▬►◄▬▬ fluconazole

Amaryl   Diflucan

Risk rating: 2
Severity: Moderate   Onset: Delayed   Likelihood: Suspected

Cause

Fluconazole may inhibit CYP2C9 metabolism of certain sulfonylureas, such as glimepiride.

Effect
Hypoglycemic effect may increase.

Nursing considerations
- Monitor blood glucose level.
- Watch for evidence of hypoglycemia: tingling of lips and tongue, nausea, vomiting, epigastric pain, lethargy, confusion, agitation, tachycardia, diaphoresis, tremor, seizures, and coma.
- Other sulfonylureas may interact with fluconazole. If you suspect an interaction, consult prescriber or pharmacist.
- If patient takes a sulfonylurea, consult prescriber about a different antifungal.
- Urge patient to monitor blood glucose level at home and to report increased episodes of hypoglycemia.

---

glimepiride ◄► salicylates
Amaryl

aspirin, choline salicylate, magnesium salicylate, salsalate, sodium salicylate, sodium thiosalicylate

Risk rating: 2
Severity: **Moderate**   Onset: **Delayed**   Likelihood: **Probable**

Cause
Salicylates reduce blood glucose level and promote insulin secretion.

Effect
Hypoglycemic effects of sulfonylureas, such as glimepiride, increase.

Nursing considerations
- Start salicylate carefully, monitoring patient for hypoglycemia.
- Consult prescriber and patient about replacing salicylate with acetaminophen or an NSAID.
- Describe signs and symptoms of hypoglycemia, including diaphoresis, fatigue, headache, hunger, irritability, malaise, nervousness, rapid heart rate, tension, and trembling.
- Instruct patient to eat a small carbohydrate snack or meal if hypoglycemia develops, preferably after checking blood glucose level.

glipizide ━━━━▶◀━━━━ alcohol
Glucotrol

Risk rating: 2
Severity: Moderate   Onset: Rapid   Likelihood: Established

Cause
Chronic alcohol use may delay absorption and elimination of sulfo-nylureas, such as glipizide.

Effect
Risk of hypoglycemia increases.

Nursing considerations
▪ Describe consequences of a disulfiram-like reaction: flushing and possible burning of face and neck, headache, nausea, and tachycardia. Explain that it typically occurs within 20 minutes of alcohol intake and lasts for 1 to 2 hours.
▪ Tell patient who takes an oral antidiabetic to avoid ingesting more alcohol than an occasional single drink.
▪ Naloxone may be used to antagonize a disulfiram-like reaction.
▪ Urge patient to have regular follow-up blood tests to monitor diabet-ic status and decrease episodes of hyperglycemia and hypoglycemia.
▪ Other sulfonylureas may interact with alcohol.

glipizide ━━━━▶◀━━━━ chloramphenicol
Glucotrol   Chloromycetin

Risk rating: 2
Severity: Moderate   Onset: Delayed   Likelihood: Suspected

Cause
Chloramphenicol reduces hepatic clearance of sulfonylureas, such as glipizide.

Effect
Prolonged sulfonylurea level may increase risk of hypoglycemia.

Nursing considerations
▪ If patient takes a sulfonylurea, start chloramphenicol carefully, and monitor patient for hypoglycemia.
▪ Describe signs and symptoms of hypoglycemia, including diaphore-sis, fatigue, headache, hunger, irritability, malaise, nervousness, rapid heart rate, tension, and trembling.
▪ Instruct patient to eat a small carbohydrate snack or meal if hypo-glycemia develops, preferably after checking blood glucose level.

glipizide ━━━━▶◀━━━━ diazoxide
Glucotrol   Hyperstat, Proglycem

Risk rating: 2
Severity: Moderate   **Onset: Delayed**   **Likelihood: Probable**

Cause
Diazoxide may decrease insulin release or stimulate release of glucose and free fatty acids by various mechanisms.

Effect
Risk of hyperglycemia increases if a patient stabilized on a sulfonylurea, such as glipizide, starts diazoxide.

Nursing considerations
■ Use these drugs together cautiously.
■ Monitor blood glucose level regularly; consult prescriber about adjustments to either drug to maintain stable glucose level.
■ Tell patient to stay alert for evidence of high blood glucose level, such as increased fatigue, thirst, eating, or urination and possible blurred vision or dry skin and mucous membranes.

glipizide ━━━━▶◀━━━━ MAO inhibitors
Glucotrol   isocarboxazid, phenelzine,
                             tranylcypromine

Risk rating: 2
Severity: Moderate   **Onset: Rapid**   **Likelihood: Suspected**

Cause
The mechanism of this interaction is unknown.

Effect
MAO inhibitors increase the hypoglycemic effects of sulfonylureas, such as glipizide.

Nursing considerations
■ If patient takes a sulfonylurea, start MAO inhibitor carefully, monitoring patient for hypoglycemia.
■ Consult prescriber about adjustments to either drug to control glucose level and mental status.
■ Describe signs and symptoms of hypoglycemia, including diaphoresis, fatigue, headache, hunger, irritability, malaise, nervousness, rapid heart rate, tension, and trembling.
■ Instruct patient to eat a small carbohydrate snack or meal if hypoglycemia develops, preferably after checking blood glucose level.

glipizide ⧓ rifamycins

Glucotrol | rifabutin, rifampin, rifapentine

Risk rating: 2
Severity: Moderate **Onset: Delayed** **Likelihood: Probable**

Cause
Rifamycins may increase hepatic metabolism of certain sulfonylureas, such as glipizide.

Effect
Risk of hyperglycemia increases.

Nursing considerations
- Use these drugs together cautiously.
- Monitor patient's blood glucose level regularly; consult prescriber about adjustments to either drug to maintain stable glucose level.
- Tell patient to stay alert for evidence of high blood glucose level: increased fatigue, thirst, eating, or urination and possible blurred vision or dry skin and mucous membranes.

glipizide ⧓ salicylates

Glucotrol | aspirin, choline salicylate, magnesium salicylate, salsalate, sodium salicylate, sodium thiosalicylate

Risk rating: 2
Severity: Moderate **Onset: Delayed** **Likelihood: Probable**

Cause
Salicylates reduce glucose level and promote insulin secretion.

Effect
Hypoglycemic effects of sulfonylureas, such as glipizide, increase.

Nursing considerations
- If patient takes a sulfonylurea, start salicylate carefully; monitor patient for hypoglycemia.
- Consult prescriber and patient about replacing salicylate with acetaminophen or an NSAID.
- Describe signs and symptoms of hypoglycemia: diaphoresis, fatigue, headache, hunger, irritability, malaise, nervousness, rapid heart rate, tension, and trembling.
- Instruct patient to eat a small carbohydrate snack or meal if hypoglycemia develops, preferably after checking blood glucose level.

glipizide ◀▶ sulfonamides

Glucotrol   sulfasalazine, sulfisoxazole

Risk rating: 2
Severity: Moderate   Onset: Delayed   Likelihood: Suspected

Cause
Sulfonamides may hinder hepatic metabolism of sulfonylureas, such as glipizide.

Effect
Prolonged sulfonylurea level increases risk of hypoglycemia.

Nursing considerations
- If patient takes a sulfonylurea, start sulfonamide carefully; monitor patient for hypoglycemia.
- Monitor patient's blood glucose level regularly; consult prescriber about adjustments to either drug to maintain stable glucose level.
- Describe signs and symptoms of hypoglycemia, including diaphoresis, fatigue, headache, hunger, irritability, malaise, nervousness, rapid heart rate, tension, and trembling.
- Instruct patient to eat a small carbohydrate snack or meal if hypoglycemia develops, preferably after checking blood glucose level.
- Glyburide doesn't interact and may be a good alternative to other sulfonylureas.

glipizide ◀▶ thiazide diuretics

Glucotrol   chlorothiazide,
                              hydrochlorothiazide,
                              indapamide, metolazone

Risk rating: 2
Severity: Moderate   Onset: Delayed   Likelihood: Probable

Cause
Thiazide diuretics may decrease insulin secretion and tissue sensitivity to insulin, and they may increase potassium loss.

Effect
Risk of hyperglycemia and hyponatremia may increase.

Nursing considerations
- Use these drugs together cautiously.
- Monitor patient's blood glucose level regularly; consult prescriber about adjustments to either drug to maintain stable glucose level.
- This interaction may occur several days to many months after dual therapy starts but is readily reversible when the diuretic stops.

■ Describe signs and symptoms of hypoglycemia, including diaphoresis, fatigue, headache, hunger, irritability, malaise, nervousness, rapid heart rate, tension, and trembling.
■ Instruct patient to eat a small carbohydrate snack or meal if hypoglycemia develops, preferably after checking blood glucose level.

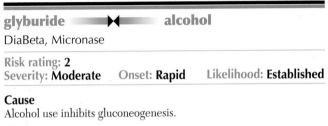

glyburide ▶◀ alcohol
DiaBeta, Micronase

Risk rating: 2
Severity: Moderate   Onset: Rapid   Likelihood: Established

Cause
Alcohol use inhibits gluconeogenesis.

Effect
Risk of hypoglycemia increases.

Nursing considerations
■ Tell patient who takes an oral antidiabetic to avoid ingesting more alcohol than an occasional single drink.
■ Urge patient to have regular follow-up blood tests to monitor diabetes and decrease episodes of hyperglycemia and hypoglycemia.
■ Sulfonylureas other than glyburide also interact with alcohol.

glyburide ▶◀ chloramphenicol
DiaBeta, Micronase   Chloromycetin

Risk rating: 2
Severity: Moderate   Onset: Delayed   Likelihood: Suspected

Cause
Chloramphenicol reduces hepatic clearance of sulfonylureas, such as glyburide.

Effect
Risk of hypoglycemia increases.

Nursing considerations
■ Start chloramphenicol carefully; monitor patient for hypoglycemia.
■ Describe signs and symptoms of hypoglycemia: diaphoresis, fatigue, headache, hunger, irritability, malaise, nervousness, rapid heart rate, tension, and trembling.
■ Instruct patient to eat a small carbohydrate snack or meal if hypoglycemia develops, preferably after checking blood glucose level.

glyburide ▬▬▬►◄ diazoxide
DiaBeta, Micronase   Hyperstat, Proglycem

Risk rating: 2
Severity: Moderate   Onset: Delayed   Likelihood: Probable

Cause
Diazoxide may decrease insulin release or stimulate release of glucose and free fatty acids by various mechanisms.

Effect
Risk of hyperglycemia increases if a patient stabilized on a sulfonylurea, such as glyburide, starts diazoxide.

Nursing considerations
■ Use these drugs together cautiously.
■ Monitor patient's blood glucose level regularly; consult prescriber about adjustments to either drug to maintain stable glucose level.
■ Tell patient to stay alert for evidence of high blood glucose level: increased fatigue, thirst, eating, or urination and possible blurred vision or dry skin and mucous membranes.

glyburide ▬▬▬►◄ MAO inhibitors
DiaBeta, Micronase   isocarboxazid, phenelzine,
                                  tranylcypromine

Risk rating: 2
Severity: Moderate   Onset: Rapid   Likelihood: Suspected

Cause
The mechanism of this interaction is unknown.

Effect
MAO inhibitors increase the hypoglycemic effects of sulfonylureas, such as glyburide.

Nursing considerations
■ Start MAO inhibitor carefully, monitoring patient for hypoglycemia.
■ Consult prescriber about adjustments to either drug to control glucose level and mental status.
■ Describe signs and symptoms of hypoglycemia, including diaphoresis, fatigue, headache, hunger, irritability, malaise, nervousness, rapid heart rate, tension, and trembling.
■ Instruct patient to eat a small carbohydrate snack or meal if hypoglycemia develops, preferably after checking blood glucose level.

glyburide ━━▶◀━━ rifamycins
DiaBeta, Micronase   rifabutin, rifampin, rifapentine

Risk rating: 2
Severity: Moderate   Onset: Delayed   Likelihood: Probable

Cause
Rifamycins may increase hepatic metabolism of certain sulfonylureas, such as glyburide.

Effect
Risk of hyperglycemia increases.

Nursing considerations
- Use these drugs together cautiously.
- Monitor patient's blood glucose level regularly; consult prescriber about adjustments to either drug to maintain stable glucose level.
- Tell patient to stay alert for evidence of high blood glucose level: increased fatigue, thirst, eating, or urination and possible blurred vision or dry skin and mucous membranes.

glyburide ━━▶◀━━ salicylates
DiaBeta, Micronase   aspirin, choline salicylate, magnesium salicylate, salsalate, sodium salicylate, sodium thiosalicylate

Risk rating: 2
Severity: Moderate   Onset: Delayed   Likelihood: Probable

Cause
Salicylates reduce glucose level and promote insulin secretion.

Effect
Hypoglycemic effects of sulfonylureas, such as glyburide, increase.

Nursing considerations
- If patient takes a sulfonylurea, start salicylate carefully, monitoring patient for hypoglycemia.
- Consult prescriber and patient about replacing salicylate with acetaminophen or an NSAID.
- Describe signs and symptoms of hypoglycemia, including diaphoresis, fatigue, headache, hunger, irritability, malaise, nervousness, rapid heart rate, tension, and trembling.
- Instruct patient to eat a small carbohydrate snack or meal if hypoglycemia develops, preferably after checking blood glucose level.

glyburide ▶◀ thiazide diuretics

DiaBeta, Micronase

chlorothiazide,
hydrochlorothiazide,
indapamide, metolazone

Risk rating: 2
Severity: **Moderate**   Onset: **Delayed**   Likelihood: **Probable**

Cause
Thiazide diuretics may decrease insulin secretion and tissue sensitivity to insulin, and they may increase potassium loss.

Effect
Risk of hyperglycemia and hyponatremia may increase.

Nursing considerations
■ Use these drugs together cautiously.
■ Monitor blood glucose level regularly, and consult prescriber about adjustments to either drug to maintain stable glucose level.
■ This interaction may occur several days to many months after dual therapy starts but is readily reversible when the diuretic stops.
■ Describe signs and symptoms of hypoglycemia, including diaphoresis, fatigue, headache, hunger, irritability, malaise, nervousness, rapid heart rate, tension, and trembling.
■ Instruct patient to eat a small carbohydrate snack or meal if hypoglycemia develops, preferably after checking blood glucose level.

haloperidol ▶◀ anticholinergics

Haldol

atropine, belladonna,
benztropine, biperiden,
dicyclomine, glycopyrrolate,
hyoscyamine, mepenzolate,
methscopolamine,
orphenadrine, oxybutynin,
procyclidine, propantheline,
scopolamine, trihexyphenidyl

Risk rating: 2
Severity: **Moderate**   Onset: **Delayed**   Likelihood: **Suspected**

Cause
The mechanism of this interaction is unknown. It may involve central cholinergic pathways rather than a true pharmacokinetic interaction.

Effect
Effects may vary and include decreased haloperidol level, worsened schizophrenic symptoms, and development of tardive dyskinesia.

Nursing considerations
◤ ALERT If patient takes haloperidol, avoid anticholinergics if possible.

▪ Watch for signs of worsening schizophrenia, including delusions, hallucinations, disorganized speech or behavior, inappropriate affect, and abnormal psychomotor activity.

▪ Watch for development of tardive dyskinesia—involuntary abnormal repetitive movements, including lip smacking, cheek puffing, chewing motions, tongue thrusting, finger flicking, and trunk twisting.

▪ Consult prescriber if adverse effects occur; anticholinergic drug may need to be stopped, or haloperidol dosage may need adjustment.

▪ Other anticholinergics may interact with haloperidol. If you suspect an interaction, consult prescriber or pharmacist.

---

haloperidol ◄► carbamazepine
Haldol
Carbatrol, Epitol, Equetro, Tegretol

Risk rating: **2**
Severity: **Moderate**   Onset: **Delayed**   Likelihood: **Suspected**

Cause
Carbamazepine may increase haloperidol hepatic metabolism; haloperidol may inhibit carbamazepine metabolism.

Effect
Haloperidol effects may decrease. Therapeutic and adverse effects of carbamazepine may increase.

Nursing considerations
▪ Assess patient for loss of haloperidol effects: psychomotor agitation, obsessive-compulsive rituals, withdrawn behavior, auditory hallucinations, delusions, and delirium.

▪ Monitor haloperidol level (therapeutic range, 5 to 20 nanograms/ml) and carbamazepine level (therapeutic range, 4 to 12 mcg/ml).

◤ ALERT Watch for signs of anorexia or subtle appetite changes, which may indicate excessive carbamazepine level.

▪ Watch for evidence of carbamazepine toxicity, including dizziness, ataxia, respiratory depression, tachycardia, arrhythmias, blood pressure changes, impaired consciousness, abnormal reflexes, nystagmus, seizures, nausea, vomiting, and urine retention.

▪ If adverse effects occur, consult prescriber; dosages of one or both drugs may need adjustment.

haloperidol ━━▶◀━━ lithium
Haldol   Eskalith

Risk rating: 1
Severity: Major   **Onset: Delayed**   **Likelihood: Suspected**

Cause
The exact mechanism of this interaction is unknown.

Effect
Patient may have altered level of consciousness, encephalopathy, extrapyramidal effects, fever, leukocytosis, and increased enzyme levels.

Nursing considerations
⚠ **ALERT** Monitor patient closely, especially the first 3 weeks.
- Watch for early evidence of neurologic toxicity, such as altered mental status, rigidity, or hyperpyrexia; treatment should be stopped promptly if such signs appear.
- Evidence of more severe neurologic toxicity includes weakness, lethargy, tremulousness, confusion, stupor, fever, severe extrapyramidal symptoms, and dystonias. Some patients may have permanent brain damage.
- Check lab studies for leukocytosis, elevated serum enzyme levels, and increased BUN level. Therapeutic lithium level is 0.6 to 1.2 mEq/L; therapeutic haloperidol level is 5 to 20 nanograms/ml.
- If an interaction occurs, alert prescriber. One or both drugs may need to be stopped. Give supportive treatment for symptoms.

haloperidol ━━▶◀━━ rifamycins
Haldol   rifabutin, rifampin

Risk rating: 2
Severity: Moderate   **Onset: Delayed**   **Likelihood: Suspected**

Cause
Haloperidol metabolism may increase.

Effect
Haloperidol level and effects may decrease.

Nursing considerations
- Watch for expected haloperidol effects if patient starts or stops a rifamycin.
- Monitor haloperidol level (therapeutic range, 5 to 20 nanograms/ml).

■ Watch for loss of haloperidol effects: psychomotor agitation, obsessive-compulsive rituals, withdrawn behavior, auditory hallucinations, delusions, and delirium.
■ Consult prescriber if haloperidol effects decline; haloperidol dosage may need adjustment.
■ Advise patient to tell prescriber about increased adverse effects.

heparin ━━━▶◀━━━ alteplase
Activase, tPA

Risk rating: 1
Severity: **Major**   Onset: **Rapid**   Likelihood: **Suspected**

Cause
The combined effect of this interaction may be greater than the sum of each individual effect.

Effect
Risk of serious bleeding is increased.

Nursing considerations
◪ ALERT Use of heparin with alteplase is contraindicated.
◪ ALERT Use of alteplase in patients with acute ischemic stroke is contraindicated if patient has a bleeding diathesis, use of heparin within 48 hours before onset of stroke, or elevated APTT. This poses an increased risk of bleeding that may cause disability or death.

heparin ━━━▶◀━━━ aspirin
Bayer

Risk rating: 2
Severity: **Moderate**   Onset: **Rapid**   Likelihood: **Probable**

Cause
Aspirin may inhibit platelet aggregation and cause bleeding; this effect may be additive to heparin anticoagulation.

Effect
Risk of bleeding increases.

Nursing considerations
■ Monitor coagulation studies.
■ Assess patient for signs of bleeding: bleeding gums, bruises on arms or legs, petechiae, epistaxis, melena, hematuria, or hematemesis.
■ Advise patient to report signs of bleeding or bruising immediately.

- Provide treatment for symptoms, as needed.
- Urge patient to tell prescriber about increased adverse effects.

hormonal contraceptives ▶◀ barbiturates
amobarbital, butabarbital, pentobarbital, phenobarbital, primidone, secobarbital

Risk rating: 1
Severity: Major   **Onset: Delayed**   **Likelihood: Suspected**

Cause
Barbiturates may induce hepatic metabolism of contraceptives and synthesis of sex-hormone–binding protein.

Effect
Risk of breakthrough bleeding and pregnancy may increase.

Nursing considerations
- Consult prescriber about increasing contraceptive dosage during barbiturate therapy.
- Consult prescriber about alternative treatments for seizures or sleep disturbance.
- Instruct patient to use barrier contraception.

hydralazine ▶◀ beta blockers
Apresoline   metoprolol, propranolol

Risk rating: 2
Severity: Moderate   **Onset: Rapid**   **Likelihood: Probable**

Cause
Hydralazine may cause transient increase in visceral blood flow and decreased first-pass hepatic metabolism of some oral beta blockers.

Effect
Effects of both drugs may increase.

Nursing considerations
- Monitor blood pressure regularly; dosage of both drugs may need adjustment based on patient's response.
- With propranolol, interaction involves only oral, immediate-release form and not extended-release or I.V. drug.
- Other beta blockers may interact with hydralazine. If you suspect an interaction, consult prescriber or pharmacist.

■ Explain that both drugs can affect blood pressure. Urge patient to report evidence of hypotension, such as light-headedness or dizziness when changing positions.

---

hydrochlorothiazide ▶◀ loop diuretics

Microzide   bumetanide, ethacrynic acid, furosemide, torsemide

Risk rating: 2
Severity: Moderate   **Onset: Rapid**   **Likelihood: Probable**

Cause
The mechanism of this interaction is unclear.

Effect
Because these drugs work synergistically, they may cause profound diuresis and serious electrolyte abnormalities.

Nursing considerations
■ These drugs may be used together for therapeutic benefit.
■ Expect increased sodium, potassium, and chloride excretion and greater diuresis during combined therapy.
■ Monitor patient for dehydration and electrolyte abnormalities.
■ Carefully adjust drugs, using small or intermittent doses.

---

hydrochlorothiazide ▶◀ sulfonylureas

Microzide   acetohexamide, chlorpropamide, glipizide, glyburide, tolazamide, tolbutamide

Risk rating: 2
Severity: Moderate   **Onset: Delayed**   **Likelihood: Probable**

Cause
Thiazide diuretics, such as hydrochlorothiazide, may decrease insulin secretion and tissue sensitivity, and may increase potassium loss.

Effect
Risk of hyperglycemia and hyponatremia may increase.

Nursing considerations
■ Use these drugs together cautiously.
■ Check patient's blood glucose level regularly, and consult prescriber about adjustments to either drug to maintain stable glucose level.

■ This interaction may occur several days to many months after dual therapy starts but is readily reversible when the diuretic stops.

■ Describe signs and symptoms of hypoglycemia, including diaphoresis, fatigue, headache, hunger, irritability, malaise, nervousness, rapid heart rate, tension, and trembling.

■ Instruct patient to eat a small carbohydrate snack or meal if hypoglycemia develops, preferably after checking blood glucose level.

hydrocortisone ▪▶◀▪ aprepitant
Cortef   Emend

Risk rating: 2
Severity: Moderate   Onset: Delayed   Likelihood: Suspected

Cause
Aprepitant may inhibit first-pass metabolism of certain corticosteroids, such as hydrocortisone.

Effect
Corticosteroid level may be increased and the half-life prolonged.

Nursing considerations
■ Corticosteroid dosage may need to be decreased.

■ When starting or stopping aprepitant, adjust corticosteroid dosage as needed.

■ Watch closely for evidence of increased corticosteroid level, such as insomnia, euphoria, increased appetite, mood changes, and increased blood glucose level.

■ Tell patient to report symptoms of increased blood glucose level: increased thirst or hunger and increased frequency of urination.

hydrocortisone ▪▶◀▪ barbiturates
Cortef   amobarbital, butabarbital,
                                          pentobarbital, phenobarbital,
                                          primidone, secobarbital

Risk rating: 2
Severity: Moderate   Onset: Delayed   Likelihood: Established

Cause
Barbiturates induce liver enzymes, which stimulate metabolism of corticosteroids, such as hydrocortisone.

Effect
Corticosteroid effects may decrease.

Nursing considerations
- Avoid giving barbiturates with corticosteroids, if possible.
- If patient takes a corticosteroid, watch for worsening symptoms when a barbiturate is started or stopped.
- Corticosteroid dosage may need to be increased.

---

hydrocortisone ▸◂ bile acid sequestrants
Cortef   cholestyramine, colestipol

Risk rating: 2
Severity: Moderate   **Onset: Delayed**   **Likelihood: Suspected**

Cause
Bile acid sequestrants disrupt GI absorption of hydrocortisone.

Effect
Hydrocortisone effects may decrease.

Nursing considerations
- If patient needs hydrocortisone, consider a different cholesterol-lowering drug.
- If drugs must be taken together, separate doses to help improve hydrocortisone absorption, although doing so has no proven effect.
- Check for expected hydrocortisone effects.
- If needed, consult prescriber about increasing hydrocortisone dosage to achieve desired effect.
- Help patient develop a plan to ensure proper dosage intervals.

---

hydrocortisone ▸◂ cholinesterase inhibitors
Cortef   ambenonium, edrophonium, neostigmine, pyridostigmine

Risk rating: 1
Severity: Major   **Onset: Delayed**   **Likelihood: Probable**

Cause
In myasthenia gravis, hydrocortisone and other corticosteroids antagonize cholinesterase inhibitors by an unknown mechanism.

Effect
Patient may develop severe muscular depression refractory to cholinesterase inhibitor.

Nursing considerations
- Corticosteroids may have long-term benefits in myasthenia gravis.
- Combined therapy may be attempted under strict supervision.

■ In myasthenia gravis, watch for severe muscle deterioration.
▶ ALERT Be prepared to provide respiratory support and mechanical ventilation if needed.
■ Consult prescriber or pharmacist about safe corticosteroid delivery to maximize improvement in muscle strength.

hydrocortisone ➤◀ estrogens

Cortef   conjugated estrogens, esterified estrogens, estradiol, estrone, estropipate, ethinyl estradiol

Risk rating: 2
Severity: Moderate   Onset: Delayed   Likelihood: Suspected

Cause
Estrogens may inhibit hepatic metabolism of corticosteroids, such as hydrocortisone.

Effect
Therapeutic and toxic corticosteroid effects may increase.

Nursing considerations
■ Assess response to corticosteroid when given with an estrogen.
■ Watch for corticosteroid toxicity, including nervousness, sleepiness, depression, psychosis, weakness, decreased hearing, edema of lower legs, skin disorders, hypertension, muscle weakness, and seizures.
■ Corticosteroid dosage may need adjustment.
■ Estrogen may continue to affect corticosteroid therapy for an unknown length of time after estrogen is stopped.
■ Other corticosteroids may interact with estrogens. If you suspect an interaction, consult prescriber or pharmacist.
■ Tell patient to report increased adverse effects.

hydrocortisone ➤◀ hydantoins

Cortef   ethotoin, fosphenytoin, phenytoin

Risk rating: 2
Severity: Moderate   Onset: Delayed   Likelihood: Established

Cause
Hydantoins induce liver enzymes, which stimulate metabolism of corticosteroids, such as hydrocortisone.

Effect
Corticosteroid effects may decrease.

Nursing considerations
- Avoid giving hydantoins with corticosteroids if possible.
- If drugs must be given together, monitor patient for decreased corticosteroid effects. Also monitor phenytoin level, and adjust dosage of either drug as needed.
- Corticosteroid effects may decrease within days of starting phenytoin and may stay decreased 3 weeks after it stops.
- Dosage of either or both drugs may need to be increased.

---

hydrocortisone ▶◀ rifamycins
Cortef   rifabutin, rifampin, rifapentine

Risk rating: 1
Severity: Major   **Onset: Delayed**   **Likelihood: Established**

Cause
Rifamycins increase hepatic metabolism of corticosteroids, such as hydrocortisone.

Effect
Corticosteroid effects may decrease.

Nursing considerations
- If possible, avoid giving rifamycins with corticosteroids.
- Monitor patient for decreased corticosteroid effects, including loss of disease control.
- Watch closely for symptom control after increasing rifamycin dose. Drug may need to be stopped to regain control of disease.
- Corticosteroid effects may decrease within days of starting rifampin and may stay decreased 2 to 3 weeks after it stops.
- Corticosteroid dose may need to be doubled after adding rifampin.

---

hydrocortisone ▶◀ salicylates
Cortef   aspirin, bismuth subsalicylate, choline salicylate, magnesium salicylate, salsalate, sodium salicylate, sodium thiosalicylate

Risk rating: 2
Severity: Moderate   **Onset: Delayed**   **Likelihood: Probable**

Cause
Hydrocortisone and other corticosteroids stimulate hepatic metabolism of salicylates and may increase renal excretion.

Effect
Salicylate level and effects decrease.

Nursing considerations
- If patient takes a salicylate and a corticosteroid, monitor salicylate efficacy and level; dosage may need adjustment.
- ◣ ALERT Giving a salicylate while tapering a corticosteroid may result in salicylate toxicity.
- Watch for evidence of salicylate toxicity, including diaphoresis, nausea, vomiting, tinnitus, hyperventilation, and CNS depression.
- Patients with renal impairment may be at greater risk.

---

ibuprofen ➤◄ aminoglycosides
Advil, Motrin

amikacin, gentamicin, kanamycin, netilmicin, streptomycin, tobramycin

Risk rating: 2
Severity: Moderate   **Onset: Delayed**   **Likelihood: Suspected**

Cause
Ibuprofen and other NSAIDs may reduce glomerular filtration rate (GFR), causing aminoglycosides to accumulate.

Effect
Aminoglycoside level in premature infants may increase.

Nursing considerations
- Before NSAID starts, aminoglycoside dose should be reduced.
- ◣ ALERT Check peak and trough aminoglycoside levels after third dose. For peak level, draw blood 30 minutes after I.V. or 60 minutes after I.M. dose. For trough level, draw blood just before a dose.
- Monitor patient's renal function.
- Although only indomethacin is known to interact with aminoglycosides, other NSAIDs probably do as well. If you suspect an interaction, consult prescriber or pharmacist.
- Other drugs cleared by GFR may have a similar interaction.

ibuprofen ━━━▶◀━━━ beta blockers

Advil, Motrin

acebutolol, atenolol, betaxolol, bisoprolol, carteolol, esmolol, metoprolol, nadolol, penbutolol, pindolol, propranolol, sotalol, timolol

Risk rating: **2**
Severity: **Moderate**   Onset: **Delayed**   Likelihood: **Probable**

Cause
Ibuprofen and other NSAIDs may inhibit renal prostaglandin synthesis, allowing pressor systems to be unopposed.

Effect
Beta blocker may not be able to lower blood pressure.

Nursing considerations
- Avoid using these drugs together if possible.
- Monitor blood pressure and related signs and symptoms of hypertension closely.
- Consult prescriber about ways to minimize interaction, such as adjusting beta blocker dosage or switching to sulindac as the NSAID.
- Explain the risks of using these drugs together, and teach patient how to monitor his blood pressure.
- Other NSAIDs may interact with beta blockers. If you suspect an interaction, consult prescriber or pharmacist.

imipenem and cilastatin ━━━▶◀━━━ cyclosporine

Primaxin

Gengraf, Neoral, Sandimmune

Risk rating: **2**
Severity: **Moderate**   Onset: **Rapid**   Likelihood: **Suspected**

Cause
Additive or synergistic toxicity may occur.

Effect
Adverse CNS effects of both drugs may increase.

Nursing considerations
- Watch for adverse CNS effects, including confusion, agitation, and tremors.
- Decreasing cyclosporine dose may decrease risk of adverse effects.
- Consider giving a different antibiotic if an interaction is suspected.

■ Adverse effects should improve after stopping imipenem and cilastatin.

---

imipramine ◀▶ azole antifungals
Tofranil   fluconazole, ketoconazole

Risk rating: 2
Severity: Moderate   **Onset: Delayed**   **Likelihood: Suspected**

Cause
Azole antifungals may inhibit metabolism of imipramine, a tricyclic antidepressant (TCA), by varying CYP pathways.

Effect
Serum TCA level and risk of toxicity may increase.

Nursing considerations
■ When starting or stopping an azole antifungal, monitor serum TCA level and adjust dosage as needed.
■ After starting an azole antifungal, check sitting and standing blood pressure for changes.
■ Assess symptoms and behavior for adverse reactions, such as increased drowsiness, dizziness, confusion, heart rate or rhythm changes, and urine retention.

---

imipramine ◀▶ fluoxetine
Tofranil   Prozac, Sarafem

Risk rating: 2
Severity: Moderate   **Onset: Delayed**   **Likelihood: Probable**

Cause
Fluoxetine may inhibit hepatic metabolism of tricyclic antidepressants (TCAs), such as imipramine.

Effect
TCA level and risk of toxicity may increase.

Nursing considerations
■ Monitor serum TCA level and watch closely for evidence of toxicity, such as increased anticholinergic effects, delirium, dizziness, drowsiness, and psychosis.
■ Report evidence of increased TCA level or toxicity; dosage may need to be decreased.
■ If TCA starts when patient already takes fluoxetine, TCA dosage may need to be decreased by up to 75% to avoid interaction.

■ Other TCAs may interact with fluoxetine. If you suspect an interaction, consult prescriber or pharmacist.

---

imipramine ▸◂ fluvoxamine
Tofranil   Luvox

Risk rating: 2
Severity: Moderate   **Onset: Delayed**   **Likelihood: Probable**

Cause
Fluvoxamine may inhibit oxidative metabolism of tricyclic antidepressants (TCAs), such as imipramine, via CYP2D6 pathway.

Effect
TCA level and risk of toxicity increase.

Nursing considerations
■ If combined use can't be avoided, TCA dosage may need to be decreased.
■ When starting or stopping fluvoxamine, monitor serum TCA level.
■ Report evidence of toxicity or increased TCA level.
■ Inhibitory effects of fluvoxamine may take up to 2 weeks to dissipate after drug is stopped.
■ Using the TCA desipramine may avoid this interaction.
■ Urge patient and family to watch for and report increased anticholinergic effects, dizziness, drowsiness, and psychosis.

---

imipramine ▸◂ levofloxacin
Tofranil   Lavequin

Risk rating: 1
Severity: Major   **Onset: Delayed**   **Likelihood: Suspected**

Cause
The mechanism of this interaction is unknown.

Effect
Life-threatening arrhythmias, including torsades de pointes, may increase.

Nursing considerations
◪ ALERT Avoid giving the quinolone levofloxacin with a tricyclic antidepressant, such as imipramine.
■ If possible, use other quinolone antibiotics that don't prolong the QTc interval or aren't metabolized by the CYP3A4 isoenzyme.

imipramine ►◄ **MAO inhibitors**
Tofranil

isocarboxazid, phenelzine,
tranylcypromine

Risk rating: 1
Severity: Major   Onset: **Rapid**   Likelihood: **Suspected**

Cause
The mechanism of this interaction is unknown.

Effect
Risk of hyperpyretic crisis, seizures, and death increases.

Nursing considerations
⚡ **ALERT** Don't give a tricyclic antidepressant (TCA), such as
imipramine, with or within 2 weeks of an MAO inhibitor.
■ Imipramine and clomipramine may be more likely than other TCAs
to interact with MAO inhibitors.
■ Watch for adverse effects, including confusion, hyperexcitability,
rigidity, seizures, increased temperature, increased pulse, increased
respiration, sweating, mydriasis, flushing, headache, coma, and DIC.

imipramine ►◄ **paroxetine**
Tofranil

Paxil

Risk rating: 2
Severity: Moderate   Onset: **Delayed**   Likelihood: **Suspected**

Cause
Paroxetine may decrease imipramine metabolism in some people and
increase it in others.

Effect
Therapeutic and toxic effects of certain tricyclic antidepressants
(TCAs), such as imipramine, may increase.

Nursing considerations
■ When starting or stopping paroxetine, monitor TCA level and adjust
dosage as needed.
■ Assess symptoms and behavior for evidence of adverse reactions,
such as increased drowsiness, dizziness, confusion, heart rate or
rhythm changes, and urine retention.
■ Watch closely for evidence of serotonin syndrome, such as delirium,
bizarre movements, and tachycardia. Alert prescriber if they occur;
TCA may need to be stopped.

■ Symptoms of serotonin syndrome may resolve within 24 hours of stopping a TCA and starting a short course of cyproheptadine.

---

imipramine ▶◀ quinolones
Tofranil

gatifloxacin, levofloxacin, moxifloxacin, sparfloxacin

Risk rating: 1
Severity: Major   **Onset: Delayed**   **Likelihood: Suspected**

Cause
The mechanism of this interaction is unknown.

Effect
Life-threatening arrhythmias, including torsades de pointes, may increase when certain tricyclic antidepressants (TCAs), such as imipramine, are used with certain quinolones.

Nursing considerations
◖ **ALERT** Sparfloxacin is contraindicated in patients taking a TCA because QTc interval may be prolonged.
◖ **ALERT** Avoid giving levofloxacin with a TCA.
■ Use gatifloxacin and moxifloxacin cautiously with TCAs.
■ If possible, use other quinolone antibiotics that don't prolong the QTc interval or aren't metabolized by the CYP3A4 isoenzyme.

---

imipramine ▶◀ rifamycins
Tofranil

rifabutin, rifampin

Risk rating: 2
Severity: Moderate   **Onset: Delayed**   **Likelihood: Suspected**

Cause
Hepatic metabolism of tricyclic antidepressants (TCAs), such as imipramine, may increase.

Effect
TCA level and efficacy may decrease.

Nursing considerations
■ When starting, stopping, or changing the dosage of a rifamycin, monitor serum TCA level to maintain therapeutic range.
■ Watch for resolution of depression as TCA dosage is adjusted to therapeutic level during rifamycin therapy.

■ Urge patient and family to watch for adverse reactions, including increased drowsiness and dizziness, for several weeks after rifamycin stops. Tell them to notify prescriber promptly.
■ Other TCAs may interact with rifamycins. If you suspect an interaction, consult prescriber or pharmacist.

---

imipramine ►◄ sertraline
Tofranil   Zoloft

Risk rating: 2
Severity: Moderate   **Onset: Delayed**   **Likelihood: Suspected**

Cause
Hepatic metabolism of imipramine, a tricyclic antidepressant (TCA), may be inhibited.

Effect
Therapeutic and toxic effects of certain TCAs may increase.

Nursing considerations
■ If possible, avoid this drug combination.
■ Watch for evidence of TCA toxicity and serotonin syndrome.
■ Signs of serotonin syndrome include delirium, bizarre movements, and tachycardia.
■ Monitor TCA level when starting or stopping sertraline.
■ If abnormalities occur, decrease TCA dosage or stop drug.

---

imipramine ►◄ sympathomimetics
Tofranil   *direct:* dobutamine, epinephrine, norepinephrine, phenylephrine
                           mixed: dopamine, ephedrine, metaraminol

Risk rating: 2
Severity: Moderate   **Onset: Rapid**   **Likelihood: Established**

Cause
Tricyclic antidepressants (TCAs), such as imipramine, increase the effects of direct-acting sympathomimetics and decrease the effects of indirect-acting sympathomimetics.

Effect
When sympathomimetic effects increase, the risk of hypertension and arrhythmias increases. When sympathomimetic effects decrease, blood pressure control decreases.

Nursing considerations
■ If possible, avoid using these drugs together.
■ Watch patient closely for hypertension and heart rhythm changes; they may warrant reduced sympathomimetic dosage.
■ If patient takes a mixed-acting sympathomimetic, watch for negative effects; dosage may need to be altered.
■ Other TCAs and sympathomimetics may interact. If you suspect an interaction, consult prescriber or pharmacist.

---

imipramine ▶◀ terbinafine
Tofranil   Lamisil

Risk rating: 2
Severity: Moderate   **Onset: Delayed**   **Likelihood: Suspected**

Cause
Hepatic metabolism of a tricyclic antidepressant (TCA), such as imipramine, may be inhibited.

Effect
Therapeutic and toxic effects of certain TCAs may increase.

Nursing considerations
■ Check for toxic TCA level; report abnormal level to prescriber.
■ TCA dosage may be decreased while patient takes terbinafine.
■ Adverse effects or toxicity may include vertigo, fatigue, loss of appetite, ataxia, muscle twitching, and trouble swallowing.
■ Terbinafine's inhibitory effects may take several weeks to dissipate after drug is stopped.
■ Describe signs and symptoms patient should look for.

---

imipramine ▶◀ valproic acid
Tofranil   divalproex sodium, valproate
                                              sodium, valproic acid

Risk rating: 2
Severity: Moderate   **Onset: Delayed**   **Likelihood: Suspected**

Cause
Valproic acid may inhibit hepatic metabolism of tricyclic antidepressants (TCAs), such as imipramine.

Effect
TCA level and effects may increase.

Nursing considerations
- Use these drugs together cautiously.
- If patient is stable on valproic acid, start TCA at reduced dosage and adjust upward slowly to address symptoms and serum level.
- If patient is stable on a TCA, monitor serum level and patient status closely when starting or stopping valproic acid.
- Explain signs and symptoms to watch for.
- Other TCAs may interact with valproic acid. If you suspect an interaction, consult prescriber or pharmacist.

---

indapamide ◄►◄ loop diuretics

Lozol

bumetanide, ethacrynic acid, furosemide, torsemide

Risk rating: 2
Severity: Moderate   **Onset: Rapid**   **Likelihood: Probable**

Cause
The mechanism of this interaction is unclear.

Effect
Because these drugs work synergistically, they may cause profound diuresis and serious electrolyte abnormalities.

Nursing considerations
- These drugs may be used together for therapeutic benefit.
- Expect increased sodium, potassium, and chloride excretion and greater diuresis during combined therapy.
- Monitor patient for dehydration and electrolyte abnormalities.
- Carefully adjust drugs, using small or intermittent doses.

---

indapamide ◄►◄ sulfonylureas

Lozol

acetohexamide, chlorpropamide, glipizide, glyburide, tolazamide, tolbutamide

Risk rating: 2
Severity: Moderate   **Onset: Delayed**   **Likelihood: Probable**

Cause
Thiazide diuretics, such as indapamide, may decrease insulin secretion and tissue sensitivity, and may increase potassium loss.

Effect
Risk of hyperglycemia and hyponatremia may increase.

Nursing considerations
- Use these drugs together cautiously.
- Monitor blood glucose level regularly; consult prescriber about adjustments to either drug to maintain stable glucose level.
- This interaction may occur several days to many months after dual therapy starts but is readily reversible when the diuretic stops.
- Describe signs and symptoms of hypoglycemia, including diaphoresis, fatigue, headache, hunger, irritability, malaise, nervousness, rapid heart rate, tension, and trembling.
- Instruct patient to eat a small carbohydrate snack or meal if hypoglycemia develops, preferably after checking blood glucose level.

---

indinavir ▶◀ atorvastatin
Crixivan   Lipitor

Risk rating: 2
Severity: Moderate   **Onset: Delayed**   **Likelihood: Suspected**

Cause
First-pass metabolism of atorvastatin by CYP3A4 in the GI tract may be inhibited.

Effect
Atorvastatin level may increase.

Nursing considerations
- Monitor patient closely if a protease inhibitor, such as indinavir, is added to atorvastatin therapy.
- ⚡ ALERT Watch for evidence of rhabdomyolysis, including dark or red urine, muscle weakness, and myalgia.
- Tell patient to immediately report unexplained muscle weakness.

---

indinavir ▶◀ azole antifungals
Crixivan   fluconazole, itraconazole, ketoconazole

Risk rating: 2
Severity: Moderate   **Onset: Delayed**   **Likelihood: Suspected**

Cause
Azole antifungals may inhibit metabolism of protease inhibitors, such as indinavir.

Effect
Protease inhibitor level may increase.

Nursing considerations
■ Protease inhibitor dosage may be decreased when therapy starts.
■ Monitor patient for increased protease inhibitor effects, including hyperglycemia, onset of diabetes, rash, GI complaints, and altered liver function tests.
■ Advise patient to report increased hunger or thirst, frequent urination, fatigue, and dry, itchy skin.
■ Tell patient not to change dosage or stop either drug without consulting prescriber.

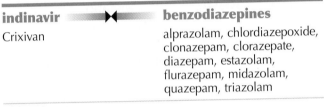

indinavir ⬦ benzodiazepines
Crixivan

alprazolam, chlordiazepoxide, clonazepam, clorazepate, diazepam, estazolam, flurazepam, midazolam, quazepam, triazolam

Risk rating: 2
Severity: Moderate   **Onset: Delayed**   **Likelihood: Suspected**

Cause
Protease inhibitors, such as indinavir, may inhibit CYP3A4 metabolism of certain benzodiazepines.

Effect
Sedative effects may be increased and prolonged, leading to severe respiratory depression.

Nursing considerations
⚠ ALERT Don't combine these benzodiazepines with protease inhibitors.
■ If patient takes any benzodiazepine–protease inhibitor combination, notify prescriber. Interaction could involve other drugs in the class.
■ Watch for evidence of oversedation and respiratory depression.
■ Teach patient and family about the risks of combining these drugs.

indinavir ◄► didanosine

Crixivan

Videx

Risk rating: 2
Severity: Moderate   **Onset: Rapid**   **Likelihood: Suspected**

Cause
Indinavir absorption may be decreased by buffers in didanosine.

Effect
Indinavir effects may decrease.

Nursing considerations
◄ **ALERT** Give indinavir and didanosine at least 1 hour apart on an empty stomach.
■ Watch for expected therapeutic effects of indinavir, including improvement in HIV symptoms.
■ Monitor lab values for an increased CD4+ T-cell count and a decreased HIV-1 RNA level.
■ Help patient develop a plan to ensure proper dosage intervals.

indinavir ◄► ergot derivatives

Crixivan

dihydroergotamine, ergonovine, ergotamine, methylergonovine

Risk rating: 1
Severity: Major   **Onset: Delayed**   **Likelihood: Probable**

Cause
Protease inhibitors, such as indinavir, may interfere with CYP3A4 metabolism of ergot derivatives.

Effect
Risk of ergot-induced peripheral vasospasm and ischemia may increase.

Nursing considerations
◄ **ALERT** Use of ergot derivatives with protease inhibitors is contraindicated.
■ Monitor patient for evidence of peripheral ischemia: pain in limb muscles while exercising and later at rest; numbness and tingling of fingers and toes; cool, pale, or cyanotic limbs; red or violet blisters on hands or feet; and gangrene.
■ Sodium nitroprusside may be used to treat ergot-induced vasospasm.

- If patient takes a protease inhibitor, consult prescriber or pharmacist about alternative treatments for migraine pain.
- Urge patient to tell prescriber about increased adverse effects.

---

indinavir ▶◀ fentanyl
Crixivan   Sublimaze

Risk rating: 1
Severity: Major   **Onset: Delayed**   **Likelihood: Suspected**

Cause
Metabolism of fentanyl in the GI tract and liver may be inhibited.

Effect
Fentanyl level may increase and half-life lengthen.

Nursing considerations
▶ ALERT If patient takes a protease inhibitor, such as indinavir, watch closely for respiratory depression if fentanyl is added.
- Because fentanyl half-life is prolonged, monitoring period should be extended, even after fentanyl is stopped.
- Keep naloxone available to treat respiratory depression.
- If fentanyl is continuously infused, dosage should be decreased.

---

indinavir ▶◀ HMG-CoA reductase inhibitors
Crixivan   lovastatin, simvastatin

Risk rating: 1
Severity: Major   **Onset: Delayed**   **Likelihood: Suspected**

Cause
Protease inhibitors, such as indinavir, may inhibit CYP3A4 metabolism of lovastatin and simvastatin.

Effect
Lovastatin or simvastatin level may increase.

Nursing considerations
- If a protease inhibitor starts, monitor patient closely.
▶ ALERT Watch for evidence of rhabdomyolysis, including dark or red urine, muscle weakness, and myalgia.
- Urge patient to immediately report unexplained muscle weakness.

indinavir 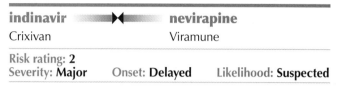 nevirapine
Crixivan   Viramune

Risk rating: 2
Severity: Major   **Onset: Delayed**   **Likelihood: Suspected**

Cause
Nevirapine may increase hepatic metabolism of protease inhibitors, such as indinavir.

Effect
Protease inhibitor level and effects decrease.

Nursing considerations
■ If nevirapine is started or stopped, monitor protease inhibitor level closely.
■ Protease inhibitor dosage may need adjustment.
■ Monitor CD4+ and T-cell counts, and tell prescriber if they decrease.
■ Urge patient to report opportunistic infections.
■ Tell patient not to change an HIV regimen without consulting prescriber.

indinavir 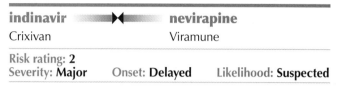 phosphodiesterase-5 inhibitors
Crixivan   sildenafil, tadalafil, vardenafil

Risk rating: 1
Severity: Major   **Onset: Rapid**   **Likelihood: Suspected**

Cause
Hepatic metabolism of the phosphodiesterase-5 (PDE-5) inhibitor is inhibited.

Effect
PDE-5 inhibitor level may increase, possibly leading to fatal hypotension.

Nursing considerations
◪ **ALERT** Warn patient about potentially fatal low blood pressure if these drugs are taken together.
◪ **ALERT** Tell patient to take PDE-5 inhibitor exactly as prescribed.
■ Dosage of PDE-5 inhibitor may be reduced and interval extended.
■ Tell patient to notify prescriber if he has dizziness, fainting, or chest pain.

indinavir ━━━━▶◀━━━━ ritonavir
Crixivan   Norvir

Risk rating: 2
Severity: Moderate   **Onset: Delayed**   **Likelihood: Probable**

Cause
Ritonavir may decrease CYP3A4 metabolism and clearance of indinavir.

Effect
Indinavir level, effects, and risk of adverse effects may increase.

Nursing considerations
⚠ **ALERT** Both drugs may need dosage adjustment.
■ Watch for increased indinavir adverse effects, including nausea, vomiting, diarrhea, and adverse renal effects.
■ Monitor patient for nephrolithiasis; patient may experience flank pain and hematuria.
■ Advise patient to drink at least six 8-ounce glasses of fluid (1.5 L) daily.
■ Help patient develop a plan to ensure proper dosage intervals.

indinavir ━━━━▶◀━━━━ St. John's wort
Crixivan

Risk rating: 1
Severity: Major   **Onset: Delayed**   **Likelihood: Suspected**

Cause
Hepatic metabolism of protease inhibitors, such as indinavir, may increase.

Effect
Protease inhibitor level and effects may decrease.

Nursing considerations
■ If patient starts or stops taking St. John's wort, monitor protease inhibitor level closely.
■ Monitor CD4+ and T-cell counts; tell prescriber if they decrease.
■ Urge patient to report opportunistic infections.
■ Tell patient not to change an HIV regimen without consulting prescriber.
■ Urge patient to tell prescribers about all drugs, supplements, and alternative therapies he uses.

indomethacin ▶◀ ACE inhibitors

Indocin

benazepril, captopril, enalapril, fosinopril, lisinopril, moexipril, perindopril, quinapril, ramipril, trandolapril

Risk rating: 2
Severity: Moderate   **Onset: Rapid**   **Likelihood: Probable**

Cause
Indomethacin inhibits synthesis of prostaglandins, which ACE inhibitors need to lower blood pressure.

Effect
ACE inhibitor's hypotensive effect will decrease.

Nursing considerations
■ **ALERT** Monitor blood pressure closely. Severe hypertension may persist until indomethacin is stopped.
■ If indomethacin can't be avoided, patient may need a different antihypertensive.
■ Other ACE inhibitors may interact with indomethacin. If you suspect an interaction, consult prescriber or pharmacist.
■ Remind patient that hypertension commonly causes no physical symptoms but sometimes may cause headache and dizziness.

indomethacin ▶◀ aminoglycosides

Indocin

amikacin, gentamicin, kanamycin, netilmicin, streptomycin, tobramycin

Risk rating: 2
Severity: Moderate   **Onset: Delayed**   **Likelihood: Suspected**

Cause
Indomethacin and other NSAIDs may reduce glomerular filtration rate (GFR), causing aminoglycosides to accumulate.

Effect
Aminoglycoside level in premature infants may increase.

Nursing considerations
■ Before NSAID starts, aminoglycoside dose should be reduced.
■ **ALERT** Check peak and trough aminoglycoside levels after third dose. For peak level, draw blood 30 minutes after I.V. or 60 minutes after I.M. dose. For trough level, draw blood just before a dose.

- Monitor patient's renal function.
- Although only indomethacin is known to interact with aminoglycosides, other NSAIDs probably do as well. If you suspect an interaction, consult prescriber or pharmacist.
- Other drugs cleared by GFR may have a similar interaction.

indomethacin ►◄ beta blockers

Indocin

acebutolol, atenolol, betaxolol, bisoprolol, carteolol, esmolol, metoprolol, nadolol, penbutolol, pindolol, propranolol, sotalol, timolol

Risk rating: 2
Severity: **Moderate**   Onset: **Delayed**   Likelihood: **Probable**

Cause
Indomethacin and other NSAIDs may inhibit renal prostaglandin synthesis, allowing pressor systems to be unopposed.

Effect
Beta blocker may not be able to lower blood pressure.

Nursing considerations
- Avoid using these drugs together if possible
- Monitor blood pressure and other evidence of hypertension closely.
- Consult prescriber about ways to minimize interaction, such as adjusting beta blocker dosage or switching to sulindac as the NSAID.
- Explain the risks of using these drugs together, and teach patient how to monitor his blood pressure.
- Other NSAIDs may interact with beta blockers. If you suspect an interaction, consult prescriber or pharmacist.

indomethacin ►◄ digoxin

Indocin

Lanoxin

Risk rating: 2
Severity: **Moderate**   Onset: **Delayed**   Likelihood: **Suspected**

Cause
Indomethacin may reduce renal digoxin elimination.

Effect
Digoxin level, effects, and adverse effects may increase.

Nursing considerations
- Interaction may not occur in patients with normal renal function.
- **⚡ ALERT** Use cautiously in preterm infants with decreased renal function. Digoxin dose may need to be reduced by 50% when indomethacin starts in these patients.
- Monitor digoxin level. Therapeutic range is 0.8 to 2 nanograms/ml.
- Monitor renal function tests and urine output.
- Monitor patient for evidence of digoxin toxicity: arrhythmias (bradycardia and AV blocks, more common in children; ventricular ectopy, more common in adults), lethargy, drowsiness, confusion, hallucinations, headaches, syncope, visual disturbances, nausea, vomiting, diarrhea, anorexia, and failure to thrive.

---

indomethacin ▶◀ losartan
Indocin   Cozaar

Risk rating: 2
Severity: Moderate   **Onset: Delayed**   **Likelihood: Suspected**

Cause
The mechanism of this interaction is unknown.

Effect
Hypotensive effect of losartan may be reduced.

Nursing considerations
- Other antihypertensives may not share this interaction.
- Monitor blood pressure closely.
- If you suspect an interaction, notify prescriber. Indomethacin may need to be stopped or a different antihypertensive considered.

---

insulin ▶◀ alcohol

Risk rating: 1
Severity: Major   **Onset: Rapid**   **Likelihood: Probable**

Cause
Alcohol enhances insulin release in response to glucose and inhibits gluconeogenesis (glucose formation).

Effect
Glucose-lowering effect of insulin may be potentiated.

Nursing considerations

- Monitor patient for evidence of hypoglycemia: tachycardia, palpitations, anxiety, diaphoresis, nausea, hunger, dizziness, restlessness, headache, confusion, tremors, and speech and motor dysfunction.
- Teach patient to avoid alcohol because it lowers the glucose level.
- Advise patient to monitor glucose level carefully if consuming alcohol.
- **ALERT** If a patient taking insulin plans to consume alcohol, advise him to drink in moderation and with food.
- Make sure patient and family can recognize hypoglycemia and respond appropriately.

---

insulin ▶◀ **beta blockers, nonselective**

carteolol, nadolol, penbutolol, pindolol, propranolol, timolol

Risk rating: 2
Severity: Moderate   **Onset: Rapid**   **Likelihood: Established**

Cause
Beta blockers lessen the sympathetic-mediated response to hypoglycemia.

Effect
Hypoglycemia may be prolonged and hypoglycemic symptoms masked.

Nursing considerations
- Nonselective beta blocker should be used cautiously in a patient with diabetes; if possible, use a selective beta blocker or one with intrinsic sympathomimetic activity, such as acebutolol, atenolol, and metoprolol.
- Watch for evidence of hypoglycemia: tachycardia, palpitations, anxiety, diaphoresis, nausea, hunger, dizziness, restlessness, headache, confusion, tremors, and speech and motor dysfunction.
- **ALERT** Hypoglycemic symptoms, such as tachycardia, may be lessened or absent in patients taking a nonselective beta blocker; other symptoms, such as dizziness and diaphoresis, will still be present.
- Monitor glucose level closely when beta blocker starts or dosage changes.
- Consult prescriber if patient continues to experience hypoglycemia; insulin dosage may need to be decreased.
- Make sure patient and family can recognize hypoglycemia and respond appropriately.

insulin ━━━━►◄━━━━ MAO inhibitors

isocarboxazid, phenelzine, tranylcypromine

Risk rating: 2
Severity: Moderate   **Onset: Delayed**   **Likelihood: Established**

Cause
MAO inhibitors stimulate insulin secretion and inhibit gluconeogenesis (glucose formation).

Effect
Hypoglycemic response to insulin may be increased and prolonged.

Nursing considerations
■ Monitor glucose level closely if MAO inhibitor starts or dosage changes.
■ The extent of MAO inhibitor effect on glucose level may not be known for several weeks.
■ Watch for evidence of hypoglycemia: tachycardia, palpitations, anxiety, diaphoresis, nausea, hunger, dizziness, restlessness, headache, confusion, tremors, and speech and motor dysfunction.
■ Consult prescriber if patient experiences hypoglycemia; insulin dosage may need to be decreased.
■ Treat hypoglycemia as needed, such as with fast-acting oral carbohydrates, parenteral glucagon, or I.V. $D_{50}W$ bolus.
■ Make sure patient and family can recognize hypoglycemia and respond appropriately.

insulin ━━━━►◄━━━━ salicylates

aspirin, bismuth subsalicylate, choline salicylate, magnesium salicylate, salsalate, sodium salicylate, sodium thiosalicylate

Risk rating: 2
Severity: Moderate   **Onset: Delayed**   **Likelihood: Probable**

Cause
Basal insulin level is increased; salicylates enhance release of insulin in response to glucose.

Effect
Glucose-lowering effect of insulin may be potentiated.

Nursing considerations
■ Monitor glucose level closely if patient who takes insulin starts a salicylate.
■ Watch for evidence of hypoglycemia: tachycardia, palpitations, anxiety, diaphoresis, nausea, hunger, dizziness, restlessness, headache, confusion, tremors, and speech and motor dysfunction.
■ Consult prescriber if patient experiences hypoglycemia; insulin dosage may need to be decreased.
■ Treat hypoglycemia as needed, such as with fast-acting oral carbohydrates, parenteral glucagon, or I.V. $D_{50}W$ bolus.
■ Urge patient to tell prescriber about increased adverse effects.
■ Make sure patient and family can recognize hypoglycemia and respond appropriately

---

irbesartan ▶◀ potassium-sparing diuretics
Avapro

amiloride, spironolactone, triamterene

Risk rating: 1
Severity: **Major**   Onset: **Delayed**   Likelihood: **Suspected**

Cause
Angiotensin II receptor antagonists, such as irbesartan, and potassium-sparing diuretics each may increase serum potassium level.

Effect
Risk of hyperkalemia may increase, especially in high-risk patients.

Nursing considerations
■ High-risk patients include elderly people and those with renal impairment, type 2 diabetes, or decreased renal perfusion; monitor these patients closely.
■ Check serum potassium, BUN, and creatinine levels regularly. If they increase, notify prescriber.
■ Advise patient to immediately report an irregular heartbeat, slow pulse, weakness, or other evidence of hyperkalemia.
■ Give patient a list of foods high in potassium; stress the need to eat them only in moderate amounts.

irinotecan ▶◀ St. John's wort
Camptosar

Risk rating: **2**
Severity: **Moderate**   Onset: **Delayed**   Likelihood: **Suspected**

Cause
The exact mechanism of this interaction is unknown. CYP3A4 hepatic metabolism of irinotecan may be altered by St. John's wort.

Effect
Irinotecan level and effects may decrease.

Nursing considerations
■ **ALERT** Those who take irinotecan shouldn't take St. John's wort.
■ If patient stops St. John's wort during irinotecan therapy, watch for severe diarrhea, nausea, vomiting, electrolyte disturbances, and hematologic toxicities.
■ Urge patient to tell prescriber about all supplements he takes.

iron salts ▶◀ levothyroxine
ferrous fumarate,   Synthroid
ferrous gluconate,
ferrous sulfate,
iron polysaccharide

Risk rating: **2**
Severity: **Moderate**   Onset: **Delayed**   Likelihood: **Suspected**

Cause
Levothyroxine absorption may decrease, probably because it forms a complex with iron salt.

Effect
Levothyroxine effects may decrease, resulting in hypothyroidism.

Nursing considerations
■ **ALERT** Separate levothyroxine and iron salts as much as possible.
■ Monitor TSH, T_3, and T_4 levels. Therapeutic range for TSH is 0.2 to 5.4 microunits/ml; for T_3, 80 to 200 nanograms/dl; and for T_4, 5.4 to 11.5 mcg/dl.
■ Levothyroxine dosage may need adjustment.
■ Watch for evidence of hypothyroidism: weakness, fatigue, weight gain, coarse dry hair, rough skin, cold intolerance, muscle aches, constipation, depression, irritability, and memory loss.
■ Explain that levothyroxine dosage may need adjustment.

■ Urge patient to tell prescriber about evidence of hypothyroidism, such as fatigue, weight gain, cold intolerance, and constipation.

---

iron salts ━━━━▶◀━━━━ mycophenolate mofetil

ferrous fumarate,
ferrous gluconate,
ferrous sulfate,
iron polysaccharide

CellCept

Risk rating: 2
Severity: Moderate   **Onset: Rapid**   **Likelihood: Suspected**

Cause
Mycophenolate mofetil absorption may decrease because drug may form a complex with iron salt in the GI tract.

Effect
Mycophenolate mofetil level and effects may decrease.

Nursing considerations
▧ **ALERT** Avoid combining iron salts with mycophenolate mofetil.
■ If you must give both, separate doses as much as possible.
■ Watch for evidence of rejection or decreased drug effect.
■ Tell patient to report signs of organ rejection: reduced urine output after kidney transplant or shortness of breath after heart transplant.
■ Help patient develop a plan to ensure proper dosage intervals.

---

iron salts ━━━━▶◀━━━━ penicillamine

ferrous fumarate,
ferrous gluconate,
ferrous sulfate,
iron polysaccharide

Cuprimine, Depen

Risk rating: 2
Severity: Moderate   **Onset: Delayed**   **Likelihood: Probable**

Cause
GI absorption of penicillamine may be decreased because of chelation with iron salts.

Effect
Penicillamine effects may decrease.

Nursing considerations
▧ **ALERT** If possible, avoid giving penicillamine with iron salts.

- If you must give both, separate doses by at least 2 hours; if penicillamine effect decreases, consult prescriber for appropriate interval.
- Give penicillamine on empty stomach, between meals, with water.
- Monitor patient for worsening symptoms of Wilson's disease: abdominal distention, jaundice, splenomegaly, arm or hand tremors, slow or stiff movements, muscle weakness, worsening speech, emotional or behavioral changes, and confusion. Or watch for worsened rheumatoid arthritis symptoms: joint pain and stiffness.
- Help patient develop a plan to ensure proper dosage intervals.

iron salts ▸◂ quinolones

ferrous fumarate, ferrous gluconate, ferrous sulfate, iron polysaccharide

ciprofloxacin, levofloxacin, lomefloxacin, norfloxacin, ofloxacin

Risk rating: 2
Severity: Moderate   **Onset: Rapid**   **Likelihood: Probable**

Cause
Formation of an iron-quinolone complex decreases GI absorption of the quinolone.

Effect
Quinolone effects decrease.

Nursing considerations
- Monitor patient for quinolone efficacy.
- Tell patient to separate quinolone dose from iron by at least 2 hours.
- Other quinolones may interact with iron.
- Help patient develop a plan to ensure proper dosage intervals.

iron salts ▸◂ tetracyclines, oral

ferrous fumarate, ferrous gluconate, ferrous sulfate, iron polysaccharide

demeclocycline, doxycycline, minocycline, oxytetracycline, tetracycline

Risk rating: 2
Severity: Moderate   **Onset: Delayed**   **Likelihood: Probable**

Cause
Tetracyclines form insoluble chelates with iron salts, which may reduce absorption of both substances.

Effect
Tetracycline and iron salt levels and effects may decrease.

Nursing considerations
⚠ ALERT If possible, avoid giving tetracyclines with iron salts.
- If they must be given together, separate doses by 3 to 4 hours.
- If you suspect an interaction, consult prescriber or pharmacist; an enteric-coated or sustained-release iron salt may reduce it.
- Monitor patient for expected therapeutic response to tetracycline.
- Assess patient for evidence of iron deficiency, including fatigue, dyspnea, tachycardia, palpitations, dizziness, and orthostatic hypotension.

---

isocarboxazid ▶◀ atomoxetine
Marplan   Strattera

Risk rating: 1
Severity: Major   **Onset: Rapid**   **Likelihood: Suspected**

Cause
Level of monoamine in the brain may change.

Effect
Possible risk increases for serious or fatal reaction resembling neuroleptic malignant syndrome.

Nursing considerations
⚠ ALERT Use of atomoxetine and an MAO inhibitor, such as isocarboxazid, together or within 2 weeks of each other is contraindicated.
- Before starting atomoxetine, ask patient when he last took an MAO inhibitor. Before starting an MAO inhibitor, ask patient when he last took atomoxetine.
- Monitor patient for hyperthermia, rapid changes in vital signs, rigidity, muscle twitching, and mental status changes.

---

isocarboxazid ▶◀ dextromethorphan
Marplan   Robitussin DM

Risk rating: 1
Severity: Major   **Onset: Rapid**   **Likelihood: Suspected**

Cause
MAO inhibitors, such as isocarboxazid, may decrease serotonin metabolism. Dextromethorphan may decrease synaptic reuptake of serotonin.

Effect
Risk of serotonin syndrome increases.

Nursing considerations
■ If possible, avoid giving these drugs together.
◪ ALERT Combined use may cause hyperpyrexia, abnormal muscle movement, hypotension, coma, and death.
■ If patient takes an MAO inhibitor, caution against taking OTC cough and cold medicines that contain dextromethorphan.

isocarboxazid ━━▶◀━━ L-tryptophan
Marplan

Risk rating: 1
Severity: Major   **Onset: Rapid**   **Likelihood: Suspected**

Cause
Giving these drugs together may cause additive serotonergic effects.

Effect
Risk of serotonin syndrome increases.

Nursing considerations
◪ ALERT Combined use of these drugs is contraindicated.
■ If given together, they may cause CNS irritability, motor weakness, shivering, muscle twitching, and altered consciousness.

isocarboxazid ━━▶◀━━ meperidine
Marplan   Demerol

Risk rating: 1
Severity: Major   **Onset: Rapid**   **Likelihood: Probable**

Cause
The mechanism of this interaction is unknown.

Effect
Risk of severe adverse reactions increases.

Nursing considerations
■ If possible, avoid giving these drugs together.
■ Monitor patient and report agitation, seizures, diaphoresis, and fever.
■ Reaction may progress to coma, apnea, and death.
■ Reaction may occur several weeks after stopping isocarboxazid, an MAO inhibitor.

ⓘ ALERT Give opioid analgesics other than meperidine cautiously. It isn't known if similar reactions occur.

---

isocarboxazid ▬▶◀▬ methylphenidates

Marplan   dexmethylphenidate,
                           methylphenidate

Risk rating: 1
Severity: Major   **Onset: Delayed**   **Likelihood: Suspected**

Cause
The mechanism of this interaction is unknown.

Effect
Risk of hypertensive crisis increases.

Nursing considerations
ⓘ ALERT Use of dexmethylphenidate with an MAO inhibitor, such as isocarboxazid, is contraindicated.
■ Don't use dexmethylphenidate within 14 days after stopping an MAO inhibitor.
■ Monitor blood pressure closely if methylphenidate is given with an MAO inhibitor.
■ Teach patient and parent to monitor and record blood pressure at home.

---

isocarboxazid ▬▶◀▬ selective 5-HT$_1$ receptor agonists

Marplan   rizatriptan, sumatriptan,
                           zolmitriptan

Risk rating: 1
Severity: Major   **Onset: Rapid**   **Likelihood: Suspected**

Cause
MAO inhibitors, subtype-A, such as isocarboxazid, may inhibit metabolism of selective 5-HT$_1$ receptor agonists.

Effect
Serum level and the risk of cardiac toxicity from certain selective 5-HT$_1$ receptor agonists may increase.

Nursing considerations
ⓘ ALERT Use of certain selective 5-HT$_1$ receptor agonists with or within 2 weeks of stopping an MAO inhibitor is contraindicated.

■ If these drugs must be used together, naratriptan is less likely to interact with an MAO inhibitor.

■ Cardiac toxicity may include coronary artery vasospasm and transient myocardial ischemia.

---

isocarboxazid ➤◄ **serotonin reuptake inhibitors**

Marplan

citalopram, escitalopram, fluoxetine, fluvoxamine, nefazodone, paroxetine, sertraline, venlafaxine

---

Risk rating: 1
Severity: Major   **Onset: Rapid**   **Likelihood: Probable**

Cause
Serotonin may accumulate rapidly in the CNS.

Effect
Risk of serotonin syndrome increases.

Nursing considerations
⚡ ALERT Don't use these drugs together.

■ Allow 1 week after stopping nefazodone or venlafaxine (2 weeks after stopping citalopram, escitalopram, fluvoxamine, paroxetine, or sertraline; 5 weeks after stopping fluoxetine) before giving an MAO inhibitor, such as isocarboxazid.

■ Allow 2 weeks after stopping an MAO inhibitor before giving a serotonin reuptake inhibitor.

■ The selective MAO type-B inhibitor selegiline has been given with fluoxetine, paroxetine, or sertraline to patients with Parkinson's disease without negative effects.

■ Describe the traits of serotonin syndrome, including CNS irritability, motor weakness, shivering, myoclonus, and altered consciousness.

■ Urge patient to promptly report adverse effects to prescriber.

isocarboxazid ◀▶ sulfonylureas

Marplan

acetohexamide, chlorpropamide, glipizide, glyburide, tolazamide, tolbutamide

Risk rating: 2
Severity: **Moderate**   Onset: **Rapid**   Likelihood: **Suspected**

Cause
The mechanism of this interaction is unknown.

Effect
MAO inhibitors, such as isocarboxazid, increase the hypoglycemic effects of sulfonylureas.

Nursing considerations
- If patient takes a sulfonylurea, start MAO inhibitor carefully, monitoring patient for hypoglycemia.
- Consult prescriber about adjustments to either drug to control glucose level and mental status.
- Describe signs and symptoms of hypoglycemia, including diaphoresis, fatigue, headache, hunger, irritability, malaise, nervousness, rapid heart rate, tension, and trembling.
- Instruct patient to eat a small carbohydrate snack or meal if hypoglycemia develops, preferably after checking blood glucose level.

isocarboxazid ◀▶ sympathomimetics

Marplan

dopamine, ephedrine, metaraminol, phenylephrine, pseudoephedrine

Risk rating: 1
Severity: **Major**   Onset: **Rapid**   Likelihood: **Established**

Cause
When MAO is inhibited, norepinephrine accumulates and is released by indirect and mixed-acting sympathomimetics, increasing the pressor response at receptor sites.

Effect
Risk of severe headaches, hypertension, high fever, and hypertensive crisis increases.

Nursing considerations
- Avoid giving indirect or mixed-acting sympathomimetics with an MAO inhibitor, such as isocarboxazid.

■ If drugs are combined, phentolamine can block epinephrine- and norepinephrine-induced vasoconstriction and reduce blood pressure.
■ Direct-acting sympathomimetics interact minimally.
⚡ ALERT Warn patient that OTC medicines, such as decongestants, may cause this interaction.

isocarboxazid ▶◀ tricyclic antidepressants

Marplan

amitriptyline, amoxapine, clomipramine, desipramine, doxepin, imipramine, nortriptyline, trimipramine

Risk rating: 1
Severity: **Major**   Onset: **Rapid**   Likelihood: **Suspected**

Cause
The mechanism of this interaction is unknown.

Effect
Risk of hyperpyretic crisis, seizures, and death increase.

Nursing considerations
⚡ ALERT Don't give a tricyclic antidepressant with or within 2 weeks of an MAO inhibitor, such as isocarboxazid.
■ Imipramine and clomipramine may be more likely to interact with MAO inhibitors.
■ Watch for adverse effects, including confusion, hyperexcitability, rigidity, seizures, increased temperature, increased pulse, increased respiration, sweating, mydriasis, flushing, headache, coma, and DIC.

isoniazid ▶◀ carbamazepine

Nydrazid

Carbatrol, Epitol, Equetro, Tegretol

Risk rating: 2
Severity: **Moderate**   Onset: **Delayed**   Likelihood: **Suspected**

Cause
Isoniazid may inhibit carbamazepine metabolism. Carbamazepine may increase isoniazid hepatotoxicity.

Effect
Risk of carbamazepine toxicity and isoniazid hepatotoxicity increase.

Nursing considerations

■ Monitor carbamazepine level; therapeutic range is 4 to 12 mcg/ml.
■ Watch for evidence of carbamazepine toxicity: dizziness, ataxia, respiratory depression, tachycardia, arrhythmias, blood pressure changes, impaired consciousness, abnormal reflexes, nystagmus, seizures, nausea, vomiting, and urine retention.
■ Carbamazepine dosage may need adjustment.
■ Monitor liver function tests. If hepatotoxicity develops, consult prescriber about stopping isoniazid.
■ Advise patient to report signs of hepatotoxicity: abdominal pain, appetite loss, fatigue, yellow skin or eye discoloration, and dark urine.

---

isoniazid ▰▰▰►◄▰▰▰ rifampin
Laniazid, Nydrazid   Rifadin

Risk rating: 1
Severity: **Major**   Onset: **Delayed**   Likelihood: **Probable**

Cause
Rifampin may alter isoniazid metabolism.

Effect
Risk of hepatotoxicity increases over either drug given alone.

Nursing considerations

■ Monitor liver function tests in patients taking both drugs.
■ Consult prescriber about increased liver enzyme levels; one or both drugs may need to be stopped.
■ Monitor patient's liver enzymes and condition even after one or both drugs are stopped because of possible severity of reaction.
■ **ALERT** Children may be more prone to hepatotoxicity.
■ Advise patient to report signs of hepatotoxicity: abdominal pain, appetite loss, fatigue, yellow skin or eye discoloration, and dark urine.

---

isosorbide dinitrate ▰►◄▰ dihydroergotamine
Isordil   D.H.E. 45

Risk rating: 2
Severity: **Moderate**   Onset: **Rapid**   Likelihood: **Suspected**

Cause
Metabolism of dihydroergotamine decreases, increasing its availability, which antagonizes coronary vasodilation caused by nitrates, such as isosorbide dinitrate.

Effect
Increased dihydroergotamine availability may increase systolic blood pressure and decrease the antianginal effects of the nitrate.

Nursing considerations
- Use these drugs together cautiously in patients with angina.
- I.V. dihydroergotamine may antagonize coronary vasodilation.
- Watch for evidence of ergotism, such as peripheral ischemia, paresthesia, headache, nausea, and vomiting.
- Teach patient to immediately report signs of peripheral ischemia, such as numbness or tingling in fingers and toes or red blisters on hands or feet. Dihydroergotamine dosage may need to be decreased.

---

isosorbide dinitrate, ◄► phosphodiesterase-5 inhibitors
isosorbide mononitrate
Imdur, Isordil

sildenafil, tadalafil, vardenafil

Risk rating: 1
Severity: Major   **Onset: Rapid**   **Likelihood: Suspected**

Cause
Phosphodiesterase-5 inhibitors potentiate hypotensive effects of nitrates, such as isosorbide.

Effect
Risk of severe hypotension increases.

Nursing considerations
⚠ **ALERT** Combined use of nitrates and erectile dysfunction (ED) drugs may be fatal and is contraindicated.
- Carefully screen patient for ED drug use before giving a nitrate.
- Even during an emergency, before giving a nitrate, find out if a patient with chest pain has taken an ED drug during the previous 24 hours.
- Monitor patient for orthostatic hypotension, dizziness, sweating, and headache.

itraconazole ▶◀ benzodiazepines

Sporanox

alprazolam, chlordiazepoxide, clonazepam, clorazepate, diazepam, estazolam, flurazepam, midazolam, quazepam, triazolam

Risk rating: 2
Severity: Moderate   Onset: Rapid   Likelihood: Established

Cause
Azole antifungals, such as itraconazole, decrease CYP3A4 metabolism of certain benzodiazepines.

Effect
Benzodiazepine effects are increased and prolonged, which may cause CNS depression and psychomotor impairment.

Nursing considerations
⚠ ALERT Use of alprazolam or triazolam with itraconazole is contraindicated.
■ Caution that the effects of this interaction may last several days after stopping the azole antifungal.
■ Explain that taking these drugs together may increase sedative effects; tell patient to report such effects promptly.
■ Explain alternative methods of inducing sleep or relieving anxiety during antifungal therapy.
■ Various azole antifungal–benzodiazepine combinations may interact. If you suspect an interaction, consult prescriber or pharmacist.

itraconazole ▶◀ cola, food, juices

Sporanox

cola, food, grapefruit juice, orange juice

Risk rating: 2
Severity: Moderate   Onset: Rapid   Likelihood: Suspected

Cause
Cola and food may increase itraconazole absorption. Grapefruit juice may decrease it. The exact mechanism of the interaction with orange juice is unknown.

Effect
Itraconazole level may increase (cola, food) or decrease (grapefruit juice, orange juice), with the latter resulting in decreased itraconazole effects.

Nursing considerations

■ Advise patient to take itraconazole capsules after meals.

◼ **ALERT** Itraconazole oral solution should be taken without food for maximum absorption.

■ Advise patient to avoid taking itraconazole with grapefruit products, orange juice, or cola.

---

itraconazole ▶◀ didanosine

Sporanox   Videx

Risk rating: 2
Severity: Moderate   **Onset: Rapid**   **Likelihood: Suspected**

Cause

Inert ingredients in chewable didanosine tablets decrease absorption of azole antifungals, such as itraconazole.

Effect

Efficacy of azole antifungal may decrease.

Nursing considerations

■ To minimize interaction, instruct patient to take antifungal drug 2 hours before didanosine.

■ Monitor patient for lack of response to antifungal drug.

■ Help patient develop a plan to ensure proper dosage intervals.

■ Other azole antifungals may interact with didanosine. If you suspect an interaction, consult prescriber or pharmacist.

---

itraconazole ▶◀ digoxin

Sporanox   Lanoxin

Risk rating: 2
Severity: Moderate   **Onset: Delayed**   **Likelihood: Established**

Cause

Renal clearance of digoxin may decrease and absorption increase.

Effect

Digoxin level, effects, and adverse effects may increase.

Nursing considerations

■ Monitor digoxin level. Therapeutic range is 0.8 to 2 nanograms/ml.

■ Watch for evidence of digoxin toxicity: arrhythmias (such as bradycardia, AV blocks, and ventricular ectopy), lethargy, drowsiness, con-

fusion, hallucinations, headaches, syncope, visual disturbances, nausea, anorexia, vomiting, and diarrhea.
■ Digoxin dosage may need reduction.
■ Azole antifungals other than itraconazole may also interact with digoxin. If you suspect an interaction, consult prescriber or pharmacist.

itraconazole ▶◀ ergot derivatives

Sporanox   dihydroergotamine, ergotamine

Risk rating: 1
Severity: Major   Onset: Delayed   Likelihood: Suspected

Cause
Itraconazole may inhibit CYP3A4 metabolism of ergot derivatives.

Effect
Risk of ergot toxicity many be increased.

Nursing considerations
❧ ALERT Use of these drugs together is contraindicated.
■ Signs of ergot toxicity include peripheral vasospasm and ischemia.
■ Caution patient to avoid ergot derivatives (for migraine, for example) while taking itraconazole; consult prescriber about alternative therapies.

itraconazole ▶◀ HMG-CoA reductase inhibitors

Sporanox

atorvastatin, fluvastatin, lovastatin, pravastatin, rosuvastatin, simvastatin

Risk rating: 2
Severity: Moderate   Onset: Rapid   Likelihood: Probable

Cause
Azole antifungals, such as itraconazole, may inhibit hepatic metabolism of HMG-CoA reductase inhibitors.

Effect
HMG-CoA reductase inhibitor level and adverse effects may increase.

Nursing considerations
■ If possible, avoid use together.
■ HMG-CoA reductase inhibitor dosage may need to be decreased.
■ Monitor serum cholesterol and lipid levels.

⚠ **ALERT** Assess patient for evidence of rhabdomyolysis, including fatigue; muscle aches and weakness; joint pain; dark, red, or cola-colored urine; weight gain; seizures; and greatly increased serum CK level.

■ Pravastatin is the HMG-CoA reductase inhibitor least affected by this interaction and may be preferable for use with an azole antifungal, if needed.

---

itraconazole ━━━►◄━━━ nisoldipine

Sporanox   Sular

Risk rating: 2
Severity: Moderate   Onset: Delayed   Likelihood: Suspected

Cause
Azole antifungals, such as itraconazole, inhibit CYP3A4, which is needed for nisoldipine metabolism.

Effect
Nisoldipine level, effects, and risk of adverse effects may increase.

Nursing considerations
■ Notify prescriber if patient takes both drugs; an alternative may be available.
■ If drugs must be taken together, watch for orthostatic hypotension, which stems from increased nisoldipine effect.
■ Tell patient to report adverse nisoldipine effects, including chest pain, dizziness, headache, weight gain, nausea, palpitations, and peripheral edema.

---

itraconazole ━━━►◄━━━ protease inhibitors

Sporanox   amprenavir, atazanavir,
                                  indinavir, lopinavir-ritonavir,
                                  nelfinavir, ritonavir, saquinavir

Risk rating: 2
Severity: Moderate   Onset: Delayed   Likelihood: Suspected

Cause
Azole antifungals, such as itraconazole, may inhibit metabolism of protease inhibitors.

Effect
Protease inhibitor level may increase.

Nursing considerations
- Protease inhibitor dosage may be decreased when therapy starts.
- Watch for increased protease inhibitor effects: hyperglycemia, onset of diabetes, rash, GI complaints, and altered liver function tests.
- Advise patient to report increased hunger or thirst, frequent urination, fatigue, and dry, itchy skin.
- Tell patient not to alter regimen without consulting prescriber.

---

itraconazole ➤◀ proton pump inhibitors

Sporanox

esomeprazole, lansoprazole, omeprazole, pantoprazole, rabeprazole

Risk rating: 2
Severity: Moderate　　**Onset: Rapid**　　Likelihood: **Suspected**

Cause
Proton pump inhibitors increase gastric pH, which may impair dissolution of azole antifungals, such as itraconazole.

Effect
Efficacy of azole antifungals may decrease.

Nursing considerations
- Notify prescriber if patient takes both drugs; an alternative may be available.
- If no alternative is possible, suggest taking the azole antifungal with an acidic beverage, such as cola.
- Monitor patient for lack of response to antifungal drug.
- If patient can't tolerate acidic beverages and antifungal therapy appears to be ineffective, antifungal dosage may need to be increased.
- Other drugs that increase gastric pH may interact with azole antifungals. If you suspect an interaction, consult prescriber or pharmacist.

---

itraconazole ➤◀ rifamycins

Sporanox

rifabutin, rifampin, rifapentine

Risk rating: 2
Severity: Moderate　　Onset: **Delayed**　　Likelihood: **Suspected**

Cause
Rifamycins may decrease the level of an azole antifungal, such as itraconazole.

Effect
Infection may recur.

Nursing considerations
■ Notify prescriber if patient takes both drugs; an alternative may be available.
■ If drugs must be taken together and the antifungal appears ineffective, antifungal dosage may need to be increased.
■ Teach patient to recognize signs and symptoms of his infection and to contact prescriber promptly if they occur.

---

itraconazole ▬▶◀▬ **selective 5-HT$_1$ receptor agonists**
Sporanox
almotriptan, eletriptan

Risk rating: 2
Severity: Moderate   Onset: Delayed   Likelihood: Suspected

Cause
Azole antifungals, such as itraconazole, inhibit CYP3A4 metabolism of certain 5-HT$_1$ receptor agonists.

Effect
Serum level and adverse effects of the selective 5-HT$_1$ receptor agonist may increase.

Nursing considerations
⚠ ALERT Don't give eletriptan within 72 hours or almotriptan within 7 days of itraconazole.
■ Adverse effects of selective 5-HT$_1$ receptor agonists may include coronary artery vasospasm, dizziness, nausea, paresthesia, and somnolence.

---

itraconazole ▬▶◀▬ **sirolimus**
Sporanox
Rapamune

Risk rating: 2
Severity: Moderate   Onset: Delayed   Likelihood: Suspected

Cause
Azole antifungals, such as itraconazole, inhibit CYP3A4, which is needed for sirolimus metabolism.

Effect
Sirolimus level, effects, and risk of adverse effects may increase.

Nursing considerations

■ Monitor trough level of sirolimus in whole blood when starting or stopping an azole antifungal. Therapeutic level varies depending on which other drugs patient receives—cyclosporine, for example.

■ Watch for signs of sirolimus toxicity, such as anemia, leukopenia, thrombocytopenia, hypokalemia, hyperlipemia, fever, interstitial lung disease, and diarrhea.

■ Other CYP3A4 inhibitors may interact with sirolimus. If you suspect an interaction, consult prescriber or pharmacist.

■ Urge patient to promptly report new onset of fever higher than 100° F (38° C), fatigue, shortness of breath, easy bruising, gum bleeding, muscle twitches, palpitations, or chest discomfort or pain.

---

itraconazole ➤◄ tolterodine
Sporanox   Detrol

Risk rating: 2
Severity: Moderate   **Onset: Delayed**   **Likelihood: Suspected**

Cause
Azole antifungals, such as itraconazole, inhibit CYP3A4, which is needed for tolterodine metabolism.

Effect
Tolterodine level, effects, and risk of toxicity may increase.

Nursing considerations
■ Tell prescriber if patient takes both drugs; an alternative may be available.

■ Watch for evidence of tolterodine overdose: dry mouth, urine retention, constipation, dizziness, and headache.

■ Explain adverse tolterodine effects and the need to report them promptly.

■ Other CYP3A4 inhibitors may interact with tolterodine. If you suspect an interaction, consult prescriber or pharmacist.

---

itraconazole ➤◄ vinca alkaloids
Sporanox   vinblastine, vincristine

Risk rating: 1
Severity: Major   **Onset: Delayed**   **Likelihood: Probable**

Cause
Azole antifungals, such as itraconazole, inhibit CYP3A4, which is needed for vinca alkaloid metabolism.

Effect
Risk of vinca alkaloid toxicity increases.

Nursing considerations
- If possible, avoid giving these drugs together.
- **ALERT** The risk of serious toxicity is increased with itraconazole.
- If use together is unavoidable, watch for evidence of toxicity, such as constipation, myalgia, hypertension, hyponatremia, and neutropenia.
- Explain adverse vinca alkaloid effects and the need to report them promptly.
- Stop azole antifungal as soon as possible.

---

ketoconazole ➤◄ benzodiazepines
Nizoral

alprazolam, chlordiazepoxide, clonazepam, clorazepate, diazepam, estazolam, flurazepam, midazolam, quazepam, triazolam

Risk rating: 2
Severity: Moderate   **Onset: Rapid**   **Likelihood: Established**

Cause
Azole antifungals, such as ketoconazole, decrease CYP3A4 metabolism of certain benzodiazepines.

Effect
Benzodiazepine effects are increased and prolonged, which may cause CNS depression and psychomotor impairment.

Nursing considerations
- **ALERT** Use of alprazolam or triazolam with ketoconazole is contraindicated.
- Caution that the effects of this interaction may last several days after stopping the azole antifungal.
- Explain that taking these drugs together may increase sedative effects; tell patient to report such effects promptly.
- Explain alternative methods of inducing sleep or relieving anxiety during antifungal therapy.
- Various azole antifungal–benzodiazepine combinations may interact. If you suspect an interaction, consult prescriber or pharmacist.

ketoconazole ▶◀ didanosine
Nizoral   Videx

Risk rating: 2
Severity: Moderate   Onset: Rapid   Likelihood: Suspected

Cause
Inert ingredients in chewable didanosine tablets decrease absorption of azole antifungals, such as ketoconazole.

Effect
Efficacy of azole antifungals may decrease.

Nursing considerations
■ To minimize interaction, instruct patient to take antifungal drug 2 hours before didanosine.
■ Monitor patient for lack of response to antifungal drug.
■ Other azole antifungals may interact with didanosine. If you suspect an interaction, consult prescriber or pharmacist.
■ Help patient develop a plan to ensure proper dosage intervals.

ketoconazole ▶◀ H₂ antagonists
Nizoral   cimetidine, famotidine,
                                 nizatidine, ranitidine

Risk rating: 2
Severity: Moderate   Onset: Delayed   Likelihood: Suspected

Cause
Ketoconazole availability may decrease because elevated gastric pH may reduce tablet dissolution.

Effect
Ketoconazole effects may decrease.

Nursing considerations
■ If possible, don't give ketoconazole, an azole antifungal, with an H_2 antagonist.
■ If combined use is needed, give 680 mg of glutamic acid hydrochloride 15 minutes before ketoconazole.
■ Watch for expected antifungal effects.
■ Explain that other drugs that increase gastric pH, such as antacids, also may decrease ketoconazole absorption.

ketoconazole ▰▰▰►◄▰▰▰ HMG-CoA reductase inhibitors
Nizoral

atorvastatin, fluvastatin, lovastatin, pravastatin, rosuvastatin, simvastatin

Risk rating: 2
Severity: Moderate   **Onset: Rapid**   Likelihood: **Probable**

Cause
Azole antifungals, such as ketoconazole, may inhibit hepatic metabolism of HMG-CoA reductase inhibitors.

Effect
HMG-CoA reductase inhibitor level and adverse effects may increase.

Nursing considerations
- If possible, avoid use together.
- If drugs must be taken together, HMG-CoA reductase inhibitor dosage may need to be decreased.
- Monitor serum cholesterol and lipid levels.
- **⚡ ALERT** Assess patient for evidence of rhabdomyolysis: fatigue; muscle aches and weakness; joint pain; dark, red, or cola-colored urine; weight gain; seizures; and greatly increased CK level.
- Pravastatin is the HMG-CoA reductase inhibitor least affected by this interaction and may be best for use with an azole antifungal.

ketoconazole ▰▰▰►◄▰▰▰ nisoldipine
Nizoral   Sular

Risk rating: 2
Severity: Moderate   **Onset: Delayed**   Likelihood: **Suspected**

Cause
Azole antifungals, such as ketoconazole, inhibit CYP3A4, which is needed for nisoldipine metabolism.

Effect
Nisoldipine level, effects, and risk of adverse effects may increase.

Nursing considerations
- Tell prescriber if patient takes both drugs; an alternative may be available.
- If drugs must be taken together, watch for orthostatic hypotension, which stems from increased nisoldipine effect.

■ Tell patient to report adverse nisoldipine effects, including chest pain, dizziness, headache, weight gain, nausea, palpitations, and peripheral edema.

---

ketoconazole ━━━▶◀ protease inhibitors

Nizoral

amprenavir, atazanavir, indinavir, lopinavir-ritonavir, nelfinavir, ritonavir, saquinavir

Risk rating: 2
Severity: Moderate   Onset: Delayed   Likelihood: Suspected

Cause
Azole antifungals, such as ketoconazole, may inhibit metabolism of protease inhibitors.

Effect
Protease inhibitor level may increase.

Nursing considerations
■ Protease inhibitor dosage may be decreased when therapy starts.
■ Monitor patient for increased protease inhibitor effects, including hyperglycemia, onset of diabetes, rash, GI complaints, and altered liver function tests.
■ Advise patient to report increased hunger or thirst, frequent urination, fatigue, and dry, itchy skin.
■ Tell patient not to change dosage or stop either drug without consulting prescriber.

---

ketoconazole ━━━▶◀ proton pump inhibitors

Nizoral

esomeprazole, lansoprazole, omeprazole, pantoprazole, rabeprazole

Risk rating: 2
Severity: Moderate   Onset: Rapid   Likelihood: Suspected

Cause
Proton pump inhibitors increase gastric pH, which may impair dissolution of azole antifungals, such as ketoconazole.

Effect
Azole antifungal efficacy may decrease.

Nursing considerations
- Tell prescriber if patient takes both drugs; an alternative may be available.
- If no alternative is possible, suggest taking the azole antifungal with an acidic beverage, such as cola.
- Monitor patient for lack of response to antifungal.
- If patient can't tolerate acidic beverages and antifungal therapy appears to be ineffective, antifungal dosage may need to be increased.
- Other drugs that increase gastric pH may interact with azole antifungals. If you suspect an interaction, consult prescriber or pharmacist.

ketoconazole ▸◀ quinine derivatives
Nizoral
quinidine, quinine

Risk rating: 2
Severity: Moderate   **Onset: Delayed**   **Likelihood: Suspected**

Cause
Hepatic CYP3A4 metabolism of quinine derivatives is inhibited.

Effect
Quinine derivative level may increase, resulting in toxicity.

Nursing considerations
- When starting or stopping ketoconazole, monitor quinidine level.
- Therapeutic range of quinidine is 2 to 6 mcg/ml. More specific assays have levels of less than 1 mcg/ml.
- Monitor ECG for conduction disturbances, prolonged QTc interval, and increased ventricular ectopy.
- Urge patient to report palpitations, chest pain, dizziness, and shortness of breath.

ketoconazole ▸◀ rifamycins
Nizoral
rifabutin, rifampin, rifapentine

Risk rating: 2
Severity: Moderate   **Onset: Delayed**   **Likelihood: Suspected**

Cause
Rifamycins may decrease level of ketoconazole, an azole antifungal. Also, ketoconazole may decease rifampin level.

Effect
Infection may recur.

Nursing considerations
- Tell prescriber if patient takes both drugs; an alternative may be available.
- If ketoconazole and rifampin must be taken together, separate doses by 12 hours.
- If drugs must be taken together and the antifungal appears ineffective, antifungal dosage may need to be increased.
- Teach patient to recognize signs and symptoms of infection and to contact prescriber promptly if they occur.

---

ketoconazole ▬▶◀▬ selective 5-HT$_1$ receptor agonists
Nizoral

almotriptan, eletriptan

Risk rating: 2
Severity: Moderate   Onset: Delayed   Likelihood: Suspected

Cause
Azole antifungals, such as ketoconazole, inhibit CYP3A4 metabolism of certain 5-HT$_1$ receptor agonists.

Effect
Serum level and adverse effects of the selective 5-HT$_1$ receptor agonist may increase.

Nursing considerations
▪ **ALERT** Don't give eletriptan within 72 hours or almotriptan within 7 days of ketoconazole.
- Adverse effects of selective 5-HT$_1$ receptor agonists may include coronary artery vasospasm, dizziness, nausea, paresthesia, and somnolence.

---

ketoconazole ▬▶◀▬ sirolimus
Nizoral

Rapamune

Risk rating: 2
Severity: Moderate   Onset: Delayed   Likelihood: Suspected

Cause
Azole antifungals, such as ketoconazole, inhibit CYP3A4, which is needed for sirolimus metabolism.

Effect
Sirolimus level, effects, and risk of toxicity may increase.

Nursing considerations
■ Monitor trough level of sirolimus in whole blood when starting or stopping an azole antifungal. Therapeutic level varies depending on which other drugs patient receives—cyclosporine, for example.
■ Watch for signs of sirolimus toxicity, such as anemia, leukopenia, thrombocytopenia, hypokalemia, hyperlipemia, fever, interstitial lung disease, and diarrhea.
■ Other CYP3A4 inhibitors may interact with sirolimus. If you suspect an interaction, consult prescriber or pharmacist.
■ Urge patient to promptly report new onset of fever higher than 100° F (38° C), fatigue, shortness of breath, easy bruising, gum bleeding, muscle twitches, palpitations, or chest discomfort or pain.

---

ketoconazole ▰▶◀▰ tolterodine
Nizoral   Detrol

Risk rating: 2
Severity: Moderate   **Onset: Delayed**   **Likelihood: Suspected**

Cause
Azole antifungals, such as ketoconazole, inhibit CYP3A4, which is needed for tolterodine metabolism.

Effect
Tolterodine level, effects, and risk of toxicity may increase.

Nursing considerations
■ Tell prescriber if patient takes both drugs; an alternative may be available.
■ Watch for evidence of tolterodine overdose, such as dry mouth, urine retention, constipation, dizziness, and headache.
■ Other CYP3A4 inhibitors may interact with tolterodine. If you suspect an interaction, consult prescriber or pharmacist.
■ Explain adverse tolterodine effects and need to report them promptly.

ketoconazole ━━━▶◀━━━ tricyclic antidepressants
Nizoral   amitriptyline, imipramine,
                                     nortriptyline

Risk rating: 2
Severity: **Moderate**   Onset: **Delayed**   Likelihood: **Suspected**

Cause
Azole antifungals, such as ketoconazole, may inhibit metabolism of
tricyclic antidepressants (TCAs) by CYP pathways.

Effect
Serum TCA level and risk of toxicity may increase.

Nursing considerations
■ When starting or stopping an azole antifungal, monitor serum TCA
level and adjust dosage as needed.
■ After starting an azole antifungal, check sitting and standing blood
pressure for changes.
■ Assess symptoms and behavior for adverse reactions, such as increased drowsiness, dizziness, confusion, heart rate or rhythm
changes, and urine retention.

ketoconazole ━━━▶◀━━━ vinca alkaloids
Nizoral   vinblastine, vincristine

Risk rating: 1
Severity: **Major**   Onset: **Delayed**   Likelihood: **Probable**

Cause
Azole antifungals, such as ketoconazole, inhibit CYP3A4, which is
needed for vinca alkaloid metabolism.

Effect
Risk of vinca alkaloid toxicity increases.

Nursing considerations
■ If possible, avoid giving these drugs together.
■ If use together is unavoidable, watch for signs of toxicity, such
as constipation, myalgia, hypertension, hyponatremia, and neutro-
penia.
■ Stop azole antifungal as soon as possible.
◢ ALERT The risk of serious toxicity is increased with ketoconazole.
■ Explain adverse vinca alkaloid effects, and tell patient to report
them promptly.

ketoprofen ■■■■▶◀■■■ aminoglycosides
Oruvail

amikacin, gentamicin,
kanamycin, netilmicin,
streptomycin, tobramycin

Risk rating: 2
Severity: Moderate   Onset: Delayed   Likelihood: Suspected

Cause
Ketoprofen and other NSAIDs may reduce glomerular filtration rate
(GFR), causing aminoglycosides to accumulate.

Effect
Aminoglycoside level in premature infants may increase.

Nursing considerations
- Before NSAID starts, aminoglycoside dose should be reduced.
- ⚡ ALERT Check peak and trough aminoglycoside levels after third
dose. For peak level, draw blood 30 minutes after I.V. or 60 minutes
after I.M. dose. For trough level, draw blood just before a dose.
- Monitor patient's renal function.
- Although only indomethacin is known to interact with aminoglyco-
sides, other NSAIDs probably do as well. If you suspect an interac-
tion, consult prescriber or pharmacist.
- Other drugs cleared by GFR may have a similar interaction.

ketorolac ■■■■▶◀■■■ aminoglycosides
Toradol

amikacin, gentamicin,
kanamycin, netilmicin,
streptomycin, tobramycin

Risk rating: 2
Severity: Moderate   Onset: Delayed   Likelihood: Suspected

Cause
Ketorolac and other NSAIDs may reduce glomerular filtration rate
(GFR), causing aminoglycosides to accumulate.

Effect
Aminoglycoside level in premature infants may increase.

Nursing considerations
- Before NSAID starts, aminoglycoside dose should be reduced.
- ⚡ ALERT Check peak and trough aminoglycoside levels after the
third dose. For peak level, draw blood 30 minutes after an I.V. or

60 minutes after an I.M. dose. For trough level, draw blood just before a dose.

- Monitor patient's renal function.
- Although only indomethacin is known to interact with aminoglycosides, other NSAIDs probably do as well. If you suspect an interaction, consult prescriber or pharmacist.
- Other drugs cleared by GFR may have a similar interaction.

---

ketorolac ■■■▶◀■■■ aspirin
Toradol   Bayer

Risk rating: 1
Severity: Major   **Onset: Delayed**   **Likelihood: Suspected**

Cause
Aspirin may displace ketorolac from protein-binding sites, increasing unbound ketorolac level.

Effect
Risk of serious ketorolac-related adverse effects increases.

Nursing considerations
◤ **ALERT** Ketorolac is contraindicated in patients taking aspirin or other NSAIDs.

- If drugs are inadvertently taken together, watch for adverse effects, such as GI bleeding, neurotoxicity, renal failure, blood dyscrasias, and hepatotoxicity.
- Ketorolac therapy isn't meant to exceed 5 days.
- Urge patient to tell prescriber and pharmacist about all drugs (prescribed and OTC) and supplements he takes.

---

ketorolac ■■■▶◀■■■ probenecid
Toradol   Probalan

Risk rating: 1
Severity: Major   **Onset: Delayed**   **Likelihood: Suspected**

Cause
Probenecid may decrease ketorolac clearance.

Effect
Ketorolac level and risk of adverse effects and toxicity may increase.

Nursing considerations
◤ **ALERT** Use of ketorolac with probenecid is contraindicated.

- Monitor patient for such adverse effects as GI bleeding, neurotoxicity, renal failure, blood dyscrasias, and hepatotoxicity.
- Monitor renal and liver function tests and hematologic and coagulation parameters.
- Ketorolac therapy isn't meant to exceed 5 days.
- Urge patient to report such adverse effects as headache, dizziness, drowsiness, increased bleeding or bruising, abdominal pain, tarry stools, hematemesis, decreased urine output, loss of appetite, fatigue, yellow skin or eye discoloration, and dark urine.

---

lamotrigine ➤◀ carbamazepine
Lamictal

Carbatrol, Epitol, Equetro, Tegretol

Risk rating: 2
Severity: Moderate   Onset: Delayed   Likelihood: Suspected

Cause
Lamotrigine metabolism may increase. Carbamazepine toxicity may increase.

Effect
Lamotrigine effects may decrease. Carbamazepine active metabolite levels and risk of carbamazepine toxicity may increase.

Nursing considerations
- Watch for expected lamotrigine effects when starting therapy in a patient taking carbamazepine.
- Lamotrigine dosage may need adjustment when starting, changing, or stopping carbamazepine therapy.
- Monitor carbamazepine level when adding lamotrigine; carbamazepine therapeutic range is 4 to 12 mcg/ml.
- Watch for evidence of carbamazepine toxicity: dizziness, ataxia, respiratory depression, tachycardia, arrhythmias, blood pressure changes, impaired consciousness, abnormal reflexes, nystagmus, seizures, nausea, vomiting, and urine retention.
- Carbamazepine dosage may need reduction.

lansoprazole ▰▰▰►◄▰▰▰ azole antifungals
Prevacid   itraconazole, ketoconazole

Risk rating: 2
Severity: Moderate   **Onset: Rapid**   **Likelihood: Suspected**

Cause
Proton pump inhibitors, such as lansoprazole, increase gastric pH, which may impair dissolution of azole antifungals.

Effect
Efficacy of azole antifungals may decrease.

Nursing considerations
■ Notify prescriber if patient takes both drugs; an alternative may be available.
■ If no alternative is possible, suggest taking the azole antifungal with an acidic beverage, such as cola.
■ Monitor patient for lack of response to antifungal drug.
■ If patient can't tolerate acidic beverages and antifungal therapy appears to be ineffective, antifungal dosage may need to be increased.
■ Other drugs that increase gastric pH may interact with azole antifungals. If you suspect an interaction, consult prescriber or pharmacist.

levodopa ▰▰▰►◄▰▰▰ iron salts
Larodopa   ferrous fumarate, ferrous gluconate, ferrous sulfate, iron polysaccharide

Risk rating: 2
Severity: Moderate   **Onset: Delayed**   **Likelihood: Probable**

Cause
Levodopa may form chelates with iron salts, which decreases levodopa absorption and serum level.

Effect
Levodopa effects may decrease.

Nursing considerations
■ Separate doses as much as possible.
■ Watch for loss of levodopa effects if iron salts are added to a stable regimen. Evidence of recurring or worsening Parkinson's symptoms may include increased tremors, muscle rigidity, bradykinesia (slowing

of voluntary movement), shuffling gait, loss of facial expression, speech disturbances, and drooling.
■ Notify prescriber about loss of symptom control.
■ Warn patient or caregiver not to change levodopa dosage without consulting prescriber.
■ Help patient develop a plan to ensure proper dosage intervals.

levodopa ▸◂ hydantoins
Larodopa   ethotoin, phenytoin

Risk rating: 2
Severity: Moderate   Onset: Delayed   Likelihood: Suspected

Cause
The exact mechanism of this interaction is unknown.

Effect
Levodopa effects may decrease.

Nursing considerations
■ Avoid this combination, if possible.
■ If these drugs are used together, watch for recurring or worsening Parkinson's symptoms: increased tremors, muscle rigidity, bradykinesia (slowing of voluntary movement), shuffling gait, loss of facial expression, speech disturbances, and drooling.
■ In patient treated for chronic manganese poisoning, watch for recurring or worsening symptoms of manganese toxicity: muscle weakness, difficulty walking, tremors, salivation, and psychological disturbances, such as irritability, aggressiveness, and hallucinations.
■ If you suspect a drug interaction, consult prescriber or pharmacist; an alternative therapy may need to be considered.
■ Warn patient or caregiver not to change levodopa dosage without consulting prescriber.

levodopa ▸◂ MAO inhibitors
Larodopa   phenelzine, tranylcypromine

Risk rating: 1
Severity: Major   Onset: Rapid   Likelihood: Established

Cause
Peripheral metabolism of levodopa-derived dopamine is inhibited, increasing level at dopamine receptors.

Effect
Risk of hypertensive reaction increases.

Nursing considerations
- If possible, avoid giving these drugs together.
- Interaction occurs within 1 hour and appears to be dose related.
- Monitor patient for flushing, light-headedness, and palpitations.
- Selegiline doesn't cause hypertensive reaction and may be used instead of other MAO inhibitors in patients taking levodopa.

---

levodopa ◄►► pyridoxine (vitamin B₆)

levodopa ▆▆▆▆◄► pyridoxine (vitamin B_6)

Larodopa   Aminoxin

Risk rating: 2
Severity: Moderate   **Onset: Rapid**   **Likelihood: Established**

Cause
Pyridoxine increases peripheral metabolism of levodopa, decreasing level available for penetration into the CNS.

Effect
Pyridoxine reduces levodopa efficacy in Parkinson's disease.

Nursing considerations
- Avoid combined use of pyridoxine and levodopa in patients taking levodopa alone.
- Watch for recurring or worsening Parkinson's symptoms: increased tremors, muscle rigidity, bradykinesia (slowing of voluntary movement), shuffling gait, loss of facial expression, speech disturbances, and drooling.
- Advise patient and caregivers that multivitamins, fortified cereals, and certain OTC drugs may contain pyridoxine.
- ◤ ALERT The effect of pyridoxine is minimal or negligible in patients taking levodopa-carbidopa combination products.

---

levofloxacin ▆▆▆◄► antiarrhythmics

Levaquin   amiodarone, bretylium, disopyramide, procainamide, quinidine, sotalol

Risk rating: 1
Severity: Major   **Onset: Delayed**   **Likelihood: Suspected**

Cause
The mechanism of this interaction is unknown.

Effect
Risk of life-threatening arrhythmias, including torsades de pointes, increases.

Nursing considerations
■ Avoid giving class IA or class III antiarrhythmics with the quinolone levofloxacin.
■ Monitor the ECG for prolonged QTc interval.
■ Tell patient to report a rapid heartbeat, shortness of breath, dizziness, fainting, and chest pain.
■ Quinolones that aren't metabolized by CYP3A4 isoenzymes or that don't prolong the QT interval may be given with antiarrhythmics.

---

levofloxacin ▶◀ erythromycin
Levaquin   E-mycin, Eryc

Risk rating: 1
Severity: Major   **Onset: Delayed**   **Likelihood: Suspected**

Cause
The mechanism of this interaction is unknown.

Effect
Risk of life-threatening arrhythmias, including torsades de pointes, increases.

Nursing considerations
■ Avoid use of levofloxacin with erythromycin because doing so may prolong the QT interval.
■ Monitor the QTc interval closely.
■ Tell patient to report palpitations, dizziness, shortness of breath, and chest pain.

---

levofloxacin ▶◀ iron salts
Levaquin   ferrous fumarate, ferrous
                                gluconate, ferrous sulfate,
                                iron polysaccharide

Risk rating: 2
Severity: Moderate   **Onset: Rapid**   **Likelihood: Probable**

Cause
Formation of an iron-quinolone complex decreases GI absorption of quinolones, such as levofloxacin.

Effect
Quinolone effects decrease.

Nursing considerations
■ Quinolones other than levofloxacin may interact with iron.

- Monitor patient for quinolone efficacy.
- Tell patient to separate quinolone dose from iron by at least 2 hours.
- Help patient develop a plan to ensure proper dosage intervals.

---

levofloxacin ▶◀ **phenothiazines**

Levaquin

chlorpromazine, fluphenazine, mesoridazine, perphenazine, prochlorperazine, promethazine, thioridazine

---

Risk rating: 1
Severity: Major   Onset: **Delayed**   Likelihood: **Suspected**

Cause
The mechanism of this interaction is unknown.

Effect
Risk of life-threatening arrhythmias, including torsades de pointes, may increase.

Nursing considerations
- Avoid giving the quinolone levofloxacin with a phenothiazine.
- Quinolones that don't prolong the QTc interval or that aren't metabolized by CYP3A4 isoenzymes may be better alternatives.

---

levofloxacin ▶◀ **tricyclic antidepressants**

Levaquin

amitriptyline, amoxapine, clomipramine, desipramine, doxepin, imipramine, nortriptyline, trimipramine

---

Risk rating: 1
Severity: Major   Onset: **Delayed**   Likelihood: **Suspected**

Cause
The mechanism of this interaction if unknown.

Effect
Life-threatening arrhythmias, including torsades de pointes, may increase when certain of these drugs are used together.

Nursing considerations
- ⚡ ALERT Avoid giving the quinolone levofloxacin with a tricyclic antidepressant.
- If possible, use other quinolone antibiotics that don't prolong the QTc interval or aren't metabolized by the CYP3A4 isoenzyme.

levothyroxine ◾▶◀◾ estrogens

Synthroid

conjugated estrogens, esterified estrogens, estradiol, estrone, estropipate, ethinyl estradiol

Risk rating: 2
Severity: Moderate   **Onset: Delayed**   **Likelihood: Probable**

Cause
Estrogen increases level of thyroxine-binding globulin. Because thyroid hormone binds to it, T_3 and T_4 levels decrease, and TSH is secreted to compensate.

Effect
In hypothyroid women, decreased T_3 and T_4 levels and increased TSH level decrease the efficacy of thyroid hormone replacement.

Nursing considerations
■ Check serum TSH, T_3, and T_4 levels about 12 weeks after a hypothyroid patient starts estrogen therapy.
■ Therapeutic range for TSH is 0.2 to 5.4 microunits/ml; for T_3, 80 to 200 nanogram/dl; and for T_4, 5.4 to 11.5 mcg/dl.
■ Watch for evidence of hypothyroidism: weakness, fatigue, weight gain, coarse dry hair, rough skin, cold intolerance, muscle aches, constipation, depression, irritability, and memory loss. Tell patient to report evidence of hypothyroidism.
■ Explain that thyroid hormone dose may need to be altered during estrogen therapy.

levothyroxine ◾▶◀◾ iron salts

Synthroid

ferrous fumarate, ferrous gluconate, ferrous sulfate, iron polysaccharide

Risk rating: 2
Severity: Moderate   **Onset: Delayed**   **Likelihood: Suspected**

Cause
Levothyroxine absorption may be decreased, probably because it forms a complex with iron salt.

Effect
Levothyroxine effects may decrease, resulting in hypothyroidism.

Nursing considerations
◆ **ALERT** Separate levothyroxine from iron salts as much as possible.

■ Monitor TSH, T_3, and T_4 levels. Therapeutic range for TSH is 0.2 to 5.4 microunits/ml; for T_3, 80 to 200 nanograms/dl; and for T_4, 5.4 to 11.5 mcg/dl.

■ Levothyroxine dosage may need adjustment.

■ Watch for evidence of hypothyroidism: weakness, fatigue, weight gain, coarse dry hair, rough skin, cold intolerance, muscle aches, constipation, depression, irritability, and memory loss. Urge patient to report such symptoms to prescriber.

---

levothyroxine ━━▶◀━━ theophyllines
Synthroid   aminophylline, theophylline

Risk rating: 2
Severity: Moderate   **Onset: Delayed**   **Likelihood: Suspected**

Cause
Thyroxine level is directly related to theophylline level. Patients who are hyperthyroid or hypothyroid may have varying interactions.

Effect
In hypothyroidism, theophylline metabolism decreases and serum level—and risk of toxicity—increase.

Nursing considerations
■ Monitor theophylline level and dosage carefully; adjust dosage as needed to avoid theophylline toxicity.

■ Normal therapeutic range is 10 to 20 mcg/ml for adults and 5 to 15 mcg/ml for children.

■ Watch for increased adverse effects of theophylline, such as tachycardia, anorexia, nausea, vomiting, diarrhea, seizures, restlessness, irritability, and headache.

■ Once a patient becomes euthyroid, theophylline clearance returns to normal.

■ Explain common side effects of theophylline and signs of toxicity, and tell patient to report them immediately to prescriber.

---

lidocaine ━━▶◀━━ beta blockers
                              atenolol, metoprolol, nadolol,
                              pindolol, propranolol

Risk rating: 2
Severity: Moderate   **Onset: Rapid**   **Likelihood: Established**

Cause
Beta blockers reduce hepatic metabolism of lidocaine.

Effect
Lidocaine level and risk of toxicity may increase.

Nursing considerations
■ Check for normal therapeutic level of lidocaine: 2 to 5 mcg/ml.
■ Assess patient for evidence of lidocaine toxicity, including dizziness, somnolence, confusion, paresthesias, and seizures.
■ Slow the I.V. bolus rate to decrease the risk of high peak level and toxic reaction.
■ Explain the warning signs of toxicity to patient and family, and tell them to contact prescriber if they have concerns.

---

lidocaine ▶◀ cimetidine
Tagamet

Risk rating: 2
Severity: Moderate   **Onset: Rapid**   **Likelihood: Established**

Cause
Hepatic metabolism of lidocaine may decrease.

Effect
Risk of lidocaine toxicity increases.

Nursing considerations
■ Ask prescriber or pharmacist about an H_2-receptor antagonist other than cimetidine, such as ranitidine or famotidine, that may be safer in combination. Monitor lidocaine level; therapeutic range is 1.5 to 6 mcg/ml.
■ Assess patient for evidence of lidocaine toxicity: dizziness, somnolence, confusion, tremors, paresthesias, seizures, hypotension, arrhythmias, respiratory depression, and coma.
■ Adjust lidocaine dosage as ordered.
■ Other H_2-receptor antagonists may interact with lidocaine. If you suspect an interaction, consult prescriber or pharmacist.

---

liothyronine ▶◀ theophyllines
Cytomel   aminophylline, theophylline

Risk rating: 2
Severity: Moderate   **Onset: Delayed**   **Likelihood: Suspected**

Cause
Thyroxine level is directly related to theophylline level. Patients who are hyperthyroid or hypothyroid may have varying interactions.

Effect

In hypothyroidism, theophylline metabolism decreases and serum level—and risk of toxicity—increase.

Nursing considerations

- Monitor theophylline level and dosage carefully; adjust dosage as needed to avoid theophylline toxicity.
- Normal therapeutic range is 10 to 20 mcg/ml for adults and 5 to 15 mcg/ml for children.
- Watch for increased adverse effects of theophylline, such as tachycardia, anorexia, nausea, vomiting, diarrhea, seizures, restlessness, irritability, and headache.
- Once a patient becomes euthyroid, theophylline clearance returns to normal.
- Explain common side effects of theophylline and signs of toxicity, and tell patient to report them immediately to prescriber.

---

liotrix ◄► estrogens

Thyrolar

conjugated estrogens, esterified estrogens, estradiol, estrone, estropipate, ethinyl estradiol

---

Risk rating: 2
Severity: Moderate   Onset: Delayed   Likelihood: Probable

Cause

Estrogen increases serum level of thyroxine-binding globulin. Because thyroid hormone binds to it, T_3 and T_4 levels decrease, and TSH is secreted to compensate.

Effect

In hypothyroid women, decreased T_3 and T_4 levels and increased TSH level decrease the efficacy of thyroid hormone replacement.

Nursing considerations

- Check serum TSH, T_3, and T_4 levels about 12 weeks after hypothyroid patient starts estrogen therapy.
- Therapeutic range for TSH is 0.2 to 5.4 microunits/ml; for T_3, 80 to 200 nanogram/dl; and for T_4, 5.4 to 11.5 mcg/dl.
- Watch for evidence of hypothyroidism: weakness, fatigue, weight gain, coarse dry hair, rough skin, cold intolerance, muscle aches, constipation, depression, irritability, and memory loss.
- Adjust thyroid hormone dose as ordered.
- Explain that thyroid hormone dose may need to be altered during estrogen therapy.
- Tell patient to report evidence of hypothyroidism, such as fatigue, weight gain, cold intolerance, and constipation.

liotrix ►◄ theophyllines
Thyrolar aminophylline, theophylline

Risk rating: 2
Severity: Moderate **Onset: Delayed** **Likelihood: Suspected**

Cause
Thyroxine level is directly related to theophylline level. Patients who are hyperthyroid or hypothyroid may have varying interactions.

Effect
In hypothyroidism, theophylline metabolism decreases and serum level—and risk of toxicity—increase.

Nursing considerations
- Monitor theophylline level and dosage carefully; adjust dosage as needed to avoid theophylline toxicity.
- Normal therapeutic range is 10 to 20 mcg/ml for adults and 5 to 15 mcg/ml for children.
- Watch for increased adverse effects of theophylline, such as tachycardia, anorexia, nausea, vomiting, diarrhea, seizures, restlessness, irritability, and headache.
- Once a patient becomes euthyroid, theophylline clearance returns to normal.
- Explain common side effects of theophylline and signs of toxicity, and tell patient to report them immediately to prescriber.

lisinopril ►◄ indomethacin
Prinivil, Zestril Indocin

Risk rating: 2
Severity: Moderate **Onset: Rapid** **Likelihood: Probable**

Cause
Indomethacin inhibits synthesis of prostaglandins, which lisinopril and other ACE inhibitors need to lower blood pressure.

Effect
ACE inhibitor's hypotensive effect will be reduced.

Nursing considerations
- **⚡ ALERT** Monitor blood pressure closely. Severe hypertension may persist until indomethacin is stopped.
- If indomethacin can't be avoided, patient may need a different antihypertensive.
- Other ACE inhibitors may interact with indomethacin. If you suspect an interaction, consult prescriber or pharmacist.

■ Remind patient that hypertension commonly causes no physical symptoms but sometimes may cause headache and dizziness.

---

lisinopril ▶◀ potassium-sparing diuretics

Prinivil, Zestril

amiloride, spironolactone, triamterene

Risk rating: 1
Severity: Major   **Onset: Delayed**   **Likelihood: Probable**

Cause
The mechanism of this interaction is unknown.

Effect
Serum potassium level may increase.

Nursing considerations
■ Use cautiously in patients at high risk for hyperkalemia, especially those with renal impairment.
■ Monitor BUN, creatinine, and serum potassium levels as needed.
■ ACE inhibitors other than lisinopril may interact with potassium-sparing diuretics. If you suspect an interaction, consult prescriber or pharmacist.
■ Urge patient to immediately report an irregular heartbeat, a slow pulse, weakness, and other evidence of hyperkalemia.

---

lithium ▶◀ ACE inhibitors

Eskalith

benazepril, captopril, enalapril, fosinopril, lisinopril, moexipril, quinapril, ramipril, trandolapril

Risk rating: 2
Severity: Moderate   **Onset: Delayed**   **Likelihood: Suspected**

Cause
The mechanism for this interaction is unknown.

Effect
Lithium level may be elevated and neurotoxicity may occur.

Nursing considerations
■ If patient takes lithium, consider an antihypertensive other than an ACE inhibitor.
■ Monitor lithium level. Steady state lithium level should be 0.6 to 1.2 mEq/L.

■ Adjust lithium dose as needed.
■ Watch for evidence of lithium toxicity, such as diarrhea, vomiting, dehydration, drowsiness, muscle weakness, tremor, fever, and ataxia.
■ Use with added caution in elderly patients and those with heart failure, renal insufficiency, or volume depletion. Dehydration may increase the effects of this interaction.

lithium ➤◀ angiotensin II receptor antagonists
Eskalith

candesartan, eprosartan, irbesartan, losartan, telmisartan, valsartan

Risk rating: 2
Severity: **Moderate**   Onset: **Delayed**   Likelihood: **Suspected**

Cause
Angiotensin II receptor antagonists may decrease lithium excretion.

Effect
Lithium level, effects, and risk of toxicity may increase.

Nursing considerations
■ If patient takes lithium, consider an antihypertensive other than an angiotensin II receptor antagonist.
■ Monitor lithium level. Steady state lithium level should be 0.6 to 1.2 mEq/L.
■ Adjust lithium dose as needed.
■ Monitor patient for evidence of lithium toxicity, such as diarrhea, vomiting, dehydration, drowsiness, muscle weakness, tremor, fever, and ataxia.

lithium ➤◀ carbamazepine
Eskalith

Carbatrol, Epitol, Equetro, Tegretol

Risk rating: 2
Severity: **Moderate**   Onset: **Delayed**   Likelihood: **Suspected**

Cause
The mechanism of this interaction is unknown.

Effect
Risk of adverse CNS effects—including lethargy, muscle weakness, ataxia, tremor, and hyperreflexia—increases.

Nursing considerations
■ Combining lithium and carbamazepine may help in treating bipolar disorder.
■ This combination may be justified if the benefits outweigh the risks; some patients can tolerate it without adverse effects.

lithium ◼	NSAIDs
Eskalith	celecoxib, diclofenac, ibuprofen, indomethacin, ketorolac, meloxicam, naproxen, piroxicam, sulindac

Risk rating: 2
Severity: Moderate   Onset: Delayed   Likelihood: Suspected

Cause
Lithium elimination may decrease because NSAIDs interfere with prostaglandin production in the kidneys.

Effect
Lithium level, effects, and risk of toxicity may increase.

Nursing considerations
■ Monitor lithium level. Steady state lithium level should be 0.6 to 1.2 mEq/L.
■ Adjust lithium dose as needed.
■ Monitor patient for evidence of lithium toxicity, such as diarrhea, vomiting, dehydration, drowsiness, muscle weakness, tremor, fever, and ataxia.
■ Expect lithium level to return to pretreatment value within 7 days of stopping the NSAID.

lithium ◼	sibutramine
Eskalith	Meridia

Risk rating: 1
Severity: Major   Onset: Rapid   Likelihood: Suspected

Cause
The serotonergic effects of these drugs may be additive.

Effect
A serotonin syndrome, including CNS irritability, motor weakness, shivering, myoclonus, and altered consciousness, may occur.

Nursing considerations
- Avoid using these drugs together.
- Monitor patient for adverse effects.
- **⚡ ALERT** If signs and symptoms of serotonin syndrome occur, provide immediate treatment.
- Although this interaction is rare, it may be fatal.

---

lithium ▶◀ thiazide diuretics

Eskalith

chlorothiazide, hydrochlorothiazide, indapamide, methyclothiazide, metolazone, polythiazide, trichlormethiazide

Risk rating: 2
Severity: Moderate   Onset: Delayed   Likelihood: Established

Cause
Thiazide diuretics may decrease lithium clearance.

Effect
Lithium level, effects, and risk of toxicity may increase.

Nursing considerations
- Despite this interaction, lithium and thiazide diuretics may be used together safely, with close monitoring of lithium level.
- Reduction in lithium clearance may depend on thiazide dose.
- Monitor lithium level, and adjust dose as needed.
- Monitor patient for evidence of lithium toxicity, such as diarrhea, vomiting, dehydration, drowsiness, muscle weakness, tremor, fever, and ataxia.

---

lomefloxacin ▶◀ didanosine

Maxaquin

Videx

Risk rating: 2
Severity: Moderate   Onset: Rapid   Likelihood: Suspected

Cause
Buffers in didanosine chewable tablets and pediatric powder for oral solution decrease GI absorption of quinolones, such as lomefloxacin.

Effect
Quinolone effects decrease.

Nursing considerations
■ Avoid use together. If it's unavoidable, give the quinolone at least 2 hours before or 6 hours after didanosine.
■ Monitor patient for improvement in infection for which quinolone was prescribed.
■ Unbuffered didanosine doesn't affect quinolone absorption.
■ Help patient develop a plan to ensure proper dosage intervals.

---

lomefloxacin ▶◀ iron salts
Maxaquin

ferrous fumarate, ferrous gluconate, ferrous sulfate, iron polysaccharide

Risk rating: 2
Severity: Moderate   **Onset: Rapid**   **Likelihood: Probable**

Cause
Formation of an iron-quinolone complex decreases GI absorption of quinolones, such as lomefloxacin.

Effect
Quinolone effects decrease.

Nursing considerations
■ Other quinolones may interact with iron.
■ Monitor patient for quinolone efficacy.
■ Tell patient to separate quinolone dose from iron by at least 2 hours.
■ Help patient develop a plan to ensure proper dosage intervals.

---

lomefloxacin ▶◀ sucralfate
Maxaquin

Carafate

Risk rating: 2
Severity: Moderate   **Onset: Rapid**   **Likelihood: Probable**

Cause
Sucralfate decreases GI absorption of quinolones, such as lomefloxacin.

Effect
Quinolone effects decrease.

Nursing considerations
■ Avoid use together. If it's unavoidable, give sucralfate at least 6 hours after the quinolone.
■ Monitor patient for resolving infection.

■ Help patient develop a plan to ensure proper dosage intervals.

lopinavir-ritonavir ►◄ azole antifungals
Kaletra   fluconazole, itraconazole,
                        ketoconazole

Risk rating: 2
Severity: Moderate   **Onset: Delayed**   **Likelihood: Suspected**

Cause
Azole antifungals may inhibit metabolism of protease inhibitors, such as lopinavir-ritonavir.

Effect
Protease inhibitor level may increase.

Nursing considerations
■ Protease inhibitor dosage may be decreased when therapy starts.
■ Monitor patient for increased protease inhibitor effects, including hyperglycemia, onset of diabetes, rash, GI complaints, and altered liver function tests.
■ Advise patient to report increased hunger or thirst, frequent urination, fatigue, and dry, itchy skin.
■ Tell patient not to change dosage or stop either drug without consulting prescriber.

lopinavir-ritonavir ►◄ benzodiazepines
Kaletra   alprazolam, chlordiazepoxide,
                        clonazepam, clorazepate,
                        diazepam, estazolam,
                        flurazepam, midazolam,
                        quazepam, triazolam

Risk rating: 2
Severity: Moderate   **Onset: Delayed**   **Likelihood: Suspected**

Cause
Protease inhibitors, such as lopinavir-ritonavir, may inhibit CYP3A4 metabolism of certain benzodiazepines.

Effect
Sedative effects may be increased and prolonged.

Nursing considerations
◪ **ALERT** Don't combine these benzodiazepines with protease inhibitors.

■ If patient takes any protease inhibitor–benzodiazepine combination, notify prescriber. Interaction could involve other drugs in the class.
■ Watch for evidence of oversedation and respiratory depression.
■ Teach patient and family about the risks of combined use.

lopinavir-ritonavir ➤◄ ergot derivatives
Kaletra

dihydroergotamine, ergonovine, ergotamine, methylergonovine

Risk rating: 1
Severity: Major   **Onset: Delayed**   **Likelihood: Probable**

Cause
Protease inhibitors, such as lopinavir-ritonavir, may interfere with CYP3A4 metabolism of ergot derivatives.

Effect
Risk of ergot-induced peripheral vasospasm and ischemia may increase.

Nursing considerations
⚡ **ALERT** Combined use of ergot derivatives and protease inhibitors is contraindicated.
■ Monitor patient for evidence of peripheral ischemia, including pain in limb muscles while exercising and later at rest; numbness and tingling of fingers and toes; cool, pale, or cyanotic limbs; red or violet blisters on hands or feet; and gangrene.
■ Sodium nitroprusside may be given for ergot-induced vasospasm.
■ If patient takes a protease inhibitor, consult prescriber and pharmacist about alternative treatments for migraine pain.
■ Urge patient to tell prescriber about increased adverse effects.

lopinavir-ritonavir ➤◄ HMG-CoA reductase inhibitors
Kaletra

atorvastatin, lovastatin, simvastatin

Risk rating: 2
Severity: Moderate   **Onset: Delayed**   **Likelihood: Suspected**

Cause
Protease inhibitors, such as lopinavir-ritonavir, may inhibit CYP3A4 metabolism of HMG-CoA reductase inhibitors.

Effect
HMG-CoA reductase inhibitor level may increase.

Nursing considerations
■ Monitor patient closely if a protease inhibitor is added to HMG-CoA reductase inhibitor therapy.

◪ ALERT Watch for evidence of rhabdomyolysis, including dark or red urine, muscle weakness, and myalgia.

■ Tell patient to immediately report unexplained muscle weakness.

---

lopinavir-ritonavir ➤◀ nevirapine
Kaletra   Viramune

Risk rating: 2
Severity: Major   Onset: Delayed   Likelihood: Suspected

Cause
Nevirapine may increase hepatic metabolism of protease inhibitors, such as lopinavir-ritonavir.

Effect
Protease inhibitor level and effects decrease.

Nursing considerations
■ If nevirapine is started or stopped, monitor protease inhibitor level.
■ Protease inhibitor dosage may need adjustment.
■ Monitor CD4+ and T-cell counts; tell prescriber if they decrease.
■ Urge patient to report opportunistic infections.
■ Tell patient not to change an HIV regimen without consulting prescriber.

---

lorazepam ➤◀ alcohol
Ativan

Risk rating: 2
Severity: Moderate   Onset: Rapid   Likelihood: Established

Cause
Alcohol inhibits hepatic enzymes, which decreases clearance and increases peak levels of benzodiazepines, such as lorazepam.

Effect
Combining a benzodiazepine and alcohol may have additive or synergistic effects.

Nursing considerations
■ Before benzodiazepine therapy starts, assess patient thoroughly for history or evidence of alcohol use.
■ Advise against consuming alcohol while taking a benzodiazepine.
■ Watch for additive CNS effects, which may suggest benzodiazepine overdose.

---

losartan ➤◀ indomethacin
Cozaar   Indocin

Risk rating: 2
Severity: Moderate   Onset: Delayed   Likelihood: Suspected

Cause
The mechanism of this interaction is unknown.

Effect
Hypotensive effect of losartan may decrease.

Nursing considerations
■ Antihypertensives other than losartan may not share this interaction.
■ Monitor blood pressure closely.
■ If you suspect an interaction, notify prescriber. Indomethacin may need to be stopped or a different antihypertensive considered.

---

losartan ➤◀ potassium-sparing diuretics
Cozaar

amiloride, spironolactone, triamterene

Risk rating: 1
Severity: Major   Onset: Delayed   Likelihood: Suspected

Cause
Both angiotensin II receptor antagonists, such as losartan, and potassium-sparing diuretics may increase the serum potassium level.

Effect
Risk of hyperkalemia may increase, especially among high-risk patients.

Nursing considerations
■ High-risk patients include elderly people and those with renal impairment, type 2 diabetes, or decreased renal perfusion; monitor these patients closely.

■ Check serum potassium, BUN, and creatinine levels regularly. If they increase, notify prescriber.
■ Advise patient to immediately report an irregular heartbeat, slow pulse, weakness, or other evidence of hyperkalemia.
■ Give patient a list of foods high in potassium; stress the need to eat them only in moderate amounts.

lovastatin ▶◀ amprenavir
Mevacor   Agenerase

Risk rating: 1
Severity: Major   **Onset: Delayed**   **Likelihood: Suspected**

Cause
Protease inhibitors, such as amprenavir, may inhibit CYP3A4 metabolism of lovastatin.

Effect
Lovastatin level may increase.

Nursing considerations
■ If a protease inhibitor is added to a regimen that includes lovastatin, monitor patient closely.
⚡ **ALERT** Watch for evidence of rhabdomyolysis, including dark or red urine, muscle weakness, and myalgia.
■ Urge patient to immediately report unexplained muscle weakness.

lovastatin ▶◀ azole antifungals
Mevacor   fluconazole, itraconazole,
                                 ketoconazole, voriconazole

Risk rating: 2
Severity: Moderate   **Onset: Rapid**   **Likelihood: Probable**

Cause
Azole antifungals may inhibit hepatic metabolism of HMG-CoA reductase inhibitors, such as lovastatin.

Effect
Lovastatin level and adverse effects may increase.

Nursing considerations
■ If possible, avoid use together.
■ Lovastatin dosage may need to be decreased.
■ Monitor serum cholesterol and lipid levels.

⚡ **ALERT** Assess patient for evidence of rhabdomyolysis, including fatigue; muscle aches and weakness; joint pain; dark, red, or cola-colored urine; weight gain; seizures; and greatly increased CK level.
■ Pravastatin is the HMG-CoA reductase inhibitor least affected by this interaction and may be preferred for use with an azole antifungal.

---

lovastatin ▶◀ bile acid sequestrants
Mevacor   cholestyramine, colestipol

Risk rating: 2
Severity: Moderate   **Onset: Delayed**   **Likelihood: Suspected**

Cause
GI absorption of HMG-CoA reductase inhibitors, such as lovastatin, may decrease.

Effect
HMG-CoA reductase inhibitor effects may decrease.

Nursing considerations
⚡ **ALERT** Separate doses of lovastatin and bile acid sequestrant by at least 4 hours.
■ If possible, give bile acid sequestrant before meals and HMG-CoA reductase inhibitor in the evening.
■ Monitor serum cholesterol and lipid levels.
■ Obtain liver function test results at start of therapy and periodically thereafter. If ALT or AST level stays three times or more above the upper limit of normal, lovastatin will need to be stopped.
■ Help patient develop a plan to ensure proper dosage intervals.

---

lovastatin ▶◀ carbamazepine
Mevacor   Carbatrol, Epitol, Equetro,
                                 Tegretol

Risk rating: 2
Severity: Moderate   **Onset: Delayed**   **Likelihood: Suspected**

Cause
Carbamazepine may increase CYP3A4 metabolism of HMG-CoA reductase inhibitors, such as lovastatin.

Effect
HMG-CoA reductase inhibitor effects may be reduced.

Nursing considerations
■ If possible, avoid use together.

- Monitor serum cholesterol and lipid levels.
- If hypercholesterolemia increases, notify prescriber.
- Pravastatin and rosuvastatin may be less likely to interact with carbamazepine and may be better choices than other HMG-CoA reductase inhibitors.
- Help patient develop a plan to ensure proper dosage intervals.

lovastatin ▶◀ cyclosporine
Mevacor   Neoral

Risk rating: 1
Severity: Major   **Onset: Delayed**   **Likelihood: Probable**

Cause
The metabolism of certain HMG-CoA reductase inhibitors, such as lovastatin, may decrease.

Effect
Plasma levels and adverse effects of HMG-CoA reductase inhibitors may increase.

Nursing considerations
- If possible, avoid use together.
- HMG-CoA reductase inhibitor dosage may need to be decreased.
- Monitor serum cholesterol and lipid levels to assess patient's response to therapy.

▶ **ALERT** Assess patient for evidence of rhabdomyolysis, including fatigue; muscle aches and weakness; joint pain; dark, red, or cola-colored urine; weight gain; seizures; and greatly increased CK level.
- Urge patient to report muscle pain, tenderness, or weakness.

lovastatin ▶◀ diltiazem
Mevacor   Cardizem

Risk rating: 2
Severity: Moderate   **Onset: Delayed**   **Likelihood: Probable**

Cause
CYP3A4 metabolism of certain HMG-CoA reductase inhibitors, such as lovastatin, may be inhibited.

Effect
HMG-CoA reductase inhibitor level may increase, raising the risk of toxicity, including myositis and rhabdomyolysis.

Nursing considerations
- If possible, avoid use together.
- **⚡ALERT** Assess patient for evidence of rhabdomyolysis, including fatigue; muscle aches and weakness; joint pain; dark, red, or cola-colored urine; weight gain; seizures; and greatly increased CK level.
- If patient may have rhabdomyolysis, notify prescriber and obtain renal function tests and serum potassium, sodium, calcium, lactic acid, and myoglobin levels.
- Pravastatin is less likely than other HMG-CoA reductase inhibitors to interact with diltiazem and may be best choice for combined use.
- Urge patient to report muscle pain, tenderness, or weakness.

---

lovastatin ◀▶ gemfibrozil
Mevacor   Lopid

Risk rating: 1
Severity: Major   **Onset: Delayed**   **Likelihood: Suspected**

Cause
The mechanism of this interaction is unknown.

Effect
Severe myopathy or rhabdomyolysis may occur.

Nursing considerations
- Avoid use together.
- If patient has severe hyperlipidemia, combined therapy may be an option, but only with careful monitoring.
- **⚡ALERT** Assess patient for evidence of rhabdomyolysis, including fatigue; muscle aches and weakness; joint pain; dark, red, or cola-colored urine; weight gain; seizures; and greatly increased CK level.
- Watch for evidence of acute renal failure, including decreased urine output, elevated BUN and creatinine levels, edema, dyspnea, tachycardia, distended neck veins, nausea, vomiting, poor appetite, weakness, fatigue, confusion, and agitation.
- Urge patient to report muscle pain, tenderness, or weakness.

lovastatin ━━━▶◀━━━ grapefruit juice
Mevacor

Risk rating: 2
Severity: Moderate   **Onset: Rapid**   **Likelihood: Suspected**

Cause
Grapefruit juice may inhibit CYP3A4 metabolism of certain HMG-CoA reductase inhibitors, such as lovastatin.

Effect
HMG-CoA reductase inhibitor level may increase, raising the risk of adverse effects.

Nursing considerations
- Avoid giving lovastatin with grapefruit juice.
- **◪ ALERT** Fluvastatin and pravastatin are metabolized by other enzymes and may be less affected by grapefruit juice.
- Caution patient to take drug with a liquid other than grapefruit juice.
- Urge patient to report muscle pain, tenderness, or weakness.

lovastatin ━━━▶◀━━━ lopinavir-ritonavir
Mevacor   Kaletra

Risk rating: 1
Severity: Major   **Onset: Delayed**   **Likelihood: Suspected**

Cause
Protease inhibitors, such as lopinavir-ritonavir, may inhibit CYP3A4 metabolism of HMG-CoA reductase inhibitors, such as lovastatin.

Effect
Lovastatin level may increase.

Nursing considerations
- Avoid using lovastatin with lopinavir-ritonavir.
- If a protease inhibitor is added to a regimen that includes lovastatin, monitor patient closely.
- **◪ ALERT** Watch for evidence of rhabdomyolysis, including dark or red urine, muscle weakness, and myalgia.
- Urge patient to immediately report unexplained muscle weakness.

lovastatin ▶◀ macrolide antibiotics

Mevacor

azithromycin, clarithromycin, erythromycin

Risk rating: 1
Severity: Major   **Onset: Delayed**   **Likelihood: Probable**

Cause
CYP3A4 metabolism of certain HMG-CoA reductase inhibitors, such as lovastatin, may be decreased.

Effect
HMG-CoA reductase inhibitor level may increase, raising the risk of severe myopathy or rhabdomyolysis.

Nursing considerations
■ If lovastatin is given with a macrolide antibiotic, watch for evidence of rhabdomyolysis, especially 5 to 21 days after macrolide starts. Evidence may include fatigue; muscle aches and weakness; joint pain; dark, red, or cola-colored urine; weight gain; seizures; and greatly increased serum CK level.
■ Fluvastatin and pravastatin are metabolized by other enzymes and may be better choices when used with macrolide antibiotic.
■ It may be safe to give atorvastatin with azithromycin.
■ Urge patient to report muscle pain, tenderness, or weakness.

lovastatin ▶◀ protease inhibitors

Mevacor

amprenavir, atazanavir, indinavir, lopinavir-ritonavir, nelfinavir, ritonavir, saquinavir

Risk rating: 1
Severity: Major   **Onset: Delayed**   **Likelihood: Suspected**

Cause
Protease inhibitors may inhibit CYP3A4 metabolism of lovastatin.

Effect
Lovastatin level may increase.

Nursing considerations
⚡ ALERT Use of lovastatin with nelfinavir is contraindicated.
■ Avoid using lovastatin with ritonavir or atazanavir.
■ If a protease inhibitor is added to a regimen that includes lovastatin, monitor patient closely.

◣ **ALERT** Watch for evidence of rhabdomyolysis, including dark or red urine, muscle weakness, and myalgia.

■ Urge patient to immediately report unexplained muscle weakness.

---

lovastatin ▸◀ rifamycins

Mevacor   rifabutin, rifampin, rifapentine

Risk rating: 2
Severity: Moderate   **Onset: Delayed**   **Likelihood: Suspected**

Cause
Rifamycins may induce CYP3A4 metabolism of HMG-CoA reductase inhibitors, such as lovastatin, in the intestine and liver.

Effect
HMG-CoA reductase inhibitor effects may decrease.

Nursing considerations
■ Assess patient for expected response to therapy. If you suspect an interaction, consult prescriber or pharmacist; patient may need a different drug.
■ Check serum cholesterol and lipid levels.
■ Obtain liver function test results at start of therapy and periodically thereafter. If ALT or AST level stays three times or more above the upper limit of normal, lovastatin will need to be stopped.
■ Withhold HMG-CoA reductase inhibitor temporarily if patient's risk of myopathy or rhabdomyolysis increases, as from sepsis, hypotension, major surgery, trauma, uncontrolled seizures, or a severe metabolic, endocrine, or electrolyte disorder.
◣ **ALERT** Pravastatin is less likely than other HMG-CoA reductase inhibitors to interact with rifamycins and may be the best choice for combined use.

---

lovastatin ▸◀ verapamil

Mevacor   Calan

Risk rating: 2
Severity: Moderate   **Onset: Delayed**   **Likelihood: Probable**

Cause
CYP3A4 metabolism of certain HMG-CoA reductase inhibitors, such as lovastatin, may decrease.

Effect
HMG-CoA reductase inhibitor level may increase, raising the risk of adverse effects.

Nursing considerations

▪ If possible, avoid giving lovastatin with verapamil. If patient must take both drugs, consult prescriber; lovastatin dosage may be decreased.

⚡ ALERT Watch for evidence of rhabdomyolysis, including fatigue; muscle aches and weakness; joint pain; dark, red, or cola-colored urine; weight gain; seizures; and greatly increased serum CK level.

▪ Fluvastatin and pravastatin are metabolized by other enzymes and may be better choices for combined use.

▪ Urge patient to report muscle pain, tenderness, or weakness.

---

magnesium salts, ➤◄ oral
magaldrate, magnesium carbonate, magnesium citrate, magnesium gluconate, magnesium hydroxide, magnesium oxide, magnesium sulfate, magnesium trisilicate

tetracyclines
doxycycline, minocycline, oxytetracycline, tetracycline

Risk rating: 2
Severity: Moderate   Onset: **Delayed**   Likelihood: **Probable**

Cause
Magnesium salts form an insoluble complex with tetracyclines that lowers tetracycline absorption.

Effect
Tetracycline level and efficacy decrease.

Nursing considerations
▪ Separate tetracyclines from magnesium salts by at least 3 to 4 hours.

▪ Monitor efficacy of tetracycline in resolving infection. Notify prescriber if infection isn't responding to treatment.

▪ Teach patients to separate tetracycline dose from magnesium-based antacids, laxatives, and supplements by 3 to 4 hours.

magnesium sulfate ■►◄■ nondepolarizing muscle relaxants

atracurium, cisatracurium, mivacurium, pancuronium, rocuronium, vecuronium

Risk rating: 2
Severity: Moderate   **Onset: Rapid**   **Likelihood: Suspected**

Cause
Magnesium probably potentiates the action of nondepolarizing muscle relaxants.

Effect
Risk of profound, severe respiratory depression increases.

Nursing considerations
- Use these drugs together cautiously.
- Nondepolarizing muscle relaxant dosage may need to be adjusted.
- Monitor patient for respiratory distress.
- Provide ventilatory support as needed.
- Make sure patient is adequately sedated when receiving a nondepolarizing muscle relaxant.

megestrol ■■■►◄■■■ dofetilide

Megace   Tikosyn

Risk rating: 1
Severity: Major   **Onset: Delayed**   **Likelihood: Suspected**

Cause
Dofetilide renal elimination may be inhibited.

Effect
Dofetilide level and risk of ventricular arrhythmias, including torsades de pointes, increase.

Nursing considerations
- **ALERT** Use of dofetilide with megestrol is contraindicated.
- Monitor ECG for prolonged QTc interval and development of ventricular arrhythmias.
- Monitor renal function every 3 months during dofetilide therapy.

■ Monitor patient for prolonged diarrhea, sweating, and vomiting during dofetilide therapy. Alert prescriber because electrolyte imbalance may increase risk of arrhythmias.
■ Urge patient to tell prescriber about increased adverse effects.

---

meperidine ➤◀ chlorpromazine
Demerol   Thorazine

Risk rating: 2
Severity: Moderate   **Onset: Rapid**   **Likelihood: Probable**

Cause
Combined use may produce additive CNS depressant and cardiovascular effects.

Effect
Excessive sedation and hypotension may occur.

Nursing considerations
■ Avoid using meperidine with phenothiazines, such as chlorpromazine.
■ These drugs have been used together to minimize opioid dosage and control nausea and vomiting, but the risks may outweigh the benefits.
■ Watch for more severe and extended respiratory depression.

---

meperidine ➤◀ MAO inhibitors
Demerol   isocarboxazid, phenelzine,
                                selegiline, tranylcypromine

Risk rating: 1
Severity: Major   **Onset: Rapid**   **Likelihood: Probable**

Cause
The mechanism of this interaction is unknown.

Effect
Risk of severe adverse reactions increases.

Nursing considerations
■ If possible, avoid giving these drugs together.
■ Monitor patient; report agitation, seizures, diaphoresis, and fever.
■ Reaction may progress to coma, apnea, and death.
■ Reaction may occur several weeks after stopping the MAO inhibitor.
◆ **ALERT** Give opioid analgesics other than meperidine cautiously. It isn't known if similar reactions occur.

meperidine ➤◄ sibutramine

Demerol   Meridia

Risk rating: 1
Severity: Major   **Onset: Rapid**   **Likelihood: Suspected**

Cause
The serotonergic effects may be additive.

Effect
Serotonin syndrome may occur.

Nursing considerations
- Avoid using these drugs together.
- Monitor patient for evidence of serotonin syndrome, including CNS irritability, motor weakness, shivering, muscle twitching, and altered consciousness.

⊠ALERT Serotonin syndrome may be fatal and warrants immediate medical attention.

metformin ➤◄ cimetidine

Glucophage   Tagamet

Risk rating: 2
Severity: Moderate   **Onset: Rapid**   **Likelihood: Suspected**

Cause
Cimetidine reduces renal clearance of metformin.

Effect
Metformin level and effects increase.

Nursing considerations
- Monitor lactic acid level; reference range is 6 to 19 mg/dl.

⊠ ALERT Advise patient to report early symptoms of lactic acidosis: malaise, myalgias, respiratory distress, increased somnolence, abdominal pain, nausea, and vomiting.

- Monitor patient for hypothermia, hypotension, and resistant bradyarrhythmias.
- Monitor blood glucose level (range, 65 to 115 mg/dl) for potential hypoglycemic response.
- Metformin dosage may need adjustment when cimetidine is started or stopped.
- H_2-receptor antagonists other than cimetidine may interact. If you suspect an interaction, consult prescriber or pharmacist.

methadone ━━━■▶◀■━━━ barbiturates

Dolophine,
Methadose

amobarbital, butabarbital,
pentobarbital, phenobarbital,
primidone, secobarbital

Risk rating: 2
Severity: Moderate   **Onset: Delayed**   **Likelihood: Suspected**

Cause
The mechanism of this interaction is unknown, but barbiturates
probably increase hepatic metabolism of methadone.

Effect
Methadone effects may be reduced, and patients on long-term therapy may notice opioid withdrawal symptoms.

Nursing considerations
■ If these drugs must be used together, monitor methadone efficacy.
■ Check methadone level regularly.
■ If methadone dosage is insufficient, it may be increased.
■ Other barbiturates interact with methadone. If you suspect an inter-
action, consult prescriber or pharmacist.

methadone ━━━■▶◀■━━━ hydantoins

Dolophine,
Methadose

ethotoin, fosphenytoin,
phenytoin

Risk rating: 2
Severity: Moderate   **Onset: Delayed**   **Likelihood: Suspected**

Cause
The mechanism of this interaction is unknown but probably involves
altered metabolic process.

Effect
Methadone level and effects may decrease.

Nursing considerations
■ Methadone dosage may need adjustment.
■ If hydantoin therapy starts while patient is taking methadone, watch
for signs of opioid withdrawal.
■ Urge patient to tell prescriber about loss of methadone effect.

methamphetamine ➡◀ MAO inhibitors
Desoxyn   phenelzine, tranylcypromine

Risk rating: 1
Severity: Major   **Onset: Rapid**   **Likelihood: Suspected**

Cause
This interaction probably stems from increased norepinephrine level at the synaptic cleft.

Effect
Anorexiant effects increase.

Nursing considerations
■ If possible, avoid giving these drugs together.
■ Headache and severe hypertension may occur rapidly if an amphetamine, such as methamphetamine, is given to patient who takes an MAO inhibitor.
⚠ **ALERT** Several deaths have resulted from hypertensive crisis and cerebral hemorrhage.
■ Monitor patient for hypotension, hyperpyrexia, and seizures.
■ Hypertensive reaction may occur for several weeks after stopping an MAO inhibitor.

methamphetamine ➡◀ SSRIs
Desoxyn   fluoxetine, fluvoxamine,
                                     paroxetine, sertraline

Risk rating: 1
Severity: Major   **Onset: Rapid**   **Likelihood: Suspected**

Cause
The mechanism of this interaction is unknown.

Effect
Sympathomimetic effects and risk of serotonin syndrome increase.

Nursing considerations
■ If these drugs must be used together, watch closely for increased CNS effects, such as anxiety, jitteriness, agitation, and restlessness.
■ Mild serotonin-like symptoms may develop, including anxiety, dizziness, restlessness, nausea, and vomiting.
■ Explain risk of interaction and need to avoid amphetamines, such as methamphetamine.

■ Describe the traits of serotonin syndrome, including CNS irritability, motor weakness, shivering, myoclonus, and altered consciousness.

---

methamphetamine ▶◀ urine alkalinizers

Desoxyn

potassium citrate, sodium acetate, sodium bicarbonate, sodium citrate, sodium lactate, tromethamine

Risk rating: 2
Severity: Moderate   Onset: Rapid   Likelihood: Established

Cause
Alkaline urine prolongs clearance of amphetamines, such as methamphetamine.

Effect
In amphetamine overdose, the toxic period is extended, increasing the risk of injury.

Nursing considerations
■ **ALERT** Avoid drugs that may alkalinize the urine, particularly during amphetamine overdose.
■ Watch for evidence of amphetamine toxicity, such as dermatoses, marked insomnia, irritability, hyperactivity, and personality changes.
■ If patient takes an anorexiant, advise against excessive use of sodium bicarbonate as an antacid.

---

methimazole ▶◀ beta blockers

Tapazole

metoprolol, propranolol

Risk rating: 2
Severity: Moderate   Onset: Delayed   Likelihood: Probable

Cause
Hyperthyroidism increases beta blocker clearance.

Effect
Beta blocker effects may increase when patient becomes euthyroid.

Nursing considerations
■ Before giving beta blocker, assess blood pressure and apical pulse.
■ Watch for increased beta blocker effects, including hypotension, bradycardia, dizziness, and lethargy.
■ When hyperthyroid patient becomes euthyroid, beta blocker dosage may need to be reduced.

■ Other beta blockers may interact with thioamines, such as methimazole. If you suspect an interaction, consult prescriber or pharmacist.
■ Caution patient not to stop a beta blocker abruptly.

---

methimazole ➤◀ theophyllines

Tapazole   aminophylline, theophylline

Risk rating: 2
Severity: Moderate   **Onset: Delayed**   **Likelihood: Suspected**

Cause
Methimazole and other thioamines increase theophylline clearance in hyperthyroid patient.

Effect
Theophylline level and effects decrease.

Nursing considerations
■ Watch closely for decreased theophylline efficacy while abnormal thyroid status continues.
◪ ALERT Assess patient for return to euthyroid state, when interaction no longer occurs.
■ Explain that hyperthyroidism and hypothyroidism can affect theophylline efficacy and toxicity; tell patient to immediately report evidence of either one.
■ Urge patients to have TSH and theophylline levels tested regularly.

---

methotrexate ➤◀ NSAIDs

Rheumatrex, Trexall   diclofenac, etodolac,
                                      fenoprofen, flurbiprofen,
                                      ibuprofen, indomethacin,
                                      ketoprofen, ketorolac,
                                      meclofenamate, nabumetone,
                                      naproxen, oxaprozin,
                                      piroxicam, sulindac, tolmetin

---

Risk rating: 1
Severity: Major   **Onset: Delayed**   **Likelihood: Suspected**

Cause
Renal clearance of methotrexate may decrease.

Effect
Methotrexate toxicity may occur.

Nursing considerations

- Monitor patient for renal impairment that may predispose him to methotrexate toxicity.
- Monitor patient for mouth sores. This may be the first outward appearance of methotrexate toxicity; however, in some patients, bone marrow suppression coincides with or precedes mouth sores.
- Methotrexate toxicity is less likely to occur with weekly low-dose methotrexate regimens for rheumatoid arthritis and other inflammatory diseases.
- Longer leucovorin rescue should be considered when giving NSAIDs and methotrexate at antineoplastic doses.
- Watch for other signs and symptoms of methotrexate toxicity, such as hematemesis, diarrhea with melena, nausea, and weakness.

---

methotrexate ▶◀ penicillins

Rheumatrex, Trexall

amoxicillin, ampicillin, carbenicillin, cloxacillin, dicloxacillin, nafcillin, oxacillin, penicillin G, penicillin V, piperacillin, ticarcillin

---

Risk rating: 1
Severity: Major   **Onset: Delayed**   **Likelihood: Suspected**

Cause
Methotrexate secretion in the renal tubules is inhibited.

Effect
Methotrexate level and risk of toxicity increase.

Nursing considerations

- Monitor patient for methotrexate toxicity, including renal failure, neutropenia, leukopenia, thrombocytopenia, increased liver function tests, and skin ulcers.
- Monitor patient for mouth sores. This may be the first outward appearance of methotrexate toxicity; however, in some patients, bone marrow suppression coincides with or precedes mouth sores.
- Obtain methotrexate level twice weekly for the first 2 weeks.
- Dose and duration of leucovorin rescue may need to be increased.

methotrexate ━━▶◀━━ probenecid

Rheumatrex, Trexall   Probalan

Risk rating: 1
Severity: Major   **Onset: Rapid**   **Likelihood: Probable**

Cause
Probenecid may impair renal excretion of methotrexate.

Effect
Methotrexate level, effects, and risk of toxicity may increase.

Nursing considerations
■ Monitor patient for methotrexate toxicity, including renal failure, neutropenia, leukopenia, thrombocytopenia, increased liver function tests, and skin ulcers.
■ Monitor patient for mouth sores. This may be the first outward appearance of methotrexate toxicity; however, in some patients, bone marrow suppression coincides with or precedes mouth sores.
■ Notify prescriber if signs of toxicity appear; the methotrexate dose may need to be reduced.

methotrexate ━━▶◀━━ salicylates

Rheumatrex, Trexall   aspirin, bismuth subsalicylate, choline salicylate, magnesium salicylate, salsalate, sodium salicylate, sodium thiosalicylate

Risk rating: 1
Severity: Major   **Onset: Rapid**   **Likelihood: Suspected**

Cause
Renal clearance and plasma protein binding of methotrexate may be decreased by salicylates.

Effect
Methotrexate toxicity may occur.

Nursing considerations
■ Monitor patient for methotrexate toxicity, including renal failure, neutropenia, leukopenia, thrombocytopenia, increased liver function tests, and skin ulcers.
■ Monitor patient for mouth sores. This may be the first outward appearance of methotrexate toxicity; however, in some patients, bone marrow suppression coincides with or precedes mouth sores.

■ Notify prescriber if signs of toxicity appear; the methotrexate dose may need to be reduced.

---

methotrexate ▸◂ sulfonamides
Rheumatrex, Trexall

sulfadiazine, sulfamethizole, sulfasalazine, sulfisoxazole, trimethoprim-sulfamethoxazole

---

Risk rating: 1
Severity: Major   **Onset: Delayed**   **Likelihood: Suspected**

Cause
Renal clearance and plasma protein binding of methotrexate may be decreased by sulfonamides. Methotrexate may induce folate deficiency, which develops into acute megaloblastic anemia when sulfonamide starts.

Effect
Methotrexate toxicity may occur. Risk of sulfonamide-induced megaloblastic anemia increases.

Nursing considerations
■ Monitor patient for methotrexate toxicity, including renal failure, neutropenia, leukopenia, thrombocytopenia, increased liver function tests, and skin ulcers.
■ Monitor patient for mouth sores. This may be the first outward appearance of methotrexate toxicity; however, in some patients, bone marrow suppression coincides with or precedes mouth sores.
■ Notify prescriber if signs of toxicity appear; the methotrexate dose may need to be reduced.
◼ ALERT Sulfamethizole may displace a highly toxic metabolite of methotrexate.

---

methotrexate ▸◂ trimethoprim
Rheumatrex, Trexall   Proloprim

Risk rating: 1
Severity: Major   **Onset: Delayed**   **Likelihood: Suspected**

Cause
Methotrexate and trimethoprim may have a synergistic effect on folate metabolism.

Effect
Methotrexate toxicity may occur.

Nursing considerations
- Avoid using methotrexate with trimethoprim if possible.
- Monitor patient for methotrexate-induced bone marrow suppression and megaloblastic anemia.
- Consider use of leucovorin to treat megaloblastic anemia and neutropenia resulting from folic acid deficiency.

---

methyldopa ▶◀ dobutamine
Aldomet   Dobutrex

Risk rating: 2
Severity: **Moderate**   Onset: **Rapid**   Likelihood: **Suspected**

Cause
The mechanism of this interaction is unknown.

Effect
Pressor response of sympathomimetics, such as dobutamine, may be increased, resulting in hypertension.

Nursing considerations
- Monitor patient's blood pressure closely.
- If patient takes methyldopa, explain that many OTC products contain drugs that can raise blood pressure. Urge patient to read labels carefully or check with prescriber before using a new product.
- Teach patient to monitor blood pressure at home.

---

methyldopa ▶◀ metaraminol
Aldomet   Aramine

Risk rating: 2
Severity: **Moderate**   Onset: **Rapid**   Likelihood: **Suspected**

Cause
The mechanism of this interaction is unknown.

Effect
Pressor response of sympathomimetics, such as metaraminol, may be increased, resulting in hypertension.

Nursing considerations
- Monitor patient's blood pressure closely.

■ If patient takes methyldopa, explain that many OTC products contain drugs that can raise blood pressure. Urge patient to read labels carefully or check with prescriber before using a new product.
■ Teach patient to monitor blood pressure at home.

methyldopa ▶◀ sympathomimetics

Aldomet

dobutamine, dopamine, ephedrine, epinephrine, metaraminol, norepinephrine, phenylephrine, pseudoephedrine

Risk rating: 2
Severity: Moderate   **Onset: Rapid**   **Likelihood: Suspected**

Cause
The mechanism of this interaction is unknown.

Effect
Pressor response of sympathomimetics may be increased, resulting in hypertension.

Nursing considerations
■ Monitor patient's blood pressure closely.
■ If patient takes methyldopa, explain that many OTC products contain drugs that can raise blood pressure. Urge patient to read labels carefully or check with prescriber before using a new product.
■ Teach patient to monitor blood pressure at home.

methylergonovine ▶◀ protease inhibitors

Methergine

amprenavir, atazanavir, indinavir, lopinavir-ritonavir, nelfinavir, ritonavir, saquinavir

Risk rating: 1
Severity: Major   **Onset: Delayed**   **Likelihood: Probable**

Cause
Protease inhibitors may interfere with CYP3A4 metabolism of ergot derivatives, such as methylergonovine.

Effect
Risk of ergot-induced peripheral vasospasm and ischemia may increase.

Nursing considerations

⚡ ALERT Use of ergot derivatives with protease inhibitors is contra-indicated.

■ Monitor patient for evidence of peripheral ischemia, including pain in limb muscles while exercising and later at rest; numbness and tingling of fingers and toes; cool, pale, or cyanotic limbs; red or violet blisters on hands or feet; and gangrene.

■ Sodium nitroprusside may be given for ergot-induced vasospasm.

■ If patient takes a protease inhibitor, consult prescriber or pharmacist about alternative treatments for migraine pain.

■ Urge patient to tell prescriber about increased adverse effects.

---

methylphenidates ▶◀ MAO inhibitors

dexmethylphenidate,
methylphenidate

isocarboxazid, phenelzine,
tranylcypromine

Risk rating: 1
Severity: Major   **Onset: Delayed**   **Likelihood: Suspected**

Cause
The mechanism of this interaction is unknown.

Effect
Risk of hypertensive crisis increases.

Nursing considerations

⚡ ALERT Use of dexmethylphenidate with MAO inhibitors is contra-indicated.

■ Don't use dexmethylphenidate within 14 days after stopping an MAO inhibitor.

■ Monitor blood pressure closely if methylphenidate is given with an MAO inhibitor.

■ Teach patient and parents to monitor blood pressure at home.

---

methylprednisolone ▶◀ aprepitant

Medrol

Emend

Risk rating: 2
Severity: Moderate   **Onset: Delayed**   **Likelihood: Suspected**

Cause
Aprepitant may inhibit first-pass metabolism of certain corticosteroids, such as methylprednisolone.

Effect
Corticosteroid level may be increased and half-life prolonged.

Nursing considerations
- Corticosteroid dosage may need to be decreased.
- When starting or stopping aprepitant, adjust corticosteroid dosage as needed.
- Watch closely for evidence of increased corticosteroid level, such as insomnia, euphoria, increased appetite, mood changes, and increased blood glucose level.
- Tell patient to report symptoms of increased blood glucose level, including increased thirst, hunger, and frequency of urination.

---

methylprednisolone ➤◄ barbiturates

Medrol

amobarbital, butabarbital, pentobarbital, phenobarbital, primidone, secobarbital

Risk rating: 2
Severity: Moderate   Onset: Delayed   Likelihood: Established

Cause
Barbiturates induce liver enzymes, which stimulate metabolism of corticosteroids, such as methylprednisolone.

Effect
Corticosteroid effects may be decreased.

Nursing considerations
- Avoid giving barbiturates with corticosteroids, if possible.
- If patient takes a corticosteroid, watch for worsening symptoms when a barbiturate is started or stopped.
- During barbiturate treatment, corticosteroid dosage may need to be increased.

---

methylprednisolone ➤◄ cholinesterase inhibitors

Medrol

ambenonium, edrophonium, neostigmine, pyridostigmine

Risk rating: 1
Severity: Major   Onset: Delayed   Likelihood: Probable

Cause
In myasthenia gravis, methylprednisolone and other corticosteroids antagonize the effects of cholinesterase inhibitors by an unknown mechanism.

Effect
Patient may develop severe muscular depression refractory to cholinesterase inhibitor.

Nursing considerations
- Corticosteroids may have long-term benefits in myasthenia gravis.
- Combined therapy may be attempted under strict supervision.
- In myasthenia gravis, monitor patient for severe muscle deterioration.

⚠ ALERT Be prepared to provide respiratory support and mechanical ventilation if needed.

- Consult prescriber or pharmacist about safe corticosteroid delivery to maximize improvement in muscle strength.

---

methylprednisolone ⤬ diltiazem
Medrol   Cardizem

Risk rating: 2
Severity: Moderate   **Onset: Delayed**   **Likelihood: Suspected**

Cause
Methylprednisolone CYP3A4 metabolism may be inhibited.

Effect
Methylprednisolone effects and risk of toxicity may increase.

Nursing considerations
- Corticosteroids other than methylprednisolone may have a similar interaction with diltiazem. If you suspect a drug interaction, consult prescriber or pharmacist.
- Monitor response to methylprednisolone.
- Monitor patient for signs of methylprednisolone toxicity, including nervousness, sleepiness, depression, psychoses, weakness, decreased hearing, leg edema, skin disorders, hypertension, muscle weakness, and seizures.
- Methylprednisolone dosage may need adjustment.
- Advise patient to report increased adverse effects.

methylprednisolone ▶◀ grapefruit juice

Medrol

Risk rating: 2
Severity: Moderate   **Onset: Delayed**   **Likelihood: Suspected**

Cause
Methylprednisolone metabolism probably is inhibited.

Effect
Methylprednisolone effects and risk of toxicity may increase.

Nursing considerations
■ Inform patient of this interaction.
■ Advise patient to take methylprednisolone with a beverage other than grapefruit juice.
■ Tell patient to report adverse effects, such as euphoria, insomnia, and GI complaints.

methylprednisolone ▶◀ hydantoins

Medrol   ethotoin, fosphenytoin,
                                phenytoin

Risk rating: 2
Severity: Moderate   **Onset: Delayed**   **Likelihood: Established**

Cause
Hydantoins induce liver enzymes, which stimulate metabolism of corticosteroids, such as methylprednisolone.

Effect
Corticosteroid effects may be decreased.

Nursing considerations
■ Avoid giving hydantoins with corticosteroids if possible.
■ Monitor patient for decreased corticosteroid effects. Also monitor phenytoin level, and adjust dosage of either drug as needed.
■ Corticosteroid effects may decrease within days of starting phenytoin and may stay decreased 3 weeks after it stops.
■ Dosage of either or both drugs may need to be increased.

methylprednisolone ▶◀ macrolide antibiotics
Medrol   clarithromycin, erythromycin

Risk rating: 2
Severity: Moderate   Onset: Delayed   Likelihood: Established

Cause
The mechanism of this interaction is unclear.

Effect
Methylprednisolone effects, including toxic effects, may increase.

Nursing considerations
■ This interaction may be used for therapeutic benefit because it may be possible to reduce methylprednisolone dosage.
■ Methylprednisolone dosage may need adjustment.
■ Monitor patient for adverse or toxic effects, such as euphoria, insomnia, peptic ulceration, and cushingoid effects.

methylprednisolone ▶◀ rifamycins
Medrol   rifabutin, rifampin, rifapentine

Risk rating: 1
Severity: Major   Onset: Delayed   Likelihood: Established

Cause
Rifamycins increase hepatic metabolism of corticosteroids, such as methylprednisolone.

Effect
Corticosteroid effects may decrease.

Nursing considerations
■ If possible, avoid giving rifamycins with corticosteroids.
■ Monitor patient for decreased corticosteroid effects, including loss of disease control.
■ Watch for symptom control after increasing rifamycin dose. Drug may need to be stopped to regain control of disease.
■ Corticosteroid effects may decrease within days of starting rifampin and may stay decreased 2 to 3 weeks after it stops.
■ Corticosteroid dose may need to be doubled after adding rifampin.

methylprednisolone ⏩⧏ salicylates

Medrol

aspirin, bismuth subsalicylate, choline salicylate, magnesium salicylate, salsalate, sodium salicylate, sodium thiosalicylate

Risk rating: 2
Severity: Moderate   Onset: Delayed   Likelihood: Probable

Cause
Methylprednisolone and other corticosteroids stimulate hepatic metabolism of salicylates and may increase renal excretion.

Effect
Salicylate level and effects decrease.

Nursing considerations
- Monitor salicylate level and efficacy; dosage may need adjustment.
- ⚠ ALERT Giving a salicylate while tapering a corticosteroid may result in salicylate toxicity.
- Watch for evidence of salicylate toxicity, including diaphoresis, nausea, vomiting, tinnitus, hyperventilation, and CNS depression.
- Patients with renal impairment may be at greater risk.

metoclopramide ⏩⧏ cyclosporine

Reglan

Gengraf, Neoral, Sandimmune

Risk rating: 2
Severity: Moderate   Onset: Delayed   Likelihood: Suspected

Cause
Metoclopramide increases gastric emptying time, which may increase cyclosporine absorption.

Effect
Cyclosporine level and risk of toxicity may increase.

Nursing considerations
- Monitor cyclosporine level closely when metoclopramide is added or stopped.
- Watch for cyclosporine toxicity, including hepatotoxicity, nephrotoxicity, nausea, vomiting, tremors, and seizures.
- Cyclosporine dosage may need reduction.

■ It isn't known whether altering the dosage or schedule of metoclo-pramide would decrease the risk or severity of the interaction.

---

metoclopramide ➤◀ digoxin
Reglan   Lanoxin

Risk rating: 2
Severity: Moderate   **Onset: Delayed**   **Likelihood: Probable**

Cause
Metoclopramide increases GI motility and may decrease digoxin ab-sorption.

Effect
Serum digoxin level and effects may decrease.

Nursing considerations
■ Monitor patient for decreased digoxin level; therapeutic range is 0.8 to 2 nanograms/ml.
■ Monitor patient for expected digoxin effects, including decreased heart rate, arrhythmia conversion, maintenance of converted rhythm, and improvement of heart failure symptoms.
■ Digoxin dosage may need adjustment if effect or level decreases.
◪ **ALERT** This interaction may not occur with high-bioavailability digoxin preparations, including capsule, elixir, and tablet with a high dissolution rate.
■ Urge patient to tell prescriber about increased adverse effects.

---

metolazone ➤◀ loop diuretics
Zaroxolyn   bumetanide, ethacrynic acid, furosemide, torsemide

Risk rating: 2
Severity: Moderate   **Onset: Rapid**   **Likelihood: Probable**

Cause
The mechanism of this interaction is unclear.

Effect
Because these drugs work synergistically, they may cause profound diuresis and serious electrolyte abnormalities.

Nursing considerations
■ This drug combination may be used for therapeutic benefit.

■ Expect increased sodium, potassium, and chloride excretion and greater diuresis.
■ Monitor patient for dehydration and electrolyte abnormalities.
■ Carefully adjust drugs, using small or intermittent doses.

---

metolazone ▶◀ sulfonylureas

Zaroxolyn

acetohexamide,
chlorpropamide,
glipizide, glyburide,
tolazamide, tolbutamide

Risk rating: 2
Severity: Moderate   **Onset: Delayed**   **Likelihood: Probable**

Cause
Metolazone and other thiazide diuretics may decrease insulin secretion and tissue sensitivity to insulin, and may increase potassium loss.

Effect
Risk of hyperglycemia and hyponatremia may increase.

Nursing considerations
■ Use these drugs together cautiously.
■ Monitor blood glucose level regularly, and consult prescriber about adjustments to either drug to maintain stable glucose level.
■ This interaction may occur several days to many months after dual therapy starts but is readily reversible when the diuretic stops.
■ Review signs and symptoms of hypoglycemia, including diaphoresis, fatigue, headache, hunger, irritability, malaise, nervousness, rapid heart rate, tension, and trembling.
■ Instruct patient to eat a small carbohydrate snack or meal if hypoglycemia develops, preferably after checking blood glucose level.

---

metoprolol ▶◀ cimetidine

Lopressor

Tagamet

Risk rating: 2
Severity: Moderate   **Onset: Rapid**   **Likelihood: Probable**

Cause
By inhibiting CYP pathway, cimetidine reduces first-pass metabolism of certain beta blockers, such as metoprolol.

Effect
Clearance of metoprolol is decreased and action increased.

Nursing considerations
- Monitor patient for severe bradycardia and hypotension.
- If interaction occurs, notify prescriber; beta blocker dosage may be decreased.
- Teach patient to monitor pulse rate. If it's significantly lower than usual, tell him to withhold beta blocker and to contact prescriber.
- Instruct patient to change positions slowly to reduce effects of orthostatic hypotension.
- Other beta blockers may interact with cimetidine. If you suspect an interaction, consult prescriber or pharmacist.

metoprolol ◄►◄ hydralazine
Lopressor   Apresoline

Risk rating: 2
Severity: Moderate   **Onset: Rapid**   **Likelihood: Probable**

Cause
Hydralazine may cause transient increase in visceral blood flow and decreased first-pass hepatic metabolism of some oral beta blockers, such as metoprolol.

Effect
Effects of both drugs may increase.

Nursing considerations
- Monitor blood pressure regularly, and tailor dosages of both drugs to patient's response.
- Other beta blockers may interact with hydralazine. If you suspect an interaction, consult prescriber or pharmacist.
- Explain that both drugs can affect blood pressure. Urge patient to report evidence of hypotension, such as light-headedness and dizziness when changing positions.

metoprolol ◄►◄ lidocaine
Lopressor

Risk rating: 2
Severity: Moderate   **Onset: Rapid**   **Likelihood: Established**

Cause
Metoprolol and other beta blockers reduce hepatic metabolism of lidocaine.

Effect
Lidocaine level and risk of toxicity may increase.

Nursing considerations
- Check for normal therapeutic level of lidocaine: 2 to 5 mcg/ml.
- Monitor patient closely for evidence of lidocaine toxicity, including dizziness, somnolence, confusion, paresthesias, and seizures.
- Slow the I.V. bolus rate to decrease risk of high peak level and toxic reaction.
- Explain warning signs of toxicity to patient and family, and tell them to contact prescriber if they have concerns.

---

metoprolol ▰▶◀ NSAIDs

Lopressor ibuprofen, indomethacin, naproxen, piroxicam

Risk rating: 2
Severity: **Moderate**   Onset: **Delayed**   Likelihood: **Probable**

Cause
NSAIDs may inhibit renal prostaglandin synthesis, allowing pressor systems to be unopposed.

Effect
Beta blockers, such as metoprolol, may not be able to lower blood pressure.

Nursing considerations
- Avoid using these drugs together if possible
- Monitor blood pressure and other evidence of hypertension closely.
- Talk with prescriber about ways to eliminate interaction, such as adjusting beta blocker dosage or switching to sulindac as the NSAID.
- Explain the risks of using these drugs together, and teach patient how to monitor his blood pressure.
- Other NSAIDs may interact with beta blockers. If you suspect an interaction, consult prescriber or pharmacist.

metoprolol 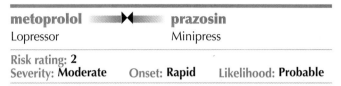 prazosin
Lopressor   Minipress

Risk rating: 2
Severity: Moderate   **Onset: Rapid**   **Likelihood: Probable**

Cause
The mechanism of this interaction is unknown.

Effect
Effect of these drugs on orthostatic hypotension is increased.

Nursing considerations
■ Assess patient's lying, sitting, and standing blood pressures closely, especially when combined use starts.
■ Adjust dosages of either drug based on patient effects.
■ To minimize effects of orthostatic hypotension, teach patient to change positions slowly.
■ Interaction is confirmed only with propranolol but may occur with other beta blockers as well.

metoprolol 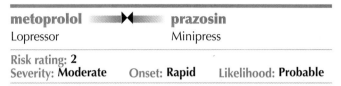 propafenone
Lopressor   Rythmol

Risk rating: 2
Severity: Moderate   **Onset: Rapid**   **Likelihood: Probable**

Cause
Propafenone inhibits first-pass metabolism of certain beta blockers, such as metoprolol, and reduces their systemic clearance.

Effect
Beta blocker effects may be increased.

Nursing considerations
■ Monitor blood pressure, pulse, and cardiac complaints.
■ Notify prescriber about abnormally low blood pressure or change in heart rate; beta blocker dosage may be decreased.
■ Tell patient to promptly report nightmares or other CNS complaints.
■ To minimize effects of orthostatic hypotension, tell patient to change positions slowly.

metoprolol ━━▶◀━━ quinidine

Lopressor

Risk rating: 2
Severity: Moderate   **Onset: Rapid**   **Likelihood: Suspected**

Cause
Quinidine may inhibit metabolism of certain beta blockers, such as metoprolol, in patients who are extensive metabolizers of debrisoquin.

Effect
Beta blocker effects may increase.

Nursing considerations
■ Monitor pulse and blood pressure more often during combined use.
■ Teach patient how to check blood pressure and pulse rate; tell him to do so regularly.
■ If pulse slows or blood pressure falls, consult prescriber. Beta blocker dosage may need to be decreased.

metoprolol ━━▶◀━━ rifamycins

Lopressor   rifabutin, rifampin, rifapentine

Risk rating: 2
Severity: Moderate   **Onset: Delayed**   **Likelihood: Probable**

Cause
Rifamycins increase hepatic metabolism of beta blockers, such as metoprolol.

Effect
Beta blocker effects are reduced.

Nursing considerations
■ Monitor blood pressure and heart rate closely to assess beta blocker efficacy.
■ If beta blocker effects are decreased, consult prescriber; dosage may need to be increased.
■ Teach patient how to monitor blood pressure and heart rate and when to contact prescriber.
■ Other beta blockers may interact with rifamycins. If you suspect an interaction, consult prescriber or pharmacist.

metoprolol ▰▰▰◄►▰▰▰ salicylates

Lopressor

aspirin, bismuth subsalicylate, choline salicylate, magnesium salicylate, salsalate, sodium salicylate, sodium thiosalicylate

Risk rating: 2
Severity: Moderate   **Onset: Rapid**   **Likelihood: Suspected**

Cause
Salicylates inhibit synthesis of prostaglandins, which metoprolol and other beta blockers need to reduce blood pressure. In patients with heart failure, the mechanism of this interaction is unknown.

Effect
Beta blocker effect is reduced.

Nursing considerations
▪ Watch closely for signs of heart failure and hypertension, and notify provider if they occur.
▪ Consult prescriber about switching patient to a different antihypertensive or antiplatelet drug.
▪ Other beta blockers may interact with salicylates. If you suspect an interaction, consult prescriber or pharmacist.
▪ Explain signs and symptoms of heart failure, and tell patient when to contact prescriber.

metoprolol ▰▰▰◄►▰▰▰ thioamines

Lopressor

methimazole, propylthiouracil

Risk rating: 2
Severity: Moderate   **Onset: Delayed**   **Likelihood: Probable**

Cause
Hyperthyroidism increases clearance of beta blockers, such as metoprolol.

Effect
Beta blocker effects may increase when patient becomes euthyroid.

Nursing considerations
▪ Before giving beta blocker, assess blood pressure and apical pulse.
▪ Watch for increased beta blocker effects, including hypotension, bradycardia, dizziness, and lethargy.

- When hyperthyroid patient becomes euthyroid, beta blocker dosage may need to be reduced.
- Other beta blockers may interact with thioamines. If you suspect an interaction, consult prescriber or pharmacist.
- Caution patient not to stop a beta blocker abruptly.

metoprolol ▶◀ verapamil
Lopressor   Calan

Risk rating: 1
Severity: Major   **Onset: Rapid**   **Likelihood: Probable**

Cause
Verapamil may inhibit metabolism of beta blockers, such as metoprolol.

Effect
Effects of both drugs may increase.

Nursing considerations
- Combination therapy is common in patients with hypertension and unstable angina.
- **ALERT** Giving these drugs together increases risk of adverse effects, including heart failure, conduction disturbances, arrhythmias, and hypotension.
- Assess patient for adverse effects, including left ventricular dysfunction and AV conduction defects.
- Risk of interaction is greater when drugs are given I.V.
- Dosages of both drugs may need to be decreased.

metronidazole ▶◀ barbiturates
Flagyl   amobarbital, butabarbital,
                                pentobarbital, phenobarbital,
                                primidone, secobarbital

Risk rating: 2
Severity: Moderate   **Onset: Delayed**   **Likelihood: Suspected**

Cause
Barbiturates may induce metronidazole metabolism, causing more rapid elimination and decreased metronidazole level.

Effect
Metronidazole effects may decrease.

Nursing considerations
■ Monitor patient receiving barbiturates with metronidazole for decreased antifungal effects.
■ Dose of metronidazole may need to be increased.

---

metronidazole ■■■►◄■■■ disulfiram
Flagyl   Antabuse

Risk rating: 2
Severity: Moderate   Onset: Delayed   Likelihood: Suspected

Cause
Excess dopaminergic activity may occur.

Effect
Acute psychosis or confusion may occur.

Nursing considerations
■ Combined use of these drugs should be avoided, if possible.
■ Watch for adverse effects, including paranoid delusions and visual and auditory hallucinations.
■ Symptoms may develop at tenth to fourteenth day of combined use.
■ Notify prescriber if acute psychosis or confusion occurs; one or both drugs may need to be stopped.
■ Symptoms may continue or increase for a few days after drugs are stopped.
■ Assure family members that full recovery usually occurs within 2 weeks.

---

mexiletine ■■■►◄■■■ theophyllines
Mexitil   aminophylline, theophylline

Risk rating: 2
Severity: Moderate   Onset: Delayed   Likelihood: Established

Cause
Mexiletine inhibits CYP metabolism of theophylline.

Effect
Theophylline level and risk of toxicity may increase.

Nursing considerations
■ When adding mexiletine, monitor theophylline level closely. Therapeutic range is 10 to 20 mcg/ml for adults and 5 to 15 mcg/ml for children.

- Interaction usually occurs within 2 days of combining these drugs. Theophylline dosage may be decreased when mexiletine starts.
- Watch for evidence of toxicity, such as ventricular tachycardia, anorexia, nausea, vomiting, diarrhea, seizures, restlessness, irritability, and headache.
- Describe adverse effects of theophylline and signs of toxicity, and tell patient to report them immediately to prescriber.

midazolam ■■■■▶◀■■■■ alcohol
Versed

Risk rating: 2
Severity: Moderate   Onset: Rapid   Likelihood: Established

Cause
Alcohol inhibits hepatic enzymes, which decreases clearance and increases peak levels of benzodiazepines, such as midazolam.

Effect
Additive or synergistic effects may occur.

Nursing considerations
- Before benzodiazepine therapy starts, assess patient thoroughly for history or evidence of alcohol use.
- Advise against consuming alcohol while taking a benzodiazepine.
- Watch for additive CNS effects, which may suggest benzodiazepine overdose.

midazolam ■■■■▶◀■■■■ azole antifungals
Versed   fluconazole, itraconazole,
                                      ketoconazole, miconazole

Risk rating: 2
Severity: Moderate   Onset: Rapid   Likelihood: Established

Cause
Azole antifungals decrease CYP3A4 metabolism of certain benzodiazepines, such as midazolam.

Effect
Benzodiazepine effects are increased and prolonged, which may cause CNS depression and psychomotor impairment.

Nursing considerations
■ If patient takes fluconazole or miconazole, talk with prescriber about giving a lower benzodiazepine dose or a drug not metabolized by CYP3A4, such as temazepam or lorazepam.
■ Caution that the effects of this interaction may last several days after stopping the azole antifungal.
■ Explain that taking these drugs together may increase sedative effects; tell patient to report such effects promptly.
■ Explain alternative methods of inducing sleep or relieving anxiety.
■ Various benzodiazepine–azole antifungal combinations may interact. If you suspect an interaction, consult prescriber or pharmacist.

midazolam ■▶◀■ grapefruit juice
Versed

Risk rating: 2
Severity: **Moderate**   Onset: **Rapid**   Likelihood: **Suspected**

Cause
Grapefruit juice inhibits first-pass CYP3A4 metabolism of certain benzodiazepines, such as midazolam.

Effect
Benzodiazepine onset is delayed and effects are increased, causing CNS depression and psychomotor impairment.

Nursing considerations
🠶 ALERT Tell patient not to take a benzodiazepine with grapefruit juice.
■ If patient uses grapefruit juice to take a benzodiazepine, explain that oversedation may last up to 72 hours.
■ This interaction is increased in patients with cirrhosis of the liver.
■ Instruct patient to tell prescriber about increased sedation or trouble walking or using limbs.

midazolam ■▶◀■ macrolide antibiotics
Versed   clarithromycin, erythromycin

Risk rating: 2
Severity: **Moderate**   Onset: **Rapid**   Likelihood: **Suspected**

Cause
Macrolide antibiotics may decrease metabolism of certain benzodiazepines, such as midazolam.

Effect
Sedative effects of benzodiazepines may be increased or prolonged.

Nursing considerations
- Consult prescriber about decreasing benzodiazepine dosage during antibiotic therapy.
- Lorazepam, oxazepam, and temazepam probably don't interact with macrolide antibiotics; substitution may be possible.
- Azithromycin doesn't alter midazolam metabolism but may delay its absorption.
- Urge patient to promptly report oversedation.

---

midazolam ━━►◄━━	nonnucleoside reverse-transcriptase inhibitors
Versed	delavirdine, efavirenz

Risk rating: 2
Severity: **Moderate**   Onset: **Delayed**   Likelihood: **Suspected**

Cause
Nonnucleoside reverse-transcriptase inhibitors may inhibit CYP3A4 metabolism of certain benzodiazepines, such as midazolam.

Effect
Sedative effects of benzodiazepines may be increased or prolonged, leading to respiratory depression.

Nursing considerations
- **⚡ ALERT** Don't combine midazolam with delavirdine or efavirenz.
- Other benzodiazepines and nonnucleoside reverse-transcriptase inhibitors may interact. If you suspect an interaction, consult prescriber or pharmacist.
- Explain the risk of oversedation and respiratory depression.
- Urge patient to promptly report any suspected interaction.

---

midazolam ━━►◄━━	protease inhibitors
Versed	amprenavir, atazanavir, indinavir, lopinavir-ritonavir, nelfinavir, ritonavir, saquinavir

Risk rating: 2
Severity: **Moderate**   Onset: **Delayed**   Likelihood: **Suspected**

Cause
Protease inhibitors may inhibit CYP3A4 metabolism of certain benzodiazepines, such as midazolam.

Effect
Sedative effects may be increased and prolonged.

Nursing considerations
⚡ **ALERT** Don't combine midazolam with protease inhibitors.
⚡ **ALERT** Midazolam is contraindicated in patients taking atazanavir.
■ If patient takes any benzodiazepine–protease inhibitor combination, notify prescriber. Interaction could involve other drugs in the class.
■ Watch for evidence of oversedation and respiratory depression.
■ Teach patient and family about risks of combined use.

| **midazolam** ➤◀ | **rifamycins** |
| Versed | rifabutin, rifampin, rifapentine |

Risk rating: 2
Severity: Moderate   **Onset: Delayed**   **Likelihood: Suspected**

Cause
Rifamycins may increase CYP3A4 metabolism of benzodiazepines, such as midazolam.

Effect
Antianxiety, sedative, and sleep-inducing effects may decrease.

Nursing considerations
■ Watch for expected benzodiazepine effects and lack of efficacy.
■ If benzodiazepine efficacy is reduced, notify prescriber; dosage may be changed.
■ Other benzodiazepines may interact with rifamycins. If you suspect an interaction, consult prescriber or pharmacist.
■ For insomnia, temazepam may be more effective because it doesn't undergo CYP3A4 metabolism.

| **minocycline** ➤◀ | **aluminum salts** |
| Minocin | aluminum carbonate, aluminum hydroxide, magaldrate |

Risk rating: 2
Severity: Moderate   **Onset: Delayed**   **Likelihood: Probable**

Cause
Formation of an insoluble chelate with aluminum may decrease absorption of tetracyclines, such as minocycline.

Effect

Tetracycline level may decline more than 50%, reducing efficacy.

Nursing considerations

- Separate doses by at least 3 hours.
- If patient must take these drugs together, notify prescriber. Minocycline dose may need adjustment.
- Monitor patient for reduced anti-infective response, including infection flare-up, fever, and malaise.
- Other tetracyclines may interact with aluminum salts. If you suspect an interaction, consult prescriber or pharmacist.
- Help patient develop a plan to ensure proper dosage intervals.

---

minocycline ━━▶◀ calcium salts

Minocin

calcium carbonate, calcium citrate, calcium gluconate, calcium lactate, tricalcium phosphate

Risk rating: 2
Severity: Moderate   Onset: **Delayed**   Likelihood: **Probable**

Cause

Calcium salts form an insoluble complex with tetracyclines, such as minocycline, that lowers tetracycline absorption.

Effect

Tetracycline level and efficacy decrease.

Nursing considerations

- Separate tetracyclines from calcium salts by at least 3 to 4 hours.
- Monitor efficacy of tetracycline. Notify prescriber if infection isn't responding to treatment.
- Doxycycline is somewhat less affected by this interaction.
- Advise against taking tetracycline with dairy products or calcium-fortified orange juice.
- Tell patient to separate tetracycline dose from calcium supplements by 3 to 4 hours.

minocycline ━━━━▶◀━━━━ iron salts

Minocin

ferrous fumarate, ferrous gluconate, ferrous sulfate, iron polysaccharide

Risk rating: 2
Severity: Moderate   **Onset: Delayed**   **Likelihood: Probable**

Cause
Minocycline and other tetracyclines form insoluble chelates with iron salts, which may reduce absorption of both substances.

Effect
Tetracycline and iron salt levels and effects may decrease.

Nursing considerations
◪ ALERT If possible, avoid giving tetracyclines with iron salts.
■ If they must be given together, separate doses by 3 to 4 hours.
■ If you suspect an interaction, consult prescriber or pharmacist; an enteric-coated or sustained-release iron salt may reduce interaction.
■ Monitor patient for expected response to tetracycline.
■ Assess patient for evidence of iron deficiency, including fatigue, dyspnea, tachycardia, palpitations, dizziness, and orthostatic hypotension.

minocycline ━━━━▶◀━━━━ magnesium salts, oral

Minocin

magaldrate, magnesium carbonate, magnesium citrate, magnesium gluconate, magnesium hydroxide, magnesium oxide, magnesium sulfate, magnesium trisilicate

Risk rating: 2
Severity: Moderate   **Onset: Delayed**   **Likelihood: Probable**

Cause
Magnesium salts form an insoluble complex with tetracyclines, such as minocycline, that lowers tetracycline absorption.

Effect
Decreased tetracycline level leads to decreased anti-infective efficacy.

Nursing considerations
■ Separate tetracyclines from magnesium salts by at least 3 to 4 hours.

■ Monitor efficacy of tetracycline. Notify prescriber if infection isn't responding to treatment.
■ Teach patient to separate tetracycline dose from magnesium-based antacids, laxatives, and supplements by 3 to 4 hours.

---

minocycline ▸◂ penicillins

Minocin

amoxicillin, ampicillin, carbenicillin, cloxacillin, dicloxacillin, nafcillin, oxacillin, penicillin G, penicillin V, piperacillin, ticarcillin

---

Risk rating: 1
Severity: Major   **Onset: Delayed**   **Likelihood: Suspected**

Cause
Minocycline and other tetracyclines may adversely affect the bactericidal activity of penicillins.

Effect
Penicillin efficacy may be reduced.

Nursing considerations
■ If possible, avoid giving tetracyclines with penicillins.
■ Monitor patient closely for lack of penicillin effect.

---

mirtazapine ▸◂ hydantoins

Remeron

ethotoin, fosphenytoin, phenytoin

Risk rating: 2
Severity: Moderate   **Onset: Delayed**   **Likelihood: Suspected**

Cause
Hydantoins may increase CYP3A3 and CYP3A4 metabolism of mirtazapine.

Effect
Mirtazapine level and effects may decrease.

Nursing considerations
■ Assess patient for expected mirtazapine effects, including improvement of depression and stabilization of mood.
■ Record mood changes, and monitor patient for suicidal tendencies.
■ If hydantoin therapy starts, mirtazapine dosage may be increased.

- If hydantoin therapy stops, watch for mirtazapine toxicity, including disorientation, drowsiness, impaired memory, tachycardia, severe hypotension, heart failure, seizures, CNS depression, and coma.
- Urge patient to tell prescriber about loss of drug effect and increased adverse effects.

---

moexipril ▶◀ indomethacin
Univasc   Indocin

Risk rating: 2
Severity: Moderate   Onset: Rapid   Likelihood: Probable

Cause
Indomethacin inhibits synthesis of prostaglandins, which moexipril and other ACE inhibitors need to lower blood pressure.

Effect
ACE inhibitor's hypotensive effect will be reduced.

Nursing considerations
⚠ **ALERT** Monitor blood pressure closely. Severe hypertension may persist until indomethacin is stopped.
- If indomethacin can't be avoided, patient may need a different antihypertensive.
- Other ACE inhibitors may interact with indomethacin. If you suspect an interaction, consult prescriber or pharmacist.
- Remind patient that hypertension commonly causes no physical symptoms but sometimes may cause headache and dizziness.

---

moexipril ▶◀ potassium-sparing diuretics
Univasc

amiloride, spironolactone, triamterene

Risk rating: 1
Severity: Major   Onset: Delayed   Likelihood: Probable

Cause
The mechanism of this interaction is unknown.

Effect
Serum potassium level may increase.

Nursing considerations
- Use cautiously in patients at high risk for hyperkalemia, especially those with renal impairment.

- Monitor BUN, creatinine, and serum potassium levels as needed.
- ACE inhibitors other than moexipril may interact with potassium-sparing diuretics. If you suspect an interaction, consult prescriber or pharmacist.
- Urge patient to immediately report an irregular heartbeat, a slow pulse, weakness, and other evidence of hyperkalemia.

---

moexipril ▶◀ salicylates

Univasc

aspirin, bismuth subsalicylate, choline salicylate, magnesium salicylate, salsalate, sodium salicylate

Risk rating: 2
Severity: **Moderate**   Onset: **Rapid**   Likelihood: **Suspected**

Cause
Salicylates inhibit synthesis of prostaglandins, which moexipril and other ACE inhibitors need to lower blood pressure.

Effect
ACE inhibitor's hypotensive effect will be reduced.

Nursing considerations
- This interaction is more likely in people with hypertension, coronary artery disease, or possibly heart failure.

---

moricizine ▶◀ cimetidine

Ethmozine

Tagamet

Risk rating: 2
Severity: **Moderate**   Onset: **Delayed**   Likelihood: **Suspected**

Cause
Cimetidine inhibits hepatic metabolism of moricizine.

Effect
Therapeutic and adverse effects of moricizine may increase.

Nursing considerations
- Monitor the ECG when starting, changing, or stopping cimetidine.
- Watch for increased moricizine toxicity: arrhythmias, vomiting, lethargy, dizziness, syncope, hypotension, worsening heart failure, respiratory failure, and coma.
- Consult prescriber for dosage adjustments.
- Urge patient to tell prescriber about increased adverse effects.

■ H_2-receptor antagonists other than cimetidine interact with moricizine. If you suspect a drug interaction, consult prescriber or pharmacist.

---

moricizine ▬▬▬►◄▬▬▬ diltiazem
Ethmozine   Cardizem

Risk rating: 2
Severity: Moderate   Onset: Delayed   Likelihood: Suspected

Cause
Moricizine metabolism may decrease; diltiazem metabolism may increase.

Effect
Therapeutic and adverse effects of moricizine may increase; therapeutic effects of diltiazem may decrease.

Nursing considerations
■ Monitor patient for expected effects of diltiazem, such as control of angina or hypertension.
■ Advise patient to report increased episodes of angina or symptoms of hypertension, including headache, dizziness, and blurred vision.
■ Monitor patient for increased moricizine adverse effects, including headache, dizziness, and paresthesia.
■ Advise the patient to avoid hazardous activities if adverse CNS reactions or blurred vision occurs. These adverse effects may be more common with increased moricizine level.
■ Dosage adjustments may be needed when either drug is started, changed, or stopped.

---

moricizine ▬▬▬►◄▬▬▬ vardenafil
Ethmozine   Levitra

Risk rating: 1
Severity: Major   Onset: Rapid   Likelihood: Suspected

Cause
The mechanism of this interaction is unknown.

Effect
QTc interval may be prolonged, particularly in patients with previous QT-interval prolongation and those taking certain antiarrhythmics, increasing the risk of such life-threatening arrhythmias as torsades de pointes.

Nursing considerations
⚡ ALERT Use of vardenafil with a class IA or class III antiarrhythmic, such as moricizine, is contraindicated.

■ Monitor ECG before and periodically after patient starts vardenafil.
■ Urge patient to report light-headedness, faintness, palpitations, and chest pain or pressure while taking vardenafil.
■ To reduce risk of adverse effects, patients age 65 and older should start with 5 mg vardenafil, half the usual starting dose.

---

moxifloxacin ◄►	**antiarrhythmics**
Avelox	amiodarone, bretylium, disopyramide, procainamide, quinidine, sotalol

Risk rating: 1
Severity: Major　　**Onset: Delayed**　　**Likelihood: Suspected**

Cause
The mechanism of this interaction is unknown.

Effect
Risk of life-threatening arrhythmias, including torsades de pointes, increases.

Nursing considerations
■ Avoid giving class IA or class III antiarrhythmics with the quinolone moxifloxacin.
■ Monitor ECG for prolonged QTc interval.
■ Quinolones that aren't metabolized by CYP3A4 isoenzymes or that don't prolong the QT interval may be given with antiarrhythmics.
■ Tell patient to report a rapid heartbeat, shortness of breath, dizziness, fainting, and chest pain.

---

moxifloxacin ◄►	**erythromycin**
Avelox	E-mycin, Eryc

Risk rating: 1
Severity: Major　　**Onset: Delayed**　　**Likelihood: Suspected**

Cause
The mechanism of this interaction is unknown.

Effect
Risk of life-threatening arrhythmias, including torsades de pointes, increases.

Nursing considerations
▪ Use erythromycin cautiously with moxifloxacin.
▪ Monitor QTc interval closely.
▪ Tell patient to report palpitations, dizziness, shortness of breath, and chest pain.

---

moxifloxacin ▶◀ phenothiazines

Avelox

chlorpromazine, fluphenazine, mesoridazine, perphenazine, prochlorperazine, promethazine, thioridazine

Risk rating: 1
Severity: Major   **Onset: Delayed**   **Likelihood: Suspected**

Cause
The mechanism of this interaction is unknown.

Effect
Risk of life-threatening arrhythmias, including torsades de pointes, may increase.

Nursing considerations
▪ Use the quinolone moxifloxacin cautiously, with increased monitoring.
▪ Quinolones that don't prolong the QTc interval or that aren't metabolized by CYP3A4 isoenzymes may be better alternatives.

---

moxifloxacin ▶◀ sucralfate

Avelox

Carafate

Risk rating: 2
Severity: Moderate   **Onset: Rapid**   **Likelihood: Probable**

Cause
Sucralfate decreases GI absorption of quinolones, such as moxifloxacin.

Effect
Quinolone effects decrease.

Nursing considerations
▪ Avoid use together. If it's unavoidable, give sucralfate at least 6 hours after the quinolone.
▪ Monitor patient for resolving infection.
▪ Help patient develop a plan to ensure proper dosage intervals.

moxifloxacin ➡️◀ tricyclic antidepressants

Avelox

amitriptyline, amoxapine, clomipramine, desipramine, doxepin, imipramine, nortriptyline, trimipramine

Risk rating: 1
Severity: Major   **Onset: Delayed**   **Likelihood: Suspected**

Cause
The mechanism of this interaction if unknown.

Effect
Life-threatening arrhythmias, including torsades de pointes, may increase when certain of these drugs are used together.

Nursing considerations
- Use the quinolone moxifloxacin cautiously with a tricyclic antidepressant.
- If possible, use other quinolone antibiotics that don't prolong the QTc interval or aren't metabolized by the CYP3A4 isoenzyme.

mycophenolate mofetil ➡️◀ iron salts

CellCept

ferrous fumarate, ferrous gluconate, ferrous sulfate, iron polysaccharide

Risk rating: 2
Severity: Moderate   **Onset: Rapid**   **Likelihood: Suspected**

Cause
Mycophenolate mofetil absorption may decrease because drug may form a complex with iron salt in the GI tract.

Effect
Mycophenolate mofetil level and effects may decrease.

Nursing considerations
- ⚡ ALERT Avoid giving iron salts with mycophenolate mofetil.
- If you must give both, separate doses as much as possible.
- Watch for evidence of rejection or decreased drug effect if iron salts are given with mycophenolate mofetil.
- Urge patient to report signs of organ rejection, such as decreased urine output in kidney transplant patients or shortness of breath in heart transplant patients.
- Help patient develop a plan to ensure proper dosage intervals.

nabumetone ◄► aminoglycosides
Relafen

amikacin, gentamicin,
kanamycin, netilmicin,
streptomycin, tobramycin

Risk rating: 2
Severity: Moderate   **Onset: Delayed**   **Likelihood: Suspected**

Cause
Nabumetone and other NSAIDs may reduce glomerular filtration rate (GFR), causing aminoglycosides to accumulate.

Effect
Aminoglycoside level in premature infants may increase.

Nursing considerations
■ Before NSAID therapy starts, aminoglycoside dose should be reduced.
◪ ALERT Check peak and trough aminoglycoside levels after third dose. For peak level, draw blood 30 minutes after I.V. or 60 minutes after I.M. dose. For trough level, draw blood just before a dose.
■ Monitor patient's renal function.
■ Although only indomethacin is known to interact with aminoglycosides, other NSAIDs probably do as well. If you suspect an interaction, consult prescriber or pharmacist.
■ Other drugs cleared by GFR may have a similar interaction.

nadolol ◄► epinephrine
Corgard

Risk rating: 1
Severity: Major   **Onset: Rapid**   **Likelihood: Established**

Cause
Alpha-receptor effects of epinephrine supersede effects of nonselective beta blockers, such as nadolol, increasing vascular resistance.

Effect
Initial marked hypertensive effect is followed by reflex bradycardia.

Nursing considerations
◪ ALERT Three days before planned use of epinephrine, stop the beta blocker. Or, if possible, don't use epinephrine.
■ If drugs must be combined, monitor blood pressure and pulse closely. If interaction occurs, give I.V. chlorpromazine, hydralazine, aminophylline, or atropine if needed.

■ Explain the risks of this interaction, and tell patient to carry medical identification at all times.
■ Other beta blockers may interact with epinephrine. If you suspect an interaction, consult prescriber or pharmacist.

---

nadolol ▶◀ ergot derivatives
Corgard   dihydroergotamine, ergotamine

Risk rating: 2
Severity: Moderate   **Onset:** Delayed   **Likelihood:** Suspected

Cause
Vasoconstriction and blockade of peripheral beta$_2$ receptors allow unopposed ergot action.

Effect
Vasoconstrictive effects of ergot derivatives increase, causing peripheral ischemia, cold limbs, and possible gangrene.

Nursing considerations
■ Watch for evidence of peripheral ischemia.
■ If needed, stop beta blocker (such as nadolol) and adjust ergot drug.
■ Other ergot derivatives may interact with beta blockers. If you suspect an interaction, consult prescriber or pharmacist.

---

nadolol ▶◀ lidocaine
Corgard

Risk rating: 2
Severity: Moderate   **Onset:** Rapid   **Likelihood:** Established

Cause
Nadolol and other beta blockers reduce hepatic metabolism of lidocaine.

Effect
Lidocaine level and risk of toxicity may increase.

Nursing considerations
■ Check for therapeutic lidocaine level: 2 to 5 mcg/ml.
■ Slow I.V. bolus rate to decrease the risk of high peak level and toxic reaction.
■ Monitor patient closely for evidence of lidocaine toxicity: dizziness, somnolence, confusion, paresthesias, and seizures.
■ Explain the warning signs of toxicity to patient and family, and tell them to contact prescriber if they have concerns.

nadolol ◄► NSAIDs

Corgard

ibuprofen, indomethacin,
naproxen, piroxicam

Risk rating: 2
Severity: Moderate   Onset: Delayed   Likelihood: Probable

Cause
NSAIDs may inhibit renal prostaglandin synthesis, allowing pressor
systems to be unopposed.

Effect
Beta blockers, such as nadolol, may not be able to lower blood pressure.

Nursing considerations
- Avoid using these drugs together if possible.
- Monitor blood pressure and other evidence of hypertension closely.
- Talk with prescriber about ways to minimize interaction, such as ad-
justing beta blocker dosage or switching to sulindac as the NSAID.
- Explain the risks of using these drugs together, and teach patient
how to monitor his blood pressure.
- Other NSAIDs may interact with beta blockers. If you suspect an
interaction, consult prescriber or pharmacist.

nadolol ◄► prazosin

Corgard

Minipress

Risk rating: 2
Severity: Moderate   Onset: Rapid   Likelihood: Probable

Cause
The mechanism of this interaction is unknown.

Effect
Effect of these drugs on orthostatic hypotension is increased.

Nursing considerations
- Assess patient's lying, sitting, and standing blood pressures closely,
especially when combined therapy starts.
- Adjust dosages of either drug based on patient effects.
- To minimize effects of orthostatic hypotension, teach patient to
change positions slowly.
- Interaction is confirmed only with propranolol but may occur with
other beta blockers as well.

nadolol ◆◀ salicylates

Corgard

aspirin, bismuth subsalicylate, choline salicylate, magnesium salicylate, salsalate, sodium salicylate, sodium thiosalicylate

Risk rating: 2
Severity: Moderate   **Onset: Rapid**   **Likelihood: Suspected**

Cause
Salicylates inhibit synthesis of prostaglandins, which nadolol and other beta blockers need to reduce blood pressure. In patients with heart failure, the mechanism of this interaction is unknown.

Effect
Beta blocker's effect will decrease.

Nursing considerations
■ Watch closely for signs of heart failure and hypertension, and notify prescriber if they occur.
■ Consult prescriber about switching patient to a different antihypertensive or antiplatelet drug.
■ Other beta blockers may interact with salicylates. If you suspect an interaction, consult prescriber or pharmacist.
■ Explain signs and symptoms of heart failure, and tell patient when to contact prescriber.

nadolol ◆◀ verapamil

Corgard

Calan

Risk rating: 1
Severity: Major   **Onset: Rapid**   **Likelihood: Probable**

Cause
Verapamil may inhibit metabolism of beta blockers, such as nadolol.

Effect
Effects of both drugs may increase.

Nursing considerations
■ Combination therapy is common in patients with hypertension and unstable angina.
■ ALERT Combining these drugs increases risk of adverse effects, including heart failure, conduction disturbances, arrhythmias, and hypotension.

- Assess patient for adverse effects, including left ventricular dysfunction and AV conduction defects.
- Risk of interaction is greater when drugs are given I.V.
- Dosages of both drugs may need to be decreased.

nafcillin ▶◀ aminoglycosides
amikacin, gentamicin, kanamycin, netilmicin, streptomycin, tobramycin

Risk rating: 2
Severity: Moderate   **Onset: Delayed**   **Likelihood: Probable**

Cause
The mechanism of this interaction is unknown.

Effect
Nafcillin and other penicillins may inactivate certain aminoglycosides, decreasing their effects.

Nursing considerations
▶ ALERT Check peak and trough aminoglycoside levels after third dose. For peak level, draw blood 30 minutes after I.V. or 60 minutes after I.M. dose. For trough level, draw blood just before a dose.
- Monitor patient's renal function.
- Penicillins affect gentamicin and tobramycin more than amikacin and netilmicin.
- Other aminoglycosides may interact with penicillins. If you suspect an interaction, consult prescriber or pharmacist.

nafcillin ▶◀ food

Risk rating: 2
Severity: Moderate   **Onset: Delayed**   **Likelihood: Suspected**

Cause
Food may delay or reduce GI absorption of penicillins, such as nafcillin.

Effect
Nafcillin efficacy may decrease.

Nursing considerations
- Food may affect nafcillin absorption and peak level.

■ Penicillin V and amoxicillin don't have this interaction and may be given without regard to meals.
■ Tell patient to take nafcillin 1 hour before or 2 hours after a meal.
■ If patient took nafcillin with food, watch for lack of drug efficacy.

---

nafcillin ◄► tetracyclines
demeclocycline, doxycycline, minocycline, tetracycline

Risk rating: 1
Severity: Major   **Onset: Delayed**   **Likelihood: Suspected**

Cause
Tetracyclines may adversely affect the bactericidal activity of penicillins, such as nafcillin.

Effect
Nafcillin efficacy may be reduced.

Nursing considerations
■ If possible, avoid giving tetracyclines with penicillins.
■ Monitor patient closely for lack of nafcillin effect.

---

naproxen ◄► aminoglycosides
Aleve
amikacin, gentamicin, kanamycin, netilmicin, streptomycin, tobramycin

Risk rating: 2
Severity: Moderate   **Onset: Delayed**   **Likelihood: Suspected**

Cause
Naproxen and other NSAIDs may reduce glomerular filtration rate (GFR), causing aminoglycosides to accumulate.

Effect
Aminoglycoside level in premature infants may increase.

Nursing considerations
■ Before NSAID starts, aminoglycoside dose should be reduced.
◆ ALERT Check peak and trough aminoglycoside levels after third dose. For peak level, draw blood 30 minutes after I.V. or 60 minutes after I.M. dose. For trough level, draw blood just before a dose.
■ Monitor patient's renal function.

■ Although only indomethacin is known to interact with aminoglycosides, other NSAIDs probably do as well. If you suspect an interaction, consult prescriber or pharmacist.

■ Other drugs cleared by GFR may have a similar interaction.

---

naproxen ▶◀	beta blockers
Aleve	acebutolol, atenolol, betaxolol, bisoprolol, carteolol, esmolol, metoprolol, nadolol, penbutolol, pindolol, propranolol, sotalol, timolol

Risk rating: 2
Severity: Moderate   **Onset: Delayed**   **Likelihood: Probable**

Cause
Naproxen and other NSAIDs may inhibit renal prostaglandin synthesis, allowing pressor systems to be unopposed.

Effect
Beta blocker may not be able to lower blood pressure.

Nursing considerations
■ Avoid using these drugs together, if possible.
■ Monitor blood pressure and other evidence of hypertension closely.
■ Consult prescriber about ways to minimize interaction, such as adjusting beta blocker dosage or switching to sulindac as the NSAID.
■ Explain the risks of using these drugs together, and teach patient how to monitor his blood pressure.
■ Other NSAIDs may interact with beta blockers. If you suspect an interaction, consult prescriber or pharmacist.

---

naratriptan ▶◀	ergot derivatives
Amerge	dihydroergotamine, ergotamine

Risk rating: 1
Severity: Major   **Onset: Rapid**   **Likelihood: Suspected**

Cause
Combined use may have additive effects.

Effect
Risk of vasospastic effects increases.

Nursing considerations
🢂 ALERT Use of these drugs within 24 hours of each other is contra-indicated.

■ Combined use may cause severe vasospastic effects, including sustained coronary artery vasospasm that triggers MI.

■ Warn patients not to mix migraine headache drugs within 24 hours of each other, but to call prescriber if a drug isn't effective.

---

naratriptan ►◄ **serotonin reuptake inhibitors**

Amerge

citalopram, fluoxetine, fluvoxamine, nefazodone, paroxetine, sertraline, venlafaxine

Risk rating: 2
Severity: Moderate   **Onset: Rapid**   **Likelihood: Suspected**

Cause
Serotonin may accumulate rapidly in the CNS.

Effect
Risk of serotonin syndrome increases.

Nursing considerations
🢂 ALERT If possible, avoid combined use of these drugs.

■ If combined use can't be avoided, start with lowest dosages possible, and assess patient closely.

■ Stop naratriptan, a selective 5-HT$_1$ receptor agonist, at the first sign of interaction, and start an antiserotonergic drug.

■ In some patients, migraine frequency may increase and antimigraine drug efficacy may decrease.

■ Describe traits of serotonin syndrome, including CNS irritability, weakness, shivering, muscle twitching, and altered consciousness.

■ State that serotonin syndrome can be fatal if not treated promptly.

---

naratriptan ►◄ **sibutramine**

Amerge   Meridia

Risk rating: 1
Severity: Major   **Onset: Rapid**   **Likelihood: Suspected**

Cause
Sibutramine inhibits serotonin reuptake, which may have an additive effect with selective 5-HT$_1$ receptor agonists, such as naratriptan.

Effect
Risk of serotonin syndrome increases.

Nursing considerations
⚠ ALERT If possible, avoid giving these drugs together.
■ If use together can't be avoided, monitor patient closely for adverse effects, which require immediate medical attention.
■ Stop the selective 5-HT$_1$ receptor agonist at the first sign of interaction, and start an antiserotonergic drug.
■ Describe the traits of serotonin syndrome, including CNS irritability, motor weakness, shivering, myoclonus, and altered consciousness.
■ Urge patient to promptly report adverse effects.

---

nefazodone ▶◀ carbamazepine
Carbatrol, Epitol, Equetro, Tegretol

Risk rating: 1
Severity: Major   **Onset: Delayed**   **Likelihood: Suspected**

Cause
Nefazodone may inhibit CYP3A4 hepatic metabolism of carbamazepine. Carbamazepine may induce nefazodone metabolism.

Effect
Carbamazepine level and risk of adverse effects may increase. Nefazodone level and effects may decrease.

Nursing considerations
⚠ ALERT Use of carbamazepine with nefazodone is contraindicated.
■ Monitor carbamazepine level; therapeutic range is 4 to 12 mcg/ml.
■ Watch for signs of anorexia or subtle appetite changes, which may indicate excessive carbamazepine level.
■ Watch for signs of carbamazepine toxicity: dizziness, ataxia, respiratory depression, tachycardia, arrhythmias, blood pressure changes, impaired consciousness, abnormal reflexes, nystagmus, seizures, nausea, vomiting, and urine retention.
■ Monitor patient for adequate nefazodone clinical effects.
■ Urge patient to tell prescriber about increased adverse effects.

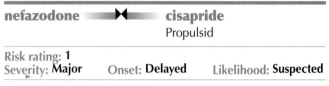

nefazodone ◄► **cisapride**
Propulsid

Risk rating: 1
Severity: **Major**   Onset: **Delayed**   Likelihood: **Suspected**

Cause
Nefazodone may inhibit CYP3A4 hepatic metabolism of cisapride.

Effect
Cisapride level and risk of cardiotoxicity may increase.

Nursing considerations
▶ ALERT Use of nefazodone with cisapride is contraindicated.
■ Combining cisapride with drugs that inhibit CYP3A4 may cause prolonged QT interval, torsades de pointes, and other life-threatening arrhythmias.
■ Cisapride is available only through a limited access program for patients who don't respond to all other standard treatments and who meet strict eligibility criteria.
■ Consult prescriber or pharmacist for alternative antidepressant if patient takes cisapride.

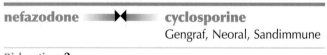

nefazodone ◄► **cyclosporine**
Gengraf, Neoral, Sandimmune

Risk rating: 2
Severity: **Moderate**   Onset: **Delayed**   Likelihood: **Probable**

Cause
Nefazodone may inhibit cyclosporine metabolism.

Effect
Cyclosporine level and risk of toxicity may increase.

Nursing considerations
■ Patient who takes cyclosporine may need an alternative antidepressant to nefazodone.
■ Monitor cyclosporine level closely when nefazodone starts or stops.
■ Toxicity may cause shakiness, headaches, tremor, hypertension, and fatigue.
■ Cyclosporine dosage may need reduction.

nefazodone ▶◀ MAO inhibitors
isocarboxazid, phenelzine, selegiline, tranylcypromine

Risk rating: 1
Severity: Major   **Onset: Rapid**   **Likelihood: Probable**

Cause
Serotonin may accumulate rapidly in the CNS.

Effect
Risk of serotonin syndrome increases.

Nursing considerations
◤ **ALERT** Don't use these drugs together.
■ Allow 1 week after stopping nefazodone before giving an MAO inhibitor. Allow 2 weeks after stopping an MAO inhibitor before giving a serotonin reuptake inhibitor, such as nefazodone.
■ The selective MAO type-B inhibitor selegiline has been given with fluoxetine, paroxetine, or sertraline to patients with Parkinson's disease without negative effects.
■ Describe the traits of serotonin syndrome, including CNS irritability, motor weakness, shivering, myoclonus, and altered consciousness.
■ Urge patient to promptly report adverse effects.

nefazodone ▶◀ selective 5-HT$_1$ receptor agonists
almotriptan, eletriptan, frovatriptan, naratriptan, rizatriptan, sumatriptan, zolmitriptan

Risk rating: 1
Severity: Major   **Onset: Rapid**   **Likelihood: Suspected**

Cause
Serotonin may accumulate rapidly in the CNS.

Effect
Risk of serotonin syndrome increases.

Nursing considerations
◤ **ALERT** If possible, avoid combined use of these drugs.
■ If combined use can't be avoided, start with lowest dosages possible, and assess patient closely.

- Stop the selective 5-HT$_1$ receptor agonist at the first sign of interaction, and start an antiserotonergic drug.
- In some patients, migraine frequency may increase and antimigraine drug efficacy may decrease when a serotonin reuptake inhibitor is started.
- Describe the traits of serotonin syndrome, including CNS irritability, motor weakness, shivering, muscle twitching, and altered consciousness.
- Explain that serotonin syndrome can be fatal if not treated immediately.

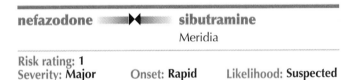

nefazodone ◀▶ sibutramine
Meridia

Risk rating: 1
Severity: Major   **Onset: Rapid**   **Likelihood: Suspected**

Cause
Serotonin may accumulate rapidly in the CNS.

Effect
Risk of serotonin syndrome increases.

Nursing considerations
⚠ **ALERT** If possible, don't give these drugs together.
- If this combination must be used, watch carefully for adverse effects, which require immediate medical attention.
- Describe the traits of serotonin syndrome, including CNS irritability, motor weakness, shivering, muscle twitching, and altered consciousness.
- Explain that serotonin syndrome can be fatal if not treated immediately.

nefazodone ◀▶ St. John's wort

Risk rating: 2
Severity: Moderate   **Onset: Rapid**   **Likelihood: Suspected**

Cause
St. John's wort may cause additive inhibition of serotonin reuptake.

Effect
Sedative-hypnotic effects of serotonin reuptake inhibitors, such as nefazodone, may increase.

Nursing considerations
⚑ ALERT Discourage use of a serotonin reuptake inhibitor with St. John's wort.
- In addition to oversedation, mild serotonin-like symptoms may occur, including anxiety, dizziness, nausea, restlessness, and vomiting.
- Inform patient about the dangers of this combination.
- Urge patient to consult prescriber before taking any herb.

---

nelfinavir ◄► azole antifungals
Viracept   fluconazole, itraconazole, ketoconazole

Risk rating: 2
Severity: Moderate   Onset: Delayed   Likelihood: Suspected

Cause
Azole antifungals may inhibit metabolism of protease inhibitors, such as nelfinavir.

Effect
Protease inhibitor level may increase.

Nursing considerations
- Protease inhibitor dosage may be decreased when therapy starts.
- Monitor patient for increased protease inhibitor effects, including hyperglycemia, onset of diabetes, rash, GI complaints, and altered liver function tests.
- Advise patient to report increased hunger or thirst, frequent urination, fatigue, and dry, itchy skin.
- Tell patient not to change dosage or stop either drug without consulting prescriber.

---

nelfinavir ◄► benzodiazepines
Viracept   alprazolam, chlordiazepoxide, clonazepam, clorazepate, diazepam, estazolam, flurazepam, midazolam, quazepam, triazolam

Risk rating: 2
Severity: Moderate   Onset: Delayed   Likelihood: Suspected

Cause
Nelfinavir and other protease inhibitors may inhibit CYP3A4 metabolism of certain benzodiazepines.

Effect
Sedative effects may be increased and prolonged.

Nursing considerations
◆ ALERT Don't combine these benzodiazepines with protease inhibitors.
■ If patient takes any protease inhibitor–benzodiazepine combination, notify prescriber. Interaction could involve other drugs in the class.
■ Watch for evidence of oversedation and respiratory depression.
■ Teach patient and family about the risks of combined use.

---

nelfinavir ▸◄	eplerenone
Viracept	Inspra

Risk rating: 1
Severity: Major   **Onset: Delayed**   **Likelihood: Suspected**

Cause
Protease inhibitors, such as nelfinavir, inhibit metabolism of eplerenone.

Effect
Eplerenone level rises, causing hyperkalemia and increasing the risk of life-threatening arrhythmias.

Nursing considerations
◆ ALERT Use of nelfinavir with eplerenone is contraindicated.
■ Potent CYP3A4 inhibitors increase the eplerenone level and the risk of hyperkalemia-induced arrhythmias—some fatal.
■ Monitor patient's serum potassium level.
■ Tell patient to report nausea, irregular heartbeat, and slowed pulse to prescriber.

---

nelfinavir ▸◄	ergot derivatives
Viracept	dihydroergotamine, ergonovine, ergotamine, methylergonovine

Risk rating: 1
Severity: Major   **Onset: Delayed**   **Likelihood: Probable**

Cause
Protease inhibitors, such as nelfinavir, may interfere with CYP3A4 metabolism of ergot derivatives.

Effect
Risk of ergot-induced peripheral vasospasm and ischemia may be increased.

Nursing considerations
⚑ ALERT Use of ergot derivatives with protease inhibitors is contraindicated.

■ Monitor patient for evidence of peripheral ischemia, including pain in limb muscles while exercising and later at rest; numbness and tingling of fingers and toes; cool, pale, or cyanotic limbs; red or violet blisters on hands or feet; and gangrene.

■ Sodium nitroprusside may be given for ergot-induced vasospasm.

■ If patient takes a protease inhibitor, consult prescriber or pharmacist about other treatments for migraine pain.

■ Urge patient to tell prescriber about increased adverse effects.

---

nelfinavir ▸◂ fentanyl
Viracept   Sublimaze

Risk rating: 1
Severity: Major   **Onset: Delayed**   **Likelihood: Suspected**

Cause
Metabolism of fentanyl in the GI tract and liver may be inhibited.

Effect
Fentanyl level may increase and half-life lengthen.

Nursing considerations
⚑ ALERT If patient takes a protease inhibitor, such as nelfinavir, watch closely for respiratory depression if fentanyl is added.

■ Because fentanyl half-life is prolonged, monitoring period should continue, even after fentanyl is stopped.

■ Keep naloxone available to treat respiratory depression.

■ If fentanyl is continuously infused, dosage should be decreased.

nelfinavir ◄► **HMG-CoA reductase inhibitors**

Viracept

atorvastatin, lovastatin, simvastatin

Risk rating: 1
Severity: Major   **Onset: Delayed**   **Likelihood: Suspected**

Cause
Protease inhibitors, such as nelfinavir, may inhibit CYP3A4 metabolism of HMG-CoA reductase inhibitors.

Effect
HMG-CoA reductase inhibitor level may increase.

Nursing considerations
◪ **ALERT** Use of nelfinavir with lovastatin or simvastatin is contraindicated.
■ Monitor patient closely if a protease inhibitor is added to HMG-CoA reductase inhibitor therapy.
◪ **ALERT** Watch for evidence of rhabdomyolysis, including dark or red urine, muscle weakness, and myalgia.
■ Urge patient to immediately report unexplained muscle weakness.

---

nelfinavir ◄► **nevirapine**

Viracept   Viramune

Risk rating: 2
Severity: Moderate   **Onset: Delayed**   **Likelihood: Suspected**

Cause
Nevirapine may increase hepatic metabolism of protease inhibitors, such as nelfinavir.

Effect
Protease inhibitor level and effects decrease.

Nursing considerations
■ If nevirapine is started or stopped, monitor protease inhibitor level.
■ Protease inhibitor dosage may need adjustment.
■ Monitor CD4+ and T-cell counts; tell prescriber if they decrease.
■ Urge patient to report opportunistic infections.
■ Tell patient not to change an HIV regimen without consulting prescriber.

nelfinavir ━━━━◄►━━━━ phosphodiesterase-5 inhibitors
Viracept

sildenafil, tadalafil, vardenafil

Risk rating: 1
Severity: Major   **Onset: Rapid**   **Likelihood: Suspected**

Cause
Phosphodiesterase-5 (PDE-5) inhibitor metabolism is inhibited.

Effect
PDE-5 inhibitor level may increase, possibly leading to fatal hypotension.

Nursing considerations
◼ **ALERT** Tell patient to take PDE-5 inhibitors exactly as prescribed.
◼ Dosage may be reduced and the interval extended if patient takes drugs together.
◼ Warn patient about potentially fatal low blood pressure if these drugs are taken together without proper precautions.
◼ Tell patient to notify prescriber if he has dizziness, fainting, or chest pain.

nelfinavir ━━━━◄►━━━━ St. John's wort
Viracept

Risk rating: 1
Severity: Major   **Onset: Delayed**   **Likelihood: Suspected**

Cause
Hepatic metabolism of protease inhibitor, such as nelfinavir, may increase.

Effect
Protease inhibitor level and effects may decrease.

Nursing considerations
◼ If patient start or stops St. John's wort, monitor protease inhibitor level closely.
◼ Monitor CD4+ and T-cell counts; tell prescriber if they decrease.
◼ Urge patient to report opportunistic infections.
◼ Tell patient not to change an HIV regimen without consulting prescriber.
◼ Urge patient to tell prescribers about all drugs, supplements, and alternative therapies he uses.

neomycin ▶◀ cephalosporins

Neo-Fradin

cefazolin, cefoperazone, cefotaxime, cefotetan, cefoxitin, ceftazidime, ceftizoxime, ceftriaxone, cefuroxime, cephradine

Risk rating: 2
Severity: Moderate   **Onset: Delayed**   **Likelihood: Suspected**

Cause
The mechanism of this interaction is unknown.

Effect
Bactericidal activity may increase against some organisms, but the risk of nephrotoxicity also may increase.

Nursing considerations
■ Assess BUN and creatinine levels.
■ Monitor urine output, and check urine for increased protein, cell, or cast levels.
■ If renal insufficiency develops, notify prescriber. Dosage may need to be reduced, or drug may need to be stopped.
■ Aminoglycosides other than neomycin may interact with cephalosporins. If you suspect an interaction, consult prescriber or pharmacist.

neomycin ▶◀ loop diuretics

Neo-Fradin

bumetanide, ethacrynic acid, furosemide, torsemide

Risk rating: 1
Severity: Major   **Onset: Rapid**   **Likelihood: Suspected**

Cause
The mechanism of this interaction is unknown.

Effect
Because of possible synergistic ototoxicity, patient may have hearing loss of varying degrees, possibly permanent.

Nursing considerations
◣ **ALERT** Patients with renal insufficiency are at increased risk for ototoxicity.
■ Perform baseline and periodic hearing function tests.
■ Aminoglycosides other than neomycin may interact with loop diuretics. If you suspect an interaction, consult prescriber or pharmacist.

■ Tell patient to immediately report ringing or roaring in the ears, muffled sounds, or noticeable changes in hearing.
■ Advise family members to stay alert for evidence of hearing loss.

---

neomycin ➤◄ nondepolarizing muscle relaxants

Neo-Fradin

atracurium, doxacurium, mivacurium, pancuronium, rocuronium, vecuronium

Risk rating: 1
Severity: Major   **Onset: Rapid**   **Likelihood: Probable**

Cause
These drugs may be synergistic.

Effect
Effects of nondepolarizing muscle relaxants may increase.

Nursing considerations
■ Give these drugs together only when needed.
■ The nondepolarizing muscle relaxant dose may need adjustment based on neuromuscular response.
■ Monitor patient for prolonged respiratory depression.
■ Provide ventilatory support as needed.

---

neostigmine ➤◄ corticosteroids

Prostigmin

betamethasone, corticotropin, cortisone, cosyntropin, dexamethasone, fludrocortisone, hydrocortisone, methylprednisolone, prednisolone, prednisone, triamcinolone

Risk rating: 1
Severity: Major   **Onset: Delayed**   **Likelihood: Probable**

Cause
In myasthenia gravis, corticosteroids antagonize the effects of cholinesterase inhibitors, such as neostigmine, by an unknown mechanism.

Effect
Patient may develop severe muscular depression refractory to cholinesterase inhibitor.

Nursing considerations
- Corticosteroids may have long-term benefits in myasthenia gravis.
- Combined therapy may be attempted under strict supervision.
- In myasthenia gravis, monitor patient for severe muscle deterioration.

⚑ ALERT Be prepared to provide respiratory support and mechanical ventilation if needed.

- Consult prescriber or pharmacist about safe corticosteroid delivery to maximize improvement in muscle strength.

---

nevirapine ▶◀ protease inhibitors

Viramune

amprenavir, indinavir, lopinavir-ritonavir, nelfinavir, ritonavir, saquinavir

Risk rating: 2
Severity: Moderate   **Onset: Delayed**   **Likelihood: Suspected**

Cause
Nevirapine may increase hepatic metabolism of protease inhibitors.

Effect
Protease inhibitor level and effects decrease.

Nursing considerations
- If nevirapine is started or stopped, monitor protease inhibitor level.
- Protease inhibitor dosage may need adjustment.
- Monitor CD4+ and T-cell counts; tell prescriber if they decrease.
- Urge patient to report opportunistic infections.
- Tell patient not to change an HIV regimen without consulting prescriber.

---

nicardipine ▶◀ cyclosporine

Cardene

Gengraf, Neoral, Sandimmune

Risk rating: 2
Severity: Moderate   **Onset: Delayed**   **Likelihood: Suspected**

Cause
Nicardipine probably inhibits cyclosporine metabolism in the liver.

Effect
Cyclosporine level and renal toxicity may increase.

Nursing considerations
- Check cyclosporine level. Trough level may be elevated.

- Monitor renal function.
- Assess patient for evidence of toxicity.
- Adjust cyclosporine dose as needed.
- If nicardipine is stopped, consider increasing cyclosporine dose to prevent rejection.

nicardipine ▶◀ grapefruit juice
Cardene

Risk rating: 2
Severity: Moderate   Onset: Delayed   Likelihood: Suspected

Cause
Grapefruit juice may inhibit nicardipine metabolism.

Effect
Nicardipine level, effects, and adverse effects may increase.

Nursing considerations
- Don't give nicardipine with grapefruit juice.
- Advise patient to take nicardipine with beverage other than grapefruit juice.
- If drug is taken with grapefruit juice, monitor patient for increased nicardipine effects, such as tachycardia.

nifedipine ▶◀ cimetidine
Procardia   Tagamet

Risk rating: 2
Severity: Moderate   Onset: Delayed   Likelihood: Suspected

Cause
Hepatic metabolism of nifedipine may be reduced.

Effect
Nifedipine effects, including adverse effects, may increase.

Nursing considerations
- Monitor patient for altered drug effects when cimetidine starts or stops or its dosage changes.
- Watch for increased adverse effects, such as hypotension, dizziness, light-headedness, syncope, peripheral edema, flushing, and nausea.
- Adjust nifedipine dose as needed.
- H_2-receptor antagonists other than cimetidine may interact with nifedipine. Calcium channel blockers other than nifedipine may inter-

act with cimetidine. If you suspect a drug interaction, consult prescriber or pharmacist.

nifedipine ▶◀ cisapride
Procardia   Propulsid

Risk rating: 2
Severity: Moderate   **Onset: Rapid**   **Likelihood: Suspected**

Cause
Enhanced GI motility caused by cisapride may increase the rate of nifedipine absorption.

Effect
Nifedipine level, effects, and adverse effects may increase.

Nursing considerations
◼ **ALERT** Because of the risk of serious arrhythmias and death, cisapride is available in the U.S. only through an investigational limited access program.
■ Monitor blood pressure closely.
■ Watch for adverse effects of nifedipine, such as dizziness, headache, light-headedness, flushing, and weakness.
■ Adjust nifedipine dose as needed.

nisoldipine ▶◀ azole antifungals
Sular   fluconazole, itraconazole, ketoconazole

Risk rating: 2
Severity: Moderate   **Onset: Delayed**   **Likelihood: Suspected**

Cause
Azole antifungals inhibit CYP3A4, which is needed for nisoldipine metabolism.

Effect
Nisoldipine level, effects, and adverse effects may increase.

Nursing considerations
■ Notify prescriber if patient takes both drugs; an alternative may be available.
■ If drugs must be taken together, watch for orthostatic hypotension from increased nisoldipine effect.

■ Tell patient to report adverse effects, such as chest pain, dizziness, headache, weight gain, nausea, palpitations, and peripheral edema.

nitrates ◄► dihydroergotamine

amyl nitrite,
isosorbide dinitrate,
nitroglycerin

D.H.E. 45

Risk rating: 2
Severity: Moderate   **Onset: Rapid**   **Likelihood: Suspected**

Cause
Metabolism of dihydroergotamine decreases, increasing its availability, which antagonizes nitrates.

Effect
Increased dihydroergotamine availability may increase systolic blood pressure and decrease the antianginal effects of nitrates.

Nursing considerations
■ Use these drugs together cautiously in patients with angina.
■ I.V. dihydroergotamine may antagonize coronary vasodilation.
■ Monitor patient for evidence of ergotism, such as peripheral ischemia, paresthesia, headache, nausea, and vomiting.
■ Teach patient to immediately report indicators of peripheral ischemia, such as numbness or tingling in fingers and toes or red blisters on hands or feet. Dihydroergotamine dosage may need to be decreased.

nitrates ◄► phosphodiesterase-5 inhibitors

amyl nitrite,
isosorbide dinitrate,
isosorbide
mononitrate,
nitroglycerin

sildenafil, tadalafil, vardenafil

Risk rating: 1
Severity: Major   **Onset: Rapid**   **Likelihood: Suspected**

Cause
Phosphodiesterase-5 (PDE-5) inhibitors potentiate the hypotensive effects of nitrates.

Effect
Risk of severe hypotension increases.

Nursing considerations

⚠ **ALERT** Use of nitrates with PDE-5 inhibitors may be fatal and is contraindicated.

■ Carefully screen patient for PDE-5 inhibitor use before giving a nitrate.

■ Even during an emergency, before giving a nitrate, find out if a patient with chest pain has taken an erectile dysfunction drug during the previous 24 hours.

■ Monitor patient for orthostatic hypotension, dizziness, sweating, and headache.

---

nitroglycerin ▶◀ alteplase

Minitran, Nitro-Dur,
NitroQuick, Nitrostat,
Nitrotab

Activase, tPA

Risk rating: 1
Severity: **Major**   Onset: **Rapid**   Likelihood: **Probable**

Cause
Nitroglycerin may enhance hepatic blood flow, thereby increasing alteplase metabolism.

Effect
Alteplase level and thrombolytic effects may decrease.

Nursing considerations
■ Don't use together, if possible.
■ If use together is unavoidable, maintain nitroglycerin at the lowest effective dose.
■ Monitor patient for inadequate thrombolytic effects.
■ Tell patient that other reperfusion therapies may be needed.

---

norepinephrine ▶◀ methyldopa

Levophed

Aldomet

Risk rating: 2
Severity: **Moderate**   Onset: **Rapid**   Likelihood: **Suspected**

Cause
The mechanism of this interaction is unknown.

Effect
Pressor response of sympathomimetics and risk of hypertension may increase.

Nursing considerations
■ Monitor patient's blood pressure closely.
■ The hypertensive response may increase two to five times over nor-epinephrine alone.

---

norepinephrine ▶◀ tricyclic antidepressants

Levophed

amitriptyline, amoxapine,
clomipramine, desipramine,
doxepin, imipramine,
nortriptyline, trimipramine

Risk rating: 2
Severity: Moderate   Onset: Rapid   Likelihood: Established

Cause
Tricyclic antidepressants (TCAs) increase the effects of direct-acting sympathomimetics, such as norepinephrine.

Effect
When sympathomimetic effects increase, the risk of hypertension and arrhythmias increases.

Nursing considerations
■ If possible, avoid using these drugs together.
■ Watch patient closely for hypertension and heart rhythm changes; they may warrant reduction of sympathomimetic dosage.
■ Other TCAs and sympathomimetics may interact. If you suspect an interaction, consult prescriber or pharmacist.

---

norfloxacin ▶◀ didanosine

Noroxin

Videx

Risk rating: 2
Severity: Moderate   Onset: Rapid   Likelihood: Suspected

Cause
Buffers in didanosine chewable tablets and pediatric powder for oral solution decrease GI absorption of quinolones, such as norfloxacin.

Effect
Quinolone effects decrease.

Nursing considerations
■ Avoid use together. If it's unavoidable, give the quinolone at least 2 hours before or 6 hours after didanosine.
■ Monitor patient for improvement in infection.

- Unbuffered didanosine doesn't affect quinolone absorption.
- Help patient develop a plan to ensure proper dosage intervals.

norfloxacin ▶◀ iron salts

Noroxin

ferrous fumarate, ferrous gluconate, ferrous sulfate, iron polysaccharide

Risk rating: 2
Severity: **Moderate**   Onset: **Rapid**   Likelihood: **Probable**

Cause
Formation of an iron-quinolone complex decreases GI absorption of quinolones, such as norfloxacin.

Effect
Quinolone effects decrease.

Nursing considerations
- Monitor patient for quinolone efficacy.
- Tell patient to separate quinolone dose from iron by at least 2 hours.
- Help patient develop a plan to ensure proper dosage intervals.
- Other quinolones may interact with iron.

norfloxacin ▶◀ milk

Noroxin

Risk rating: 2
Severity: **Moderate**   Onset: **Rapid**   Likelihood: **Suspected**

Cause
GI absorption of certain quinolones, such as norfloxacin, decreases.

Effect
Quinolone effects may decrease.

Nursing considerations
- Advise patient not to take drug with milk and to lengthen the time as much as possible between milk ingestion and the quinolone dose.
- This interaction doesn't affect all quinolones.
- Monitor patient for quinolone efficacy.

norfloxacin ▶◀ sucralfate

Noroxin   Carafate

Risk rating: 2
Severity: Moderate   Onset: Rapid   Likelihood: Probable

Cause
GI absorption of quinolones, such as norfloxacin, decreases.

Effect
Quinolone effects decrease.

Nursing considerations
- Avoid use together. If it's unavoidable, give sucralfate at least 6 hours after the quinolone.
- Monitor patient for resolving infection.
- Help patient develop a plan to ensure proper dosage intervals.

nortriptyline ▶◀ azole antifungals

Pamelor   fluconazole, ketoconazole

Risk rating: 2
Severity: Moderate   Onset: Delayed   Likelihood: Suspected

Cause
Azole antifungals may inhibit metabolism of nortriptyline and other tricyclic antidepressants (TCAs) by CYP pathways.

Effect
TCA level and risk of toxicity may increase.

Nursing considerations
- When starting or stopping an azole antifungal, monitor serum TCA level and adjust dosage as needed.
- After starting an azole antifungal, check sitting and standing blood pressure for changes.
- Assess symptoms and behavior for evidence of adverse reactions, such as increased drowsiness, dizziness, confusion, heart rate or rhythm changes, and urine retention.

nortriptyline ▶◀ cimetidine

Pamelor   Tagamet

Risk rating: 2
Severity: Moderate   **Onset: Rapid**   **Likelihood: Probable**

Cause
Cimetidine may interfere with metabolism of tricyclic antidepressants (TCAs), such as nortriptyline.

Effect
TCA level and bioavailability increase.

Nursing considerations
■ When starting or stopping cimetidine, monitor serum TCA level and adjust dosage as needed.
■ Tell prescriber if TCA level or effect increases; dosage may need to be decreased.
■ If needed, consult prescriber about possible change from cimetidine to ranitidine.
■ Urge patient and family to watch for and report increased anticholinergic effects, dizziness, drowsiness, and psychosis.

nortriptyline ▶◀ MAO inhibitors

Pamelor   isocarboxazid, phenelzine,
                                 tranylcypromine

Risk rating: 1
Severity: Major   **Onset: Rapid**   **Likelihood: Suspected**

Cause
The mechanism of this interaction is unknown.

Effect
Risk of hyperpyretic crisis, seizures, and death increases.

Nursing considerations
⚡ **ALERT** Don't give a tricyclic antidepressant (TCA), such as nortriptyline, with or within 2 weeks of an MAO inhibitor.
■ Watch for adverse effects, including confusion, hyperexcitability, rigidity, seizures, increased temperature, increased pulse, increased respiration, sweating, mydriasis, flushing, headache, coma, and DIC.

nortriptyline ▶◀ quinolones

Pamelor

gatifloxacin, levofloxacin, moxifloxacin, sparfloxacin

Risk rating: 1
Severity: **Major**   Onset: **Delayed**   Likelihood: **Suspected**

Cause
The mechanism of this interaction if unknown.

Effect
Life-threatening arrhythmias, including torsades de pointes, may increase when certain of these drugs are used together.

Nursing considerations
◪ ALERT Sparfloxacin is contraindicated in patients taking a tricyclic antidepressant (TCA), such as nortriptyline, because QTc interval may be prolonged.
◪ ALERT Avoid giving levofloxacin with a TCA.
■ Use gatifloxacin and moxifloxacin cautiously with a TCA.
■ If possible, use other quinolones that don't prolong the QTc interval or aren't metabolized by the CYP3A4 isoenzyme.

nortriptyline ▶◀ rifamycins

Pamelor

rifabutin, rifampin

Risk rating: 2
Severity: **Moderate**   Onset: **Delayed**   Likelihood: **Suspected**

Cause
Hepatic metabolism of tricyclic antidepressants (TCAs), such as nortriptyline, may increase.

Effect
TCA level and efficacy may decrease.

Nursing considerations
■ When starting or stopping a rifamycin or changing its dosage, monitor serum TCA level to maintain therapeutic range.
■ Watch for resolution of depression as TCA dosage is adjusted to therapeutic level during rifamycin therapy.
■ Urge patient and family to watch for and promptly report adverse reactions, including increased drowsiness and dizziness, for several weeks after rifamycin stops.

■ Other TCAs may interact with rifamycins. If you suspect an interaction, consult prescriber or pharmacist.

---

nortriptyline ▶◀ SSRIs

| Pamelor | fluoxetine, fluvoxamine, paroxetine, sertraline |

Risk rating: 2

| Severity: **Moderate** | Onset: **Delayed** | Likelihood: **Probable** fluoxetine, fluvoxamine **Suspected** paroxetine, sertraline |

Cause
Certain SSRIs may decrease metabolism of nortriptyline and other tricyclic antidepressants (TCAs) in some people and increase it in others.

Effect
Therapeutic and toxic effects of certain TCAs may increase.

Nursing considerations
■ If possible, avoid this drug combination.
■ Monitor serum TCA level and watch closely for evidence of toxicity, such as drowsiness, dizziness, confusion, delirium, heart rate or rhythm changes, urine retention, and psychosis.
■ Report evidence of increased TCA level or serotonin syndrome; dosage may need to be decreased or drug stopped.
■ Symptoms of serotonin syndrome may resolve within 24 hours of stopping a TCA and starting a short course of an antiserotonergic drug.
■ Inhibitory effects of fluvoxamine may take several weeks to dissipate after drug is stopped.
■ Other TCAs may interact. If you suspect an interaction, consult prescriber or pharmacist.

nortriptyline ▶◀ sympathomimetics

Pamelor

direct: dobutamine, epinephrine, norepinephrine, phenylephrine
mixed: dopamine, ephedrine, metaraminol

Risk rating: 2
Severity: **Moderate**   Onset: **Rapid**   Likelihood: **Established**

Cause
Tricyclic antidepressants (TCAs), such as nortriptyline, increase the effects of direct-acting sympathomimetics and decrease the effects of indirect-acting sympathomimetics.

Effect
When sympathomimetic effects increase, the risk of hypertension and arrhythmias increases. When sympathomimetic effects decrease, blood pressure control decreases.

Nursing considerations
- If possible, avoid using these drugs together.
- Watch patient closely for hypertension and heart rhythm changes; they may warrant reduction of sympathomimetic dosage.
- If patient takes a mixed-acting sympathomimetic, watch for negative effects; dosage may need to be altered.
- Other TCAs and sympathomimetics may interact. If you suspect an interaction, consult prescriber or pharmacist.

nortriptyline ▶◀ terbinafine

Pamelor   Lamisil

Risk rating: 2
Severity: **Moderate**   Onset: **Delayed**   Likelihood: **Suspected**

Cause
Hepatic metabolism of tricyclic antidepressants (TCAs), such as nortriptyline, may be inhibited.

Effect
Therapeutic and toxic effects of certain TCAs may increase.

Nursing considerations
- Check for toxic TCA level, and report abnormal level.
- TCA dosage may need to be decreased.

- Adverse effects or toxicity may include vertigo, fatigue, loss of appetite, ataxia, muscle twitching, or trouble swallowing.
- Terbinafine's inhibitory effects may take several weeks to dissipate after drug is stopped.
- Describe signs and symptoms patient should look for.

---

nortriptyline ▸◀ valproic acid

Pamelor

divalproex sodium, valproate sodium, valproic acid

Risk rating: 2
Severity: **Moderate**   Onset: **Delayed**   Likelihood: **Suspected**

Cause
Valproic acid may inhibit hepatic metabolism of tricyclic antidepressants (TCAs), such as nortriptyline.

Effect
TCA level and adverse effects may increase.

Nursing considerations
- Use these drugs together cautiously.
- If patient is stable on valproic acid, start TCA at reduced dosage and adjust upward slowly to address symptoms and serum level.
- If patient is stable on a TCA, monitor serum level and patient status closely when starting or stopping valproic acid.
- Explain signs and symptoms to watch for.
- Other TCAs may interact with valproic acid. If you suspect an interaction, consult prescriber or pharmacist.

---

ofloxacin ▸◀ didanosine

Floxin

Videx

Risk rating: 2
Severity: **Moderate**   Onset: **Rapid**   Likelihood: **Suspected**

Cause
Buffers in didanosine chewable tablets and pediatric powder for oral solution decrease GI absorption of quinolones, such as ofloxacin.

Effect
Quinolone effects decrease.

Nursing considerations
- Avoid use together. If it's unavoidable, give the quinolone at least 2 hours before or 6 hours after didanosine.

- Monitor patient for improvement in infection.
- Unbuffered didanosine doesn't affect quinolone absorption.
- Help patient develop a plan to ensure proper dosage intervals.

---

ofloxacin ◄►► iron salts
Floxin   ferrous fumarate, ferrous
                                    gluconate, ferrous sulfate,
                                    iron polysaccharide

Risk rating: 2
Severity: Moderate   **Onset: Rapid**   **Likelihood: Probable**

Cause
Formation of an iron-quinolone complex decreases GI absorption of quinolone antibiotics, such as ofloxacin.

Effect
Quinolone effects decrease.

Nursing considerations
- Other quinolones may interact with iron.
- Monitor patient for quinolone efficacy.
- Tell patient to separate quinolone dose from iron by at least 2 hours.
- Help patient develop a plan to ensure proper dosage intervals.

---

ofloxacin ◄►► sucralfate
Floxin   Carafate

Risk rating: 2
Severity: Moderate   **Onset: Rapid**   **Likelihood: Probable**

Cause
Sucralfate decreases GI absorption of quinolones, such as ofloxacin.

Effect
Quinolone effects decrease.

Nursing considerations
- Avoid use together. If it's unavoidable, give sucralfate at least 6 hours after the quinolone.
- Monitor patient for resolving infection.
- Help patient develop a plan to ensure proper dosage intervals.

olmesartan 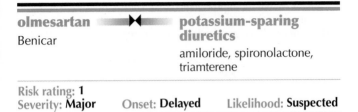 potassium-sparing diuretics
Benicar

amiloride, spironolactone, triamterene

Risk rating: 1
Severity: Major   Onset: **Delayed**   Likelihood: **Suspected**

Cause
Both angiotensin II receptor antagonists, such as olmesartan, and potassium-sparing diuretics may increase serum potassium level.

Effect
Risk of hyperkalemia may increase, especially among high-risk patients.

Nursing considerations
■ High-risk patients include elderly people and those with renal impairment, type 2 diabetes, or decreased renal perfusion; monitor these patients closely.
■ Check serum potassium, BUN, and creatinine levels regularly. If they increase, notify prescriber.
■ Advise patient to immediately report an irregular heartbeat, slow pulse, weakness, or other evidence of hyperkalemia.
■ Give patient a list of foods high in potassium; stress the need to eat them only in moderate amounts.

omeprazole 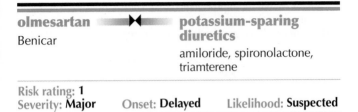 azole antifungals
Prilosec

itraconazole, ketoconazole

Risk rating: 2
Severity: Moderate   Onset: **Rapid**   Likelihood: **Suspected**

Cause
Proton pump inhibitors, such as omeprazole, increase gastric pH, which may impair dissolution of azole antifungals.

Effect
Efficacy of azole antifungals may decrease.

Nursing considerations
■ Notify prescriber if patient takes both drugs; an alternative may be available.
■ If no alternative is possible, suggest taking the azole antifungal with an acidic beverage, such as cola.
■ Monitor patient for lack of response to antifungal drug.

■ If patient can't tolerate acidic beverages and antifungal therapy appears to be ineffective, antifungal dosage may need to be increased.
■ Other drugs that increase gastric pH may interact with azole antifungals. If you suspect an interaction, consult prescriber or pharmacist.

omeprazole ▶◀ St. John's wort
Prilosec

Risk rating: 2
Severity: **Moderate**   Onset: **Delayed**   Likelihood: **Suspected**

Cause
St. John's wort may increase omeprazole metabolism.

Effect
Omeprazole level and effects may decrease.

Nursing considerations
■ Discourage use of St. John's wort while taking omeprazole.
■ If use together is unavoidable, monitor patient for loss of GI symptom control.
■ Tell patient not to change the omeprazole regimen without consulting prescriber.

orlistat ▶◀ cyclosporine
Xenical   Gengraf, Neoral, Sandimmune

Risk rating: 1
Severity: **Major**   Onset: **Delayed**   Likelihood: **Probable**

Cause
Orlistat may decrease cyclosporine absorption.

Effect
Cyclosporine level may decrease.

Nursing considerations
■ Avoid orlistat in patients being treated with cyclosporine.
■ If drugs are used together, monitor cyclosporine level.
■ Increasing the cyclosporine dose may not result in elevated level.

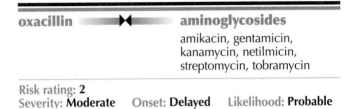

oxacillin ▶◀ **aminoglycosides**
amikacin, gentamicin,
kanamycin, netilmicin,
streptomycin, tobramycin

Risk rating: **2**
Severity: **Moderate**   Onset: **Delayed**   Likelihood: **Probable**

Cause
Oxacillin and other penicillins may inactivate certain aminoglycosides.

Effect
Aminoglycoside effects may decrease.

Nursing considerations
◣ **ALERT** Check peak and trough aminoglycoside levels after third dose. For peak level, draw blood 30 minutes after I.V. or 60 minutes after I.M. dose. For trough level, draw blood just before a dose.
■ Monitor patient's renal function.
■ Other aminoglycosides may interact with penicillins. If you suspect an interaction, consult prescriber or pharmacist.
■ Penicillins affect gentamicin and tobramycin more than amikacin.

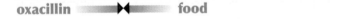

oxacillin ▶◀ **food**

Risk rating: **2**
Severity: **Moderate**   Onset: **Delayed**   Likelihood: **Suspected**

Cause
Food may delay or reduce GI absorption of penicillins, including oxacillin.

Effect
Oxacillin efficacy may decrease.

Nursing considerations
■ Food may affect penicillin absorption and peak level.
■ Penicillin V and amoxicillin don't have this interaction and may be given without regard to meals.
■ Tell patient to take oxacillin 1 hour before or 2 hours after a meal.
■ If patient takes oxacillin with food, watch for lack of drug effect.

oxacillin 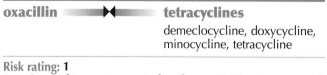 tetracyclines

demeclocycline, doxycycline,
minocycline, tetracycline

Risk rating: 1
Severity: Major   **Onset: Delayed**   **Likelihood: Suspected**

Cause
Tetracyclines may adversely affect the bactericidal activity of penicillins, such as oxacillin.

Effect
Oxacillin efficacy may be reduced.

Nursing considerations
- If possible, avoid giving tetracyclines with penicillins.
- Monitor patient closely for lack of penicillin effect.

---

oxaprozin 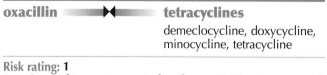 aminoglycosides

Daypro

amikacin, gentamicin,
kanamycin, netilmicin,
streptomycin, tobramycin

Risk rating: 2
Severity: Moderate   **Onset: Delayed**   **Likelihood: Suspected**

Cause
NSAIDs, including oxaprozin, may reduce glomerular filtration rate (GFR), causing aminoglycosides to accumulate.

Effect
Aminoglycoside level in premature infants may increase.

Nursing considerations
- Before NSAID starts, aminoglycoside dose should be reduced.
- **⚡ ALERT** Check peak and trough aminoglycoside levels after third dose. For peak level, draw blood 30 minutes after I.V. or 60 minutes after I.M. dose. For trough level, draw blood just before a dose.
- Monitor patient's renal function.
- Although only indomethacin is known to interact with aminoglycosides, other NSAIDs probably do as well. If you suspect an interaction, consult prescriber or pharmacist.
- Other drugs cleared by GFR may have a similar interaction.

oxazepam 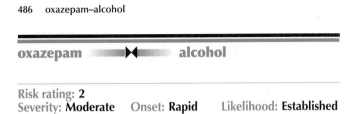 alcohol

Risk rating: 2
Severity: Moderate **Onset: Rapid** **Likelihood: Established**

Cause
Alcohol inhibits hepatic enzymes, which decreases clearance and increases peak levels of benzodiazepines, such as oxazepam.

Effect
Additive or synergistic effects may occur.

Nursing considerations
- Before benzodiazepine therapy starts, assess patient thoroughly for history or evidence of alcohol use.
- Advise against consuming alcohol while taking a benzodiazepine.
- Watch for additive CNS effects, which may suggest benzodiazepine overdose.

oxybutynin 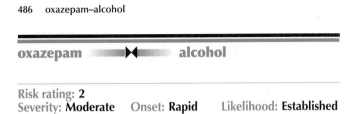 phenothiazines

Ditropan

chlorpromazine, fluphenazine, mesoridazine, perphenazine, prochlorperazine, promethazine, thioridazine, trifluoperazine

Risk rating: 2
Severity: Moderate **Onset: Delayed** **Likelihood: Suspected**

Cause
Oxybutynin and other anticholinergics may antagonize phenothiazines. Also, phenothiazine metabolism may increase.

Effect
Phenothiazine efficacy may decrease.

Nursing considerations
- Data regarding this interaction conflict.
- Monitor patient for decreased phenothiazine efficacy.
- Phenothiazine dosage may need adjustment.
- Anticholinergic effects may increase.
- Monitor patient for adynamic ileus, hyperpyrexia, hypoglycemia, and neurologic changes.

pancuronium ▶◀ aminoglycosides
amikacin, gentamicin, kanamycin, neomycin, netilmicin, streptomycin, tobramycin

Risk rating: 1
Severity: Major   **Onset: Rapid**   **Likelihood: Probable**

Cause
These drugs may be synergistic.

Effect
Effects of nondepolarizing muscle relaxant, such as pancuronium, may increase.

Nursing considerations
- Give these drugs together only when needed.
- Nondepolarizing muscle relaxant dosage may need adjustment based on neuromuscular response.
- Monitor patient for prolonged respiratory depression.
- Provide ventilatory support as needed.

pancuronium ▶◀ carbamazepine
Carbatrol, Epitol, Equetro, Tegretol

Risk rating: 2
Severity: Moderate   **Onset: Rapid**   **Likelihood: Probable**

Cause
The mechanism of this interaction is unknown.

Effect
Effects or duration of a nondepolarizing muscle relaxant, such as pancuronium, may decrease.

Nursing considerations
- Monitor patient for decreased efficacy of muscle relaxant.
- Dosage of nondepolarizing muscle relaxant may be increased.
- Make sure patient is adequately sedated when receiving a nondepolarizing muscle relaxant.

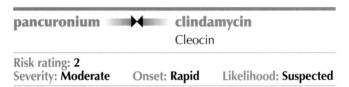

pancuronium ◄ clindamycin
Cleocin

Risk rating: 2
Severity: Moderate   **Onset: Rapid**   **Likelihood: Suspected**

Cause
Clindamycin may potentiate the actions of nondepolarizing muscle relaxants, such as pancuronium.

Effect
Nondepolarizing muscle relaxant action may increase.

Nursing considerations
- If possible, avoid using clindamycin or other lincosamides with nondepolarizing muscle relaxants.
- Monitor patient for respiratory distress.
- Combined use may lead to profound, severe respiratory depression.
- Provide ventilatory support as needed.
- Cholinesterase inhibitors or calcium may help reverse drug effects.
- Make sure patient is adequately sedated when receiving a nondepolarizing muscle relaxant.

pancuronium ◄ magnesium sulfate

Risk rating: 2
Severity: Moderate   **Onset: Rapid**   **Likelihood: Suspected**

Cause
Magnesium probably potentiates the action of nondepolarizing muscle relaxants, such as pancuronium.

Effect
Risk of profound, severe respiratory depression increases.

Nursing considerations
- Use these drugs together cautiously.
- Nondepolarizing muscle relaxant dosage may need to be adjusted.
- Monitor patient for respiratory distress.
- Provide ventilatory support as needed.
- Make sure patient is adequately sedated when receiving a nondepolarizing muscle relaxant.

pancuronium 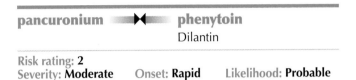 phenytoin
Dilantin

Risk rating: 2
Severity: **Moderate**   Onset: **Rapid**   Likelihood: **Probable**

Cause
Phenytoin has effects at prejunctional sites similar to those of nondepolarizing muscle relaxants, such as pancuronium. Also, phenytoin alters the metabolism of pancuronium.

Effect
Effects or duration of nondepolarizing muscle relaxant may decrease.

Nursing considerations
■ Monitor patient for decreased efficacy of the nondepolarizing muscle relaxant.
■ Dosage of nondepolarizing muscle relaxant may need to be increased.
■ Atracurium may be a suitable alternative to pancuronium because this interaction may not occur in all patients.
■ Make sure patient is adequately sedated when receiving a nondepolarizing muscle relaxant.

pancuronium 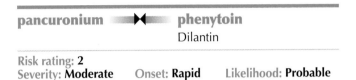 polypeptide antibiotics
bacitracin, polymyxin B, vancomycin

Risk rating: 2
Severity: **Moderate**   Onset: **Rapid**   Likelihood: **Probable**

Cause
Polypeptide antibiotics may act synergistically with nondepolarizing muscle relaxants, such as pancuronium.

Effect
Neuromuscular blockade may increase.

Nursing considerations
■ If possible, avoid using polypeptide antibiotics with nondepolarizing muscle relaxants.
■ Monitor neuromuscular function closely.
■ Dosage of nondepolarizing muscle relaxant may need adjustment.
■ Provide ventilatory support, as needed.
■ Make sure patient is adequately sedated when receiving a nondepolarizing muscle relaxant.

pancuronium 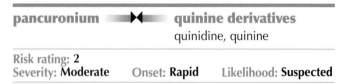 quinine derivatives
quinidine, quinine

Risk rating: **2**
Severity: **Moderate**   Onset: **Rapid**   Likelihood: **Suspected**

Cause
Quinine derivatives may act synergistically with nondepolarizing muscle relaxants, such as pancuronium.

Effect
Effects of nondepolarizing muscle relaxants may increase.

Nursing considerations
◣ ALERT This interaction may be life-threatening. Monitor neuromuscular function closely.
■ Intensity and duration of neuromuscular blockade may be affected.
■ Dosage of nondepolarizing muscle relaxant may need adjustment.
■ Provide ventilatory support, as needed.
■ Make sure patient is adequately sedated when receiving a nondepolarizing muscle relaxant.

pancuronium theophyllines
aminophylline, theophylline

Risk rating: **2**
Severity: **Moderate**   Onset: **Rapid**   Likelihood: **Suspected**

Cause
These drugs may act antagonistically.

Effect
Neuromuscular blockade may be reversed.

Nursing considerations
■ Monitor patient closely for lack of drug effect.
■ Dosage of nondepolarizing muscle relaxant may need adjustment.
■ This interaction is dose dependent.
■ Make sure patient is adequately sedated when receiving a nondepolarizing muscle relaxant.

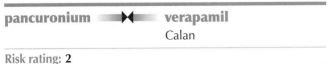

pancuronium ◄► verapamil
Calan

Risk rating: 2
Severity: **Moderate**   Onset: **Rapid**   Likelihood: **Suspected**

Cause
This interaction may stem from a blockade of calcium channels in skeletal muscle.

Effect
Effects of nondepolarizing muscle relaxants, such as pancuronium, may increase.

Nursing considerations
- Avoid using verapamil with nondepolarizing muscle relaxants.
- Watch for prolonged respiratory depression.
- Provide ventilatory support, as needed.
- Dosage of nondepolarizing muscle relaxant may be decreased.

pantoprazole ◄► azole antifungals
Protonix   itraconazole, ketoconazole

Risk rating: 2
Severity: **Moderate**   Onset: **Rapid**   Likelihood: **Suspected**

Cause
Proton pump inhibitors, such as pantoprazole, increase gastric pH, which may impair dissolution of azole antifungals.

Effect
Efficacy of azole antifungals may decrease.

Nursing considerations
- Notify prescriber if patient takes both drugs; an alternative may be available.
- If no alternative is possible, suggest taking the azole antifungal with an acidic beverage, such as cola.
- Monitor patient for lack of response to antifungal drug.
- If patient can't tolerate acidic beverages and antifungal therapy appears to be ineffective, antifungal dosage may need to be increased.
- Other drugs that increase gastric pH may interact with azole antifungals. If you suspect an interaction, consult prescriber or pharmacist.

paroxetine ▰▰▰ ◄► ▰▰▰ amitriptyline
Paxil

Risk rating: 2
Severity: Moderate   **Onset: Delayed**   **Likelihood: Suspected**

Cause
Paroxetine may decrease metabolism of tricyclic antidepressants (TCAs), such as amitriptyline, in some people and increase it in others.

Effect
Therapeutic and toxic effects of certain TCAs may increase.

Nursing considerations
■ When starting or stopping paroxetine, monitor TCA level and adjust dosage as needed.
■ Assess symptoms and behavior for evidence of adverse reactions, such as increased drowsiness, dizziness, confusion, heart rate or rhythm changes, and urine retention.
■ Watch closely for evidence of serotonin syndrome, such as delirium, bizarre movements, and tachycardia. Alert prescriber if they occur; TCA may need to be stopped.

paroxetine ▰▰▰ ◄► ▰▰▰ MAO inhibitors
Paxil   isocarboxazid, phenelzine,
                             selegiline, tranylcypromine

Risk rating: 2
Severity: Major   **Onset: Rapid**   **Likelihood: Probable**

Cause
Serotonin may accumulate rapidly in the CNS.

Effect
Risk of serotonin syndrome increases.

Nursing considerations
◩ ALERT Don't use these drugs together.
■ Allow 2 weeks after stopping paroxetine before giving an MAO inhibitor. Allow 2 weeks after stopping an MAO inhibitor before giving an SSRI, such as paroxetine.
■ Describe traits of serotonin syndrome, including CNS irritability, motor weakness, shivering, myoclonus, and altered consciousness.
■ Urge patient to promptly report adverse effects.

paroxetine ▶◀ phenothiazines

Paxil

chlorpromazine, fluphenazine, mesoridazine, perphenazine, prochlorperazine, promethazine, thioridazine, trifluoperazine

Risk rating: 2
Severity: Moderate   Onset: Delayed   Likelihood: Probable

Cause
The metabolism of phenothiazines is decreased.

Effect
Phenothiazine level, effects, and adverse effects may increase.

Nursing considerations
◪ **ALERT** Thioridazine is contraindicated in patients taking paroxetine. Life-threatening arrhythmias may occur.
■ The initial phenothiazine dose should be reduced in patients taking paroxetine.
■ If patient takes a phenothiazine, watch closely for response when starting, stopping, or changing the dose of paroxetine.
■ Phenothiazine dosage may need adjustment.
■ Monitor patient for adverse CNS effects, such as sedation, extrapyramidal effects, and impaired psychomotor performance and memory.

paroxetine ▶◀ propafenone

Paxil

Rythmol

Risk rating: 2
Severity: Moderate   Onset: Delayed   Likelihood: Suspected

Cause
Certain serotonin reuptake inhibitors, such as paroxetine, may inhibit CYP2D6 metabolism of propafenone.

Effect
Propafenone level and risk of adverse effects may increase.

Nursing considerations
■ Monitor cardiac function closely.
■ Citalopram doesn't inhibit CYP2D6 and may be a safer choice.
■ Tell the patient to promptly report dizziness, drowsiness, ataxia, tremor, palpitations, chest pain, edema, dyspnea, and other new symptoms to the prescriber.

paroxetine ▬▶◀▬ selective 5-HT$_1$ receptor agonists
Paxil

almotriptan, eletriptan, frovatriptan, naratriptan, rizatriptan, sumatriptan, zolmitriptan

Risk rating: 2
Severity: Moderate   **Onset: Rapid**   **Likelihood: Suspected**

Cause
Serotonin may accumulate rapidly in the CNS.

Effect
Risk of serotonin syndrome increases.

Nursing considerations
■ **ALERT** If possible, avoid combined use of these drugs.
■ Start with lowest dosages possible, and assess patient closely.
■ Stop the selective 5-HT$_1$ receptor agonist at the first sign of interaction, and start an antiserotonergic drug.
■ In some patients, migraine frequency may increase and antimigraine drug efficacy may decrease when an SSRI, such as paroxetine, is started.
■ Describe traits of serotonin syndrome: CNS irritability, motor weakness, shivering, muscle twitching, and altered consciousness.
■ Explain that serotonin syndrome can be fatal if not treated immediately.

paroxetine ▬▶◀▬ sibutramine
Paxil

Meridia

Risk rating: 1
Severity: Major   **Onset: Rapid**   **Likelihood: Suspected**

Cause
Serotonin may accumulate rapidly in the CNS.

Effect
Risk of serotonin syndrome increases.

Nursing considerations
■ **ALERT** If possible, don't give these drugs together.
■ Watch carefully for adverse effects, which require immediate medical attention.

■ Describe traits of serotonin syndrome: CNS irritability, motor weakness, shivering, muscle twitching, and altered consciousness.
■ Explain that serotonin syndrome can be fatal if not treated immediately.

---

paroxetine ▶◀ St. John's wort
Paxil

Risk rating: 2
Severity: **Moderate**   Onset: **Rapid**   Likelihood: **Suspected**

Cause
St. John's wort may cause additive inhibition of serotonin reuptake.

Effect
Sedative-hypnotic effects of SSRIs, such as paroxetine, may increase.

Nursing considerations
⚑ ALERT Discourage use of an SSRI with St. John's wort.
■ In addition to oversedation, mild serotonin-like symptoms may occur, including anxiety, dizziness, nausea, restlessness, and vomiting.
■ Inform patient about the dangers of this combination.
■ Urge patient to consult prescriber before taking any herb.

---

paroxetine ▶◀ sympathomimetics
Paxil

amphetamine,
dextroamphetamine,
methamphetamine,
phentermine

Risk rating: 1
Severity: **Major**   Onset: **Rapid**   Likelihood: **Suspected**

Cause
The mechanism of this interaction is unknown.

Effect
Sympathomimetic effects and the risk of serotonin syndrome increase.

Nursing considerations
■ If these drugs must be used together, watch closely for increased CNS effects, such as anxiety, jitteriness, agitation, and restlessness.
■ Mild serotonin-like symptoms may develop, including anxiety, dizziness, restlessness, nausea, and vomiting.
■ Explain risk of interaction and need to avoid sympathomimetics.

■ Describe traits of serotonin syndrome, including CNS irritability, motor weakness, shivering, myoclonus, and altered consciousness.

---

paroxetine ▶◀ tricyclic antidepressants
Paxil   amitriptyline, desipramine,
                         imipramine, nortriptyline

Risk rating: 2
Severity: Moderate   Onset: Delayed   Likelihood: Suspected

Cause
Paroxetine may decrease tricyclic antidepressant (TCA) metabolism in some people and increase it in others.

Effect
Therapeutic and toxic effects of certain TCAs may increase.

Nursing considerations
■ When starting or stopping paroxetine, monitor TCA level and adjust dosage as needed.
■ Assess symptoms and behavior for evidence of adverse reactions, such as increased drowsiness, dizziness, confusion, heart rate or rhythm changes, and urine retention.
■ Watch closely for evidence of serotonin syndrome, such as delirium, bizarre movements, and tachycardia. Alert prescriber if they occur; TCA may need to be stopped.
■ Symptoms of serotonin syndrome may resolve within 24 hours of stopping a TCA and starting a short course of antiserotonergic drug.
◨ ALERT Other TCAs may have this interaction.

---

penbutolol ▶◀ epinephrine
Levatol   Adrenalin

Risk rating: 1
Severity: Major   Onset: Rapid   Likelihood: Established

Cause
Alpha-receptor effects of epinephrine supersede effects of nonselective beta blockers, such as penbutolol, increasing vascular resistance.

Effect
Initial marked hypertensive effect is followed by reflex bradycardia.

Nursing considerations
◨ ALERT Three days before planned use of epinephrine, stop the beta blocker. Or, if possible, don't use epinephrine.

- If drugs must be used together, monitor blood pressure and pulse closely. If interaction occurs, give I.V. chlorpromazine, hydralazine, aminophylline, or atropine if needed.
- Explain the risks of this interaction, and tell patient to carry medical identification at all times.
- Other beta blockers may interact with epinephrine. If you suspect an interaction, consult prescriber or pharmacist.

penbutolol ▶◀ ergot derivatives

Levatol   dihydroergotamine, ergotamine

Risk rating: 2
Severity: Moderate   Onset: Delayed   Likelihood: Suspected

Cause
Vasoconstriction and blockade of peripheral beta$_2$ receptors allows unopposed ergot action.

Effect
Vasoconstrictive effects of ergot derivatives are increased, causing peripheral ischemia, cold limbs, and possible gangrene.

Nursing considerations
- Watch for evidence of peripheral ischemia.
- If needed, stop beta blocker and adjust ergot derivative.
- Other ergot derivatives may interact with beta blockers. If you suspect an interaction, consult prescriber or pharmacist.

penbutolol ▶◀ NSAIDs

Levatol   ibuprofen, indomethacin, naproxen, piroxicam

Risk rating: 2
Severity: Moderate   Onset: Delayed   Likelihood: Probable

Cause
NSAIDs may inhibit renal prostaglandin synthesis, allowing pressor systems to be unopposed.

Effect
Penbutolol and other beta blockers may not be able to lower blood pressure.

Nursing considerations
- Avoid using these drugs together if possible.

- Monitor blood pressure and related signs and symptoms of hypertension closely.
- Consult prescriber about ways to minimize interaction, such as adjusting beta blocker dosage or switching to sulindac as the NSAID.
- Explain the risks of using these drugs together, and teach patient how to monitor his blood pressure.
- Other NSAIDs may interact with beta blockers. If you suspect an interaction, consult prescriber or pharmacist.

penbutolol ➡️◀ prazosin

Levatol   Minipress

Risk rating: 2
Severity: Moderate   **Onset: Rapid**   **Likelihood: Probable**

Cause
The mechanism of this interaction is unknown.

Effect
Effect of these drugs on orthostatic hypotension increases.

Nursing considerations
- Assess patient's lying, sitting, and standing blood pressures closely, especially when combined therapy starts.
- Adjust dosages of either drug as needed.
- To minimize effects of orthostatic hypotension, teach patient to change positions slowly.
- Interaction is confirmed only with propranolol but may occur with penbutolol and other beta blockers as well.

penbutolol ➡️◀ salicylates

Levatol   aspirin, bismuth subsalicylate, choline salicylate, magnesium salicylate, salsalate, sodium salicylate, sodium thiosalicylate

Risk rating: 2
Severity: Moderate   **Onset: Rapid**   **Likelihood: Suspected**

Cause
Salicylates inhibit synthesis of prostaglandins, which penbutolol and other beta blockers need to reduce blood pressure. In patients with heart failure, the mechanism of this interaction is unknown.

Effect
Beta blocker's effect decreases.

Nursing considerations
■ Watch closely for signs of heart failure and hypertension, and notify prescriber if they occur.
■ Consult prescriber about switching patient to a different antihypertensive or antiplatelet drug.
■ Other beta blockers may interact with salicylates. If you suspect an interaction, consult prescriber or pharmacist.
■ Explain signs and symptoms of heart failure, and tell patient when to contact prescriber.

---

penbutolol	▶◀	theophyllines
Levatol		aminophylline, theophylline

Risk rating: 2
Severity: Moderate   **Onset: Rapid**   **Likelihood: Probable**

Cause
Theophylline clearance may be reduced up to 50%.

Effect
Theophylline efficacy may decrease.

Nursing considerations
■ When a nonselective beta blocker, such as penbutolol, starts, watch for decreased theophylline efficacy.
■ Monitor serum theophylline level closely, and notify prescriber about subtherapeutic level.
■ Normal therapeutic range for theophylline is 10 to 20 mcg/ml for adults and 5 to 15 mcg/ml for children.
■ Selective beta blockers may be preferred for patients who take theophylline, but interaction still occurs with high doses of beta blocker.
■ Other beta blockers may interact with theophyllines. If you suspect an interaction, consult prescriber or pharmacist.

---

penbutolol	▶◀	verapamil
Levatol		Calan

Risk rating: 1
Severity: Major   **Onset: Rapid**   **Likelihood: Probable**

Cause
Verapamil may inhibit metabolism of beta blockers, such as penbutolol.

Effect
Effects of both drugs may be increased.

Nursing considerations
■ Combined use is common in patients with hypertension and unstable angina.

⚡ ALERT Giving these drugs together increases risk of adverse effects, including heart failure, conduction disturbances, arrhythmias, and hypotension.

■ Assess patient for adverse effects, including left ventricular dysfunction and AV conduction defects.

■ Risk of interaction is greater when drugs are given I.V.

■ Dosages of both drugs may need to be decreased.

---

penicillins ◄►◄ aminoglycosides

penicillins	aminoglycosides
ampicillin, oxacillin, nafcillin, penicillin G, piperacillin, ticarcillin	amikacin, gentamicin, kanamycin, netilmicin, streptomycin, tobramycin

Risk rating: 2
Severity: Moderate   Onset: Delayed   Likelihood: Probable

Cause
The mechanism of this interaction is unknown.

Effect
Penicillins may inactivate certain aminoglycosides.

Nursing considerations
⚡ ALERT Check peak and trough aminoglycoside levels after third dose. For peak level, draw blood 30 minutes after I.V. or 60 minutes after I.M. dose. For trough level, draw blood just before a dose.

■ Monitor patient's renal function.

■ Other aminoglycosides may interact with penicillins. If you suspect an interaction, consult prescriber or pharmacist.

■ Penicillins affect gentamicin and tobramycin more than amikacin and netilmicin.

penicillins ◄ food

ampicillin, cloxacillin,
dicloxacillin, nafcillin,
oxacillin, penicillin G

Risk rating: 2
Severity: Moderate   **Onset: Delayed**   **Likelihood: Suspected**

Cause
Food may delay or reduce GI absorption of penicillins.

Effect
Penicillin efficacy may decrease.

Nursing considerations
- Food may affect penicillin absorption and peak level.
- Penicillin V and amoxicillin don't have this interaction and may be given without regard to meals.
- If patient took penicillin with food, watch for lack of drug effect.
- Tell patient to take penicillin 1 hour before or 2 hours after a meal.

penicillins ◄ tetracyclines

amoxicillin, ampi-
cillin, carbenicillin,
cloxacillin,
dicloxacillin,
nafcillin, oxacillin,
penicillin G,
penicillin V, pipera-
cillin, ticarcillin

demeclocycline, doxycycline,
minocycline, tetracycline

Risk rating: 1
Severity: Major   **Onset: Delayed**   **Likelihood: Suspected**

Cause
Tetracyclines may adversely affect bactericidal activity of penicillins.

Effect
Penicillin efficacy may be reduced.

Nursing considerations
- If possible, avoid giving tetracyclines with penicillins.
- Monitor patient closely for lack of penicillin effect.

pentobarbital ━━▶◀━━ alcohol
Nembutal

Risk rating: 1
Severity: **Major**   Onset: **Rapid**   Likelihood: **Established**

Cause
Acute alcohol intake inhibits hepatic metabolism of barbiturates, such as pentobarbital. Chronic alcohol use increases barbiturate clearance, probably by inducing liver enzymes.

Effect
Acute alcohol intake with barbiturates can cause impaired hand-eye coordination, additive CNS effects, and death. Chronic alcohol use with barbiturates may cause drug tolerance and an increased risk of adverse effects, including death.

Nursing considerations
◪ **ALERT** Because of the risk of serious adverse effects, including death, alcohol and barbiturates shouldn't be combined.
■ Before barbiturate therapy starts, assess patient thoroughly for history or evidence of alcohol use.
■ Watch for additive CNS effects, which may suggest barbiturate overdose.

pentobarbital ━━▶◀━━ beta blockers
Nembutal   metoprolol, propranolol

Risk rating: 2
Severity: **Moderate**   Onset: **Rapid**   Likelihood: **Probable**

Cause
Increased enzyme induction and first-pass hepatic metabolism of certain beta blockers reduce their availability.

Effect
Beta blocker efficacy may be reduced.

Nursing considerations
■ Assess beta blocker efficacy by monitoring blood pressure, apical pulse, and presence of chest pain or headache, as appropriate.
■ If patient has increased angina, rhythm problems, or blood pressure problems when the barbiturate starts, notify prescriber promptly. Beta blocker dosage may be increased.

■ Other beta blockers may interact with barbiturates, such as pentobarbital. If you suspect an interaction, consult prescriber or pharmacist.

■ Explain the potential interaction between these drugs and the need to tell prescriber about any problems.

pentobarbital ◄► corticosteroids

Nembutal

betamethasone, corticotropin, cortisone, cosyntropin, dexamethasone, fludrocortisone, hydrocortisone, methylprednisolone, prednisolone, prednisone, triamcinolone

Risk rating: 2
Severity: Moderate   Onset: Delayed   Likelihood: Established

Cause
Pentobarbital and other barbiturates induce liver enzymes, which stimulate corticosteroid metabolism.

Effect
Corticosteroid effects may decrease.

Nursing considerations
■ Avoid giving barbiturates with corticosteroids, if possible.
■ Watch for worsening symptoms when a barbiturate starts or stops.
■ Corticosteroid dosage may increase.

pentobarbital ◄► hormonal contraceptives

Nembutal

Risk rating: 2
Severity: Moderate   Onset: Delayed   Likelihood: Suspected

Cause
Pentobarbital and other barbiturates may induce hepatic metabolism of contraceptives and synthesis of sex-hormone–binding protein.

Effect
Risk of breakthrough bleeding and pregnancy may increase.

Nursing considerations
■ Consult prescriber about increasing contraceptive dosage during barbiturate therapy.

- Consult prescriber about alternative treatments for seizures or sleep disturbance.
- Instruct patient to also use barrier contraception.

---

pentobarbital ▶◀ methadone
Nembutal   Dolophine, Methadose

Risk rating: 2
Severity: Moderate   **Onset: Delayed**   **Likelihood: Suspected**

Cause
Pentobarbital and other barbiturates probably increase hepatic metabolism of methadone.

Effect
Methadone effects may be reduced, and patients on long-term therapy may notice opioid withdrawal symptoms.

Nursing considerations
- If these drugs must be used together, monitor methadone efficacy.
- Check serum methadone level regularly.
- If methadone dosage is insufficient, it may be increased.
- Other barbiturates interact with methadone. If you suspect an interaction, consult prescriber or pharmacist.

---

pentobarbital ▶◀ theophyllines
Nembutal   aminophylline, theophylline

Risk rating: 2
Severity: Moderate   **Onset: Delayed**   **Likelihood: Suspected**

Cause
Pentobarbital and other barbiturates may stimulate theophylline clearance by inducing CYP.

Effect
Theophylline level and efficacy may decrease.

Nursing considerations
- Monitor patient closely to determine theophylline efficacy.
- Monitor serum theophylline level regularly. Normal therapeutic range is 10 to 20 mcg/ml for adults and 5 to 15 mcg/ml for children.
- Theophylline dosage may need to be increased.
- Dyphylline undergoes renal elimination and may not be affected by this interaction.

perindopril ◄►◄ indomethacin

Aceon   Indocin

Risk rating: 2
Severity: Moderate   **Onset: Rapid**   **Likelihood: Probable**

Cause
Indomethacin inhibits synthesis of prostaglandins, which perindopril and other ACE inhibitors need to lower blood pressure.

Effect
ACE inhibitor's hypotensive effect is reduced.

Nursing considerations
⚠ **ALERT** Monitor blood pressure closely. Severe hypertension may persist until indomethacin is stopped.
- If indomethacin can't be avoided, patient may need a different antihypertensive.
- Other ACE inhibitors may interact with indomethacin. If you suspect an interaction, consult prescriber or pharmacist.
- Remind patient that hypertension commonly causes no physical symptoms but sometimes may cause headache and dizziness.

perindopril ◄►◄ potassium-sparing diuretics

Aceon

amiloride, spironolactone, triamterene

Risk rating: 1
Severity: Major   **Onset: Delayed**   **Likelihood: Probable**

Cause
The mechanism of this interaction is unknown.

Effect
Serum potassium level may increase.

Nursing considerations
- Use cautiously in patients at high risk for hyperkalemia, especially those with renal impairment.
- Monitor BUN, creatinine, and serum potassium levels as needed.
- ACE inhibitors other than perindopril may interact with potassium-sparing diuretics. If you suspect an interaction, consult prescriber or pharmacist.
- Urge patient to immediately report an irregular heartbeat, a slow pulse, weakness, and other evidence of hyperkalemia.

perindopril  salicylates

Aceon

aspirin, bismuth subsalicylate, choline salicylate, magnesium salicylate, salsalate, sodium salicylate

Risk rating: 2
Severity: **Moderate**   Onset: **Rapid**   Likelihood: **Suspected**

Cause
Salicylates inhibit synthesis of prostaglandins, which perindopril and other ACE inhibitors need to lower blood pressure.

Effect
ACE inhibitor's hypotensive effect is reduced.

Nursing considerations
▪ This interaction is more likely in people with hypertension, coronary artery disease, or possibly heart failure.

perphenazine ▬▬▶◀▬▬ alcohol

Risk rating: 2
Severity: **Moderate**   Onset: **Rapid**   Likelihood: **Probable**

Cause
The mechanism of this interaction is unknown. It may be that these substances produce CNS depression by working on different sites in the brain. Also, alcohol may lower resistance to neurotoxic effects of phenothiazines, such as perphenazine.

Effect
CNS depression may increase.

Nursing considerations
▪ Watch for extrapyramidal reactions, such as dystonic reactions, and acute akathisia and restlessness.
▪ If patient takes a phenothiazine, warn that alcohol may worsen CNS depression and impair psychomotor skills.
▪ Discourage alcohol intake during phenothiazine therapy.

perphenazine ◄► anticholinergics

atropine, belladonna,
benztropine, biperiden,
dicyclomine, hyoscyamine,
oxybutynin, propantheline,
scopolamine

Risk rating: 2
Severity: Moderate   **Onset: Delayed**   **Likelihood: Suspected**

Cause
Anticholinergics may antagonize phenothiazines, such as perphenazine. Also, phenothiazine metabolism may increase.

Effect
Phenothiazine efficacy may decrease.

Nursing considerations
- Data regarding this interaction conflict.
- Monitor patient for decreased phenothiazine efficacy.
- Phenothiazine dosage may need adjustment.
- Anticholinergic side effects may increase.
- Monitor patient for adynamic ileus, hyperpyrexia, hypoglycemia, and neurologic changes.

---

perphenazine ◄► quinolones

gatifloxacin, levofloxacin,
moxifloxacin, sparfloxain

Risk rating: 1
Severity: Major   **Onset: Delayed**   **Likelihood: Suspected**

Cause
The mechanism of this interaction is unknown.

Effect
Risk of life-threatening arrhythmias, including torsades de pointes, may increase.

Nursing considerations
🔌 **ALERT** Sparfloxacin is contraindicated in patients taking drugs that prolong the QTc interval, including perphenazine and other phenothiazines.
- Avoid giving levofloxacin.
- Use gatifloxacin and moxifloxacin cautiously, with increased monitoring.

■ Quinolones that don't prolong the QTc interval or that aren't metabolized by CYP3A4 isoenzymes may be better alternatives.

---

phenelzine ◄►► **anorexiants**
Nardil   amphetamine, benzphetamine, dextroamphetamine, methamphetamine, phentermine

Risk rating: 1
Severity: Major   **Onset: Rapid**   **Likelihood: Suspected**

Cause
This interaction probably stems from increased norepinephrine levels at the synaptic cleft.

Effect
Anorexiant effects increase.

Nursing considerations
■ If possible, avoid giving these drugs together.
■ Headache and severe hypertension may occur rapidly if amphetamine is given to patient who takes an MAO inhibitor, such as phenelzine.
▶ ALERT Several deaths have resulted from hypertensive crisis and resulting cerebral hemorrhage.
■ Monitor patient for hypotension, hyperpyrexia, and seizures.
■ Hypertensive reaction may occur for several weeks after stopping an MAO inhibitor.

---

phenelzine ◄►► **atomoxetine**
Nardil   Strattera

Risk rating: 1
Severity: Major   **Onset: Rapid**   **Likelihood: Suspected**

Cause
Level of monoamine in the brain may change.

Effect
Risk of serious or fatal reaction resembling neuroleptic malignant syndrome may increase.

Nursing considerations
▶ ALERT Use of atomoxetine and an MAO inhibitor, such as phenelzine, together or within 2 weeks of each other is contraindicated.

■ Before starting atomoxetine, ask patient when he last took an MAO inhibitor. Before starting an MAO inhibitor, ask patient when he last took atomoxetine.

■ Monitor patient for hyperthermia, rapid changes in vital signs, rigidity, muscle twitching, and mental status changes.

phenelzine ▶◀ dextromethorphan
Nardil   Robitussin DM

Risk rating: 1
Severity: Major   **Onset: Rapid**   **Likelihood: Suspected**

Cause
MAO inhibitors, such as phenelzine, may decrease serotonin metabolism. Dextromethorphan may decrease synaptic reuptake of serotonin.

Effect
Risk of serotonin syndrome increases.

Nursing considerations
■ If possible, avoid giving these drugs together.

◪ **ALERT** Combined use may cause hyperpyrexia, abnormal muscle movement, hypotension, coma, and death.

■ If patient takes an MAO inhibitor, caution against taking OTC cough and cold medicines that contain dextromethorphan.

phenelzine ▶◀ foods that contain amines
Nardil

aged, fermented, and overripe foods and drinks: broad beans, caviar, fermented sausage, liver, pickled herring, red wines, various cheeses, yeast extract

Risk rating: 1
Severity: Major   **Onset: Rapid**   **Likelihood: Established**

Cause
MAO inhibition interferes with metabolism of tyramine and other amines in certain foods.

Effect
Risk of marked hypertension increases.

Nursing considerations
- Give patient a list of foods to avoid while taking an MAO inhibitor, such as phenelzine.
- Urge patient to avoid high-amine foods for 4 or more weeks after stopping an MAO inhibitor.
- Monitor blood pressure closely because marked hypertension, hypertensive crisis, and hemorrhagic stroke are possible.
- If patient takes an MAO inhibitor, explain that yeast-containing supplements and cocoa-containing chocolates may cause this interaction.

---

phenelzine ▰▰▰►◄▰▰▰ levodopa
Nardil   Larodopa

Risk rating: 1
Severity: **Major**   Onset: **Rapid**   Likelihood: **Established**

Cause
Peripheral metabolism of levodopa-derived dopamine is inhibited, increasing level at dopamine receptors.

Effect
Risk of hypertensive reaction increases.

Nursing considerations
- If possible, avoid giving these drugs together.
- If they're given together, interaction occurs within 1 hour and appears to be dose related.
- Monitor patient for flushing, light-headedness, and palpitations.
- Selegiline doesn't cause hypertensive reaction and may be used instead of phenelzine and other MAO inhibitors in patients taking levodopa.

---

phenelzine ▰▰▰►◄▰▰▰ L-tryptophan
Nardil

Risk rating: 1
Severity: **Major**   Onset: **Rapid**   Likelihood: **Suspected**

Cause
Giving these drugs together may cause additive serotonergic effects.

Effect
Risk of serotonin syndrome increases.

Nursing considerations
- ◣ ALERT Combined use of these drugs is contraindicated.

■ They may cause CNS irritability, motor weakness, shivering, muscle twitching, and altered consciousness.

phenelzine ━━━━▶◀━━━━ meperidine
Nardil   Demerol

Risk rating: 1
Severity: Major   **Onset: Rapid**   **Likelihood: Probable**

Cause
The mechanism of this interaction is unknown.

Effect
Risk of severe adverse reactions increases.

Nursing considerations
■ If possible, avoid giving these drugs together.
■ If given together, monitor patient and report agitation, seizures, diaphoresis, and fever.
■ Reaction may progress to coma, apnea, and death.
■ Reaction may occur several weeks after stopping an MAO inhibitor, such as phenelzine.
◪ ALERT Give opioid analgesics other than meperidine cautiously. It isn't known if similar reactions occur.

phenelzine ━━━━▶◀━━━━ methylphenidates
Nardil   dexmethylphenidate,
                                methylphenidate

Risk rating: 1
Severity: Major   **Onset: Delayed**   **Likelihood: Suspected**

Cause
The mechanism of this interaction is unknown.

Effect
Risk of hypertensive crisis increases.

Nursing considerations
◪ ALERT Use of dexmethylphenidate with MAO inhibitors, such as phenelzine, is contraindicated.
■ Don't use dexmethylphenidate within 14 days after stopping an MAO inhibitor.
■ Monitor blood pressure closely.
■ Teach patient and parents to monitor blood pressure at home.

phenelzine ▬▶◀▬	**selective 5-HT$_1$ receptor agonists**
Nardil	rizatriptan, sumatriptan, zolmitriptan

Risk rating: 1
Severity: Major   **Onset: Rapid**   **Likelihood: Suspected**

Cause
Monoamine oxidase subtype-A may inhibit metabolism of selective 5-HT$_1$ receptor agonists.

Effect
Serum level of—and risk of cardiac toxicity from—certain selective 5-HT$_1$ receptor agonists may increase.

Nursing considerations
◼ **ALERT** Use of certain selective 5-HT$_1$ receptor agonists with or within 2 weeks of stopping an MAO inhibitor, such as phenelzine, is contraindicated.
◼ If these drugs must be used together, naratriptan is less likely to interact with an MAO inhibitor.
◼ Cardiac toxicity may include coronary artery vasospasm and transient myocardial ischemia.

phenelzine ▬▶◀▬	**serotonin reuptake inhibitors**
Nardil	citalopram, escitalopram, fluoxetine, fluvoxamine, nefazodone, paroxetine, sertraline, venlafaxine

Risk rating: 1
Severity: Major   **Onset: Rapid**   **Likelihood: Probable**

Cause
Serotonin may accumulate rapidly in the CNS.

Effect
Risk of serotonin syndrome increases.

Nursing considerations
◼ **ALERT** Don't use these drugs together.
◼ Allow 1 week after stopping nefazodone or venlafaxine (2 weeks after stopping citalopram, escitalopram, fluvoxamine, paroxetine, or ser-

traline; 5 weeks after stopping fluoxetine) before giving an MAO inhibitor, such as phenelzine.

■ Allow 2 weeks after stopping an MAO inhibitor before giving a serotonin reuptake inhibitor.

■ The selective MAO type-B inhibitor selegiline has been given with fluoxetine, paroxetine, or sertraline to patients with Parkinson's disease without negative effects.

■ Describe the traits of serotonin syndrome, including CNS irritability, motor weakness, shivering, myoclonus, and altered consciousness.

■ Urge patient to promptly report adverse effects to prescriber.

---

phenelzine ━━━━━━ ▶◀ ━━━━━━ sulfonylureas
Nardil

acetohexamide,
chlorpropamide,
glipizide, glyburide,
tolazamide, tolbutamide

Risk rating: 2
Severity: Moderate   Onset: **Rapid**   Likelihood: **Suspected**

Cause
The mechanism of this interaction is unknown.

Effect
Phenelzine and other MAO inhibitors increase the hypoglycemic effects of sulfonylureas.

Nursing considerations
■ If patient takes a sulfonylurea, start MAO inhibitor carefully, monitoring patient for hypoglycemia.

■ Consult prescriber about adjustments to either drug to control glucose level and mental status.

■ Describe signs and symptoms of hypoglycemia: diaphoresis, fatigue, headache, hunger, irritability, malaise, nervousness, rapid heart rate, tension, and trembling.

■ Instruct patient to eat a small carbohydrate snack or meal if hypoglycemia develops, preferably after checking blood glucose level.

phenelzine ━━▶◀━━ sympathomimetics

Nardil

dopamine, ephedrine, metaraminol, phenylephrine, pseudoephedrine

Risk rating: 1
Severity: Major   **Onset: Rapid**   **Likelihood: Established**

Cause
When MAO is inhibited, as by phenelzine and other MAO inhibitors, norepinephrine accumulates and is released by indirect and mixed-acting sympathomimetics, increasing the pressor response at receptor sites.

Effect
Risk of severe headaches, hypertension, high fever, and hypertensive crisis increases.

Nursing considerations
■ Avoid giving indirect or mixed-acting sympathomimetics with an MAO inhibitor.
■ Phentolamine can be administered to block epinephrine- and norepinephrine-induced vasoconstriction and reduce blood pressure.
■ Direct-acting sympathomimetics interact minimally.
◤ ALERT Warn patient that OTC medicines, such as decongestants, may cause this interaction.

phenelzine ━━▶◀━━ tricyclic antidepressants

Nardil

amitriptyline, amoxapine, clomipramine, desipramine, doxepin, imipramine, nortriptyline, trimipramine

Risk rating: 1
Severity: Major   **Onset: Rapid**   **Likelihood: Suspected**

Cause
The mechanism of this interaction is unknown.

Effect
Risk of hyperpyretic crisis, seizures, and death increase.

Nursing considerations
◤ ALERT Don't give a tricyclic antidepressant with or within 2 weeks of an MAO inhibitor, such as phenelzine.
■ Imipramine and clomipramine may be more likely to interact with MAO inhibitors.

■ Watch for adverse effects, including confusion, hyperexcitability, rigidity, seizures, increased temperature, increased pulse, increased respiration, sweating, mydriasis, flushing, headache, coma, and DIC.

phenobarbital ▶◀ alcohol
Luminal

Risk rating: 1
Severity: **Major**   Onset: **Rapid**   Likelihood: **Established**

Cause
Acute alcohol intake inhibits hepatic metabolism of barbiturates, such as phenobarbital. Chronic alcohol use increases barbiturate clearance, probably by inducing liver enzymes.

Effect
Acute alcohol intake with barbiturates can cause impaired hand-eye coordination, additive CNS effects, and death. Chronic alcohol use with barbiturates may cause drug tolerance and an increased risk of adverse effects, including death.

Nursing considerations
■ **ALERT** Because of the risk of serious adverse effects, including death, alcohol and barbiturates shouldn't be combined.
■ Before barbiturate therapy starts, assess patient thoroughly for history or evidence of alcohol use.
■ Watch for additive CNS effects, which may suggest barbiturate overdose.
■ Other barbiturates interact with alcohol. If you suspect an interaction, consult prescriber or pharmacist.
■ When a barbiturate starts, stress the high risk of consuming alcohol.

phenobarbital ▶◀ beta blockers
Luminal   metoprolol, propranolol

Risk rating: 2
Severity: **Moderate**   Onset: **Rapid**   Likelihood: **Probable**

Cause
Increased enzyme induction and first-pass hepatic metabolism of certain beta blockers reduce their availability.

Effect
Beta blocker efficacy may be reduced.

Nursing considerations
■ Assess beta blocker efficacy by monitoring blood pressure, apical pulse, and presence of chest pain or headache, as appropriate.
■ If patient has increased angina, rhythm problems, or blood pressure problems when phenobarbital or another barbiturate starts, notify prescriber promptly. Beta blocker dosage may be increased.
■ Other beta blockers may interact with barbiturates. If you suspect an interaction, consult prescriber or pharmacist.
■ Explain the potential interaction between these drugs and the need to tell prescriber about any problems.

phenobarbital ▶◀	corticosteroids
Luminal	betamethasone, corticotropin, cortisone, cosyntropin, dexamethasone, fludrocortisone, hydrocortisone, methylprednisolone, prednisolone, prednisone, triamcinolone

Risk rating: 2
Severity: **Moderate**   Onset: **Delayed**   Likelihood: **Established**

Cause
Phenobarbital and other barbiturates induce liver enzymes, which stimulate corticosteroid metabolism.

Effect
Corticosteroid effects may decrease.

Nursing considerations
■ Avoid giving barbiturates with corticosteroids, if possible.
■ If patient takes a corticosteroid, watch for worsening symptoms when a barbiturate is started or stopped.
■ During barbiturate treatment, corticosteroid dosage may increase.

phenobarbital ▶◀	hormonal contraceptives
Luminal	

Risk rating: 2
Severity: **Moderate**   Onset: **Delayed**   Likelihood: **Suspected**

Cause
Phenobarbital and other barbiturates may induce hepatic metabolism of contraceptives and synthesis of sex-hormone–binding protein.

Effect
Risk of breakthrough bleeding and pregnancy may increase.

Nursing considerations
■ Consult prescriber about increasing contraceptive dosage during barbiturate therapy.
■ Consult prescriber about alternative treatments for seizures or sleep disturbance.
■ Instruct patient to also use barrier contraception.

phenobarbital ▶◀ methadone
Luminal   Dolophine, Methadose

Risk rating: 2
Severity: Moderate   Onset: Delayed   Likelihood: Suspected

Cause
Phenobarbital and other barbiturates probably increase hepatic metabolism of methadone.

Effect
Methadone effects may be reduced, and patients on long-term therapy may notice opioid withdrawal symptoms.

Nursing considerations
■ Monitor methadone efficacy.
■ Check serum methadone level regularly.
■ If methadone dosage is insufficient, it may be increased.
■ Other barbiturates interact with methadone. If you suspect an interaction, consult prescriber or pharmacist.

phenobarbital ▶◀ theophyllines
Luminal   aminophylline, theophylline

Risk rating: 2
Severity: Moderate   Onset: Delayed   Likelihood: Suspected

Cause
Phenobarbital and other barbiturates may stimulate theophylline clearance by inducing CYP.

Effect
Theophylline level and efficacy may decrease.

Nursing considerations
■ Monitor patient closely to determine theophylline efficacy.

■ Monitor serum theophylline level regularly. Normal therapeutic range is 10 to 20 mcg/ml for adults and 5 to 15 mcg/ml for children.
■ When a barbiturate is added, theophylline dosage may be increased.
■ Dyphylline undergoes renal elimination and may not be affected by this interaction.

---

phentermine ▶◀ MAO inhibitors
Adipex-P   phenelzine, tranylcypromine

Risk rating: 1
Severity: Major   **Onset: Rapid**   **Likelihood: Suspected**

Cause
This interaction probably stems from increased norepinephrine level at the synaptic cleft.

Effect
Anorexiant effects increase.

Nursing considerations
■ If possible, avoid giving these drugs together.
■ Headache and severe hypertension may occur rapidly if amphetamine, such as phentermine, is given to patient who takes an MAO inhibitor.
⚠ ALERT Death may result from hypertensive crisis and resulting cerebral hemorrhage.
■ Monitor patient for hypotension, hyperpyrexia, and seizures.
■ Hypertensive reaction may occur for several weeks after stopping an MAO inhibitor.

---

phentermine ▶◀ SSRIs
Adipex-P   fluoxetine, fluvoxamine,
                                  paroxetine, sertraline

Risk rating: 1
Severity: Major   **Onset: Rapid**   **Likelihood: Suspected**

Cause
The mechanism of this interaction is unknown.

Effect
Sympathomimetic effects and risk of serotonin syndrome increase.

Nursing considerations
■ Watch closely for increased CNS effects, such as anxiety, jitteriness, agitation, and restlessness.

- Mild serotonin-like symptoms may develop, including anxiety, dizziness, restlessness, nausea, and vomiting.
- Explain the risk of interaction and the need to avoid amphetamines, such as phentermine.
- Describe the traits of serotonin syndrome, including CNS irritability, motor weakness, shivering, myoclonus, and altered consciousness.

---

phenylephrine ➤◀ MAO inhibitors
Neo-Synephrine
isocarboxazid, phenelzine, tranylcypromine

Risk rating: 1
Severity: Major   **Onset: Rapid**   **Likelihood: Established**

Cause
When MAO is inhibited, norepinephrine accumulates and is released by indirect and mixed-acting sympathomimetics, such as phenylephrine, increasing the pressor response at receptor sites.

Effect
Risk of severe headaches, hypertension, high fever, and hypertensive crisis increases.

Nursing considerations
- Avoid giving indirect or mixed-acting sympathomimetics with an MAO inhibitor.
- Phentolamine can be administered to block epinephrine- and norepinephrine-induced vasoconstriction and reduce blood pressure.
- Direct-acting sympathomimetics interact minimally.

⚠ ALERT Warn patient that OTC medicines, such as decongestants, may cause this interaction.

---

phenylephrine ➤◀ methyldopa
Neo-Synephrine
Aldomet

Risk rating: 2
Severity: Moderate   **Onset: Rapid**   **Likelihood: Suspected**

Cause
The mechanism of this interaction is unknown.

Effect
Pressor response of sympathomimetics, such as phenylephrine, may be increased, resulting in hypertension.

Nursing considerations
- Monitor patient's blood pressure closely.
- If patient takes methyldopa, explain that many OTC products contain drugs that can raise blood pressure. Urge patient to read labels carefully or check with prescriber before using a new product.
- Teach patient to monitor blood pressure at home.

---

phenylephrine ▶◀ tricyclic antidepressants

Neo-Synephrine

amitriptyline, amoxapine, clomipramine, desipramine, doxepin, imipramine, nortriptyline, trimipramine

Risk rating: 2
Severity: Moderate   **Onset: Rapid**   **Likelihood: Established**

Cause
Tricyclic antidepressants (TCAs) increase the effects of direct-acting sympathomimetics, such as phenylephrine.

Effect
When sympathomimetic effects increase, the risk of hypertension and arrhythmias increases.

Nursing considerations
- If possible, avoid using these drugs together.
- Watch patient closely for hypertension and heart rhythm changes; they may warrant reduction of sympathomimetic dosage.
- Other TCAs and sympathomimetics may interact. If you suspect an interaction, consult prescriber or pharmacist.

---

phenytoin ▶◀ acetaminophen

Dilantin

Acephen, Neopap, Tylenol

Risk rating: 2
Severity: Moderate   **Onset: Delayed**   **Likelihood: Suspected**

Cause
Phenytoin may induce hepatic microsomal enzymes, accelerating the metabolism of acetaminophen.

Effect
An abnormally high rate of acetaminophen metabolism may lead to higher level of hepatotoxic metabolites, increasing the risk of hepatic impairment.

Nursing considerations
■ Hydantoins other than phenytoin may have a similar interaction with acetaminophen. Discuss concerns with prescriber.

▌ **ALERT** The hepatotoxic risk is greatest after acetaminophen overdose in a patient who uses phenytoin regularly.

■ No special monitoring or dosage adjustment is required at the usual therapeutic dosages.

■ Advise patient who takes phenytoin to avoid regular use of acetaminophen.

■ Tell patient to notify prescriber about abdominal pain, yellowing of skin or eyes, or darkened urine.

---

phenytoin ━━━━▶◀━━━━ **antineoplastics**

Dilantin

bleomycin, carboplatin, carmustine, cisplatin, methotrexate, vinblastine

---

Risk rating: 2
Severity: Moderate   **Onset: Delayed**   **Likelihood: Suspected**

Cause
Phenytoin absorption may be decreased or metabolism may be increased.

Effect
Phenytoin level and effects may decrease.

Nursing considerations
■ Monitor phenytoin level closely. Dosage may need to be adjusted.

■ Therapeutic range for phenytoin is 10 to 20 mcg/ml.

■ Toxic effects can occur at therapeutic level. Adjust the measured level for hypoalbuminemia or renal impairment, which can increase free drug level.

■ Monitor patient for seizure activity.

■ Carefully monitor phenytoin level between courses of chemotherapy. Phenytoin dose may need to be reduced.

■ Signs and symptoms of phenytoin toxicity include nystagmus, slurred speech, ataxia, blurred or double vision, confusion, drowsiness, and lethargy.

phenytoin ━━━▶◀━━━ cimetidine

Dilantin   Tagamet

Risk rating: 2
Severity: Moderate   Onset: Delayed   Likelihood: Established

Cause
The hepatic metabolism of phenytoin is inhibited.

Effect
Phenytoin level and risk of toxicity may increase.

Nursing considerations
- Hydantoins other than phenytoin may have a similar interaction with cimetidine.
- Monitor phenytoin level closely. Dosage may need to be adjusted.
- The therapeutic range for phenytoin is 10 to 20 mcg/ml.
- Toxic effects can occur at therapeutic level. Adjust the measured level for hypoalbuminemia or renal impairment, which can increase free drug level.
- Signs and symptoms of phenytoin toxicity include nystagmus, slurred speech, ataxia, blurred or double vision, confusion, drowsiness, and lethargy.
- Ranitidine and felodipine may be better alternatives to use than cimetidine.

phenytoin ━━━▶◀━━━ corticosteroids

Dilantin   betamethasone, corticotropin, cortisone, cosyntropin, dexamethasone, fludrocortisone, hydrocortisone, methylprednisolone, prednisolone, prednisone, triamcinolone

Risk rating: 2
Severity: Moderate   Onset: Delayed   Likelihood: Established

Cause
Phenytoin and other hydantoins induce liver enzymes, which stimulate corticosteroid metabolism. Dexamethasone may enhance hepatic clearance of phenytoin.

Effect
Corticosteroid effects may decrease.

Nursing considerations
- Avoid giving hydantoins with corticosteroids if possible.
- Monitor patient for decreased corticosteroid effects. Also monitor phenytoin level, and adjust dosage of either drug as needed.
- Corticosteroid effects may decrease within days of starting phenytoin and may stay decreased 3 weeks after it stops.
- Dosage of either or both drugs may need to be increased.

---

phenytoin ▸◂ disulfiram
Dilantin   Antabuse

Risk rating: 2
Severity: Moderate   **Onset: Rapid**   **Likelihood: Established**

Cause
Disulfiram inhibits hepatic metabolism of the hydantoin phenytoin and may also interfere with the rate of elimination.

Effect
Phenytoin level, effects, and risk of toxicity may increase.

Nursing considerations
- Other hydantoins may have a similar interaction with disulfiram. If you suspect a drug interaction, consult prescriber or pharmacist.
- Monitor phenytoin level; therapeutic range is 10 to 20 mcg/ml.
- Monitor patient for signs of phenytoin toxicity, including drowsiness, nausea, vomiting, nystagmus, ataxia, dysarthria, tremor, slurred speech, hypotension, arrhythmias, respiratory depression, and coma.
- Watch for loss of phenytoin effects (for example, loss of seizure control) if disulfiram therapy is stopped.
- Adjust phenytoin dose as ordered.

---

phenytoin ▸◂ dopamine
Dilantin   Intropin

Risk rating: 1
Severity: Major   **Onset: Rapid**   **Likelihood: Suspected**

Cause
Hypotension may result from phenytoin-induced myocardial depression and dopamine-related depletion of catecholamines.

Effect
Profound, life-threatening hypotension may occur.

Nursing considerations
■ Use together with extreme caution and frequent blood pressure monitoring.

⚡ **ALERT** Life-threatening hypotension can occur in a few minutes of coadministration. Cardiac arrest and death may occur.
■ Stop phenytoin infusion at the first sign of hypotension.
■ It isn't known if phenytoin reacts similarly to sympathomimetics other than dopamine. Use cautiously.

---

phenytoin ▶◀ **doxycycline**

Dilantin   Vibramycin

Risk rating: 2
Severity: Moderate   **Onset: Delayed**   **Likelihood: Probable**

Cause
Phenytoin induces doxycycline metabolism. In addition, doxycycline may be displaced from plasma proteins.

Effect
Doxycycline elimination may increase and effects decrease.

Nursing considerations
■ Monitor patient for expected doxycycline effects (absence of infection) when given with the hydantoin phenytoin.
■ Doxycycline dose may need to be doubled to maintain therapeutic serum level.
■ Consult prescriber or pharmacist about using a tetracycline (other than doxycycline) that doesn't interact with phenytoin.
■ Urge patient to tell prescriber if signs and symptoms don't improve.
■ Other hydantoins may have a similar interaction with doxycycline. If you suspect an interaction, consult prescriber or pharmacist.

---

phenytoin ▶◀ **estrogens**

Dilantin   conjugated estrogens, esterified estrogens, estradiol, estrone, estropipate, ethinyl estradiol

---

Risk rating: 2
Severity: Moderate   **Onset: Delayed**   **Likelihood: Suspected**

Cause
Phenytoin may induce hepatic metabolism of estrogens. Estrogens may increase water retention, worsen seizures, and alter phenytoin protein-binding.

Effect
Risk of spotting, breakthrough bleeding, and pregnancy increases. Seizure control may decrease.

Nursing considerations
- Estrogen dose may need to be altered to obtain cycle control.
- **ALERT** Advise patient that breakthrough bleeding, spotting, and amenorrhea are signs of contraceptive failure.
- Although unconfirmed, seizures may worsen in patients who take estrogens.
- Monitor patient for increased seizure activity when estrogen therapy starts.
- Hydantoins other than phenytoin may interact with estrogens. If you suspect an interaction, consult prescriber or pharmacist.
- If patient takes phenytoin, suggest a nonhormonal contraceptive.

---

phenytoin ▶◀ fluvoxamine
Dilantin   Luvox

Risk rating: 2
Severity: Moderate   **Onset: Delayed**   **Likelihood: Suspected**

Cause
Fluvoxamine may inhibit CYP2C9 and CYP2C19 metabolism of hydantoins, such as phenytoin.

Effect
Hydantoin level and risk of toxic effects may increase.

Nursing considerations
- Monitor serum hydantoin level. Therapeutic range for phenytoin is 10 to 20 mcg/ml.
- Hydantoin dosage may need adjustment.
- When fluvoxamine starts, watch for hydantoin toxicity: drowsiness, nausea, vomiting, nystagmus, ataxia, dysarthria, tremor, slurred speech, hypotension, arrhythmias, respiratory depression, and coma.
- When fluvoxamine stops, watch for loss of anticonvulsant effect and increased seizure activity.

phenytoin ▶◀ folic acid
Dilantin   Folvite

Risk rating: 2
Severity: Moderate   **Onset: Delayed**   **Likelihood: Suspected**

Cause
The mechanism of this interaction is unknown but probably involves altered metabolic process.

Effect
Level and effects of hydantoins, such as phenytoin, may decrease.

Nursing considerations
■ Monitor hydantoin level. Therapeutic range for phenytoin is 10 to 20 mcg/ml.
■ Hydantoin dosage may need adjustment.
■ If folic acid is started during hydantoin therapy, watch for loss of anticonvulsant effect and increased seizure activity.
■ If folic acid is stopped during hydantoin therapy, watch for signs of hydantoin toxicity, such as drowsiness, nausea, vomiting, nystagmus, ataxia, dysarthria, tremor, slurred speech, hypotension, arrhythmias, respiratory depression, and coma.
■ Urge patient to tell prescriber about increased adverse effects.

phenytoin ▶◀ isoniazid
Dilantin   Nydrazid

Risk rating: 2
Severity: Moderate   **Onset: Delayed**   **Likelihood: Established**

Cause
Hepatic microsomal enzyme metabolism of phenytoin is inhibited.

Effect
Phenytoin level, effects, and risk of toxicity increase.

Nursing considerations
■ Monitor phenytoin level closely. Dosage may need to be adjusted. Therapeutic range for phenytoin is 10 to 20 mcg/ml.
■ Toxic effects can occur at therapeutic level. Adjust the measured level for hypoalbuminemia or renal impairment, which can increase free drug level.
■ Signs and symptoms of phenytoin toxicity include nystagmus, slurred speech, ataxia, blurred or double vision, confusion, drowsiness, and lethargy.

■ If patient's phenytoin level has been stabilized with isoniazid and isoniazid stops, watch for loss of seizure control.

■ Hydantoins other than phenytoin may have a similar interaction with isoniazid.

phenytoin ▶◀ methadone
Dilantin   Dolophine, Methadose

Risk rating: 2
Severity: Moderate   Onset: Delayed   Likelihood: Suspected

Cause
The mechanism of this interaction is unknown but probably involves altered metabolic process.

Effect
Level and effects of methadone may decrease.

Nursing considerations
■ Methadone dosage may need adjustment.

■ If phenytoin is started during methadone therapy, watch for signs and symptoms of opioid withdrawal.

■ Urge patient to tell prescriber about return of withdrawal symptoms.

phenytoin ▶◀ mirtazapine
Dilantin   Remeron

Risk rating: 2
Severity: Moderate   Onset: Delayed   Likelihood: Suspected

Cause
Phenytoin and other hydantoins may increase CYP3A3 and CYP3A4 metabolism of mirtazapine.

Effect
Mirtazapine level and effects may decrease.

Nursing considerations
■ Assess patient for expected mirtazapine effects, including improvement of depression and stabilization of mood.

■ Record mood changes, and monitor patient for suicidal tendencies.

■ If a hydantoin starts, mirtazapine dosage may need to be increased.

- If a hydantoin stops, watch for mirtazapine toxicity, including disorientation, drowsiness, impaired memory, tachycardia, severe hypotension, heart failure, seizures, CNS depression, and coma.
- Urge patient to tell prescriber about loss of drug effect and increased adverse effects.

---

phenytoin ━━━▶◀━━━ **nondepolarizing muscle relaxants**

Dilantin

atracurium, cisatracurium, mivacurium, pancuronium, rocuronium, vecuronium

Risk rating: 2
Severity: Moderate   **Onset: Rapid**   **Likelihood: Probable**

Cause
Phenytoin has effects at prejunctional sites similar to those of nondepolarizing muscle relaxants. Also, phenytoin alters the metabolism of pancuronium.

Effect
Effect or duration of nondepolarizing muscle relaxant may decrease.

Nursing considerations
- Monitor patient for decreased efficacy of the muscle relaxant.
- Dosage of nondepolarizing muscle relaxant may need to increase.
- Atracurium may be a suitable alternative because this interaction may not occur in all patients.
- Make sure patient is adequately sedated when receiving a nondepolarizing muscle relaxant.

---

phenytoin ━━━▶◀━━━ **quetiapine**

Dilantin   Seroquel

Risk rating: 2
Severity: Moderate   **Onset: Delayed**   **Likelihood: Suspected**

Cause
Quetiapine metabolism increases.

Effect
Pharmacologic response to quetiapine may decrease.

Nursing considerations
■ Monitor patient for loss of symptom control for bipolar disorder or schizophrenia.
■ The dose of quetiapine may need to be changed when starting, stopping, or changing the dose of phenytoin.
■ Tell patient that, although no serious side effects have been noted from this interaction, he should report unusual or bothersome adverse effects to prescriber.

phenytoin ▶◀ sertraline
Dilantin   Zoloft

Risk rating: 2
Severity: **Moderate**   Onset: **Delayed**   Likelihood: **Suspected**

Cause
Sertraline may inhibit metabolism of hydantoins, such as phenytoin.

Effect
Hydantoin level, effects, and risk of toxicity may increase.

Nursing considerations
■ Monitor hydantoin level. Therapeutic range for phenytoin is 10 to 20 mcg/ml.
■ Hydantoin dosage may need adjustment.
■ If sertraline starts during hydantoin therapy, watch for evidence of hydantoin toxicity, including drowsiness, nausea, vomiting, nystagmus, ataxia, dysarthria, tremor, slurred speech, hypotension, arrhythmias, respiratory depression, and coma.
■ If sertraline stops during hydantoin therapy, watch for decreased anticonvulsant effect and increased seizure activity.
■ Urge patient to tell prescriber about loss of drug effect and increased adverse effects.

phenytoin ▶◀ sulfadiazine
Dilantin

Risk rating: 2
Severity: **Moderate**   Onset: **Delayed**   Likelihood: **Probable**

Cause
Sulfadiazine may inhibit hepatic metabolism of hydantoins, such as phenytoin.

Effect
Hydantoin level, effects, and risk of toxicity may increase.

Nursing considerations
■ Monitor hydantoin level. Therapeutic range for phenytoin is 10 to 20 mcg/ml.
■ Hydantoin dosage may need adjustment.
■ If sulfadiazine starts during hydantoin therapy, watch for evidence of hydantoin toxicity, including drowsiness, nausea, vomiting, nystagmus, ataxia, dysarthria, tremor, slurred speech, hypotension, arrhythmias, respiratory depression, and coma.
■ If sulfadiazine stops during hydantoin therapy, watch for decreased anticonvulsant effect and increased seizure activity.
■ Consult prescriber and pharmacist about other anti-infective drugs if patient takes a hydantoin.

---

phenytoin ◄► theophyllines
Dilantin   aminophylline, theophylline

Risk rating: 2
Severity: Moderate   **Onset: Delayed**   **Likelihood: Probable**

Cause
Metabolism of both drugs increases.

Effect
Theophylline or phenytoin efficacy may decrease.

Nursing considerations
■ Monitor levels of both drugs carefully. Normal phenytoin level is 10 to 20 mcg/ml. Normal theophylline level is 10 to 20 mcg/ml for adults and 5 to 15 mcg/ml for children.
■ Assess patient for recurrence of seizures and increased respiratory distress, and report findings to prescriber promptly; dosages may need adjustment.
■ Interaction typically occurs within 5 days of starting combined use.

---

phenytoin ◄► ticlopidine
Dilantin   Ticlid

Risk rating: 2
Severity: Moderate   **Onset: Delayed**   **Likelihood: Probable**

Cause
Ticlopidine may inhibit hepatic metabolism of hydantoins, such as phenytoin.

Effect
Hydantoin level may increase, raising the risk of adverse effects.

Nursing considerations
■ Monitor hydantoin level. Therapeutic range for phenytoin is 10 to 20 mcg/ml.
■ Hydantoin level may increase gradually over a month.
■ Hydantoin dosage may need adjustment.
■ If ticlopidine starts during hydantoin therapy, monitor patient for adverse CNS effects of hydantoins, including vertigo, ataxia, and somnolence.
■ If ticlopidine stops during hydantoin therapy, watch for decreased anticonvulsant effect and increased seizure activity.

---

phenytoin ▶◀ warfarin
Dilantin   Coumadin

Risk rating: 2
Severity: Moderate   Onset: Delayed   Likelihood: Suspected

Cause
Phenytoin level may increase and half-life lengthen. Phenytoin may increase PT when added to warfarin therapy.

Effect
Risk of phenytoin toxicity and severe bleeding increases.

Nursing considerations
■ Monitor patient for signs or symptoms of phenytoin toxicity or for altered anticoagulant effects.
■ Therapeutic range for phenytoin is 10 to 20 mcg/ml.
■ Toxic effects can occur at therapeutic level. Adjust the measured level for hypoalbuminemia or renal impairment, which can increase free drug level.
■ Signs and symptoms of phenytoin toxicity include nystagmus, slurred speech, ataxia, blurred or double vision, confusion, drowsiness, and lethargy.
■ Monitor phenytoin level 7 to 10 days after therapy starts or changes.
■ Tell patient to report unusual bruising or bleeding.

---

pimozide ▶◀ aprepitant
Orap   Emend

Risk rating: 1
Severity: Major   Onset: Delayed   Likelihood: Suspected

Cause
Aprepitant may inhibit CYP3A4 metabolism of pimozide.

Effect
Risk of life-threatening arrhythmias may increase.

Nursing considerations
⚠ ALERT Combined use of these drugs is contraindicated.
- Arrhythmias are related to prolonged QT interval, a known risk of pimozide.
- Interaction warning is based on pharmokinetics of these drugs, not actual patient studies.

---

pimozide ━━━━▶◀ azole antifungals
Orap   itraconazole, ketoconazole

Risk rating: 1
Severity: Major   **Onset: Delayed**   **Likelihood: Suspected**

Cause
Azole antifungals may inhibit CYP3A4 metabolism of pimozide.

Effect
Risk of life-threatening arrhythmias may increase.

Nursing considerations
⚠ ALERT Combined use of these drugs is contraindicated.
- Arrhythmias are related to prolonged QT interval, a known risk of pimozide.
- Interaction warning is based on pharmokinetics of these drugs, not actual patient studies.

---

pimozide ━━━━▶◀ macrolide antibiotics
Orap   clarithromycin, erythromycin

Risk rating: 1
Severity: Major   **Onset: Delayed**   **Likelihood: Probable**

Cause
Macrolide antibiotics may inhibit CYP3A4 metabolism of pimozide.

Effect
Risk of life-threatening arrhythmias may increase.

Nursing considerations
⚠ ALERT Combined use of these drugs is contraindicated.
- Arrhythmias are related to prolonged QT interval, a known risk of pimozide.

◥ **ALERT** People with normal baseline ECG and no history have died from pimozide blood levels 2.5 times the upper limit of normal from this interaction.

---

pimozide ▶◀ **nefazodone**
Orap

Risk rating: 1
Severity: **Major**   Onset: **Delayed**   Likelihood: **Suspected**

Cause
Nefazodone may inhibit CYP3A4 metabolism of pimozide.

Effect
Risk of life-threatening arrhythmias may increase.

Nursing considerations
◥ **ALERT** Combined use of these drugs is contraindicated.
■ Arrhythmias are related to prolonged QT interval, a known risk of pimozide.
■ Interaction warning is based on pharmokinetics of these drugs, not actual patient studies.

---

pimozide ▶◀ **protease inhibitors**
Orap   amprenavir, indinavir,
                          nelfinavir, ritonavir, saquinavir

Risk rating: 1
Severity: **Major**   Onset: **Delayed**   Likelihood: **Suspected**

Cause
Protease inhibitors may inhibit CYP3A4 metabolism of pimozide.

Effect
Risk of life-threatening arrhythmias may increase.

Nursing considerations
◥ **ALERT** Combined use of these drugs is contraindicated.
■ Arrhythmias are related to prolonged QT interval, a known risk of pimozide.
■ Interaction warning is based on pharmokinetics of these drugs, not actual patient studies.

pimozide ━━━━►◄━━━━ SSRIs

Orap   citalopram, sertraline

Risk rating: 1
Severity: Major   **Onset: Delayed**   **Likelihood: Suspected**

Cause
The mechanism of this interaction is unknown.

Effect
Risk of life-threatening arrhythmias, including torsades de pointes, may increase.

Nursing considerations
⚠ ALERT Combined use of these drugs is contraindicated.
■ Arrhythmias are related to prolonged QT interval, a known risk of pimozide.
■ Interaction warning is based on actual patient experience with these drugs as well as pharmacokinetics.

pimozide ━━━━►◄━━━━ telithromycin

Orap   Ketek

Risk rating: 1
Severity: Major   **Onset: Delayed**   **Likelihood: Suspected**

Cause
CYP3A4 hepatic metabolism of pimozide may be inhibited.

Effect
Pimozide level and risk of life-threatening arrhythmias, including torsades de pointes, may increase.

Nursing considerations
⚠ ALERT Use of pimozide with telithromycin is contraindicated.
■ Arrhythmias are related to prolonged QT interval, a known risk of pimozide.
■ Interaction warning is based on pharmokinetics of these drugs, not actual patient studies.

pimozide ━━━━▶◀━━━━ voriconazole
Orap   Vfend

Risk rating: 1
Severity: Major   **Onset: Delayed**   **Likelihood: Suspected**

Cause
Voriconazole may inhibit CYP3A4 metabolism of pimozide.

Effect
Risk of life-threatening arrhythmias may increase.

Nursing considerations
◪ ALERT Combined use of these drugs is contraindicated.
■ Arrhythmias are related to prolonged QT interval, a known risk of
pimozide.
■ Interaction warning is based on pharmokinetics of these drugs, not
actual patient studies.

pimozide ━━━━▶◀━━━━ zileuton
Orap   Zyflo

Risk rating: 1
Severity: Major   **Onset: Delayed**   **Likelihood: Suspected**

Cause
Zileuton may inhibit CYP3A4 metabolism of pimozide.

Effect
Risk of life-threatening arrhythmias may increase.

Nursing considerations
◪ ALERT Combined use of these drugs is contraindicated.
■ Arrhythmias are related to prolonged QT interval, a known risk of
pimozide.
■ Interaction warning is based on known pharmokinetics of these
drugs, not actual patient studies.

pimozide ━━━━▶◀━━━━ ziprasidone
Orap   Geodon

Risk rating: 1
Severity: Major   **Onset: Delayed**   **Likelihood: Suspected**

Cause
Ziprasidone may have additive effects on QT-interval prolongation.

Effect
Risk of life-threatening arrhythmias, including torsades de pointes, may increase.

Nursing considerations
◖ ALERT Combined use of these drugs is contraindicated.

■ Arrhythmias are related to prolonged QT interval, a known risk of pimozide.

■ Interaction warning is based on known pharmokinetics of these drugs, not actual patient studies.

---

pindolol ▶◀ epinephrine
Visken   Adrenalin

Risk rating: 1
Severity: Major   **Onset: Rapid**   **Likelihood: Established**

Cause
Alpha-receptor effects of epinephrine supersede the effects of non-selective beta blockers, such as pindolol, increasing vascular resistance.

Effect
Initial marked hypertensive effect is followed by reflex bradycardia.

Nursing considerations
◖ ALERT Three days before planned use of epinephrine, stop the beta blocker. Or, if possible, don't use epinephrine.

■ Monitor blood pressure and pulse closely. If interaction occurs, give I.V. chlorpromazine, hydralazine, aminophylline, or atropine if needed.

■ Explain the risks of this interaction, and tell patient to carry medical identification at all times.

■ Other beta blockers may interact with epinephrine. If you suspect an interaction, consult prescriber or pharmacist.

---

pindolol ▶◀ ergot derivatives
Visken   dihydroergotamine, ergotamine

Risk rating: 2
Severity: Moderate   **Onset: Delayed**   **Likelihood: Suspected**

Cause
Vasoconstriction and blockade of peripheral beta$_2$ receptors allows unopposed ergot action.

Effect
Vasoconstrictive effects of ergot derivatives are increased, causing peripheral ischemia, cold limbs, and possible gangrene.

Nursing considerations
- Watch for evidence of peripheral ischemia.
- If needed, stop pindolol, a beta blocker, and adjust ergot derivative.
- Other ergot derivatives may interact with beta blockers. If you suspect an interaction, consult prescriber or pharmacist.

---

pindolol 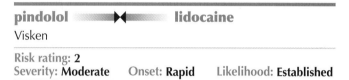 lidocaine
Visken

Risk rating: 2
Severity: Moderate   **Onset: Rapid**   **Likelihood: Established**

Cause
Pindolol and other beta blockers reduce hepatic metabolism of lidocaine.

Effect
Lidocaine level and risk of toxicity may increase.

Nursing considerations
- Check for normal therapeutic level of lidocaine: 2 to 5 mcg/ml.
- Monitor patient closely for evidence of lidocaine toxicity, including dizziness, somnolence, confusion, paresthesias, and seizures.
- Slow I.V. bolus rate to decrease risk of high peak level and toxic reaction.
- Explain warning signs of toxicity to patient and family, and tell them to contact prescriber if they have concerns.

---

pindolol NSAIDs
Visken   ibuprofen, indomethacin, naproxen, piroxicam

Risk rating: 2
Severity: Moderate   **Onset: Delayed**   **Likelihood: Probable**

Cause
NSAIDs may inhibit renal prostaglandin synthesis, allowing pressor systems to be unopposed.

Effect

Pindolol and other beta blockers may not be able to lower blood pressure.

Nursing considerations

- Avoid using these drugs together if possible.
- Monitor blood pressure and related signs and symptoms of hypertension closely.
- Consult prescriber about ways to minimize interaction, such as adjusting beta blocker dosage or switching to sulindac as the NSAID.
- Explain the risks of using these drugs together, and teach patient how to monitor his blood pressure.
- Other NSAIDs may interact with beta blockers. If you suspect an interaction, consult prescriber or pharmacist.

---

pindolol ▸◂	phenothiazines
Visken	chlorpromazine, thioridazine

Risk rating: 1
Severity: **Major**   Onset: **Delayed**   Likelihood: **Probable**

Cause

Pindolol inhibits thioridazine metabolism.

Effect

Effects of both drugs and the risk of serious adverse reactions may increase.

Nursing considerations

- **⚠ ALERT** Use of thioridazine with pindolol is contraindicated.
- Educate patient and family about the risk of drug interaction.
- Beta blockers other than pindolol may interact with phenothiazines. If you suspect an interaction, consult prescriber or pharmacist.

---

pindolol ▸◂	prazosin
Visken	Minipress

Risk rating: 2
Severity: **Moderate**   Onset: **Rapid**   Likelihood: **Probable**

Cause

The mechanism of this interaction is unknown.

Effect

Effect of these drugs on orthostatic hypotension is increased.

Nursing considerations
- Assess patient's lying, sitting, and standing blood pressures closely, especially when combined therapy starts.
- Adjust dosages of either drug to patient effects.
- To minimize effects of orthostatic hypotension, teach patient to change positions slowly.
- Interaction is confirmed only with propranolol but may occur with pindolol and other beta blockers as well.

---

pindolol ▶◀ salicylates

Visken

aspirin, bismuth subsalicylate, choline salicylate, magnesium salicylate, salsalate, sodium salicylate, sodium thiosalicylate

Risk rating: 2
Severity: Moderate   **Onset: Rapid**   **Likelihood: Suspected**

Cause
Salicylates inhibit synthesis of prostaglandins, which pindolol and other beta blockers need to reduce blood pressure. In patients with heart failure, the mechanism of this interaction is unknown.

Effect
Beta blocker's effect is reduced.

Nursing considerations
- Watch closely for signs of heart failure and hypertension, and notify provider if they occur.
- Talk with prescriber about switching patient to a different antihypertensive or antiplatelet drug.
- Other beta blockers may interact with salicylates. If you suspect an interaction, consult prescriber or pharmacist.
- Explain signs and symptoms of heart failure, and tell patient when to contact prescriber.

---

pindolol ▶◀ theophyllines

Visken   aminophylline, theophylline

Risk rating: 2
Severity: Moderate   **Onset: Rapid**   **Likelihood: Probable**

Cause
Theophylline clearance may be reduced up to 50%.

Effect
Theophylline efficacy may decrease.

Nursing considerations
■ When therapy starts with a nonselective beta blocker, such as pindolol, watch for decreased theophylline efficacy.

■ Monitor serum theophylline level closely, and notify prescriber about subtherapeutic level.

■ Normal therapeutic range for theophylline is 10 to 20 mcg/ml for adults and 5 to 15 mcg/ml for children.

■ Selective beta blockers may be preferred for patients who take theophylline, but the interaction will still occur with high doses of beta blockers.

■ Other beta blockers may interact with theophyllines. If you suspect an interaction, consult prescriber or pharmacist.

---

pindolol ◄►◄ verapamil
Visken   Calan

Risk rating: **1**
Severity: **Major**   Onset: **Rapid**   Likelihood: **Probable**

Cause
Verapamil may inhibit metabolism of beta blockers, such as pindolol.

Effect
Effects of both drugs may be increased.

Nursing considerations
↘ **ALERT** Giving these drugs together increases risk of adverse effects, including heart failure, conduction disturbances, arrhythmias, and hypotension.

■ Combination therapy is, in general, effective and acceptable in patients with hypertension and unstable angina.

■ Monitor patient for adverse effects, including left ventricular dysfunction and AV conduction defects.

■ Risk of interaction is greater when drugs are given I.V.

■ Dosages of both drugs may need to be decreased.

piperacillin ━━▶◀━━ aminoglycosides

amikacin, gentamicin,
kanamycin, netilmicin,
streptomycin, tobramycin

Risk rating: 2
Severity: Moderate   Onset: **Delayed**   Likelihood: **Probable**

Cause
The mechanism of this interaction is unknown.

Effect
Piperacillin and other penicillins may inactivate certain aminoglycosides, decreasing their effects.

Nursing considerations
▶ **ALERT** Check peak and trough aminoglycoside levels after third dose. For peak level, draw blood 30 minutes after I.V. or 60 minutes after I.M. dose. For trough level, draw blood just before a dose.
- Monitor patient's renal function.
- Other aminoglycosides may interact with penicillins. If you suspect an interaction, consult prescriber or pharmacist.

piperacillin ━━▶◀━━ tetracyclines

demeclocycline, doxycycline,
minocycline, tetracycline

Risk rating: 1
Severity: Major   Onset: **Delayed**   Likelihood: **Suspected**

Cause
Tetracyclines may adversely affect the bactericidal activity of penicillins, such as piperacillin.

Effect
Penicillin efficacy may be reduced.

Nursing considerations
- If possible, avoid giving tetracyclines with penicillins.
- Monitor patient closely for lack of penicillin effect.

piroxicam ⧓ aminoglycosides

Feldene

amikacin, gentamicin, kanamycin, netilmicin, streptomycin, tobramycin

Risk rating: 2
Severity: Moderate **Onset: Delayed** **Likelihood: Suspected**

Cause
Piroxicam and other NSAIDs may reduce glomerular filtration rate (GFR), causing aminoglycosides to accumulate.

Effect
Aminoglycoside level in premature infants may increase.

Nursing considerations
- Before NSAID starts, aminoglycoside dose should be reduced.

ALERT Check peak and trough aminoglycoside levels after third dose. For peak level, draw blood 30 minutes after I.V. or 60 minutes after I.M. dose. For trough level, draw blood just before a dose.

- Monitor patient's renal function.
- Although only indomethacin is known to interact with aminoglycosides, other NSAIDs probably do as well. If you suspect an interaction, consult prescriber or pharmacist.
- Other drugs cleared by GFR may have a similar interaction.

piroxicam ⧓ beta blockers

Feldene

acebutolol, atenolol, betaxolol, bisoprolol, carteolol, esmolol, metoprolol, nadolol, penbutolol, pindolol, propranolol, sotalol, timolol

Risk rating: 2
Severity: Moderate **Onset: Delayed** **Likelihood: Probable**

Cause
Piroxicam and other NSAIDs may inhibit renal prostaglandin synthesis, allowing pressor systems to be unopposed.

Effect
Beta blocker may not be able to lower blood pressure.

Nursing considerations
- Avoid using these drugs together if possible.
- Monitor blood pressure and other evidence of hypertension closely.

■ Talk with prescriber about ways to minimize interaction, such as adjusting beta blocker dosage or switching to sulindac as the NSAID.
■ Explain the risks of using these drugs together, and teach patient how to monitor his blood pressure.
■ Other NSAIDs may interact with beta blockers. If you suspect an interaction, consult prescriber or pharmacist.

---

polymyxin B ◄► nondepolarizing muscle relaxants

atracurium, pancuronium, vecuronium

Risk rating: 2
Severity: Moderate   **Onset: Rapid**   **Likelihood: Probable**

Cause
Polymyxin B and other polypeptide antibiotics may act synergistically with nondepolarizing muscle relaxants.

Effect
Neuromuscular blockade may increase.

Nursing considerations
■ If possible, avoid using polypeptide antibiotics with nondepolarizing muscle relaxants.
■ Monitor neuromuscular function closely.
■ Dosage of nondepolarizing muscle relaxant may need adjustment.
■ Provide ventilatory support, as needed.
■ Make sure patient is adequately sedated when receiving a nondepolarizing muscle relaxant.

---

polythiazide ◄► loop diuretics

Renese

bumetanide, ethacrynic acid, furosemide, torsemide

Risk rating: 2
Severity: Moderate   **Onset: Rapid**   **Likelihood: Probable**

Cause
The mechanism of this interaction is unclear.

Effect
Because these drugs work synergistically, they may cause profound diuresis and serious electrolyte abnormalities.

Nursing considerations

- This drug combination may be used for therapeutic benefit.
- Expect increased sodium, potassium, and chloride excretion and greater diuresis.
- Monitor patient for dehydration and electrolyte abnormalities.
- Carefully adjust drugs, using small or intermittent doses.

---

potassium preparations ▶◀	potassium-sparing diuretics
potassium acetate, potassium bicarbonate, potassium chloride, potassium citrate, potassium gluconate, potassium iodine, potassium phosphate	amiloride, spironolactone, triamterene

Risk rating: **1**
Severity: **Major**   Onset: **Delayed**   Likelihood: **Established**

Cause
This interaction reduces renal elimination of potassium ions.

Effect
Risk of severe hyperkalemia increases.

Nursing considerations
▌ **ALERT** Don't use this combination unless patient has severe hypokalemia that isn't responding to either drug class alone.
- To avoid hyperkalemia, monitor potassium level when therapy starts and often thereafter.
- Tell patient to avoid high-potassium foods, such as citrus juices, bananas, spinach, broccoli, beans, potatoes, and salt substitutes.
- Urge patient to immediately report palpitations, chest pain, nausea, vomiting, paresthesias, muscle weakness, and other signs of potassium overload.

pravastatin ▶◀ azole antifungals
Pravachol

fluconazole, itraconazole,
ketoconazole, voriconazole

Risk rating: 2
Severity: **Moderate**   Onset: **Rapid**   Likelihood: **Probable**

Cause
Azole antifungals may inhibit hepatic metabolism of HMG-CoA reductase inhibitors, such as pravastatin.

Effect
Pravastatin level and adverse effects may increase.

Nursing considerations
- If possible, avoid use together.
- Pravastatin dosage may need to be decreased.
- Monitor serum cholesterol and lipid levels to assess patient's response to therapy.
- ◪ ALERT Assess patient for evidence of rhabdomyolysis, including fatigue; muscle aches and weakness; joint pain; dark, red, or cola-colored urine; weight gain; seizures; and greatly increased serum CK level.
- Pravastatin is the HMG-CoA reductase inhibitor least affected by this interaction and may be preferable for use with azole antifungals.

pravastatin ▶◀ bile acid sequestrants
Pravachol

cholestyramine, colestipol

Risk rating: 2
Severity: **Moderate**   Onset: **Delayed**   Likelihood: **Suspected**

Cause
GI absorption of HMG-CoA reductase inhibitor, such as pravastatin, may decrease.

Effect
Pravastatin effects may decrease.

Nursing considerations
- ◪ ALERT Separate pravastatin and bile acid sequestrant by at least 4 hours.
- If possible, give bile acid sequestrant before meals and HMG-CoA reductase inhibitor in the evening.
- Monitor serum cholesterol and lipid levels.

■ Obtain liver function test results at start of therapy and periodically thereafter. If ALT or AST level stays three times or more above the upper limit of normal, pravastatin will need to be stopped.
■ Help patient develop a plan to ensure proper dosage intervals.

pravastatin ⧓ cyclosporine

Pravachol — Neoral

Risk rating: **1**
Severity: **Major** Onset: **Delayed** Likelihood: **Probable**

Cause
Metabolism of certain HMG-CoA reductase inhibitors, such as pravastatin, may decrease.

Effect
Pravastatin level and adverse effects may increase.

Nursing considerations
■ If possible, avoid use together.
■ Pravastatin dosage may need to be decreased.
■ Monitor serum cholesterol and lipid levels.
ALERT Assess patient for evidence of rhabdomyolysis, including fatigue; muscle aches and weakness; joint pain; dark, red, or cola-colored urine; weight gain; seizures; and greatly increased CK level.
■ Urge patient to report muscle pain, tenderness, or weakness.

pravastatin ⧓ gemfibrozil

Pravachol — Lopid

Risk rating: **1**
Severity: **Major** Onset: **Delayed** Likelihood: **Suspected**

Cause
The mechanism of this interaction is unknown.

Effect
Severe myopathy or rhabdomyolysis may occur.

Nursing considerations
■ Avoid use together.
■ If patient has severe hyperlipidemia, combined therapy may be an option, but only with careful monitoring.
ALERT Assess patient for evidence of rhabdomyolysis, including fatigue; muscle aches and weakness; joint pain; dark, red, or cola-colored urine; weight gain; seizures; and greatly increased CK level.

■ Watch for evidence of acute renal failure, including decreased urine output, elevated BUN and creatinine levels, edema, dyspnea, tachycardia, distended neck veins, nausea, vomiting, poor appetite, weakness, fatigue, confusion, and agitation.

■ Urge patient to report muscle pain, tenderness, or weakness.

pravastatin ▶◀ rifamycins

Pravachol

rifabutin, rifampin, rifapentine

Risk rating: 2
Severity: Moderate   Onset: Delayed   Likelihood: Suspected

Cause
Rifamycins may induce CYP3A4 metabolism of pravastatin and other HMG-CoA reductase inhibitors in the intestine and liver.

Effect
Pravastatin effects may decrease.

Nursing considerations
■ Assess patient for expected response to therapy. If you suspect an interaction, consult prescriber or pharmacist.

■ Check serum cholesterol and lipid levels.

■ Obtain liver function test results at start of therapy and periodically thereafter. If ALT or AST level stays three times or more above the upper limit of normal, pravastatin will need to be stopped.

◼ ALERT Withhold HMG-CoA reductase inhibitor temporarily if patient's risk of myopathy or rhabdomyolysis increases, as from sepsis, hypotension, major surgery, trauma, uncontrolled seizures, or a severe metabolic, endocrine, or electrolyte disorder.

■ Pravastatin is the HMG-CoA reductase inhibitor least likely to interact with rifamycins and may be the best choice for combined use.

prazosin ▶◀ beta blockers

Minipress

acebutolol, atenolol, betaxolol, bisoprolol, carteolol, esmolol, metoprolol, nadolol, penbutolol, pindolol, propranolol, sotalol, timolol

Risk rating: 2
Severity: Moderate   Onset: Rapid   Likelihood: Probable

Cause
The mechanism of this interaction is unknown.

Effect
Effect of these drugs on orthostatic hypotension increases.

Nursing considerations
■ Assess patient's lying, sitting, and standing blood pressures closely, especially when combined therapy starts.
■ Adjust dosages of either drug based on patient effects.
■ To minimize effects of orthostatic hypotension, teach patient to change positions slowly.
■ Interaction is confirmed only with propranolol but may occur with other beta blockers as well.

---

prednisolone, ▶◀ **barbiturates**
prednisone   amobarbital, butabarbital, pentobarbital, phenobarbital, primidone, secobarbital

Risk rating: 2
Severity: Moderate   Onset: Delayed   Likelihood: Established

Cause
Barbiturates induce liver enzymes, which stimulate metabolism of corticosteroids, such as prednisolone and prednisone.

Effect
Corticosteroid effects may be decreased.

Nursing considerations
■ Avoid giving barbiturates with corticosteroids, if possible.
■ If patient takes a corticosteroid, watch for worsening symptoms when a barbiturate is started or stopped.
■ During barbiturate treatment, corticosteroid dosage may need to be increased.

---

prednisolone, ▶◀ **cholinesterase**
prednisone   **inhibitors**
                                 ambenonium, edrophonium, neostigmine, pyridostigmine

Risk rating: 1
Severity: Major   Onset: Delayed   Likelihood: Probable

Cause
In myasthenia gravis, prednisolone, prednisone, and other cortico-steroids antagonize the effects of cholinesterase inhibitors.

Effect

Patient may develop severe muscular depression refractory to cholinesterase inhibitor.

Nursing considerations

- Corticosteroids may have long-term benefits in myasthenia gravis.
- Combined therapy may be attempted under strict supervision.
- In myasthenia gravis, monitor patient for severe muscle deterioration.

⚠ ALERT Be prepared to provide respiratory support and mechanical ventilation if needed.

- Consult prescriber or pharmacist about safe corticosteroid delivery to maximize improvement in muscle strength.

---

prednisolone, prednisone ▶◀ estrogens

conjugated estrogens, esterified estrogens, estradiol, estrone, estropipate, ethinyl estradiol

Risk rating: 2
Severity: Moderate   Onset: Delayed   Likelihood: Suspected

Cause

Estrogens may inhibit hepatic metabolism of corticosteroids, such as prednisolone and prednisone.

Effect

Therapeutic and toxic corticosteroid effects may increase.

Nursing considerations

- Assess patient's response to corticosteroid.
- Watch for evidence of corticosteroid toxicity: nervousness, sleepiness, depression, psychosis, weakness, decreased hearing, leg edema, skin disorders, hypertension, muscle weakness, and seizures.
- If given with estrogens, corticosteroid dosage may need adjustment.
- Estrogen may continue to affect corticosteroid therapy for an unknown length of time after estrogen is stopped.
- Other corticosteroids may interact with estrogens. If you suspect an interaction, consult prescriber or pharmacist.
- Tell patient to report increased adverse effects.

prednisolone, prednisone ➤◀ hydantoins
ethotoin, fosphenytoin, phenytoin

Risk rating: 2
Severity: Moderate   **Onset: Delayed**   **Likelihood: Established**

Cause
Hydantoins induce liver enzymes, which stimulate metabolism of corticosteroids, such as prednisolone and prednisone.

Effect
Corticosteroid effects may decrease.

Nursing considerations
- Avoid giving hydantoins with corticosteroids if possible.
- Monitor patient for decreased corticosteroid effects. Also monitor phenytoin level, and adjust dosage of either drug as needed.
- Corticosteroid effects may decrease within days of starting phenytoin and may stay decreased 3 weeks after it stops.
- Dosage of either or both drugs may need to be increased.

prednisolone, prednisone ➤◀ rifamycins
rifabutin, rifampin, rifapentine

Risk rating: 1
Severity: Major   **Onset: Delayed**   **Likelihood: Established**

Cause
Rifamycins increase hepatic metabolism of corticosteroids, such as prednisolone and prednisone.

Effect
Corticosteroid effects may decrease.

Nursing considerations
- If possible, avoid giving rifamycins with corticosteroids.
- Monitor patient for decreased corticosteroid effects, including loss of disease control.
- Monitor patient closely for symptom control after increasing rifamycin dose. Drug may need to be stopped to regain control of disease.
- Corticosteroid effects may decrease within days of starting rifampin and may stay decreased 2 to 3 weeks after it stops.
- Corticosteroid dose may need to be doubled after adding rifampin.

prednisolone, prednisone ⧓ salicylates

aspirin, bismuth subsalicylate, choline salicylate, magnesium salicylate, salsalate, sodium salicylate, sodium thiosalicylate

Risk rating: **2**
Severity: **Moderate** Onset: **Delayed** Likelihood: **Probable**

Cause
Prednisolone, prednisone, and other corticosteroids stimulate hepatic metabolism of salicylates and may increase renal excretion.

Effect
Salicylate level and effects decrease.

Nursing considerations
- Monitor salicylate level and efficacy; dosage may need adjustment.

ALERT Giving a salicylate while tapering a corticosteroid may result in salicylate toxicity.

- Watch for evidence of salicylate toxicity, including diaphoresis, nausea, vomiting, tinnitus, hyperventilation, and CNS depression.
- Patients with renal impairment may be at greater risk.

primidone ⧓ alcohol

Mysoline

Risk rating: **1**
Severity: **Major** Onset: **Rapid** Likelihood: **Established**

Cause
Acute alcohol intake inhibits hepatic metabolism of barbiturates, such as primidone. Chronic alcohol use increases barbiturate clearance, probably by inducing liver enzymes.

Effect
Acute alcohol intake with barbiturates can cause impaired hand-eye coordination, additive CNS effects, and death. Chronic alcohol use with barbiturates may cause drug tolerance, a need for increased barbiturate dosage, and an increased risk of adverse effects, including death.

Nursing considerations
ALERT Because of the risk of serious adverse effects, including death, alcohol and barbiturates shouldn't be combined.

■ Before barbiturate therapy starts, assess patient thoroughly for history or evidence of alcohol use.
■ Watch for additive CNS effects, which may suggest barbiturate overdose.

---

primidone ▶◀ beta blockers

Mysoline   metoprolol, propranolol

Risk rating: 2
Severity: Moderate   **Onset: Rapid**   **Likelihood: Probable**

Cause
Increased enzyme induction and first-pass hepatic metabolism of certain beta blockers reduce their availability.

Effect
Beta blocker efficacy may be reduced.

Nursing considerations
■ Assess beta blocker efficacy by monitoring blood pressure, apical pulse, and presence of chest pain or headache, as appropriate.
■ If patient has increased angina, rhythm problems, or blood pressure problems when starting a barbiturate, such as primidone, notify prescriber promptly. Beta blocker dosage may be increased.
■ Other beta blockers may interact with barbiturates. If you suspect an interaction, consult prescriber or pharmacist.
■ Explain the potential interaction between these drugs and the need to tell prescriber about any problems.

---

primidone ▶◀ corticosteroids

Mysoline   betamethasone, corticotropin, cortisone, cosyntropin, dexamethasone, fludrocortisone, hydrocortisone, methylprednisolone, prednisolone, prednisone, triamcinolone

Risk rating: 2
Severity: Moderate   **Onset: Delayed**   **Likelihood: Established**

Cause
Primidone and other barbiturates induce liver enzymes, which stimulate corticosteroid metabolism.

Effect
Corticosteroid effects may decrease.

Nursing considerations
- Avoid giving barbiturates with corticosteroids, if possible.
- If patient takes a corticosteroid, watch for worsening symptoms when a barbiturate is started or stopped.
- During barbiturate treatment, corticosteroid dosage may need to be increased.

---

primidone ▶◀ hormonal contraceptives
Mysoline

Risk rating: 1
Severity: Major   **Onset: Delayed**   **Likelihood: Suspected**

Cause
Primidone and other barbiturates may induce hepatic metabolism of contraceptives and synthesis of sex-hormone–binding protein.

Effect
Risk of breakthrough bleeding and pregnancy may increase.

Nursing considerations
- Consult prescriber about increasing contraceptive dosage during barbiturate therapy.
- Consult prescriber about alternative treatments for seizures or sleep disturbance.
- Instruct patient to also use barrier contraception.

---

primidone ▶◀ methadone
Mysoline   Dolophine, Methadose

Risk rating: 2
Severity: Moderate   **Onset: Delayed**   **Likelihood: Suspected**

Cause
Primidone and other barbiturates probably increase hepatic metabolism of methadone.

Effect
Methadone effects may be reduced, and patients on long-term therapy may notice opioid withdrawal symptoms.

Nursing considerations
- If these drugs must be used together, monitor methadone efficacy.
- Check serum methadone level regularly.
- If methadone dosage is insufficient, it may be increased.

■ Other barbiturates interact with methadone. If you suspect an interaction, consult prescriber or pharmacist.

---

primidone ■■■■►◄■■■■ theophyllines
Mysoline   aminophylline, theophylline

Risk rating: 2
Severity: Moderate   Onset: Delayed   Likelihood: Suspected

Cause
Primidone and other barbiturates may stimulate theophylline clearance by inducing CYP.

Effect
Theophylline level and efficacy may decrease.

Nursing considerations
■ Monitor patient closely to determine theophylline efficacy.
■ Monitor serum theophylline level regularly. Normal therapeutic range is 10 to 20 mcg/ml for adults and 5 to 15 mcg/ml for children.
■ When a barbiturate is added to regimen, theophylline dosage may need to be increased.
■ Dyphylline, a theophylline, undergoes renal elimination and may not be affected by this interaction.

---

probenecid ■■■■►◄■■■■ methotrexate
Probalan   Rheumatrex, Trexall

Risk rating: 1
Severity: Major   Onset: Rapid   Likelihood: Probable

Cause
Probenecid may impair excretion of methotrexate by the kidneys.

Effect
Methotrexate level, effects, and toxicity may increase.

Nursing considerations
■ Monitor patient for methotrexate toxicity, including renal failure, neutropenia, leukopenia, thrombocytopenia, increased liver function tests, and skin ulcers.
■ Check patient for mouth sores. This may be the first outward appearance of methotrexate toxicity; however, in some patients, bone marrow suppression coincides with or precedes mouth sores.
■ Notify prescriber if signs of toxicity appear; the methotrexate dose may need to be reduced.

probenecid ◄►► salicylates

Probalan

aspirin, bismuth subsalicylate,
choline salicylate, magnesium
salicylate, salsalate, sodium
salicylate, sodium
thiosalicylate

Risk rating: 2
Severity: **Moderate**   Onset: **Delayed**   Likelihood: **Probable**

Cause
The mechanism of this interaction is unknown. It may stem from altered renal filtration of uric acid.

Effect
Combined use inhibits uricosuric action of both drugs.

Nursing considerations
◼ **ALERT** Typically, combining probenecid and a salicylate is contraindicated.

◼ Occasional use of aspirin at low doses may not interfere with uricosuric action of probenecid.

◼ Monitor serum urate level; the usual goal of probenecid therapy is about 6 mg/dl.

◼ **ALERT** Remind patient to carefully read the labels of OTC medicines because many contain salicylates.

◼ If an analgesic or antipyretic is needed during probenecid therapy, suggest acetaminophen.

◼ Advise patient to maintain adequate fluid intake to prevent formation of uric acid kidney stones.

procainamide ◄►► cimetidine

Pronestyl

Tagamet

Risk rating: 2
Severity: **Moderate**   Onset: **Rapid**   Likelihood: **Established**

Cause
Cimetidine may reduce procainamide renal clearance.

Effect
Procainamide level and risk of toxicity may increase.

Nursing considerations
◼ **ALERT** Avoid combined use if possible.

■ Monitor levels of procainamide and its active metabolite NAPA. Therapeutic range for procainamide is 4 to 8 mcg/ml; therapeutic level of NAPA is 10 to 30 mcg/ml.

■ Monitor patient for increased adverse effects, including severe hypotension, widening QRS complex, arrhythmias, seizures, oliguria, confusion, lethargy, nausea, and vomiting.

■ Procainamide dosage may need adjustment.

■ H_2-receptor antagonists other than cimetidine may interact. If you suspect an interaction, consult prescriber or pharmacist.

procainamide ▶◀ quinolones

Pronestyl   gatifloxacin, levofloxacin,
                                    moxifloxacin, sparfloxacin

Risk rating: 1
Severity: Major   **Onset: Delayed**   **Likelihood: Suspected**

Cause
The mechanism of this interaction is unknown.

Effect
Risk of life-threatening arrhythmias, including torsades de pointes, increases.

Nursing considerations
⚠ **ALERT** Giving sparfloxacin with antiarrhythmics, such as procainamide, is contraindicated.

■ Quinolones that aren't metabolized by CYP3A4 isoenzymes or that don't prolong the QT interval may be given with antiarrhythmics.

■ Avoid giving class IA or class III antiarrhythmics with gatifloxacin, levofloxacin, and moxifloxacin.

■ Monitor ECG for prolonged QTc interval.

■ Tell patient to report a rapid heartbeat, shortness of breath, dizziness, fainting, and chest pain.

procainamide ▶◀ vardenafil

Pronestyl   Levitra

Risk rating: 1
Severity: Major   **Onset: Rapid**   **Likelihood: Suspected**

Cause
The mechanism of this interaction is unknown.

Effect
QTc interval may be prolonged, particularly in patients with previous QT-interval prolongation and those taking certain antiarrhythmics (such as procainamide), increasing the risk of such life-threatening arrhythmias as torsades de pointes.

Nursing considerations
🚩 ALERT Avoid use of vardenafil with a class IA or class III antiarrhythmic.
■ Monitor ECG before and periodically after patient starts vardenafil.
■ Urge patient to report light-headedness, faintness, palpitations, and chest pain or pressure while taking vardenafil.
■ To reduce risk of adverse effects, patients age 65 and older should start with 5 mg vardenafil, half the usual starting dose.

---

prochlorperazine ➤◀ dofetilide
Compazine   Tikosyn

Risk rating: 1
Severity: Major   **Onset: Delayed**   **Likelihood: Suspected**

Cause
Dofetilide renal elimination may be inhibited.

Effect
Dofetilide level and risk of ventricular arrhythmias, including torsades de pointes, may increase.

Nursing considerations
🚩 ALERT Use of dofetilide with prochlorperazine is contraindicated.
■ Watch ECG for prolonged QTc interval and ventricular arrhythmias.
■ Monitor renal function and QTc interval every 3 months during dofetilide therapy.
■ Consult prescriber or pharmacist for alternative to prochlorperazine to control nausea, vomiting, and psychoses.

---

prochlorperazine, ➤◀ alcohol
promethazine
Compazine, Phenergan

Risk rating: 2
Severity: Moderate   **Onset: Rapid**   **Likelihood: Probable**

Cause
The mechanism of this interaction is unknown. It may be that these substances produce CNS depression by working on different sites in

the brain. Also, alcohol may lower resistance to neurotoxic effects of phenothiazines, such as prochlorperazine and promethazine.

Effect
CNS depression may increase.

Nursing considerations
■ Watch for extrapyramidal reactions, such as dystonic reactions, acute akathisia, and restlessness.
■ If patient takes a phenothiazine, warn that alcohol may worsen CNS depression and impair psychomotor skills.
■ Discourage patient from drinking alcohol when taking a pheno-thiazine.

---

prochlorperazine, promethazine ◄►◄ anticholinergics

Compazine, Phenergan

atropine, belladonna, benztropine, biperiden, dicyclomine, hyoscyamine, oxybutynin, propantheline, scopolamine

Risk rating: 2
Severity: Moderate   Onset: Delayed   Likelihood: Suspected

Cause
Anticholinergics may antagonize phenothiazines, such as prochlor-perazine and promethazine. Also, phenothiazine metabolism may increase.

Effect
Phenothiazine efficacy may decrease.

Nursing considerations
■ Data regarding this interaction conflict.
■ Monitor patient for decreased phenothiazine efficacy.
■ The phenothiazine dosage may need adjustment.
■ Anticholinergic effects may increase.
■ Monitor patient for adynamic ileus, hyperpyrexia, hypoglycemia, and neurologic changes.

prochlorperazine, ━━►◄━━ quinolones
promethazine
Compazine, Phenergan

gatifloxacin, levofloxacin,
moxifloxacin, sparfloxacin

Risk rating: 1
Severity: **Major**   Onset: **Delayed**   Likelihood: **Suspected**

Cause
The mechanism of this interaction is unknown.

Effect
Risk of life-threatening arrhythmias, including torsades de pointes,
may increase.

Nursing considerations
■ **ALERT** Sparfloxacin is contraindicated in patients taking drugs that
prolong the QTc interval, including prochlorperazine, promethazine,
and other phenothiazines.
■ Avoid giving levofloxacin.
■ Use gatifloxacin and moxifloxacin cautiously, with increased monitoring.
■ Quinolones that don't prolong the QTc interval or that aren't metabolized by CYP3A4 isoenzymes may be better alternatives.

propafenone ━━━►◄━━━ beta blockers
Rythmol

metoprolol, propranolol

Risk rating: 2
Severity: **Moderate**   Onset: **Rapid**   Likelihood: **Probable**

Cause
Propafenone inhibits first-pass metabolism of certain beta blockers
and reduces their systemic clearance.

Effect
Beta blocker effects may increase.

Nursing considerations
■ Monitor blood pressure, pulse, and cardiac complaints.
■ Notify prescriber about abnormally low blood pressure or change in
heart rate; beta blocker dosage may be decreased.
■ If patient takes metoprolol and propafenone, tell him to promptly
report nightmares or other CNS complaints.
■ To minimize effects of orthostatic hypotension, tell patient to
change positions slowly.

propafenone 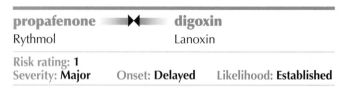 digoxin
Rythmol   Lanoxin

Risk rating: 1
Severity: **Major**   Onset: **Delayed**   Likelihood: **Established**

Cause
Exact cause of this interaction is unknown; decreased digoxin distribution and renal and nonrenal clearance of digoxin may be involved.

Effect
Digoxin level and risk of toxicity may increase.

Nursing considerations
■ Monitor digoxin level. Therapeutic range is 0.8 to 2 nanograms/ml.
■ Monitor ECG for signs of digoxin toxicity: arrhythmias (such as bradycardia and AV blocks), ventricular ectopy, and shortened QTc interval.
■ Watch for other signs of digoxin toxicity, including lethargy, drowsiness, confusion, hallucinations, headaches, syncope, visual disturbances, nausea, anorexia, failure to thrive, vomiting, and diarrhea.
■ Digoxin dosage may need adjustment if propafenone starts or stops.

propafenone 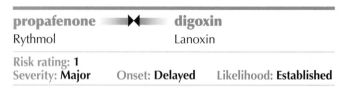 rifamycins
Rythmol   rifabutin, rifampin, rifapentine

Risk rating: 2
Severity: **Moderate**   Onset: **Delayed**   Likelihood: **Probable**

Cause
Rifamycins may enhance hepatic metabolism of propafenone.

Effect
Propafenone clearance is increased, and effects may decrease.

Nursing considerations
■ Consult prescriber about alternative anti-infective drug for patients stabilized on propafenone.
■ If this combination can't be avoided, monitor propafenone level and watch for loss of effect.
■ Propafenone dosage may need adjustment while patient takes a rifamycin.
■ This effect was seen less readily with I.V. propafenone than with the oral dosage form.

propafenone ▬▬►◄ SSRIs

Rythmol

fluoxetine, paroxetine, sertraline

Risk rating: 2
Severity: **Moderate**   Onset: **Delayed**   Likelihood: **Suspected**

Cause
Certain serotonin reuptake inhibitors may inhibit CYP2D6 metabolism of propafenone.

Effect
Serum propafenone level and risk of adverse effects may increase.

Nursing considerations
- Monitor cardiac function closely during combined therapy.
- Citalopram doesn't inhibit CYP2D6 and may be a safer choice than these SSRIs.
- Tell patient to promptly report dizziness, drowsiness, ataxia, tremor, palpitations, chest pain, edema, dyspnea, and other new symptoms.

propantheline ▬▬►◄ phenothiazines

chlorpromazine, fluphenazine, mesoridazine, perphenazine, prochlorperazine, promethazine, thioridazine, trifluoperazine

Risk rating: 2
Severity: **Moderate**   Onset: **Delayed**   Likelihood: **Suspected**

Cause
Propantheline and other anticholinergics may antagonize phenothiazines. Also, phenothiazine metabolism may increase.

Effect
Phenothiazine efficacy may decrease.

Nursing considerations
- Data regarding this interaction conflict.
- Monitor patient for decreased phenothiazine efficacy.
- Phenothiazine dosage may need adjustment.
- Anticholinergic effects may increase.

■ Monitor patient for adynamic ileus, hyperpyrexia, hypoglycemia, and neurologic changes.

propoxyphene ▬►◄▬ carbamazepine

Darvon

Carbatrol, Epitol, Equetro, Tegretol

Risk rating: 2
Severity: Moderate   **Onset: Rapid**   **Likelihood: Suspected**

Cause
Hepatic metabolism of carbamazepine is inhibited, decreasing drug clearance.

Effect
Carbamazepine level and risk of toxicity may increase.

Nursing considerations
⚠ ALERT Avoid combined use if possible.
■ Consult prescriber or pharmacist about alternative analgesics.
■ Monitor carbamazepine level; therapeutic range is 4 to 12 mcg/ml.
■ Monitor patient for signs of carbamazepine toxicity, including dizziness, ataxia, respiratory depression, tachycardia, arrhythmias, blood pressure changes, impaired consciousness, abnormal reflexes, nystagmus, seizures, nausea, vomiting, and urine retention.
■ Carbamazepine dosage may need adjustment.

propranolol ▬►◄▬ barbiturates

Inderal

amobarbital, butabarbital, pentobarbital, phenobarbital, primidone, secobarbital

Risk rating: 2
Severity: Moderate   **Onset: Rapid**   **Likelihood: Probable**

Cause
Increased enzyme induction and first-pass hepatic metabolism of certain beta blockers, such as propranolol, reduce their availability.

Effect
Beta blocker efficacy may be reduced.

Nursing considerations
■ Assess beta blocker efficacy by monitoring blood pressure, apical pulse, and presence of chest pain or headache, as appropriate.

■ If patient has increased angina, rhythm problems, or blood pressure problems when barbiturate starts, notify prescriber promptly. Beta blocker dosage may be increased.

■ Other beta blockers may interact with barbiturates. If you suspect an interaction, consult prescriber or pharmacist.

■ Explain the potential interaction between these drugs and the need to tell prescriber about any problems.

propranolol ▶◀ cimetidine
Inderal   Tagamet

Risk rating: 2
Severity: Moderate   Onset: Rapid   Likelihood: Probable

Cause
By inhibiting CYP, cimetidine reduces first-pass metabolism of certain beta blockers, such as propranolol.

Effect
Clearance of propranolol is decreased, increasing its action.

Nursing considerations
■ Monitor patient for severe bradycardia and hypotension.

■ If interaction occurs, notify prescriber; beta blocker dosage may be decreased.

■ Teach patient to monitor pulse rate. If it's significantly lower than usual, tell him to withhold beta blocker and to contact prescriber.

■ Instruct patient to change positions slowly to reduce effects of orthostatic hypotension.

■ Other beta blockers may interact with cimetidine. If you suspect an interaction, consult prescriber or pharmacist.

propranolol ▶◀ epinephrine
Inderal   Adrenalin

Risk rating: 1
Severity: Major   Onset: Rapid   Likelihood: Established

Cause
Alpha-receptor effects of epinephrine supersede the effects of nonselective beta blockers, such as propranolol, increasing vascular resistance.

Effect
Initial marked hypertensive effect is followed by reflex bradycardia.

Nursing considerations
⚡ **ALERT** Three days before planned use of epinephrine, stop the beta blocker. Or, if possible, don't use epinephrine.
■ Monitor blood pressure and pulse. If interaction occurs, give I.V. chlorpromazine, hydralazine, aminophylline, or atropine if needed.
■ Explain the risks of this interaction, and tell patient to carry medical identification at all times.
■ Other beta blockers may interact with epinephrine. If you suspect an interaction, consult prescriber or pharmacist.

---

propranolol ➤◄ ergot derivatives
Inderal   dihydroergotamine, ergotamine

Risk rating: 2
Severity: Moderate   Onset: Delayed   Likelihood: Suspected

Cause
Vasoconstriction and blockade of peripheral beta$_2$ receptors allows unopposed ergot action.

Effect
Vasoconstrictive effects of ergot derivatives increase, causing peripheral ischemia, cold extremities, and possible gangrene.

Nursing considerations
■ Watch for evidence of peripheral ischemia.
■ If needed, stop propranolol and adjust ergot derivative.
■ Other ergot derivatives may interact with propranolol and other beta blockers. If you suspect an interaction, consult prescriber or pharmacist.

---

propranolol ➤◄ hydralazine
Inderal   Apresoline

Risk rating: 2
Severity: Moderate   Onset: Rapid   Likelihood: Probable

Cause
Hydralazine may cause transient increase in visceral blood flow and decreased first-pass hepatic metabolism of some oral beta blockers, such as propranolol.

Effect
Effects of both drugs may increase.

Nursing considerations
■ Monitor blood pressure regularly, and tailor dosages of both drugs to patient's response.
■ With propranolol, interaction involves only oral, immediate-release form and not extended-release or I.V. drug.
■ Other beta blockers may interact with hydralazine. If you suspect an interaction, consult prescriber or pharmacist.
■ Explain that both drugs can affect blood pressure. Urge patient to report evidence of hypotension, such as light-headedness or dizziness when changing positions.

propranolol ▶◀ lidocaine
Inderal

Risk rating: 2
Severity: Moderate   **Onset: Rapid**   **Likelihood: Established**

Cause
Propranolol and other beta blockers reduce hepatic metabolism of lidocaine.

Effect
Lidocaine level and risk of toxicity may increase.

Nursing considerations
■ Check for normal therapeutic level of lidocaine: 2 to 5 mcg/ml.
■ Monitor patient closely for evidence of lidocaine toxicity, including dizziness, somnolence, confusion, paresthesias, and seizures.
■ Slow the I.V. bolus rate to decrease the risk of high peak level and toxic reaction.
■ Explain the warning signs of toxicity to patient and family, and tell them to contact prescriber if they have concerns.

propranolol ▶◀ NSAIDs
Inderal   ibuprofen, indomethacin,
                                     naproxen, piroxicam

Risk rating: 2
Severity: Moderate   **Onset: Delayed**   **Likelihood: Probable**

Cause
NSAIDs may inhibit renal prostaglandin synthesis, allowing pressor systems to be unopposed.

Effect
Propranolol and other beta blockers may not be able to lower blood pressure.

Nursing considerations
- Avoid using these drugs together if possible.
- Monitor blood pressure and related signs and symptoms of hypertension closely.
- Talk with prescriber about ways to minimize interaction, such as adjusting beta blocker dosage or switching to sulindac as the NSAID.
- Explain the risks of using these drugs together, and teach patient how to monitor his blood pressure.
- Other NSAIDs may interact with beta blockers. If you suspect an interaction, consult prescriber or pharmacist.

---

propranolol ➤◄ phenothiazines
Inderal   chlorpromazine, thioridazine

Risk rating: 1
Severity: Major   **Onset: Delayed**   **Likelihood: Probable**

Cause
Chlorpromazine may inhibit first-pass hepatic metabolism of propranolol. Propranolol inhibits thioridazine metabolism.

Effect
Effects of both drugs and the risk of serious adverse reactions may increase.

Nursing considerations
⚠ ALERT Use of thioridazine with propranolol is contraindicated.
- Assess patient for fatigue, lethargy, dizziness, nausea, heart failure, and agranulocytosis, all adverse reactions to propranolol.
- Educate patient and family about the risk of drug interactions.
- Beta blockers other than propranolol may interact with phenothiazines. If you suspect an interaction, consult prescriber or pharmacist.

---

propranolol ➤◄ prazosin
Inderal   Minipress

Risk rating: 2
Severity: Moderate   **Onset: Rapid**   **Likelihood: Probable**

Cause
The mechanism of this interaction is unknown.

Effect
Effect of these drugs on orthostatic hypotension is increased.

Nursing considerations
■ Assess patient's lying, sitting, and standing blood pressures closely, especially when concurrent therapy starts.
■ Adjust dosages of either drug based on patient effects.
■ To minimize effects of orthostatic hypotension, teach patient to change positions slowly.
■ Interaction is confirmed only with propranolol but may occur with other beta blockers as well.

propranolol ◖━━━▶◀ propafenone
Inderal   Rythmol

Risk rating: 2
Severity: Moderate   **Onset: Rapid**   **Likelihood: Probable**

Cause
Propafenone inhibits first-pass metabolism of certain beta blockers, such as propranolol, and reduces their systemic clearance.

Effect
Beta blocker effects may be increased.

Nursing considerations
■ Monitor blood pressure, pulse, and cardiac complaints.
■ Notify prescriber about abnormally low blood pressure or change in heart rate; beta blocker dosage may be decreased.
■ To minimize effects of orthostatic hypotension, tell patient to change positions slowly.

propranolol ◖━━━▶◀ quinidine
Inderal

Risk rating: 2
Severity: Moderate   **Onset: Rapid**   **Likelihood: Suspected**

Cause
Quinidine may inhibit metabolism of certain beta blockers, such as propranolol, in patients who are extensive metabolizers of debrisoquin.

Effect
Beta blocker effects may be increased.

Nursing considerations
- Monitor pulse and blood pressure more often during combined use.
- If pulse slows or blood pressure falls, consult prescriber. Beta blocker dosage may need to be decreased.
- Teach patient how to check blood pressure and pulse rate; tell him to do so regularly.

---

propranolol ▶◀ rifamycins
Inderal   rifabutin, rifampin, rifapentine

Risk rating: 2
Severity: **Moderate**   Onset: **Delayed**   Likelihood: **Probable**

Cause
Rifamycins increase hepatic metabolism of beta blockers, such as propranolol.

Effect
Beta blocker effects are reduced.

Nursing considerations
- Monitor blood pressure and heart rate closely to assess beta blocker efficacy.
- If beta blocker effects are decreased, consult prescriber; dosage may need to be increased.
- Teach patient how to monitor blood pressure and heart rate and when to contact prescriber.
- Other beta blockers may interact with rifamycins. If you suspect an interaction, consult prescriber or pharmacist.

---

propranolol ▶◀ salicylates
Inderal   aspirin, bismuth subsalicylate, choline salicylate, magnesium salicylate, salsalate, sodium salicylate, sodium thiosalicylate

Risk rating: 2
Severity: **Moderate**   Onset: **Rapid**   Likelihood: **Suspected**

Cause
Salicylates inhibit synthesis of prostaglandins, which propranolol and other beta blockers need to reduce blood pressure. In patients with heart failure, the mechanism of this interaction is unknown.

Effect
Beta blocker effects decrease.

Nursing considerations
■ Watch closely for signs of heart failure and hypertension, and notify provider if they occur.
■ Consult prescriber about a different antihypertensive or antiplatelet drug.
■ Other beta blockers may interact with salicylates. If you suspect an interaction, consult prescriber or pharmacist.
■ Explain signs and symptoms of heart failure, and tell patient when to contact prescriber.

---

propranolol ▶◀ thioamines
Inderal   methimazole, propylthiouracil

Risk rating: 2
Severity: Moderate   **Onset: Delayed**   **Likelihood: Probable**

Cause
Hyperthyroidism increases clearance of beta blockers, such as propranolol.

Effect
Beta blocker effects may increase when patient becomes euthyroid.

Nursing considerations
■ Before giving beta blocker, assess blood pressure and apical pulse.
■ Watch for increased beta blocker effects, including hypotension, bradycardia, dizziness, and lethargy.
■ When hyperthyroid patient becomes euthyroid, beta blocker dosage may need to be reduced.
■ Other beta blockers may interact with thioamines. If you suspect an interaction, consult prescriber or pharmacist.
■ Caution patient not to stop a beta blocker abruptly.

---

propranolol ▶◀ verapamil
Inderal   Calan

Risk rating: 1
Severity: Major   **Onset: Rapid**   **Likelihood: Probable**

Cause
Verapamil may inhibit metabolism of beta blockers, such as propranolol.

Effect
Effects of both drugs may be increased.

Nursing considerations
- Combination therapy is common in patients with hypertension and unstable angina.
- **⚠ ALERT** Giving these drugs together increases risk of adverse effects, including heart failure, conduction disturbances, arrhythmias, and hypotension.
- Assess patient for increased risk of adverse effects, including left ventricular dysfunction and AV conduction defects.
- Risk of interaction is greater when drugs are given I.V.
- Monitor cardiac function.
- Dosages of both drugs may need to be decreased.

---

propylthiouracil ➤◀ beta blockers
metoprolol, propranolol

Risk rating: 2
Severity: Moderate   Onset: Delayed   Likelihood: Probable

Cause
Hyperthyroidism increases clearance of beta blockers.

Effect
Beta blocker effects may increase when patient becomes euthyroid.

Nursing considerations
- Before giving beta blocker, assess blood pressure and apical pulse.
- Watch for increased beta blocker effects including hypotension, bradycardia, dizziness, and lethargy.
- When hyperthyroid patient becomes euthyroid, beta blocker dosage may need to be reduced.
- Other beta blockers may interact with thioamines, such as propylthiouracil. If you suspect an interaction, consult prescriber or pharmacist.
- Caution patient not to stop a beta blocker abruptly.

propylthiouracil ➡◀ theophyllines
aminophylline, theophylline

Risk rating: **2**
Severity: **Moderate**   Onset: **Delayed**   Likelihood: **Suspected**

Cause
Propylthiouracil and other thioamines increase theophylline clearance when patient is in hyperthyroid state.

Effect
Theophylline level and effects decrease.

Nursing considerations
■ Watch closely for decreased theophylline efficacy while abnormal thyroid status continues.
◪ ALERT Assess patient for return to euthyroid state, when interaction no longer occurs.
■ Explain that hyperthyroidism and hypothyroidism can affect theophylline efficacy and toxicity; tell patient to immediately report evidence of either one to prescriber.
■ To prevent this interaction, urge patients to have TSH and theophylline levels tested regularly.

pseudoephedrine ➡◀ MAO inhibitors
Sudafed
isocarboxazid, phenelzine, tranylcypromine

Risk rating: **1**
Severity: **Major**   Onset: **Rapid**   Likelihood: **Established**

Cause
When MAO is inhibited, norepinephrine accumulates and is released by indirect-acting sympathomimetics, such as pseudoephedrine, increasing the pressor response at receptor sites.

Effect
Risk of severe headaches, hypertension, high fever, and hypertensive crisis increases.

Nursing considerations
■ Avoid giving indirect-acting sympathomimetic with MAO inhibitor.
◪ ALERT Warn patient that OTC medicines, such as decongestants, may cause this interaction.

pyridostigmine ▶◀ corticosteroids

Mestinon

betamethasone, corticotropin, cortisone, cosyntropin, dexamethasone, fludrocortisone, hydrocortisone, methylprednisolone, prednisolone, prednisone, triamcinolone

Risk rating: 1
Severity: Major   **Onset: Delayed**   **Likelihood: Probable**

Cause
In myasthenia gravis, corticosteroids antagonize cholinesterase inhibitors, such as pyridostigmine, by an unknown mechanism.

Effect
Patient may develop severe muscular depression refractory to cholinesterase inhibitor.

Nursing considerations
■ Corticosteroids may have long-term benefits in myasthenia gravis.
■ Combined therapy may be attempted under strict supervision.
■ In myasthenia gravis, monitor patient for severe muscle deterioration.
⚠ ALERT Be prepared to provide respiratory support and mechanical ventilation if needed.
■ Consult prescriber or pharmacist about safe corticosteroid delivery to maximize improvement in muscle strength.

quazepam ▶◀ alcohol

Doral

Risk rating: 2
Severity: Moderate   **Onset: Rapid**   **Likelihood: Established**

Cause
Alcohol inhibits hepatic enzymes, which decreases clearance and increases peak levels of benzodiazepines, such as quazepam.

Effect
Additive or synergistic effects may occur.

Nursing considerations
■ Advise against consuming alcohol while taking a benzodiazepine.

■ Before benzodiazepine therapy starts, assess patient thoroughly for history or evidence of alcohol use.
■ Watch for additive CNS effects, which may suggest benzodiazepine overdose.

---

quazepam ▶◀ azole antifungals
Doral

fluconazole, itraconazole, ketoconazole, miconazole

Risk rating: 2
Severity: Moderate **Onset: Rapid** **Likelihood: Established**

Cause
Azole antifungals decrease CYP3A4 metabolism of certain benzodiazepines, such as quazepam.

Effect
Benzodiazepine effects are increased and prolonged, which may cause CNS depression and psychomotor impairment.

Nursing considerations
■ Various benzodiazepine–azole antifungal combinations may interact. If you suspect an interaction, consult prescriber or pharmacist.
■ If patient takes fluconazole or miconazole, consult prescriber about giving a lower benzodiazepine dose or a drug not metabolized by CYP3A4, such as temazepam or lorazepam.
■ Caution that the effects of this interaction may last several days after stopping the azole antifungal.
■ Explain that taking these drugs together may increase sedative effects; tell patient to report such effects promptly.

---

quazepam ▶◀ protease inhibitors
Doral

amprenavir, atazanavir, indinavir, lopinavir-ritonavir, nelfinavir, ritonavir, saquinavir

Rating: 2
Severity: Moderate **Onset: Delayed** **Likelihood: Suspected**

Cause
Protease inhibitors may inhibit CYP3A4 metabolism of certain benzodiazepines, such as quazepam.

Effect
Sedative effects may be increased and prolonged, leading to severe respiratory depression.

Nursing considerations
⚡ **ALERT** Don't combine quazepam with protease inhibitors.
- If patient takes any benzodiazepine–protease inhibitor combination, notify prescriber. Interaction could involve other drugs in the class.
- Watch for evidence of oversedation and respiratory depression.
- Teach patient and family about the risks of using these drugs together.

---

quazepam ▸◂ rifamycins
Doral   rifabutin, rifampin, rifapentine

Risk rating: 2
Severity: **Moderate**   Onset: **Delayed**   Likelihood: **Suspected**

Cause
Rifamycins may increase CYP3A4 metabolism of benzodiazepines, such as quazepam.

Effect
Antianxiety, sedative, and sleep-inducing effects of benzodiazepines may decrease.

Nursing considerations
- Watch for expected benzodiazepine effects and lack of efficacy.
- If benzodiazepine efficacy is reduced, notify prescriber; dosage may be changed.
- Other benzodiazepines may interact with rifamycins. If you suspect an interaction, consult prescriber or pharmacist.
- For insomnia, temazepam may be more effective because it doesn't undergo CYP3A4 metabolism.

---

quinapril ▸◂ indomethacin
Accupril   Indocin

Risk rating: 2
Severity: **Moderate**   Onset: **Rapid**   Likelihood: **Probable**

Cause
Indomethacin inhibits synthesis of prostaglandins, which quinapril and other ACE inhibitors need to lower blood pressure.

Effect
ACE inhibitor's hypotensive effect will be reduced.

Nursing considerations
⚠ ALERT Monitor blood pressure closely. Severe hypertension may persist until indomethacin is stopped.
■ If indomethacin can't be avoided, patient may need a different antihypertensive.
■ Other ACE inhibitors may interact with indomethacin. If you suspect an interaction, consult prescriber or pharmacist.
■ Remind patient that hypertension commonly causes no physical symptoms but sometimes may cause headache and dizziness.

---

quinapril ━━━━━◄►━━━━━ **potassium-sparing diuretics**
Accupril

amiloride, spironolactone, triamterene

Risk rating: 1
Severity: Major   Onset: **Delayed**   Likelihood: **Probable**

Cause
The mechanism of this interaction is unknown.

Effect
Serum potassium level may increase.

Nursing considerations
■ Use cautiously in patients at high risk for hyperkalemia, especially those with renal impairment.
■ Monitor BUN, creatinine, and serum potassium levels as needed.
■ ACE inhibitors other than quinapril may interact with potassium-sparing diuretics. If you suspect an interaction, consult prescriber or pharmacist.
■ Urge patient to immediately report an irregular heartbeat, a slow pulse, weakness, and other evidence of hyperkalemia.

quinapril ━━━▶◀━━━ salicylates

Accupril

aspirin, bismuth subsalicylate, choline salicylate, magnesium salicylate, salsalate, sodium salicylate

Risk rating: 2
Severity: Moderate   **Onset: Rapid**   **Likelihood: Suspected**

Cause
Salicylates inhibit synthesis of prostaglandins, which quinapril and other ACE inhibitors need to lower blood pressure.

Effect
ACE inhibitor's hypotensive effect will be reduced.

Nursing considerations
■ This interaction is more likely in people with hypertension, coronary artery disease, or possibly heart failure.

quinidine ━━━▶◀━━━ amiloride

Midamor

Risk rating: 1
Severity: Major   **Onset: Delayed**   **Likelihood: Suspected**

Cause
This interaction may result from a synergistic increase in myocardial sodium channel blockade.

Effect
Quinidine effects may be reversed, contributing to a proarrhythmic state.

Nursing considerations
■ If possible, avoid combining quinidine and amiloride.
■ If unavoidable, monitor ECG closely.
■ Therapeutic range of quinidine is 2 to 6 mcg/ml. More specific assays have levels of less than 1 mcg/ml.
■ Monitor patient for loss of arrhythmia control.
■ Advise patient to report palpitations, shortness of breath, dizziness or fainting, and chest pain.

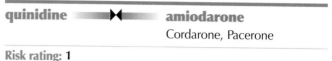

quinidine ◄► **amiodarone**
Cordarone, Pacerone

Risk rating: 1
Severity: Major   **Onset: Rapid**   **Likelihood: Probable**

Cause
The mechanism of this interaction is unknown.

Effect
Risk of potentially fatal arrhythmias increases.

Nursing considerations
- If possible, avoid combining quinidine and amiodarone.
- If unavoidable, monitor ECG closely for prolonged QTc interval, increasing ventricular ectopy, and torsades de pointes.
- Therapeutic range of quinidine is 2 to 6 mcg/ml. More specific assays have levels of less than 1 mcg/ml.
- Monitor patient for signs and symptoms of quinidine toxicity, including GI irritation, arrhythmias, hypotension, vertigo, and rash.
- Advise patient to report palpitations, shortness of breath, dizziness or fainting, and chest pain.
- If amiodarone is stopped in a patient stabilized on combined therapy, quinidine dosage may need to be increased.

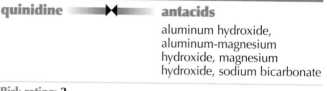

quinidine ◄► **antacids**
aluminum hydroxide,
aluminum-magnesium
hydroxide, magnesium
hydroxide, sodium bicarbonate

Risk rating: 2
Severity: Moderate   **Onset: Delayed**   **Likelihood: Suspected**

Cause
Interaction may result from a pH-related decrease in urinary quinidine excretion.

Effect
Quinidine level and risk of toxicity may increase.

Nursing considerations
- Monitor quinidine level closely during combined use.
- Therapeutic range of quinidine is 2 to 6 mcg/ml. More specific assays have levels of less than 1 mcg/ml.
- Monitor patient for evidence of quinidine toxicity, including GI irritation, arrhythmias, hypotension, vertigo, and rash.

■ Advise patient to report palpitations, shortness of breath, dizziness or fainting, and chest pain.
■ Aluminum-only antacid may be a suitable alternative.

---

quinidine ━━►◄━━ **barbiturates**
amobarbital, butabarbital, pentobarbital, phenobarbital, primidone, secobarbital

Risk rating: 2
Severity: Moderate   **Onset: Delayed**   **Likelihood: Probable**

Cause
Metabolic clearance of quinidine is increased.

Effect
Barbiturates decrease quinidine level and reduce elimination half-life.

Nursing considerations
■ Closely monitor quinidine level if barbiturate is started or stopped.
■ Therapeutic range of quinidine is 2 to 6 mcg/ml. More specific assays have levels of less than 1 mcg/ml.
■ Monitor patient for loss of arrhythmia control.
■ Advise patient to report palpitations, shortness of breath, dizziness or fainting, and chest pain.

---

quinidine ━━►◄━━ **beta blockers**
atenolol, metoprolol, propranolol, timolol

Risk rating: 2
Severity: Moderate   **Onset: Rapid**   **Likelihood: Suspected**

Cause
Quinidine may inhibit metabolism of certain beta blockers in patients who are extensive metabolizers of debrisoquin.

Effect
Beta blocker effects may increase.

Nursing considerations
■ Monitor pulse and blood pressure more often during combined use.
■ If pulse slows or blood pressure falls, consult prescriber. Beta blocker dosage may need to be decreased.

■ Teach patient how to check blood pressure and pulse rate; tell him to do so regularly.
■ If patient uses timolol eye drops, warn about possible systemic effects, including slow pulse and low blood pressure; urge patient to notify prescriber promptly if they occur.

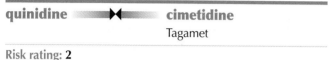

quinidine   cimetidine
Tagamet

Risk rating: 2
Severity: Moderate   **Onset: Delayed**   **Likelihood: Probable**

Cause
Interaction may result from increased quinidine absorption, decreased quinidine metabolism, or both.

Effect
Quinidine effects and risk of toxicity increase.

Nursing considerations
■ If possible, use of quinidine with cimetidine should be avoided.
■ Monitor quinidine level closely; dose may need to be reduced.
■ Therapeutic range of quinidine is 2 to 6 mcg/ml. More specific assays have levels of less than 1 mcg/ml.
■ **ALERT** Monitor patient for evidence of quinidine toxicity, including GI irritation, arrhythmias, hypotension, vertigo, and rash.
■ Advise patient to report palpitations, shortness of breath, dizziness or fainting, and chest pain.

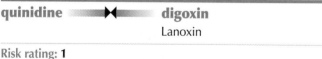

quinidine   digoxin
Lanoxin

Risk rating: 1
Severity: Major   **Onset: Delayed**   **Likelihood: Established**

Cause
Total renal and biliary digoxin clearance and distribution decrease.

Effect
Digoxin level and risk of toxicity may increase.

Nursing considerations
■ Monitor digoxin level. Therapeutic range is 0.8 to 2 nanograms/ml.
■ For some patients, digoxin toxicity may occur even within therapeutic range.

■ Watch for evidence of digoxin toxicity, including arrhythmias (such as bradycardia, AV blocks, and ventricular ectopy), lethargy, drowsiness, confusion, hallucinations, headaches, syncope, visual disturbances, nausea, anorexia, vomiting, and diarrhea.

■ Digoxin dosage may need adjustment (up to 50% reduction in some patients) if quinidine is started.

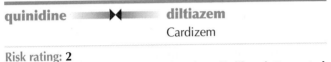

quinidine ▶◀ diltiazem
Cardizem

Risk rating: 2
Severity: Moderate   **Onset: Delayed**   **Likelihood: Suspected**

Cause
Hepatic metabolism of quinidine may be inhibited.

Effect
Quinidine effects, including toxic effects, may increase.

Nursing considerations
■ Check serum quinidine level; therapeutic range is 2 to 6 mcg/ml.
■ Monitor ECG for widened QRS complexes, prolonged QT and PR intervals, and ventricular arrhythmias, including torsades de pointes.
■ Watch for evidence of quinidine toxicity: hypotension, seizures, ataxia, anuria, respiratory distress, irritability, and hallucinations.
■ Advise patient that adverse GI effects, especially diarrhea, may be an indicator of quinidine toxicity. Tell patient to alert prescriber.
■ Adjust the quinidine dosage as ordered.

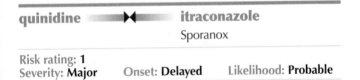

quinidine ▶◀ itraconazole
Sporanox

Risk rating: 1
Severity: Major   **Onset: Delayed**   **Likelihood: Probable**

Cause
Itraconazole may inhibit the CYP3A4 metabolism and renal excretion of quinidine.

Effect
Increased quinidine level may cause serious arrhythmias.

Nursing considerations
■ **ALERT** Use of quinidine with itraconazole is contraindicated.
■ **ALERT** Monitor patient for evidence of quinidine toxicity, including GI irritation, arrhythmias, hypotension, vertigo, and rash.

■ Advise patient to report palpitations, shortness of breath, dizziness or fainting, and chest pain.

---

quinidine ◀▶ phenytoin
Dilantin

Risk rating: 2
Severity: Moderate **Onset: Delayed** **Likelihood: Suspected**

Cause
Phenytoin stimulates the hepatic enzyme system, which increases quinidine metabolism.

Effect
Quinidine level decreases.

Nursing considerations
■ Monitor quinidine level during combined use.
■ Therapeutic range of quinidine is 2 to 6 mcg/ml. More specific assays have levels of less than 1 mcg/ml.
■ Monitor patient for loss of arrhythmia control if phenytoin starts.
■ Tell patient to report palpitations, shortness of breath, dizziness or fainting, and chest pain.
■ If patient's quinidine level is stable on combined therapy, and phenytoin is stopped, monitor patient for toxicity.
◤ ALERT Quinidine toxicity may cause GI irritation, arrhythmias, hypotension, vertigo, and rash.

---

quinidine ◀▶ protease inhibitors
nelfinavir, ritonavir

Risk rating: 1
Severity: Major **Onset: Delayed** **Likelihood: Suspected**

Cause
CYP3A4 metabolism of quinidine may be inhibited.

Effect
Quinidine level and risk of toxicity may increase.

Nursing considerations
◤ ALERT Use of ritonavir or nelfinavir with quinidine is contraindicated.
■ Monitor ECG for prolonged QT interval and arrhythmias.
◤ ALERT Quinidine toxicity may cause GI irritation, arrhythmias, hypotension, vertigo, and rash.

quinidine ━━━►◄━━━ quinolones
gatifloxacin, levofloxacin, moxifloxacin, sparfloxacin

Risk rating: 1
Severity: Major   **Onset: Delayed**   **Likelihood: Suspected**

Cause
The mechanism of this interaction is unknown.

Effect
Risk of life-threatening arrhythmias, including torsades de pointes, increases.

Nursing considerations
⚠ **ALERT** Giving sparfloxacin with antiarrhythmics, such as quinidine, is contraindicated.
■ Quinolones that aren't metabolized by CYP3A4 isoenzymes or that don't prolong the QT interval may be given with antiarrhythmics.
■ Avoid giving class IA or class III antiarrhythmics with gatifloxacin, levofloxacin, and moxifloxacin.
■ Monitor ECG for prolonged QTc interval.
■ Tell patient to report a rapid heartbeat, shortness of breath, dizziness, fainting, and chest pain.

quinidine ━━━►◄━━━ verapamil
Calan

Risk rating: 1
Severity: Major   **Onset: Rapid**   **Likelihood: Suspected**

Cause
Verapamil may interfere with quinidine clearance and prolong its half-life.

Effect
Serious cardiac events may result.

Nursing considerations
■ Use together only when there are no other alternatives.
■ Monitor patient for hypotension, bradycardia, ventricular tachycardia, and AV block.
■ Tell patient to report diaphoresis, dizziness or fainting, blurred vision, palpitations, shortness of breath, and chest pain.
■ Notify prescriber if arrhythmias occur. One or both drugs may need to be stopped.

■ The complications of this interaction may be noticed in a little as 1 day or after as long as 5 months of combined use.

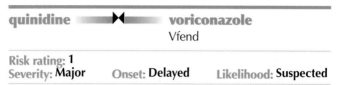

quinidine voriconazole
Vfend

Risk rating: 1
Severity: Major   **Onset:** Delayed   **Likelihood:** Suspected

Cause
Voriconazole may inhibit CYP3A4 metabolism of quinidine.

Effect
Life-threatening arrhythmias, including torsades de pointes, may occur.

Nursing considerations
◣ **ALERT** Use of quinidine with voriconazole is contraindicated.
◣ **ALERT** Quinidine toxicity may cause GI irritation, arrhythmias, hypotension, vertigo, and rash.
■ Monitor ECG for prolonged QT interval and arrhythmias.

quinine derivatives ketoconazole
quinidine, quinine   Nizoral

Risk rating: 2
Severity: Moderate   **Onset:** Delayed   **Likelihood:** Suspected

Cause
Hepatic CYP3A4 metabolism of quinine derivative is inhibited.

Effect
Quinine derivative level may increase, resulting in toxicity.

Nursing considerations
■ When starting or stopping ketoconazole, monitor quinidine level.
■ Therapeutic range of quinidine is 2 to 6 mcg/ml. More specific assays have levels of less than 1 mcg/ml.
■ Monitor ECG for conduction disturbances, prolonged QTc interval, and increased ventricular ectopy.
■ Urge patient to report palpitations, chest pain, dizziness, and shortness of breath.

quinine derivatives ▶◀ nondepolarizing muscle relaxants
quinidine, quinine

atracurium, pancuronium, vecuronium

Risk rating: 2
Severity: Moderate   **Onset: Rapid**   **Likelihood: Suspected**

Cause
Quinine derivatives may act synergistically with nondepolarizing muscle relaxants.

Effect
Effects of nondepolarizing muscle relaxants may increase.

Nursing considerations
◤ **ALERT** This interaction may be life-threatening. Monitor neuromuscular function closely.
■ The intensity and duration of neuromuscular blockade may be affected.
■ The dosage of nondepolarizing muscle relaxant may need adjustment.
■ Provide ventilatory support, as needed.
■ Make sure patient is adequately sedated when receiving a nondepolarizing muscle relaxant.

quinine derivatives ▶◀ rifamycins
quinidine, quinine   rifabutin, rifampin, rifapentine

Risk rating: 2
Severity: Moderate   **Onset: Delayed**   **Likelihood: Probable**

Cause
Rifamycins are potent inducers of hepatic enzymes and increase quinidine clearance.

Effect
Quinine derivative level and effects may decrease.

Nursing considerations
■ Therapeutic range of quinidine is 2 to 6 mcg/ml. More specific assays have levels of less than 1 mcg/ml.
■ Monitor patient for loss of arrhythmia control.
■ If rifamycin is added to a stable quinidine regimen, rifamycin dosage may be increased.
◤ **ALERT** Stopping a rifamycin during quinidine therapy may cause dose-related toxicity. Monitor quinidine level and ECG closely.

- Enzyme induction may persist for several days after rifamycin stops.
- Urge patient to report palpitations, chest pain, dizziness, and shortness of breath.

rabeprazole ▶◀ azole antifungals
Aciphex   itraconazole, ketoconazole

Risk rating: 2
Severity: Moderate   **Onset: Rapid**   **Likelihood: Suspected**

Cause
Proton pump inhibitors, such as rabeprazole, increase gastric pH, which may impair dissolution of azole antifungals.

Effect
Efficacy of azole antifungals may decrease.

Nursing considerations
- Tell prescriber if patient takes both drugs; options may be available.
- If no alternative is possible, suggest taking the azole antifungal with an acidic beverage, such as cola.
- Monitor patient for lack of response to antifungal drug.
- If patient can't tolerate acidic beverages and antifungal therapy appears to be ineffective, antifungal dosage may need to be increased.
- Other drugs that increase gastric pH may interact with azole antifungals. If you suspect an interaction, consult prescriber or pharmacist.

ramipril ▶◀ indomethacin
Altase   Indocin

Risk rating: 2
Severity: Moderate   **Onset: Rapid**   **Likelihood: Probable**

Cause
Indomethacin inhibits synthesis of prostaglandins, which ramipril and other ACE inhibitors need to lower blood pressure.

Effect
ACE inhibitor's hypotensive effect will decrease.

Nursing considerations
⚡ ALERT Monitor blood pressure closely. Severe hypertension may persist until indomethacin is stopped.
- If indomethacin can't be avoided, patient may need a different antihypertensive.

■ Other ACE inhibitors may interact with indomethacin. If you suspect an interaction, consult prescriber or pharmacist.
■ Remind patient that hypertension commonly causes no physical symptoms but sometimes may cause headache and dizziness.

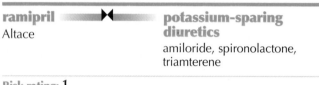

ramipril
Altace

potassium-sparing diuretics
amiloride, spironolactone, triamterene

Risk rating: 1
Severity: Major   **Onset: Delayed**   **Likelihood: Probable**

Cause
The mechanism of this interaction is unknown.

Effect
Serum potassium level may increase.

Nursing considerations
■ Use cautiously in patients at high risk for hyperkalemia, especially those with renal impairment.
■ Monitor BUN, creatinine, and serum potassium levels as needed.
■ ACE inhibitors other than ramipril may interact with potassium-sparing diuretics. If you suspect an interaction, consult prescriber or pharmacist.
■ Urge patient to immediately report an irregular heartbeat, a slow pulse, weakness, and other evidence of hyperkalemia.

ramipril
Altace

salicylates
aspirin, bismuth subsalicylate, choline salicylate, magnesium salicylate, salsalate, sodium salicylate

Risk rating: 2
Severity: Moderate   **Onset: Rapid**   **Likelihood: Suspected**

Cause
Salicylates inhibit synthesis of prostaglandins, which ramipril and other ACE inhibitors need to lower blood pressure.

Effect
ACE inhibitor's hypotensive effect will be reduced.

Nursing considerations
■ This interaction is more likely in people with hypertension, coronary artery disease, and possibly heart failure.

---

repaglinide ▸◂ macrolide antibiotics
Prandin   clarithromycin, erythromycin

Risk rating: 2
Severity: Moderate   **Onset: Delayed**   **Likelihood: Suspected**

Cause
Certain macrolide antibiotics may inhibit repaglinide metabolism.

Effect
Repaglinide level and effects, including adverse effects, may increase.

Nursing considerations
■ Monitor blood glucose level closely when starting or stopping a macrolide antibiotic.
■ Adjust repaglinide dose as needed.
■ Monitor patient for evidence of hypoglycemia, including hunger, dizziness, shakiness, sweating, confusion, and light-headedness.
■ Advise patient to carry glucose tablets or another simple sugar in case of hypoglycemia.
■ Make sure patient and family know what to do about hypoglycemia.

---

rifamycins ▸◂ azole antifungals
rifabutin, rifampin,   fluconazole, itraconazole,
rifapentine   ketoconazole, miconazole

Risk rating: 2
Severity: Moderate   **Onset: Delayed**   **Likelihood: Suspected**

Cause
Rifamycins may decrease azole antifungal levels. Also, ketoconazole may decease rifampin level.

Effect
Infection may recur.

Nursing considerations
■ Notify prescriber if patient takes both drugs; an alternative may be available.
■ If drugs must be taken together and the antifungal appears ineffective, antifungal dosage may need to be increased.

■ Teach patient to recognize signs and symptoms of his infection and to contact prescriber promptly if they occur.
■ If ketoconazole and rifampin must be taken together, separate doses by 12 hours.

---

rifamycins ▶◀ benzodiazepines

| rifabutin, rifampin, rifapentine | alprazolam, chlordiazepoxide, clonazepam, clorazepate, diazepam, estazolam, flurazepam, midazolam, quazepam, triazolam |

Risk rating: 2
Severity: Moderate   Onset: Delayed   Likelihood: Suspected

Cause
Rifamycins may increase CYP3A4 metabolism of benzodiazepines.

Effect
Antianxiety, sedative, and sleep-inducing effects of benzodiazepines may be decreased.

Nursing considerations
■ Watch for expected benzodiazepine effects and lack of efficacy.
■ If benzodiazepine efficacy is reduced, notify prescriber; dosage may be changed.
■ Other benzodiazepines may interact with rifamycins. If you suspect an interaction, consult prescriber or pharmacist.
■ For insomnia, temazepam may be more effective because it doesn't undergo CYP3A4 metabolism.

---

rifamycins ▶◀ beta blockers

| rifabutin, rifampin, rifapentine | bisoprolol, metoprolol, propranolol |

Risk rating: 2
Severity: Moderate   Onset: Delayed   Likelihood: Probable

Cause
Rifamycins increase hepatic metabolism of beta blockers.

Effect
Beta blocker effects are reduced.

Nursing considerations

■ Monitor blood pressure and heart rate closely to assess beta blocker efficacy.

■ If beta blocker effects are decreased, consult prescriber; dosage may need to be increased.

■ Teach patient how to monitor blood pressure and heart rate and when to contact prescriber.

■ Other beta blockers may interact with rifamycins. If you suspect an interaction, consult prescriber or pharmacist.

rifamycins ▶◀ corticosteroids

rifabutin, rifampin, rifapentine

betamethasone, cortisone, dexamethasone, fludrocortisone, hydrocortisone, methylprednisolone, prednisolone, prednisone, triamcinolone

Risk rating: 1
Severity: Major   **Onset: Delayed**   **Likelihood: Established**

Cause
Rifamycins increase hepatic metabolism of corticosteroid.

Effect
Corticosteroid effects may be decreased.

Nursing considerations

■ If possible, avoid giving rifamycins with corticosteroids.

■ Monitor patient for decreased corticosteroid effects, including loss of disease control.

■ Monitor patient closely for symptom control after increasing rifamycin dose. Drug may need to be stopped to regain control of disease.

■ Corticosteroid effects may decrease within days of starting rifampin and may stay decreased 2 to 3 weeks after it stops.

■ Corticosteroid dose may need to be doubled after adding rifampin.

rifamycins ▶◀ estrogens

rifabutin, rifampin, rifapentine

conjugated estrogens, esterified estrogens, estradiol, estrone, estropipate, ethinyl estradiol

Risk rating: 2
Severity: Moderate   Onset: **Delayed**   Likelihood: **Suspected**

Cause
Rifamycins induce hepatic metabolism of estrogens, leading to increased estrogen elimination and decreased estrogen levels.

Effect
Estrogen efficacy may be reduced.

Nursing considerations
■ If patient takes a rifamycin and estrogen, watch for menstrual disturbances, such as spotting, intermenstrual bleeding, and amenorrhea.
■ Estrogen dose may need to be increased during rifamycin therapy; consult prescriber or pharmacist.
■ If patient takes a rifamycin anti-infective, suggest using a nonhormonal contraceptive.
■ Explain that contraception may fail during combined therapy.
■ Urge patient to take the full course of rifamycin anti-infective exactly as prescribed to minimize risk of continued infection.

rifamycins ▶◀ HMG-CoA reductase inhibitors

rifabutin, rifampin, rifapentine

atorvastatin, fluvastatin, lovastatin, pravastatin, simvastatin

Risk rating: 2
Severity: Moderate   Onset: **Delayed**   Likelihood: **Suspected**

Cause
Rifamycins may induce CYP3A4 metabolism of HMG-CoA reductase inhibitors in the intestine and liver.

Effect
HMG-CoA reductase inhibitor effects may decrease.

Nursing considerations
■ Assess patient for expected response to therapy. If you suspect an

interaction, consult prescriber or pharmacist; patient may need a different drug.

■ Check serum cholesterol and lipid levels.

■ Obtain liver function test results at start of therapy and periodically thereafter. If ALT or AST level stays three times or more above the upper limit of normal, HMG-CoA reductase inhibitor will need to be stopped.

■ Withhold HMG-CoA reductase inhibitor temporarily if patient's risk of myopathy or rhabdomyolysis increases, as from sepsis, hypotension, major surgery, trauma, uncontrolled seizures, or a severe metabolic, endocrine, or electrolyte disorder.

⚡ **ALERT** Pravastatin is less likely to interact with rifamycins and may be the best choice for combined use.

---

rifamycins ═══►◄═══ macrolide antibiotics

rifabutin, rifampin, rifapentine

clarithromycin, erythromycin

Risk rating: 2
Severity: Moderate   **Onset: Delayed**   **Likelihood: Suspected**

Cause
Rifamycin metabolism may be inhibited and macrolide antibiotic metabolism may increase.

Effect
Adverse effects of rifamycins may increase. Antimicrobial effects of macrolide antibiotics may decrease.

Nursing considerations
■ Monitor patient for increased rifamycin adverse effects, such as abdominal pain, anorexia, nausea, vomiting, diarrhea, and rash.

■ Monitor patient for decreased response to macrolide antibiotic.

■ When given together, rifabutin and clarithromycin usually cause nausea, vomiting, and diarrhea. This interaction doesn't occur with azithromycin or dirithromycin; these drugs may be better choices.

■ Giving azithromycin or clarithromycin with rifabutin may increase the risk of neutropenia.

rifamycins ▶◀ quinine derivatives

rifabutin, rifampin,
rifapentine

quinidine, quinine

Risk rating: 2
Severity: Moderate   **Onset: Delayed**   **Likelihood: Probable**

Cause
Rifamycins are potent inducers of hepatic enzymes and increase
quinidine clearance.

Effect
Quinine derivative level and effects may decrease.

Nursing considerations
■ Therapeutic range of quinidine is 2 to 6 mcg/ml. More specific as-
says have levels of less than 1 mcg/ml.
■ Monitor patient for loss of arrhythmia control.
■ If rifamycin is added to a stable quinidine regimen, rifamycin
dosage may be increased.
◤ **ALERT** Stopping a rifamycin during quinidine therapy may cause
dose-related toxicity. Monitor quinidine level and ECG closely.
■ Enzyme induction may persist for several days after rifamycin stops.
■ Urge patient to report palpitations, chest pain, dizziness, and short-
ness of breath.

rifamycins ▶◀ sulfonylureas

rifabutin, rifampin,
rifapentine

acetohexamide, chlorpropamide, glipizide, glyburide,
tolazamide, tolbutamide

Risk rating: 2
Severity: Moderate   **Onset: Delayed**   **Likelihood: Probable**

Cause
Rifamycins may increase hepatic metabolism of certain sulfonylureas.

Effect
Risk of hyperglycemia increases.

Nursing considerations
■ Use these drugs together cautiously.
■ Monitor blood glucose level regularly, and consult prescriber about
adjustments to either drug to maintain stable glucose level.
■ Tell patient to stay alert for increased fatigue, thirst, eating, or urination and possible blurred vision or dry skin and mucous membranes
as evidence of high blood glucose level.

rifamycins ▶◀ theophyllines

rifabutin, rifampin, rifapentine

aminophylline, theophylline

Risk rating: 2
Severity: Moderate   **Onset: Delayed**   **Likelihood: Established**

Cause
Rifamycins may induce GI and hepatic metabolism of theophyllines.

Effect
Theophylline efficacy may decrease.

Nursing considerations
■ Monitor serum theophylline level closely. Therapeutic range is 10 to 20 mcg/ml for adults and 5 to 15 mcg/ml for children.
■ After a rifamycin is started, watch for increased pulmonary signs and symptoms.
■ Tell patient to immediately report all concerns about drug efficacy to prescriber; dosage may need adjustment.

rifamycins ▶◀ tricyclic antidepressants

rifabutin, rifampin

amitriptyline, amoxapine, clomipramine, desipramine, doxepin, imipramine, nortriptyline, trimipramine

Risk rating: 2
Severity: Moderate   **Onset: Delayed**   **Likelihood: Suspected**

Cause
Metabolism of tricyclic antidepressants (TCAs) in the liver may increase.

Effect
TCA level and efficacy may decrease.

Nursing considerations
■ When starting, stopping, or changing the dosage of a rifamycin, monitor serum TCA level to maintain therapeutic range.
■ Watch for resolution of depression as TCA dosage is adjusted to therapeutic level during rifamycin therapy.
■ Urge patient and family to watch for adverse reactions, including increased drowsiness and dizziness, for several weeks after rifamycin stops. Tell them to notify prescriber promptly if reactions occur.
■ Other TCAs may interact with rifamycins. If you suspect an interaction, consult prescriber or pharmacist.

risperidone ▶◀ SSRIs

Risperdal

fluoxetine, paroxetine,
sertraline

Risk rating: 1
Severity: Major   **Onset: Rapid**   **Likelihood: Suspected**

Cause
SSRIs may inhibit CYP2D6 metabolism of risperidone.

Effect
Risperidone level and risk of adverse reactions and rapid accumulation of serotonin in the CNS may increase.

Nursing considerations
- Monitor patient carefully if SSRI therapy starts or stops or if the dosage changes during risperidone therapy.
- Assess patient for CNS irritability, increased muscle tone, muscle twitching or jerking, and changes in level of consciousness.
- Advise patient not to alter the dose of either drug without the advice of his prescriber.
- Average doses of fluoxetine and paroxetine may cause this interaction; higher doses of sertraline (greater than 100 mg daily) are needed.

ritonavir ▶◀ azole antifungals

Norvir

fluconazole, itraconazole,
ketoconazole

Risk rating: 2
Severity: Moderate   **Onset: Delayed**   **Likelihood: Suspected**

Cause
Azole antifungals may inhibit metabolism of protease inhibitors, such as ritonavir.

Effect
Protease inhibitor level may increase.

Nursing considerations
- Protease inhibitor dosage may be decreased when therapy starts.
- Monitor patient for increased protease inhibitor effects, including hyperglycemia, onset of diabetes, rash, GI complaints, and altered liver function tests.
- Advise patient to report increased hunger or thirst, frequent urination, fatigue, and dry, itchy skin.

■ Tell patient not to change dosage or stop either drug without consulting prescriber.

---

ritonavir ▶◀ benzodiazepines

Norvir

alprazolam, chlordiazepoxide, clonazepam, clorazepate, diazepam, estazolam, flurazepam, midazolam, quazepam, triazolam

Risk rating: 2
Severity: Moderate   Onset: Delayed   Likelihood: Suspected

Cause
Protease inhibitors, such as ritonavir, may inhibit CYP3A4 metabolism of certain benzodiazepines.

Effect
Sedative effects of benzodiazepines may be increased and prolonged, leading to severe respiratory depression.

Nursing considerations
⊠ ALERT Don't combine these benzodiazepines with protease inhibitors.
⊠ ALERT Midazolam and triazolam are contraindicated in patients taking ritonavir.
■ If patient takes any protease inhibitor–benzodiazepine combination, notify prescriber. Interaction could involve other drugs in the class.
■ Watch for evidence of oversedation and respiratory depression.
■ Teach patient and family about the risks of combining these drugs.

---

ritonavir ▶◀ bupropion

Norvir

Wellbutrin

Risk rating: 2
Severity: Moderate   Onset: Delayed   Likelihood: Suspected

Cause
Ritonavir may inhibit bupropion metabolism.

Effect
Large increases in serum bupropion level may occur.

Nursing considerations
⊠ ALERT Use of ritonavir with bupropion is contraindicated.
■ Risk of bupropion toxicity–induced seizures increases.

■ Increased seizure risk is associated with high bupropion doses.
■ Assess patient for increased risk of seizures, including history of head trauma, seizures, CNS tumor, and use of other drugs that lower the seizure threshold.

ritonavir ◄► clozapine
Norvir   Clozaril

Risk rating: 1
Severity: Major   **Onset: Delayed**   **Likelihood: Suspected**

Cause
Ritonavir may inhibit metabolism of clozapine.

Effect
Clozapine level and risk of toxicity may increase.

Nursing considerations
■◗ ALERT Using clozapine with ritonavir is contraindicated.
■ Increased clozapine dose may increase risk of seizures.
■ Monitor patient for signs and symptoms of clozapine toxicity, including agranulocytosis, ECG changes, and seizures.
■ Monitor ECG. Clozapine-induced ECG changes should normalize after drug is stopped.

ritonavir ◄► eplerenone
Norvir   Inspra

Risk rating: 1
Severity: Major   **Onset: Delayed**   **Likelihood: Suspected**

Cause
Protease inhibitors, such as ritonavir, inhibit eplerenone metabolism.

Effect
Eplerenone level rises, causing hyperkalemia and increasing the risk of life-threatening arrhythmias.

Nursing considerations
■◗ ALERT Use of ritonavir with eplerenone is contraindicated.
■ Potent CYP3A4 inhibitors increase eplerenone level and the risk of hyperkalemia-induced arrhythmias—some fatal.
■ Monitor patient's serum potassium level.
■ Tell patient to report nausea, irregular heartbeat, or slowed pulse to prescriber.

ritonavir ▶◀ ergot derivatives

Norvir

dihydroergotamine,
ergonovine, ergotamine,
methylergonovine

Risk rating: 1
Severity: Major   **Onset: Delayed**   **Likelihood: Probable**

Cause
Protease inhibitors, such as ritonavir, may interfere with CYP3A4
metabolism of ergot derivatives.

Effect
Risk of ergot-induced peripheral vasospasm and ischemia may increase.

Nursing considerations
◤ ALERT Use of ergot derivatives with protease inhibitors is contraindicated.

■ Monitor patient for evidence of peripheral ischemia, including pain
in limb muscles while exercising and later at rest; numbness and tingling of fingers and toes; cool, pale, or cyanotic limbs; red or violet
blisters on hands or feet; and gangrene.

■ Sodium nitroprusside may be given for ergot-induced vasospasm.

■ If patient takes a protease inhibitor, consult prescriber or pharmacist about alternative treatments for migraine pain.

ritonavir ▶◀ fentanyl

Norvir

Sublimaze

Risk rating: 1
Severity: Major   **Onset: Delayed**   **Likelihood: Suspected**

Cause
Metabolism of fentanyl in the GI tract and liver may be inhibited.

Effect
Fentanyl level may increase and half-life lengthen.

Nursing considerations
◤ ALERT If patient takes a protease inhibitor, such as ritonavir, watch
closely for respiratory depression when fentanyl is added.

■ Because fentanyl half-life is prolonged, monitoring period should be
extended, even after fentanyl is stopped.

■ Keep naloxone available to treat respiratory depression.

■ If fentanyl is continuously infused, dosage should be decreased.

ritonavir ◄► HMG-CoA reductase inhibitors

Norvir

atorvastatin, lovastatin, simvastatin

Risk rating: 1 lovastatin, simvastatin
2 atorvastatin

Severity: Major **Onset: Delayed** **Likelihood: Suspected**
lovastatin,
simvastatin
Moderate
atorvastatin

Cause

Protease inhibitors, such as ritonavir, may inhibit metabolism of HMG-CoA reductase inhibitors.

Effect

HMG-CoA reductase inhibitor level may increase.

Nursing considerations

- Avoid giving lovastatin or simvastatin with ritonavir or atazanavir.
- Monitor patient closely if a protease inhibitor is added to HMG-CoA reductase inhibitor therapy.
- ✎ ALERT Watch for evidence of rhabdomyolysis, including dark or red urine, muscle weakness, and myalgia.
- This interaction may be more likely with combined use of ritonavir and saquinavir.
- Tell patient to immediately report unexplained muscle weakness.

ritonavir ◄► nevirapine

Norvir

Viramune

Risk rating: 2
Severity: Major **Onset: Delayed** **Likelihood: Suspected**

Cause

Nevirapine may increase hepatic metabolism of protease inhibitors, such as ritonavir.

Effect

Protease inhibitor level and effects decrease.

Nursing considerations

- If nevirapine is started or stopped, monitor protease inhibitor level closely.

- Protease inhibitor dosage may need adjustment.
- Monitor CD4+ and T-cell counts; tell prescriber if they decrease.
- Urge patient to report opportunistic infections.
- Tell patient not to change an HIV regimen without consulting prescriber.

---

ritonavir ▬▬▬►◄▬▬▬	phosphodiesterase-5 inhibitors
Norvir	sildenafil, tadalafil, vardenafil

Risk rating: 1
Severity: Major   **Onset: Rapid**   **Likelihood: Suspected**

Cause
Phosphodiesterase-5 (PDE-5) inhibitor metabolism is inhibited.

Effect
PDE-5 inhibitor level may increase, possibly leading to fatal hypotension.

Nursing considerations
◪ ALERT Tell patient to take PDE-5 inhibitors exactly as prescribed.
- Dosage of PDE-5 inhibitor may be reduced and interval lengthened.
- Warn patient about potentially fatal low blood pressure if these drugs are taken together.
- Tell patient to notify prescriber about dizziness, fainting, or chest pain if drugs are used together.

---

ritonavir ▬▬▬►◄▬▬▬	propafenone
Norvir	Rythmol

Risk rating: 1
Severity: Major   **Onset: Delayed**   **Likelihood: Suspected**

Cause
Ritonavir may inhibit CYP2D6 metabolism of propafenone.

Effect
Propafenone level and risk of toxicity may increase.

Nursing considerations
◪ ALERT Use of ritonavir with propafenone is contraindicated.
- Monitor patient for new or worsened arrhythmias, including an increase in premature ventricular contractions, ventricular tachycardia, ventricular fibrillation, and torsades de pointes.

■ Monitor ECG for AV block and QTc interval prolongation.
■ Advise patient to report a rapid heartbeat, shortness of breath, dizziness or fainting, and chest pain.

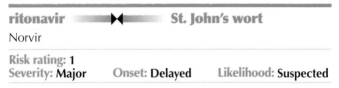

ritonavir ◄►◄ St. John's wort

Norvir

Risk rating: 1
Severity: Major   **Onset: Delayed**   **Likelihood: Suspected**

Cause
Hepatic metabolism of protease inhibitors, such as ritonavir, may increase.

Effect
Protease inhibitor level and effects may decrease.

Nursing considerations
■ If patient starts or stops taking St. John's wort, monitor protease inhibitor level closely.
■ Monitor CD4+ and T-cell counts; tell prescriber if they decrease.
■ Urge patient to report opportunistic infections.
■ Tell patient not to change an HIV regimen without consulting prescriber.
■ Urge patient to tell prescribers about all drugs, supplements, and alternative therapies he uses.

rizatriptan ►◄ ergot derivatives

Maxalt   dihydroergotamine, ergotamine

Risk rating: 1
Severity: Major   **Onset: Rapid**   **Likelihood: Suspected**

Cause
Combined use may have additive effects.

Effect
Risk of vasospastic effects increases.

Nursing considerations
◄ ALERT Use of these drugs within 24 hours of each other is contraindicated. Combined use may cause severe vasospastic effects, including sustained coronary artery vasospasm that triggers MI.
◄ ALERT Similarly, use of another selective 5-HT_1 receptor agonist

(such as frovatriptan, naratriptan, sumatriptan, or zolmitriptan) within 24 hours of rizatriptan is contraindicated.

■ Warn patients not to mix migraine headache drugs within 24 hours of each other, but to call the prescriber if a drug isn't effective.

rizatriptan ▶◀ MAO inhibitors

Maxalt

isocarboxazid, phenelzine, tranylcypromine

Risk rating: 1
Severity: **Major**   Onset: **Rapid**   Likelihood: **Suspected**

Cause
MAO inhibitors, subtype-A, may inhibit metabolism of selective $5-HT_1$ receptor agonists, such as rizatriptan.

Effect
Serum level of—and risk of cardiac toxicity from—certain selective $5-HT_1$ receptor agonists may increase.

Nursing considerations
◼ ALERT Use of certain selective $5-HT_1$ receptor agonists with or within 2 weeks of stopping an MAO inhibitor is contraindicated.
■ If these drugs must be used together, naratriptan is less likely to interact with an MAO inhibitor.
■ Cardiac toxicity may include coronary artery vasospasm and transient myocardial ischemia.

rizatriptan ▶◀ serotonin reuptake inhibitors

Maxalt

citalopram, fluoxetine, fluvoxamine, nefazodone, paroxetine, sertraline, venlafaxine

Risk rating: 1
Severity: **Major**   Onset: **Rapid**   Likelihood: **Suspected**

Cause
Serotonin may accumulate rapidly in the CNS.

Effect
Risk of serotonin syndrome increases.

Nursing considerations
◼ ALERT If possible, avoid combined use of these drugs.

- Start with lowest dosages possible, and assess patient closely.
- Stop the selective 5-HT$_1$ receptor agonist at the first sign of interaction, and start an antiserotonergic drug.
- In some patients, migraine frequency may increase and antimigraine drug efficacy may decrease when a serotonin reuptake inhibitor is started.
- Describe the traits of serotonin syndrome: CNS irritability, motor weakness, shivering, muscle twitching, and altered consciousness.
- Explain that serotonin syndrome can be fatal if not treated immediately.

rizatriptan ◄►► sibutramine
Maxalt   Meridia

Risk rating: 1
Severity: Major   **Onset: Rapid**   **Likelihood: Suspected**

Cause
Sibutramine inhibits serotonin reuptake, which may have an additive effect with drugs that have serotonergic activity.

Effect
Risk of serotonin syndrome increases.

Nursing considerations
⚠ ALERT If possible, avoid giving these drugs together.
- If use together can't be avoided, monitor patient closely for adverse effects, which require immediate medical attention.
- Stop rizatriptan, a selective 5-HT$_1$ receptor agonist, at the first sign of interaction, and start an antiserotonergic drug.
- Describe the traits of serotonin syndrome, including CNS irritability, motor weakness, shivering, myoclonus, and altered consciousness.
- Urge patient to promptly report adverse effects.

rocuronium ◄►► aminoglycosides
Zemuron   amikacin, gentamicin,
                                kanamycin, neomycin,
                                streptomycin, tobramycin

Risk rating: 1
Severity: Major   **Onset: Rapid**   **Likelihood: Probable**

Cause
These drugs may be synergistic.

Effect
Effects of nondepolarizing muscle relaxants, such as rocuronium, may increase.

Nursing considerations
■ The nondepolarizing muscle relaxant dose may need adjustment based on neuromuscular response.
■ Monitor patient for prolonged respiratory depression.
■ Provide ventilatory support as needed.

---

rocuronium ▶◀ carbamazepine
Zemuron   Carbatrol, Epitol, Equetro, Tegretol

Risk rating: 2
Severity: Moderate   **Onset: Rapid**   **Likelihood: Probable**

Cause
The mechanism of this interaction is unknown.

Effect
Effects or duration of a nondepolarizing muscle relaxant, such as rocuronium, may decrease.

Nursing considerations
■ Monitor patient for decreased efficacy of muscle relaxant.
■ Dosage of the nondepolarizing muscle relaxant may need to be increased.
■ Make sure patient is adequately sedated when receiving a nondepolarizing muscle relaxant.

---

rocuronium ▶◀ clindamycin
Zemuron   Cleocin

Risk rating: 2
Severity: Moderate   **Onset: Rapid**   **Likelihood: Suspected**

Cause
Clindamycin may potentiate the actions of nondepolarizing muscle relaxants, such as rocuronium.

Effect
Effects of the nondepolarizing muscle relaxant may increase.

Nursing considerations
■ If possible, avoid using clindamycin or other lincosamides with nondepolarizing muscle relaxants.

- Monitor patient for respiratory distress.
- Combined use may lead to profound, severe respiratory depression.
- Provide ventilatory support as needed.
- Cholinesterase inhibitors or calcium may be useful in reversing drug effects.
- Make sure patient is adequately sedated when receiving a nondepolarizing muscle relaxant.

---

rocuronium ▶◀ magnesium sulfate
Zemuron

Risk rating: 2
Severity: Moderate   **Onset: Rapid**   **Likelihood: Suspected**

Cause
Magnesium probably potentiates the action of nondepolarizing muscle relaxants, such as rocuronium.

Effect
Risk of profound respiratory depression increases.

Nursing considerations
- Use these drugs together cautiously.
- The nondepolarizing muscle relaxant dosage may need to be adjusted.
- Monitor patient for respiratory distress.
- Provide ventilatory support as needed.
- Make sure patient is adequately sedated when receiving a nondepolarizing muscle relaxant.

---

rocuronium ▶◀ phenytoin
Zemuron   Dilantin

Risk rating: 2
Severity: Moderate   **Onset: Rapid**   **Likelihood: Probable**

Cause
Phenytoin has effects at prejunctional sites similar to those of nondepolarizing muscle relaxants, such as rocuronium.

Effect
Effect or duration of the nondepolarizing muscle relaxant may decrease.

Nursing considerations
- Monitor patient for decreased efficacy of the muscle relaxant.

■ The dosage of nondepolarizing muscle relaxant may need to be increased.

■ Atracurium may be a suitable alternative because this interaction may not occur in all patients.

■ Make sure patient is adequately sedated when receiving a nondepolarizing muscle relaxant.

rosuvastatin ▶◀ azole antifungals

Crestor

fluconazole, itraconazole, ketoconazole, voriconazole

Risk rating: 2
Severity: Moderate   **Onset: Rapid**   **Likelihood: Probable**

Cause
Azole antifungals may inhibit hepatic metabolism of HMG-CoA reductase inhibitors, such as rosuvastatin.

Effect
HMG-CoA reductase inhibitor level and adverse effects may increase.

Nursing considerations
■ If possible, avoid use together.

■ If drugs must be taken together, HMG-CoA reductase inhibitor dosage may need to be decreased.

■ Monitor serum cholesterol and lipid levels.

⚡ **ALERT** Assess patient for evidence of rhabdomyolysis, including fatigue; muscle aches and weakness; joint pain; dark, red, or cola-colored urine; weight gain; seizures; and greatly increased CK level.

■ Pravastatin is the HMG-CoA reductase inhibitor least affected by this interaction and may be preferable for use with azole antifungals.

rosuvastatin ▶◀ bile acid sequestrants

Crestor

cholestyramine, colestipol

Risk rating: 2
Severity: Moderate   **Onset: Delayed**   **Likelihood: Suspected**

Cause
GI absorption of HMG-CoA reductase inhibitors, such as rosuvastatin, may decrease.

Effect
HMG-CoA reductase inhibitor effects may decrease.

Nursing considerations
⚠ **ALERT** Separate doses of HMG-CoA reductase inhibitor and bile acid sequestrant by at least 4 hours.
■ If possible, give bile acid sequestrant before meals and HMG-CoA reductase inhibitor in the evening.
■ Monitor serum cholesterol and lipid levels.
■ Obtain liver function test results at start of therapy and periodically thereafter. If ALT or AST level stays three times or more above the upper limit of normal, rosuvastatin will need to be stopped.
■ Help patient develop a plan to ensure proper dosage intervals.

---

rosuvastatin ➤◀ **cyclosporine**

Crestor   Neoral

Risk rating: 1
Severity: Major   **Onset: Delayed**   **Likelihood: Probable**

Cause
Metabolism of certain HMG-CoA reductase inhibitors, such as rosuvastatin, may decrease.

Effect
Plasma level and adverse effects of HMG-CoA reductase inhibitors may increase.

Nursing considerations
⚠ **ALERT** If possible, avoid use together.
■ HMG-CoA reductase inhibitor dosage may need to be decreased.
■ Monitor serum cholesterol and lipid levels.
■ Assess patient for evidence of rhabdomyolysis, including fatigue; muscle aches and weakness; joint pain; dark, red, or cola-colored urine; weight gain; seizures; and greatly increased CK level.
■ Urge patient to report muscle pain, tenderness, or weakness.

---

rosuvastatin ➤◀ **gemfibrozil**

Crestor   Lopid

Risk rating: 1
Severity: Major   **Onset: Delayed**   **Likelihood: Suspected**

Cause
The mechanism of this interaction is unknown.

Effect
Severe myopathy or rhabdomyolysis may occur.

Nursing considerations
■ Avoid use together.
■ If patient has severe hyperlipidemia, combined therapy may be an option, but only with careful monitoring.
⚠ **ALERT** Assess patient for evidence of rhabdomyolysis, including fatigue; muscle aches and weakness; joint pain; dark, red, or cola-colored urine; weight gain; seizures; and greatly increased CK level.
■ Watch for evidence of acute renal failure, including decreased urine output, elevated BUN and creatinine levels, edema, dyspnea, tachycardia, distended neck veins, nausea, vomiting, poor appetite, weakness, fatigue, confusion, and agitation.
■ Urge patient to report muscle pain, tenderness, or weakness.

---

saquinavir ━━━►◄━━━ azole antifungals
Fortovase

fluconazole, itraconazole, ketoconazole

Risk rating: 2
Severity: Moderate   **Onset: Delayed**   **Likelihood: Suspected**

Cause
Azole antifungals may inhibit metabolism of protease inhibitors, such as saquinavir.

Effect
Protease inhibitor plasma level may increase.

Nursing considerations
■ Protease inhibitor dosage may be decreased when therapy starts.
■ Monitor patient for increased protease inhibitor effects, including hyperglycemia, onset of diabetes, rash, GI complaints, and altered liver function tests.
■ Advise patient to report increased hunger or thirst, frequent urination, fatigue, and dry, itchy skin.
■ Tell patient not to change dosage or stop either drug without consulting prescriber.

saquinavir ▰▰▰▶◀ **benzodiazepines**

alprazolam, chlordiazepoxide, clonazepam, clorazepate, diazepam, estazolam, flurazepam, midazolam, quazepam, triazolam

Risk rating: 2
Severity: Moderate   Onset: Delayed   Likelihood: Suspected

Cause
Protease inhibitors, such as saquinavir, may inhibit CYP3A4 metabolism of certain benzodiazepines.

Effect
Sedative effects of benzodiazepines may be increased and prolonged, leading to severe respiratory depression.

Nursing considerations
◣ **ALERT** Don't combine these benzodiazepines with protease inhibitors.
◣ **ALERT** Midazolam and triazolam are contraindicated in patients taking saquinavir.
▪ If patient takes any protease inhibitor–benzodiazepine combination, notify prescriber. Interaction could involve other drugs in the class.
▪ Watch for evidence of oversedation and respiratory depression.
▪ Teach patient and family about the risks of combining these drugs.

saquinavir ▰▰▰▶◀ **ergot derivatives**

Fortovase

dihydroergotamine, ergonovine, ergotamine, methylergonovine

Risk rating: 1
Severity: Major   Onset: Delayed   Likelihood: Probable

Cause
Protease inhibitors, such as saquinavir, may interfere with CYP3A4 metabolism of ergot derivatives.

Effect
Risk of ergot-induced peripheral vasospasm and ischemia may increase.

Nursing considerations
◣ **ALERT** Combining ergot derivatives and protease inhibitors is contraindicated.

■ Monitor patient for evidence of peripheral ischemia, including pain in limb muscles while exercising and later at rest; numbness and tingling of fingers and toes; cool, pale, or cyanotic limbs; red or violet blisters on hands or feet; and gangrene.

■ Sodium nitroprusside may be given for ergot-induced vasospasm.

■ If patient takes a protease inhibitor, consult prescriber or pharmacist about alternative treatments for migraine pain.

■ Advise patient to tell prescriber about increased adverse effects.

saquinavir ◄►◄ fentanyl
Fortovase   Sublimaze

Risk rating: 1
Severity: Major   **Onset: Delayed**   **Likelihood: Suspected**

Cause
Metabolism of fentanyl in the GI tract and liver may be inhibited.

Effect
Fentanyl level may increase and half-life lengthen.

Nursing considerations
⚑ ALERT If patient takes a protease inhibitor, such as saquinavir, watch closely for respiratory depression when fentanyl is added.

■ Because fentanyl half-life is prolonged, monitoring period should be extended, even after fentanyl is stopped.

■ Keep naloxone available to treat respiratory depression.

■ If fentanyl is continuously infused, dosage should be decreased.

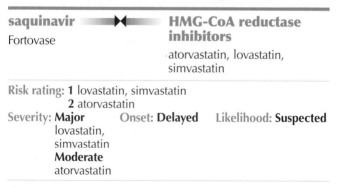

saquinavir ◄►◄ HMG-CoA reductase inhibitors
Fortovase   atorvastatin, lovastatin, simvastatin

Risk rating: 1 lovastatin, simvastatin
              2 atorvastatin
Severity: Major   **Onset: Delayed**   **Likelihood: Suspected**
          lovastatin,
          simvastatin
          Moderate
          atorvastatin

Cause
Protease inhibitors, such as saquinavir, may inhibit CYP3A4 metabolism of HMG-CoA reductase inhibitors.

Effect
HMG-CoA reductase inhibitor level may increase.

Nursing considerations
■ If a protease inhibitor is added to lovastatin, monitor patient closely.
■ With atorvastatin, interaction may be more likely with combined use of ritonavir and saquinavir.
◤ ALERT Watch for evidence of rhabdomyolysis, including dark or red urine, muscle weakness, and myalgia.
■ Urge patient to immediately report unexplained muscle weakness.

---

saquinavir ▶◀ nevirapine
Fortovase   Viramune

Risk rating: 2
Severity: Moderate   Onset: Delayed   Likelihood: Suspected

Cause
Nevirapine may increase hepatic metabolism of protease inhibitors, such as saquinavir.

Effect
Protease inhibitor level and effects decrease.

Nursing considerations
■ If nevirapine is started or stopped, monitor protease inhibitor level.
■ Protease inhibitor dosage may need adjustment.
■ Monitor CD4+ and T-cell counts; tell prescriber if they decrease.
■ Urge patient to report opportunistic infections.
■ Tell patient not to change an HIV regimen without consulting prescriber.

---

saquinavir ▶◀ phosphodiesterase-5 inhibitors
Fortovase   sildenafil, tadalafil, vardenafil

Risk rating: 1
Severity: Major   Onset: Rapid   Likelihood: Suspected

Cause
Phosphodiesterase-5 (PDE-5) inhibitor metabolism is inhibited.

Effect
PDE-5 inhibitor level may increase, possibly leading to fatal hypotension.

Nursing considerations
- Tell patient to take PDE-5 inhibitors exactly as prescribed.
- PDE-5 inhibitor dosage will be reduced and interval lengthened.
- **ALERT** Warn patient about potentially fatal low blood pressure.
- Tell patient to notify his prescriber about dizziness, fainting, or chest pain if drugs are used together.

saquinavir ▶◀ St. John's wort
Fortovase

Risk rating: 1
Severity: Major   **Onset: Delayed**   **Likelihood: Suspected**

Cause
Hepatic metabolism of protease inhibitors, such as saquinavir, may increase.

Effect
Protease inhibitor level and effects may decrease.

Nursing considerations
- If patient starts or stops taking St. John's wort, monitor protease inhibitor level closely.
- Monitor CD4+ and T-cell counts; tell prescriber if they decrease.
- Urge patient to report opportunistic infections.
- Tell patient not to change an HIV regimen without consulting prescriber.
- Urge patient to tell prescribers about all drugs, supplements, and alternative therapies he uses.

saquinavir mesylate ▶◀ grapefruit juice
Invirase

Risk rating: 2
Severity: Moderate   **Onset: Delayed**   **Likelihood: Suspected**

Cause
Grapefruit juice may inhibit CYP3A4 GI metabolism of saquinavir.

Effect
Saquinavir level may increase.

Nursing considerations
- Avoid giving saquinavir with grapefruit juice.
- Teach patient to separate grapefruit products as much as possible from saquinavir doses.

■ This interaction was tested on Invirase, the mesylate capsule form of saquinavir, not on Fortovase, the soft gelatin capsule form. The interaction isn't likely with Fortovase, which has greater bioavailability.

---

secobarbital ➤◀ alcohol

Seconal

Risk rating: 1
Severity: **Major**   Onset: **Rapid**   Likelihood: **Established**

Cause
Acute alcohol intake inhibits hepatic metabolism of barbiturates, such as secobarbital. Chronic alcohol use increases barbiturate clearance, probably by inducing liver enzymes.

Effect
Acute alcohol intake with barbiturates can cause impaired hand-eye coordination, additive CNS effects, and death. Chronic alcohol use with barbiturates may cause drug tolerance and an increased risk of adverse effects, including death.

Nursing considerations
�︎ ALERT Because of the risk of serious adverse effects and death, alcohol and barbiturates shouldn't be combined.
■ Before barbiturate therapy starts, assess patient thoroughly for history or evidence of alcohol use.
■ Watch for additive CNS effects, which may suggest barbiturate overdose.

---

secobarbital ➤◀ beta blockers

Seconal   metoprolol, propranolol

Risk rating: 2
Severity: **Moderate**   Onset: **Rapid**   Likelihood: **Probable**

Cause
Increased enzyme induction and first-pass hepatic metabolism of certain beta blockers reduce their availability.

Effect
Beta blocker efficacy may be reduced.

Nursing considerations
■ Assess beta blocker efficacy by monitoring blood pressure, apical pulse, and presence of chest pain or headache, as appropriate.

■ If patient has increased angina, rhythm problems, or blood pressure problems when starting a barbiturate, such as secobarbital, notify prescriber promptly. Beta blocker dosage may be increased.
■ Other beta blockers may interact with barbiturates. If you suspect an interaction, consult prescriber or pharmacist.
■ Explain the potential interaction between these drugs and the need to tell prescriber about any problems.

secobarbital ▶◀ corticosteroids

Seconal

betamethasone, corticotropin, cortisone, cosyntropin, dexamethasone, fludrocortisone, hydrocortisone, methylprednisolone, prednisolone, prednisone, triamcinolone

Risk rating: 2
Severity: Moderate   **Onset: Delayed**   **Likelihood: Established**

Cause
Secobarbital and other barbiturates induce liver enzymes, which stimulate corticosteroid metabolism.

Effect
Corticosteroid effects may be decreased.

Nursing considerations
■ Avoid giving barbiturates with corticosteroids, if possible.
■ If patient takes a corticosteroid, watch for worsening symptoms when a barbiturate is started or stopped.
■ Corticosteroid dosage may need to be increased.

secobarbital ▶◀ hormonal contraceptives

Seconal

Risk rating: 1
Severity: Major   **Onset: Delayed**   **Likelihood: Suspected**

Cause
Secobarbital and other barbiturates may induce hepatic metabolism of contraceptives and synthesis of sex-hormone–binding protein.

Effect
Risk of breakthrough bleeding and pregnancy may increase.

Nursing considerations
- Talk with prescriber about increasing contraceptive dosage during barbiturate therapy.
- Talk with prescriber about alternative treatments for seizures or sleep disturbance.
- Instruct patient to also use barrier contraception.

---

secobarbital ➤◄ methadone
Seconal   Dolophine, Methadose

Risk rating: 2
Severity: Moderate   **Onset: Delayed**   **Likelihood: Suspected**

Cause
The mechanism of this interaction is unknown, but secobarbital and other barbiturates may increase hepatic metabolism of methadone.

Effect
Methadone effects may be reduced, and patients receiving long-term therapy may notice opioid withdrawal symptoms.

Nursing considerations
- If these drugs must be used together, monitor methadone efficacy.
- Check serum methadone level regularly.
- If methadone dosage is insufficient, it may be increased.
- Other barbiturates interact with methadone. If you suspect an interaction, consult prescriber or pharmacist.

---

secobarbital ➤◄ theophyllines
Seconal   aminophylline, theophylline

Risk rating: 2
Severity: Moderate   **Onset: Delayed**   **Likelihood: Suspected**

Cause
Barbiturates may stimulate theophylline clearance by inducing the CYP pathway.

Effect
Theophylline level and efficacy may decrease.

Nursing considerations
- Monitor patient closely to determine theophylline efficacy.
- Monitor serum theophylline level regularly. Therapeutic range is 10 to 20 mcg/ml for adults and 5 to 15 mcg/ml for children.

■ When a barbiturate is added to regimen, theophylline dosage may need to be increased.

■ Dyphylline undergoes renal elimination and may not be affected by this interaction.

selegiline ▶◀ meperidine
Eldepryl   Demerol

Risk rating: 1
Severity: **Major**   Onset: **Rapid**   Likelihood: **Probable**

Cause
The mechanism of this interaction is unknown.

Effect
Risk of severe adverse reactions increases.

Nursing considerations
■ If possible, avoid giving these drugs together.
■ Monitor patient and report agitation, seizures, diaphoresis, and fever.
◼ ALERT Reaction may progress to coma, apnea, and death.
■ Reaction may occur several weeks after stopping an MAO inhibitor, such as selegiline.
◼ ALERT Give opioid analgesics other than meperidine cautiously. It isn't known if similar reactions occur.

selegiline ▶◀ serotonin reuptake inhibitors
Eldepryl

citalopram, escitalopram, fluoxetine, fluvoxamine, nefazodone, paroxetine, sertraline, venlafaxine

Risk rating: 1
Severity: **Major**   Onset: **Rapid**   Likelihood: **Probable**

Cause
Serotonin may accumulate rapidly in the CNS.

Effect
Risk of serotonin syndrome increases.

Nursing considerations
◼ ALERT Don't use these drugs together.
■ Allow 1 week after stopping nefazodone or venlafaxine (2 weeks after stopping citalopram, escitalopram, fluvoxamine, paroxetine, or ser-

traline; 5 weeks after stopping fluoxetine) before giving an MAO inhibitor, such as selegiline.
■ Allow 2 weeks after stopping an MAO inhibitor before giving a serotonin reuptake inhibitor.
■ A selective MAO type-B inhibitor, selegiline has been given with fluoxetine, paroxetine, or sertraline to patients with Parkinson's disease without negative effects.
■ Describe the traits of serotonin syndrome, including CNS irritability, motor weakness, shivering, myoclonus, and altered consciousness.
■ Urge patient to promptly report adverse effects.

---

sertraline ▶◀	hydantoins
Zoloft	ethotoin, fosphenytoin, phenytoin

Risk rating: 2
Severity: Moderate   **Onset: Delayed**   **Likelihood: Suspected**

Cause
Sertraline may inhibit hydantoin metabolism.

Effect
Hydantoin level and effects may be increased, along with risk of toxic effects.

Nursing considerations
■ Monitor serum hydantoin level. Therapeutic range for phenytoin is 10 to 20 mcg/ml.
■ Hydantoin dosage may need adjustment.
■ **⚠ ALERT** If sertraline starts during hydantoin therapy, watch for evidence of hydantoin toxicity, including drowsiness, nausea, vomiting, nystagmus, ataxia, dysarthria, tremor, slurred speech, hypotension, arrhythmias, respiratory depression, and coma.
■ If sertraline stops during hydantoin therapy, watch for decreased anticonvulsant effect and increased seizure activity.
■ Urge patient to tell prescriber about loss of drug effect and increased adverse effects.

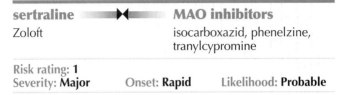

sertraline ━━━━▶◀━━━━ MAO inhibitors
Zoloft   isocarboxazid, phenelzine,
                                      tranylcypromine

Risk rating: 1
Severity: Major   **Onset: Rapid**   **Likelihood: Probable**

Cause
Serotonin may accumulate rapidly in the CNS.

Effect
Risk of serotonin syndrome increases.

Nursing considerations
◾ ALERT Don't use these drugs together.
■ Allow 2 weeks after stopping sertraline before giving an MAO inhibitor. Allow 2 weeks after stopping an MAO inhibitor before giving an SSRI, such as sertraline.
■ The selective MAO type-B inhibitor selegiline has been given with fluoxetine, paroxetine, or sertraline to patients with Parkinson's disease without negative effects.
■ Describe the traits of serotonin syndrome, including CNS irritability, motor weakness, shivering, myoclonus, and altered consciousness.
■ Urge patient to promptly report adverse effects.

sertraline ━━━━▶◀━━━━ propafenone
Zoloft   Rythmol

Risk rating: 2
Severity: Moderate   **Onset: Delayed**   **Likelihood: Suspected**

Cause
Certain serotonin reuptake inhibitors, such as sertraline, may inhibit CYP2D6 metabolism of propafenone.

Effect
Propafenone level and risk of adverse effects may increase.

Nursing considerations
■ Monitor cardiac function closely.
■ Citalopram doesn't inhibit CYP2D6 and may be a safer choice than sertraline.
■ Tell patient to promptly report dizziness, drowsiness, ataxia, tremor, palpitations, chest pain, edema, dyspnea, and other new symptoms.

| sertraline | ▶◀ | selective 5-HT$_1$ receptor |
| Zoloft | | agonists |

almotriptan, eletriptan, frovatriptan, naratriptan, rizatriptan, sumatriptan, zolmitriptan

Risk rating: 1
Severity: Major   **Onset: Rapid**   **Likelihood: Suspected**

Cause
Serotonin may accumulate rapidly in the CNS.

Effect
Risk of serotonin syndrome increases.

Nursing considerations
▪ If possible, avoid combined use of these drugs.
▪ Start with lowest dosages possible, and assess patient closely.
▪ Stop the selective 5-HT$_1$ receptor agonist at the first sign of interaction, and start an antiserotonergic.
▪ In some patients, migraine frequency may increase and antimigraine drug efficacy may decrease when an SSRI, such as sertraline, is started.
▪ Describe the traits of serotonin syndrome: CNS irritability, motor weakness, shivering, muscle twitching, and altered consciousness.
▪ Explain that serotonin syndrome can be fatal if not treated immediately.

| sertraline | ▶◀ | sibutramine |
| Zoloft | | Meridia |

Risk rating: 1
Severity: Major   **Onset: Rapid**   **Likelihood: Suspected**

Cause
Serotonin may accumulate rapidly in the CNS.

Effect
Risk of serotonin syndrome increases.

Nursing considerations
◨ ALERT If possible, don't give these drugs together.
▪ Watch carefully for adverse effects, which require immediate medical attention.

■ Describe the traits of serotonin syndrome: CNS irritability, motor weakness, shivering, muscle twitching, and altered consciousness.
■ Explain that serotonin syndrome can be fatal if not treated immediately.

---

sertraline ▶◀ St. John's wort
Zoloft

Risk rating: 2
Severity: Moderate   **Onset: Rapid**   **Likelihood: Suspected**

Cause
St. John's wort may cause additive inhibition of serotonin reuptake.

Effect
Sedative-hypnotic effects of SSRIs, such as sertraline, may increase.

Nursing considerations
⚑ ALERT Discourage use of an SSRI with St. John's wort.
■ In addition to oversedation, mild serotonin-like symptoms may occur, including anxiety, dizziness, nausea, restlessness, and vomiting.
■ Inform patient about the dangers of this combination.
■ Urge patient to consult prescriber before taking any herb.

---

sertraline ▶◀ sympathomimetics
Zoloft   amphetamine, dextroamphetamine, methamphetamine, phentermine

Risk rating: 1
Severity: Major   **Onset: Rapid**   **Likelihood: Suspected**

Cause
The mechanism of this interaction is unknown.

Effect
Sympathomimetic effects and the risk of serotonin syndrome increase.

Nursing considerations
■ If these drugs must be used together, watch closely for increased CNS effects, such as anxiety, jitteriness, agitation, and restlessness.
■ Mild serotonin-like symptoms may develop, including anxiety, dizziness, restlessness, nausea, and vomiting.
■ Inform patient of the risk of interaction and the need to avoid sympathomimetics.

■ Describe the traits of serotonin syndrome, including CNS irritability, motor weakness, shivering, myoclonus, and altered consciousness.

---

sertraline ▶◀ tricyclic antidepressants
Zoloft

amitriptyline, amoxapine, clomipramine, desipramine, doxepin, imipramine, nortriptyline, trimipramine

---

Risk rating: 2
Severity: Moderate   Onset: Delayed   Likelihood: Suspected

Cause
Hepatic metabolism of tricyclic antidepressants (TCAs) by CYP2D6 may be inhibited.

Effect
Therapeutic and toxic effects of certain TCAs may increase.

Nursing considerations
■ If possible, avoid this drug combination.
■ **ALERT** Watch for evidence of TCA toxicity and serotonin syndrome.
■ Signs of serotonin syndrome include delirium, bizarre movements, and tachycardia.
■ Monitor serum TCA level when starting or stopping sertraline.
■ If abnormalities occur, decrease TCA dosage or stop drug.

---

sibutramine ▶◀ ergot derivatives
Meridia

dihydroergotamine, ergotamine

Risk rating: 1
Severity: Major   Onset: Rapid   Likelihood: Suspected

Cause
Drugs may have additive serotonergic effects.

Effect
Risk of serotonin syndrome may increase.

Nursing considerations
■ **ALERT** If possible, avoid giving an ergot derivative with sibutramine.
■ Watch for evidence of serotonin syndrome, including excitement, hypomania, restlessness, loss of consciousness, confusion, disorientation, anxiety, agitation, motor weakness, myoclonus, tremor, hemibal-

lismus, hyperreflexia, ataxia, dysarthria, incoordination, hyperthermia, shivering, papillary dilation, diaphoresis, emesis, hypertension, and tachycardia.
■ If serotonin syndrome occurs, stop these drugs and provide supportive care as needed.
■ Other ergot derivatives may interact with sibutramine. If you suspect an interaction, consult prescriber or pharmacist.
■ Advise patient to tell prescriber about increased adverse effects.

sibutramine ▸◂ lithium

Meridia   Eskalith

Risk rating: 1
Severity: Major   **Onset: Rapid**   **Likelihood: Suspected**

Cause
Serotonergic effects of these drugs may be additive.

Effect
Serotonin syndrome, including CNS irritability, motor weakness, shivering, myoclonus, and altered consciousness, may occur.

Nursing considerations
■ Use of these drugs together isn't recommended.
■ If used together, monitor patient for adverse effects.
◗ ALERT If signs and symptoms of serotonin syndrome occur, provide immediate treatment. Although rare, interaction may be fatal.

sibutramine ▸◂ meperidine

Meridia   Demerol

Risk rating: 1
Severity: Major   **Onset: Rapid**   **Likelihood: Suspected**

Cause
Serotonergic effects may be additive.

Effect
Serotonin syndrome may occur.

Nursing considerations
■ Use of these drugs together isn't recommended.
■ Monitor patient for serotonin syndrome: CNS irritability, motor weakness, shivering, muscle twitching, and altered consciousness.
◗ ALERT If serotonin syndrome occurs, immediate medical attention is required. Serotonin syndrome may be fatal.

sibutramine ▬▶◀ selective 5-HT$_1$ receptor agonists

Meridia

naratriptan, rizatriptan, sumatriptan, zolmitriptan

Risk rating: 1
Severity: Major   **Onset: Rapid**   **Likelihood: Suspected**

Cause
Sibutramine inhibits serotonin reuptake, which may have an additive effect with drugs that have serotonergic activity.

Effect
Risk of serotonin syndrome increases.

Nursing considerations
⚡ ALERT If possible, avoid giving these drugs together.
■ Monitor patient closely for adverse effects, which require immediate medical attention.
■ Stop the selective 5-HT$_1$ receptor agonist at the first sign of interaction, and start an antiserotonergic drug.
■ Describe the traits of serotonin syndrome, including CNS irritability, motor weakness, shivering, myoclonus, and altered consciousness.
■ Urge patient to promptly report adverse effects.

sibutramine ▬▶◀ serotonin reuptake inhibitors

Meridia

fluoxetine, fluvoxamine, nefazodone, paroxetine, sertraline, venlafaxine

Risk rating: 1
Severity: Major   **Onset: Rapid**   **Likelihood: Suspected**

Cause
Serotonin may accumulate rapidly in the CNS.

Effect
Risk of serotonin syndrome increases.

Nursing considerations
⚡ ALERT If possible, don't give these drugs together.
■ Watch carefully for adverse effects, which require immediate medical attention.
■ Describe the traits of serotonin syndrome: CNS irritability, motor weakness, shivering, muscle twitching, and altered consciousness.

■ Explain that serotonin syndrome can be fatal if not treated immediately.

sildenafil ▬▬►◄▬▬ amprenavir
Viagra   Agenerase

Risk rating: 1
Severity: Major   **Onset: Rapid**   **Likelihood: Suspected**

Cause
Sildenafil metabolism is inhibited.

Effect
Sildenafil level may increase, possibly leading to fatal hypotension.

Nursing considerations
■ Tell patient to take sildenafil exactly as prescribed.
■ Dosage may be reduced to 25 mg and an interval of at least 48 hours may be needed.
◪ ALERT Warn patient about potentially fatal low blood pressure.
■ Tell patient to notify prescriber about dizziness, fainting, or chest pain.

sildenafil ▬▬►◄▬▬ nitrates
Viagra   amyl nitrite, isosorbide
                                dinitrate, isosorbide
                                mononitrate, nitroglycerin

Risk rating: 1
Severity: Major   **Onset: Rapid**   **Likelihood: Suspected**

Cause
Sildenafil potentiates hypotensive effects of nitrates.

Effect
Risk of severe hypotension increases.

Nursing considerations
◪ ALERT Use of nitrates with sildenafil may be fatal and is contraindicated.
■ Carefully screen patient for sildenafil use before giving a nitrate. Even during an emergency, before giving a nitrate, find out if a patient with chest pain has taken sildenafil during previous 24 hours.
■ Monitor patient for orthostatic hypotension, dizziness, sweating, and headache.

sildenafil ▶◀ protease inhibitors

Viagra   amprenavir, indinavir,
                                nelfinavir, ritonavir, saquinavir

Risk rating: 1
Severity: Major   **Onset: Rapid**   **Likelihood: Suspected**

Cause
Sildenafil metabolism is inhibited.

Effect
Sildenafil level may increase, possibly leading to fatal hypotension.

Nursing considerations
- Tell patient to take sildenafil exactly as prescribed.
- Dosage may be reduced to 25 mg and an interval of at least 48 hours may be needed.
- **ALERT** Warn patient about potentially fatal low blood pressure.
- Tell patient to notify prescriber about dizziness, fainting, or chest pain.

---

simvastatin ▶◀ azole antifungals

Zocor   fluconazole, itraconazole,
                                ketoconazole, voriconazole

Risk rating: 2
Severity: Moderate   **Onset: Rapid**   **Likelihood: Probable**

Cause
Azole antifungals may inhibit hepatic metabolism of HMG-CoA reductase inhibitors, such as simvastatin.

Effect
Sinvastatin level and adverse effects may increase.

Nursing considerations
- If possible, avoid use together.
- HMG-CoA reductase inhibitor dosage may need to be decreased.
- Monitor serum cholesterol and lipid levels.
- **ALERT** Assess patient for evidence of rhabdomyolysis, including fatigue; muscle aches and weakness; joint pain; dark, red, or cola-colored urine; weight gain; seizures; and greatly increased CK level.
- Pravastatin is the HMG-CoA reductase inhibitor least affected by this interaction and may be preferable for use with azole antifungals.

simvastatin ━━━▶◀━━━ bile acid sequestrants
Zocor   cholestyramine, colestipol

Risk rating: 2
Severity: Moderate   Onset: Delayed   Likelihood: Suspected

Cause
GI absorption of HMG-CoA reductase inhibitor, such as simvastatin, may decrease.

Effect
Simvastatin effects may decrease.

Nursing considerations
▶ **ALERT** Separate doses of HMG-CoA reductase inhibitor and bile acid sequestrant by at least 4 hours.
■ If possible, give bile acid sequestrant before meals and HMG-CoA reductase inhibitor in the evening.
■ Monitor serum cholesterol and lipid levels.
■ Obtain liver function test results at start of therapy and periodically thereafter. If ALT or AST level stays three times or more above the upper limit of normal, simvastatin will need to be stopped.
■ Help patient develop a daily plan to ensure proper dosage intervals.

simvastatin ━━━▶◀━━━ carbamazepine
Zocor   Carbatrol, Epitol, Equetro, Tegretol

Risk rating: 2
Severity: Moderate   Onset: Delayed   Likelihood: Suspected

Cause
Carbamazepine may increase CYP3A4 metabolism of HMG-CoA reductase inhibitors, such as simvastatin.

Effect
Simvastatin effects may be reduced.

Nursing considerations
■ If possible, avoid use together.
■ Monitor serum cholesterol and lipid levels.
■ If hypercholesterolemia increases, notify prescriber.
■ Pravastatin and rosuvastatin may be less likely to interact with carbamazepine and may be better choices than simvastatin.
■ Help patient develop a plan to ensure proper dosage intervals.

simvastatin ➤◄ cyclosporine
Zocor   Neoral

Risk rating: 1
Severity: Major   **Onset: Delayed**   **Likelihood: Probable**

Cause
Metabolism of certain HMG-CoA reductase inhibitors, such as simvastatin, may decrease.

Effect
Simvastatin level and adverse effects may increase.

Nursing considerations
- If possible, avoid use together.
- HMG-CoA reductase inhibitor dosage may need to be decreased.
- Monitor serum cholesterol and lipid levels.

⚡ ALERT Assess patient for evidence of rhabdomyolysis, including fatigue; muscle aches and weakness; joint pain; dark, red, or cola-colored urine; weight gain; seizures; and greatly increased CK level.
- Urge patient to report muscle pain, tenderness, or weakness.

simvastatin ➤◄ diltiazem
Zocor   Cardizem

Risk rating: 2
Severity: Moderate   **Onset: Delayed**   **Likelihood: Probable**

Cause
CYP3A4 metabolism of certain HMG-CoA reductase inhibitors, such as simvastatin, may be inhibited.

Effect
HMG-CoA reductase inhibitor level may increase, raising the risk of toxicity, including myositis and rhabdomyolysis.

Nursing considerations
- If possible, avoid use together.

⚡ ALERT Assess patient for evidence of rhabdomyolysis, including fatigue; muscle aches and weakness; joint pain; dark, red, or cola-colored urine; weight gain; seizures; and greatly increased CK level.

⚡ ALERT If patient may have rhabdomyolysis, notify prescriber and obtain renal function tests and serum potassium, sodium, calcium, lactic acid, and myoglobin levels.

■ Pravastatin is less likely to interact with diltiazem than other HMG-CoA reductase inhibitors and may be best choice for combined use.
■ Urge patient to report muscle pain, tenderness, or weakness.

simvastatin ▸◂ gemfibrozil

Zocor   Lopid

Risk rating: 1
Severity: Major   **Onset: Delayed**   **Likelihood: Suspected**

Cause
The mechanism of this interaction is unknown.

Effect
Severe myopathy or rhabdomyolysis may occur.

Nursing considerations
■ Avoid use together.
■ If patient has severe hyperlipidemia, combined therapy may be an option, but only with careful monitoring.
◤ **ALERT** Assess patient for evidence of rhabdomyolysis, including fatigue; muscle aches and weakness; joint pain; dark, red, or cola-colored urine; weight gain; seizures; and greatly increased CK level.
■ Watch for evidence of acute renal failure, including decreased urine output, elevated BUN and creatinine levels, edema, dyspnea, tachycardia, distended neck veins, nausea, vomiting, poor appetite, weakness, fatigue, confusion, and agitation.
■ Urge patient to report muscle pain, tenderness, or weakness.

simvastatin ▸◂ grapefruit juice

Zocor

Risk rating: 2
Severity: Moderate   **Onset: Rapid**   **Likelihood: Suspected**

Cause
Grapefruit juice may inhibit CYP3A4 metabolism of certain HMG-CoA reductase inhibitors, such as simvastatin.

Effect
HMG-CoA reductase inhibitor level may increase, raising the risk of adverse effects.

Nursing considerations
■ Caution patient to take drug with liquid other than grapefruit juice.

⚠ ALERT Watch for evidence of rhabdomyolysis, including fatigue; muscle aches and weakness; joint pain; dark, red, or cola-colored urine; weight gain; seizures; and greatly increased CK level.
- Fluvastatin and pravastatin are metabolized by other enzymes and may be less affected by grapefruit juice.
- Urge patient to report muscle pain, tenderness, or weakness.

---

simvastatin ➤◀ macrolide antibiotics

Zocor   azithromycin, clarithromycin, erythromycin

Risk rating: 1
Severity: Major   Onset: Delayed   Likelihood: Probable

Cause
CYP3A4 metabolism of certain HMG-CoA reductase inhibitors, such as simvastatin, may decrease.

Effect
HMG-CoA reductase inhibitor level may increase, raising the risk of severe myopathy or rhabdomyolysis.

Nursing considerations
⚠ ALERT Watch for evidence of rhabdomyolysis, especially 5 to 21 days after macrolide starts. Evidence may include fatigue; muscle aches and weakness; joint pain; dark, red, or cola-colored urine; weight gain; seizures; and greatly increased CK level.
- Fluvastatin and pravastatin are metabolized by other enzymes and may be better choices when used with macrolide antibiotics.
- Urge patient to report muscle pain, tenderness, or weakness.

---

simvastatin ➤◀ protease inhibitors

Zocor   amprenavir, atazanavir, indinavir, lopinavir-ritonavir, nelfinavir, ritonavir, saquinavir

Risk rating: 1
Severity: Major   Onset: Delayed   Likelihood: Suspected

Cause
First-pass metabolism of simvastatin by CYP3A4 in the GI tract may be inhibited.

Effect
Simvastatin level may increase.

Nursing considerations
◪ **ALERT** Use of nelfinavir with simvastatin is contraindicated.
▪ Avoid giving simvastatin and ritonavir together.
▪ If a protease inhibitor is added to simvastatin, monitor patient closely.
◪ **ALERT** Watch for evidence of rhabdomyolysis, including dark or red urine, muscle weakness, and myalgia.
▪ Urge patient to immediately report unexplained muscle weakness.

---

simvastatin ▶◀ rifamycins

Zocor   rifabutin, rifampin, rifapentine

Risk rating: 2
Severity: Moderate   **Onset: Delayed**   **Likelihood: Suspected**

Cause
Rifamycins may induce CYP3A4 metabolism of HMG-CoA reductase inhibitors, such as simvastatin, in the intestine and liver.

Effect
HMG-CoA reductase inhibitor effects may decrease.

Nursing considerations
▪ Assess patient for expected response to therapy. If you suspect an interaction, consult prescriber; patient may need a different drug.
▪ Check serum cholesterol and lipid levels.
▪ Obtain liver function test results at start of therapy and periodically thereafter. If ALT or AST level stays three times or more above the upper limit of normal, simvastatin will need to be stopped.
▪ Withhold HMG-CoA reductase inhibitor temporarily if patient's risk of myopathy or rhabdomyolysis increases, as from sepsis, hypotension, major surgery, trauma, uncontrolled seizures, or a severe metabolic, endocrine, or electrolyte disorder.
▪ Pravastatin is less likely to interact with rifamycins and may be the best choice for combined use.

---

simvastatin ▶◀ verapamil

Zocor   Calan

Risk rating: 2
Severity: Moderate   **Onset: Delayed**   **Likelihood: Probable**

Cause
CYP3A4 metabolism of certain HMG-CoA reductase inhibitors, such as simvastatin, may decrease.

Effect
HMG-CoA reductase inhibitor level may increase, raising the risk of adverse effects.

Nursing considerations
- If possible, avoid giving simvastatin with verapamil. If patient must take both drugs, consult prescriber; HMG-CoA reductase inhibitor dosage may be decreased.
- **⚠ ALERT** Watch for evidence of rhabdomyolysis, including fatigue; muscle aches and weakness; joint pain; dark, red, or cola-colored urine; weight gain; seizures; and greatly increased CK level.
- Fluvastatin and pravastatin are metabolized by other enzymes and may be better choices for combined use.
- Urge patient to report muscle pain, tenderness, or weakness.

---

sirolimus ◀▶	azole antifungals
Rapamune	fluconazole, itraconazole, ketoconazole

Risk rating: 2
Severity: Moderate   **Onset: Delayed**   **Likelihood: Suspected**

Cause
Azole antifungals inhibit CYP3A4, which is needed for sirolimus metabolism.

Effect
Sirolimus level, effects, and risk of toxicity may increase.

Nursing considerations
- Monitor trough level of sirolimus in whole blood when starting or stopping an azole antifungal. Therapeutic level varies depending on which other drugs patient receives—cyclosporine, for example.
- Watch for signs of sirolimus toxicity, such as anemia, leukopenia, thrombocytopenia, hypokalemia, hyperlipemia, fever, interstitial lung disease, and diarrhea.
- Other CYP3A4 inhibitors may interact with sirolimus. If you suspect an interaction, consult prescriber or pharmacist.
- Urge patient to promptly report new onset of fever over 100° F (38° C), fatigue, shortness of breath, easy bruising, gum bleeding, muscle twitches, palpitations, or chest discomfort or pain.

sirolimus 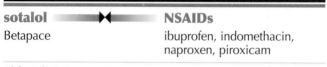 cyclosporine

Rapamune   Gengraf, Neoral, Sandimmune

Risk rating: 2
Severity: Moderate   **Onset: Delayed**   **Likelihood: Probable**

Cause
The mechanism of this interaction is unknown.

Effect
Sirolimus level and risk of toxicity may increase.

Nursing considerations
■ Give sirolimus 4 hours after cyclosporine.
■ Monitor patient for evidence of sirolimus toxicity, such as anxiety, headache, hypertension, and thrombocytopenia.
■ Sirolimus level may decrease when cyclosporine is stopped.
■ Sirolimus dosage may be increased if cyclosporine is stopped.

sotalol 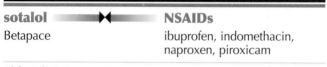 NSAIDs

Betapace   ibuprofen, indomethacin, naproxen, piroxicam

Risk rating: 2
Severity: Moderate   **Onset: Delayed**   **Likelihood: Probable**

Cause
NSAIDs may inhibit renal prostaglandin synthesis, allowing pressor systems to be unopposed.

Effect
Beta blockers, such as sotalol, may not be able to lower blood pressure.

Nursing considerations
■ Avoid using these drugs together if possible.
■ Monitor blood pressure and other evidence of hypertension closely.
■ Talk with prescriber about ways to minimize interaction, such as adjusting beta blocker dosage or switching to sulindac as the NSAID.
■ Explain risks of using these drugs together, and teach patient how to monitor his blood pressure.
■ Other NSAIDs may interact with beta blockers. If you suspect an interaction, consult prescriber or pharmacist.

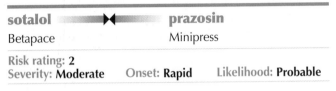

sotalol ▶◀ prazosin
Betapace   Minipress

Risk rating: 2
Severity: Moderate   **Onset: Rapid**   **Likelihood: Probable**

Cause
The mechanism of this interaction is unknown.

Effect
Effect of these drugs on orthostatic hypotension is increased.

Nursing considerations
■ Assess patient's lying, sitting, and standing blood pressures closely, especially when combined therapy starts.
■ Adjust dosages of either drug based on patient effects.
■ To minimize effects of orthostatic hypotension, teach patient to change positions slowly.
■ Interaction is confirmed only with propranolol but may occur with beta blockers other than sotalol as well.

sotalol ▶◀ quinolones
Betapace   gatifloxacin, levofloxacin, moxifloxacin, sparfloxacin

Risk rating: 1
Severity: Major   **Onset: Delayed**   **Likelihood: Suspected**

Cause
The mechanism of this interaction is unknown.

Effect
Risk of life-threatening arrhythmias, including torsades de pointes, increases.

Nursing considerations
⚡ **ALERT** Giving sparfloxacin with an antiarrhythmic, such as sotalol, is contraindicated.
■ Quinolones that aren't metabolized by CYP3A4 isoenzymes or that don't prolong the QT interval may be given with antiarrhythmics.
■ Avoid giving class IA or class III antiarrhythmics with gatifloxacin, levofloxacin, and moxifloxacin.
■ Monitor ECG for prolonged QTc interval.
■ Tell patient to report a rapid heartbeat, shortness of breath, dizziness, fainting, and chest pain.

sotalol ◄►► vardenafil
Betapace   Levitra

Risk rating: 1
Severity: Major   **Onset: Rapid**   **Likelihood: Suspected**

Cause
The mechanism of this interaction is unknown.

Effect
QTc interval may be prolonged, particularly in patients with previous
QT-interval prolongation and those taking certain antiarrhythmics,
increasing the risk of such life-threatening arrhythmias as torsades de
pointes.

Nursing considerations
⚠ ALERT Use of vardenafil with a class IA or class III antiarrhythmic,
such as sotalol, is contraindicated.
■ Monitor patient's ECG before and periodically after patient starts
taking vardenafil.
■ Urge patient to report light-headedness, faintness, palpitations, and
chest pain or pressure while taking vardenafil.
■ To reduce risk of adverse effects, patients age 65 and older should
start with 5 mg vardenafil, half the usual starting dose.

sotalol ◄►► verapamil
Betapace   Calan

Risk rating: 1
Severity: Major   **Onset: Rapid**   **Likelihood: Probable**

Cause
Verapamil may inhibit metabolism of beta blockers, such as sotalol.

Effect
Effects of both drugs may be increased.

Nursing considerations
■ Combination therapy is common in patients with hypertension and
unstable angina.
⚠ ALERT Giving these drugs together increases risk of adverse ef-
fects, including heart failure, conduction disturbances, arrhythmias,
and hypotension.
■ Assess patient for adverse effects, including left ventricular dysfunc-
tion and AV conduction defects.
■ Risk of interaction is greater when drugs are given I.V.
■ Dosages of both drugs may need to be decreased.

sparfloxacin ▶◀ antiarrhythmics

Zagam

amiodarone, bretylium,
disopyramide, procainamide,
quinidine, sotalol

Risk rating: 1
Severity: Major　　**Onset: Delayed**　　**Likelihood: Suspected**

Cause
The mechanism of this interaction is unknown.

Effect
Risk of life-threatening arrhythmias, including torsades de pointes,
increases.

Nursing considerations
◤ ALERT Giving the quinolone sparfloxacin with antiarrhythmics is
contraindicated.
■ Quinolones that aren't metabolized by CYP3A4 isoenzymes or that
don't prolong the QT interval may be given with antiarrhythmics.
■ Monitor ECG for prolonged QTc interval.
■ Tell patient to report a rapid heartbeat, shortness of breath, dizziness, fainting, and chest pain.

sparfloxacin ▶◀ erythromycin

Zagam

E-mycin, Eryc

Risk rating: 1
Severity: Major　　**Onset: Delayed**　　**Likelihood: Suspected**

Cause
The mechanism of this interaction is unknown.

Effect
Risk of life-threatening arrhythmias, including torsades de pointes,
increases.

Nursing considerations
◤ ALERT Use of sparfloxacin with erythromycin is contraindicated.
■ Monitor QTc interval closely.
■ Tell patient to report palpitations, dizziness, shortness of breath, and
chest pain.

sparfloxacin ━━━▶◀━━━ tricyclic antidepressants

Zagam

amitriptyline, amoxapine, clomipramine, desipramine, doxepin, imipramine, nortriptyline, trimipramine

Risk rating: 1
Severity: Major   **Onset: Delayed**   **Likelihood: Suspected**

Cause
The mechanism of this interaction if unknown.

Effect
Life-threatening arrhythmias, including torsades de pointes, may increase when certain of these drugs are used together.

Nursing considerations
◼ **ALERT** The quinolone sparfloxacin is contraindicated in patients taking a tricyclic antidepressant because the QTc interval may be prolonged.
■ If possible, use other quinolone antibiotics that don't prolong the QTc interval or aren't metabolized by the CYP3A4 isoenzyme.

spironolactone ━━━▶◀━━━ ACE inhibitors

Aldactone

benazepril, captopril, enalapril, fosinopril, lisinopril, moexipril, perindopril, quinapril, ramipril, trandolapril

Risk rating: 1
Severity: Major   **Onset: Delayed**   **Likelihood: Probable**

Cause
The mechanism of this interaction is unknown.

Effect
Serum potassium level may increase.

Nursing considerations
■ Use cautiously in patients at high risk for hyperkalemia.
■ Monitor BUN, creatinine, and serum potassium levels as needed.
■ Other ACE inhibitors may interact with potassium-sparing diuretics, such as spironolactone. If you suspect an interaction, consult prescriber or pharmacist.
■ Urge patient to immediately report an irregular heartbeat, a slow pulse, weakness, and other evidence of hyperkalemia.

spironolactone ▰▰▶◀▰▰ angiotensin II receptor antagonists
Aldactone

candesartan, eprosartan, irbesartan, losartan, olmesartan, telmisartan, valsartan

Risk rating: 1
Severity: Major   **Onset: Delayed**   **Likelihood: Suspected**

Cause
Both angiotensin II receptor antagonists and potassium-sparing diuretics, such as spironolactone, may increase serum potassium level.

Effect
Risk of hyperkalemia may increase, especially among high-risk patients.

Nursing considerations
▪ High-risk patients include elderly people and those with renal impairment, type 2 diabetes, or decreased renal perfusion; monitor these patients closely.
▪ Check serum potassium, BUN, and creatinine levels regularly. If they increase, notify prescriber.
▪ Advise patient to immediately report an irregular heartbeat, slow pulse, weakness, or other evidence of hyperkalemia.
▪ Give patient a list of foods high in potassium; stress the need to eat them only in moderate amounts.

spironolactone ▰▰▶◀▰▰ digoxin
Aldactone   Lanoxin

Risk rating: 2
Severity: Moderate   **Onset: Rapid**   **Likelihood: Suspected**

Cause
Spironolactone may lessen digoxin's ability to increase the strength of myocardial contraction. Spironolactone may also decrease renal clearance of digoxin, resulting in increased serum level.

Effect
Positive inotropic effect of digoxin may decrease. Serum digoxin level may increase.

Nursing considerations
▪ Monitor patient for expected digoxin effects, especially in heart failure patients.
▪ Monitor digoxin level. Therapeutic range is 0.8 to 2 nanograms/ml.

⚠ ALERT Spironolactone may interfere with determination of serum digoxin level, causing falsely elevated digoxin level.
■ Digoxin dosage may need adjustment during spironolactone therapy; remember the possibility of a falsely elevated level.

---

spironolactone ◄►◄ potassium preparations

Aldactone

potassium acetate, potassium bicarbonate, potassium chloride, potassium citrate, potassium gluconate, potassium iodine, potassium phosphate

Risk rating: 1
Severity: Major   **Onset: Delayed**   **Likelihood: Established**

Cause
Renal elimination of potassium ions is decreased.

Effect
Risk of severe hyperkalemia increases.

Nursing considerations
⚠ ALERT Don't use this combination unless the patient has severe hypokalemia that isn't responding to either drug class alone.
■ To avoid hyperkalemia, monitor potassium level when therapy starts and frequently thereafter.
■ Tell patient to avoid high-potassium foods, such as citrus juices, bananas, spinach, broccoli, beans, potatoes, and salt substitutes.
■ Urge patient to immediately report palpitations, chest pain, nausea, vomiting, paresthesias, muscle weakness, and other signs of potassium overload.

---

streptomycin ◄►◄ cephalosporins

cefazolin, cefoperazone, cefotaxime, cefotetan, cefoxitin, ceftazidime, ceftizoxime, ceftriaxone, cefuroxime, cephradine

Risk rating: 2
Severity: Moderate   **Onset: Delayed**   **Likelihood: Suspected**

Cause
The mechanism of this interaction is unknown.

Effect
Bactericidal activity may increase against some organisms, but the risk of nephrotoxicity also may increase.

Nursing considerations
⚡ ALERT Check peak and trough streptomycin (aminoglycoside) levels after third dose. For peak level, draw blood 30 minutes after I.V. or 60 minutes after I.M. dose. For trough level, draw blood just before a dose.

■ Assess BUN and creatinine levels.

■ Monitor urine output, and check urine for increased protein, cell, or cast levels.

■ If renal insufficiency develops, notify prescriber. Dosage may need to be reduced, or drug may need to be stopped.

■ Other aminoglycosides may interact with cephalosporins. If you suspect an interaction, consult prescriber or pharmacist.

---

streptomycin ➤◀ loop diuretics
bumetanide, ethacrynic acid, furosemide, torsemide

Risk rating: 1
Severity: Major **Onset: Rapid** **Likelihood: Suspected**

Cause
The mechanism of this interaction is unknown.

Effect
Synergistic ototoxicity may cause hearing loss of varying degrees, possibly permanent.

Nursing considerations
⚡ ALERT Patients with renal insufficiency are at increased risk for ototoxicity.

■ Perform baseline and periodic hearing function tests.

■ Aminoglycosides other than streptomycin may interact with loop diuretics. If you suspect an interaction, consult prescriber or pharmacist.

■ Tell patient to immediately report ringing or roaring in the ears, muffled sounds, or any noticeable changes in hearing.

■ Advise family members to stay alert for evidence of hearing loss.

streptomycin ▬▶◀▬ nondepolarizing muscle relaxants

atracurium, mivacurium, pancuronium, rocuronium, vecuronium

Risk rating: 1
Severity: Major   **Onset: Rapid**   **Likelihood: Probable**

Cause
These drugs may be synergistic.

Effect
Effects of nondepolarizing muscle relaxants may increase.

Nursing considerations
- Give these drugs together only when needed.
- The nondepolarizing muscle relaxant dose may need adjustment based on neuromuscular response.
- Monitor patient for prolonged respiratory depression.
- Provide ventilatory support as needed.

streptomycin ▬▶◀▬ NSAIDs

diclofenac, etodolac, fenoprofen, flurbiprofen, ibuprofen, indomethacin, ketoprofen, ketorolac, meclofenamate, nabumetone, naproxen, oxaprozin, piroxicam, sulindac, tolmetin

Risk rating: 2
Severity: Moderate   **Onset: Delayed**   **Likelihood: Suspected**

Cause
NSAIDs may reduce glomerular filtration rate (GFR), causing streptomycin and other aminoglycosides to accumulate.

Effect
Aminoglycoside level in premature infants may increase.

Nursing considerations
- Before NSAID starts, aminoglycoside dose should be reduced.
- ◤ ALERT Check peak and trough aminoglycoside levels after third dose. For peak level, draw blood 30 minutes after I.V. or 60 minutes after I.M. dose. For trough level, draw blood just before a dose.

- Monitor patient's renal function.
- Although only indomethacin is known to interact with aminoglycosides, other NSAIDs probably do as well. If you suspect an interaction, consult prescriber or pharmacist.
- Other drugs cleared by GFR may have a similar interaction.

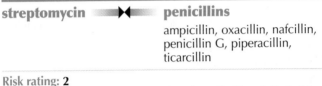

streptomycin ▸◂ penicillins

ampicillin, oxacillin, nafcillin, penicillin G, piperacillin, ticarcillin

Risk rating: 2
Severity: Moderate   **Onset: Delayed**   **Likelihood: Probable**

Cause
The mechanism of this interaction is unknown.

Effect
Penicillins may inactivate certain aminoglycosides, such as streptomycin, decreasing their effects.

Nursing considerations
⚠ ALERT Check peak and trough aminoglycoside levels after third dose. For peak level, draw blood 30 minutes after I.V. or 60 minutes after I.M. dose. For trough level, draw blood just before a dose.
- Monitor patient's renal function.
- Other aminoglycosides may interact with penicillins. If you suspect an interaction, consult prescriber or pharmacist.

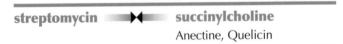

streptomycin ▸◂ succinylcholine

Anectine, Quelicin

Risk rating: 2
Severity: Moderate   **Onset: Rapid**   **Likelihood: Probable**

Cause
Streptomycin and other aminoglycosides may stabilize the postjunctional membrane and disrupt prejunctional calcium influx and acetylcholine output, thereby causing a synergistic interaction with succinylcholine.

Effect
Aminoglycosides potentiate the neuromuscular effects of succinylcholine.

Nursing considerations
■ After succinylcholine use, delay aminoglycoside delivery as long as possible after adequate respirations return.
■ If drugs must be given together, use extreme caution, and monitor respiratory status closely.
N ALERT Patients with renal impairment and those receiving amino-glycosides by peritoneal instillation have an increased risk of prolonged neuromuscular blockade.
■ If respiratory depression occurs, patient may need mechanical ventilation. Give I.V. calcium or a cholinesterase inhibitor if needed.

---

sucralfate ━━━►◄━━━ penicillamine
Carafate   Cuprimine, Depen

Risk rating: 2
Severity: Moderate   Onset: Delayed   Likelihood: Probable

Cause
Formation of a physical or chemical complex with aluminum may decrease GI absorption of penicillamine.

Effect
Penicillamine efficacy may be reduced.

Nursing considerations
■ Separate administration times.
■ If patient must take these drugs together, notify prescriber. Penicillamine dose may need adjustment.
■ Monitor patient for reduced penicillamine efficacy.
■ Help patient develop a plan to ensure proper dosage intervals.

---

sucralfate ━━━►◄━━━ quinolones
Carafate   ciprofloxacin, lomefloxacin, moxifloxacin, norfloxacin, ofloxacin

Risk rating: 2
Severity: Moderate   Onset: Rapid   Likelihood: Probable

Cause
Sucralfate decreases GI absorption of quinolone.

Effect
Quinolone effects decrease.

Nursing considerations
- Avoid use together. If it's unavoidable, give sucralfate at least 6 hours after the quinolone.
- Monitor patient for resolving infection.
- Help patient develop a plan to ensure proper dosage intervals.

---

sulfadiazine ◄► hydantoins
ethotoin, fosphenytoin, phenytoin

Risk rating: 2
Severity: **Moderate**   Onset: **Delayed**   Likelihood: **Probable**

Cause
Sulfadiazine may inhibit hepatic metabolism of hydantoins.

Effect
Hydantoin level and effects may be increased, along with risk of toxic effects.

Nursing considerations
- Monitor serum hydantoin level. Therapeutic range for phenytoin is 10 to 20 mcg/ml.
- Hydantoin dosage may need adjustment.
- **⚡ ALERT** If sulfadiazine starts during hydantoin therapy, watch for evidence of hydantoin toxicity, including drowsiness, nausea, vomiting, nystagmus, ataxia, dysarthria, tremor, slurred speech, hypotension, arrhythmias, respiratory depression, and coma.
- If sulfadiazine stops during hydantoin therapy, watch for decreased anticonvulsant effect and increased seizure activity.
- Consult prescriber or pharmacist about other anti-infective drugs if patient takes a hydantoin.

---

sulfasalazine ◄► sulfonylureas
Azulfidine

acetohexamide, chlorpropamide, glipizide, tolazamide, tolbutamide

Risk rating: 2
Severity: **Moderate**   Onset: **Delayed**   Likelihood: **Suspected**

Cause
Sulfasalazine and other sulfonamides may hinder hepatic metabolism of sulfonylureas.

Effect
Prolonged sulfonylurea level increases risk of hypoglycemia.

Nursing considerations
■ If patient takes a sulfonylurea, start sulfonamide treatment carefully, watching for hypoglycemia.
■ Monitor blood glucose level regularly, and consult prescriber about adjustments to either drug to maintain stable glucose level.
■ Glyburide doesn't interact and may be a good alternative to other sulfonylureas.
■ Describe signs and symptoms of hypoglycemia, including diaphoresis, fatigue, headache, hunger, irritability, malaise, nervousness, rapid heart rate, tension, and trembling.
■ Instruct patient to eat a small carbohydrate snack or meal if hypoglycemia develops, preferably after checking blood glucose level.

---

sulfinpyrazone ▶◀ acetaminophen
Anturane   Acephen, Neopap, Tylenol

Risk rating: 2
Severity: Moderate   **Onset: Delayed**   **Likelihood: Suspected**

Cause
Sulfinpyrazone may induce hepatic microsomal enzymes, accelerating the metabolism of acetaminophen.

Effect
Abnormally high rate of acetaminophen metabolism may lead to higher levels of hepatotoxic metabolites, increasing the risk of hepatic impairment.

Nursing considerations
◪ ALERT The hepatotoxic risk is greatest after acetaminophen overdose in a patient who uses sulfinpyrazone regularly.
■ No special monitoring or dosage adjustment is needed at usual therapeutic dosages.
■ Advise patient who is taking sulfinpyrazone to avoid long-term use of acetaminophen.
■ Tell patient to notify prescriber about abdominal pain, yellowing of the skin or eyes, or dark urine.

sulfinpyrazone ➤◄ salicylates

Anturane

aspirin, bismuth subsalicylate, choline salicylate, magnesium salicylate, salsalate, sodium salicylate

Risk rating: 2
Severity: Moderate   Onset: Delayed   Likelihood: Established

Cause
Salicylates block the effect of sulfinpyrazone on tubular reabsorption of uric acid, and they displace sulfinpyrazone from plasma protein-binding sites, decreasing sulfinpyrazone level.

Effect
Uricosuric effects of sulfinpyrazone are inhibited.

Nursing considerations
⚠ ALERT Typically, use of sulfinpyrazone with a salicylate is contraindicated.
■ Monitor serum urate level; the usual goal of sulfinpyrazone therapy is about 6 mg/dl.
■ Occasional use of aspirin at low doses may not interfere with the uricosuric action of sulfinpyrazone.
⚠ ALERT Remind patient to carefully read the labels of OTC medicines because many contain salicylates.
■ If an analgesic or antipyretic is needed during sulfinpyrazone therapy, suggest acetaminophen.
■ Advise patient to maintain adequate fluid intake to prevent formation of uric acid kidney stones.

sulfisoxazole ➤◄ sulfonylureas

Gantrisin

acetohexamide, chlorpropamide, glipizide, tolazamide, tolbutamide

Risk rating: 2
Severity: Moderate   Onset: Delayed   Likelihood: Suspected

Cause
Sulfisoxazole and other sulfonamides may hinder hepatic metabolism of sulfonylureas.

Effect
Prolonged sulfonylurea level increases risk of hypoglycemia.

Nursing considerations
■ If patient takes a sulfonylurea, start sulfonamide treatment carefully, monitoring patient for hypoglycemia.
■ Monitor blood glucose level regularly, and consult prescriber about adjustments to either drug to maintain stable glucose level.
■ Glyburide doesn't interact and may be a good alternative to other sulfonylureas.
■ Describe signs and symptoms of hypoglycemia, including diaphoresis, fatigue, headache, hunger, irritability, malaise, nervousness, rapid heart rate, tension, and trembling.
■ Instruct patient to eat a small carbohydrate snack or meal if hypoglycemia develops, preferably after checking blood glucose level.

---

sulindac ▶◀ aminoglycosides
Clinoril

amikacin, gentamicin, kanamycin, netilmicin, streptomycin, tobramycin

Risk rating: 2
Severity: Moderate   Onset: Delayed   Likelihood: Suspected

Cause
Sulindac and other NSAIDs may reduce glomerular filtration rate (GFR), causing aminoglycosides to accumulate.

Effect
Aminoglycoside level in premature infants may increase.

Nursing considerations
■ Before NSAID starts, aminoglycoside dose should be reduced.
◤ **ALERT** Check peak and trough aminoglycoside levels after third dose. For peak level, draw blood 30 minutes after I.V. or 60 minutes after I.M. dose. For trough level, draw blood just before a dose.
■ Monitor patient's renal function.
■ Although only indomethacin is known to interact with aminoglycosides, other NSAIDs probably do as well. If you suspect an interaction, consult prescriber or pharmacist.
■ Other drugs cleared by GFR may have a similar interaction.

sumatriptan ▸◂ ergot derivatives

Imitrex   dihydroergotamine, ergotamine

Risk rating: 1
Severity: Major   **Onset: Rapid**   **Likelihood: Suspected**

Cause
Combined use may have additive effects.

Effect
Risk of vasospastic effects increases.

Nursing considerations
⚠ **ALERT** Use of these drugs or any two selective 5-HT$_1$ receptor agonists within 24 hours of each other is contraindicated.
■ Combined use may cause severe vasospastic effects, including sustained coronary artery vasospasm that triggers MI.
■ Warn patient not to mix migraine headache drugs within 24 hours of each other, but to call prescriber if a drug isn't effective.

sumatriptan ▸◂ MAO inhibitors

Imitrex   isocarboxazid, phenelzine,
                                 tranylcypromine

Risk rating: 1
Severity: Major   **Onset: Rapid**   **Likelihood: Suspected**

Cause
MAO inhibitors, subtype-A, may inhibit metabolism of selective 5-HT$_1$ receptor agonists, such as sumatriptan.

Effect
Serum level of—and risk of cardiac toxicity from—certain selective 5-HT$_1$ receptor agonists may increase.

Nursing considerations
⚠ **ALERT** Use of certain selective 5-HT$_1$ receptor agonists with or within 2 weeks of stopping an MAO inhibitor is contraindicated.
■ If these drugs must be used together, naratriptan is less likely than sumatriptan to interact with an MAO inhibitor.
■ Cardiac toxicity may include coronary artery vasospasm and transient myocardial ischemia.

sumatriptan ▶◀ serotonin reuptake inhibitors

Imitrex

citalopram, fluoxetine, fluvoxamine, nefazodone, paroxetine, sertraline, venlafaxine

Risk rating: 1
Severity: Major   **Onset: Rapid**   **Likelihood: Suspected**

Cause
Serotonin may accumulate rapidly in the CNS.

Effect
Risk of serotonin syndrome increases.

Nursing considerations
◼ **ALERT** If possible, avoid combined use of these drugs.
■ Start with lowest dosages possible, and assess patient closely.
■ Stop the selective 5-HT$_1$ receptor agonist, such as sumatriptan, at the first sign of interaction, and notify prescriber.
■ In some patients, migraine frequency may increase and antimigraine drug efficacy may decrease when a serotonin reuptake inhibitor is started.
■ Describe the traits of serotonin syndrome: CNS irritability, motor weakness, shivering, muscle twitching, and altered consciousness.
■ Explain that serotonin syndrome can be fatal if not treated immediately.

sumatriptan ▶◀ sibutramine

Imitrex   Meridia

Risk rating: 1
Severity: Major   **Onset: Rapid**   **Likelihood: Suspected**

Cause
Sibutramine inhibits serotonin reuptake, which may have an additive effect with selective 5-HT$_1$ receptor agonists, such as sumatriptan.

Effect
Risk of serotonin syndrome increases.

Nursing considerations
◼ **ALERT** If possible, avoid giving these drugs together.
■ Monitor patient closely for adverse effects, which require immediate medical attention.

■ Stop the selective 5-HT$_1$ receptor agonist at the first sign of interaction, and notify prescriber.
■ Describe the traits of serotonin syndrome, including CNS irritability, motor weakness, shivering, myoclonus, and altered consciousness.
■ Urge patient to promptly report adverse effects.

---

tacrolimus ➤◄ azole antifungals

Prograf

fluconazole, itraconazole, ketoconazole, miconazole

Risk rating: **2**
Severity: **Moderate**   Onset: **Delayed**   Likelihood: **Probable**

Cause
Azole antifungals inhibit tacrolimus metabolism in the liver and GI tract.

Effect
Tacrolimus level and risk of adverse effects may increase.

Nursing considerations
■ Monitor renal function and mental status closely.
■ Check tacrolimus level often. Normal trough level is 6 to 10 mcg/L.
■ Tacrolimus dosage may need to be decreased when patient takes an azole antifungal.
■ Signs of toxicity often occur within 3 days of combined use
◪ **ALERT** Watch for renal failure, nephrotoxicity, hyperkalemia, hyperglycemia, delirium, and other changes in mental status.

---

tacrolimus ➤◄ diltiazem

Prograf

Cardizem

Risk rating: **2**
Severity: **Moderate**   Onset: **Delayed**   Likelihood: **Suspected**

Cause
Tacrolimus CYP3A4 hepatic metabolism may be inhibited.

Effect
Tacrolimus level and risk of toxicity may increase.

Nursing considerations
■ Monitor serum tacrolimus level; therapeutic range for liver transplants is 5 to 20 nanograms/ml; for kidney transplants, it's 7 to

20 nanograms/ml for the first 3 months and 5 to 15 nanograms/ml through 1 year.
■ Watch for evidence of tacrolimus toxicity: delirium, confusion, agitation, tremor, adverse GI effects, and abnormal renal function tests.
■ Tacrolimus dosage may need adjustment when diltiazem is started or stopped or when its dosage is changed.
■ Diltiazem may have similar effects on cyclosporine and sirolimus.

tacrolimus ▸◂ hydantoins
Prograf   fosphenytoin, phenytoin

Risk rating: 2
Severity: Moderate   Onset: Delayed   Likelihood: Suspected

Cause
CYP3A4 metabolism of tacrolimus may increase.

Effect
Tacrolimus level may decrease. Phenytoin level may increase.

Nursing considerations
■ Monitor levels of both drugs. Expected trough level of tacrolimus is 6 to 10 mcg/L; expected phenytoin level is 10 to 20 mcg/ml.
■ Watch closely for signs of neurotoxicity or syncope; adjust doses of both drugs as needed.
■ This effect may occur with fosphenytoin as well.
■ If one drug is stopped, continue to monitor serum level of remaining drug; dosage may need to be changed.

tacrolimus ▸◂ macrolide antibiotics
Prograf   clarithromycin, erythromycin, troleandomycin

Risk rating: 2
Severity: Moderate   Onset: Delayed   Likelihood: Suspected

Cause
Certain macrolide antibiotics inhibit CYP3A4 metabolism of tacrolimus.

Effect
Tacrolimus level and risk of toxicity may increase.

Nursing considerations
■ If possible, use a different class of antibiotic.

- Monitor tacrolimus level and renal function test results. Expected trough level of tacrolimus is 6 to 10 mcg/L.
- This effect occurs in children and adults.
- Tacrolimus may need to be stopped temporarily because reduced dosages may not prevent renal changes.
- Other macrolide antibiotics may interact.

tacrolimus ▶◀ rifamycins

Prograf   rifabutin, rifampin, rifapentine

Risk rating: 1
Severity: Major   Onset: Delayed   Likelihood: Probable

Cause
Rifamycins increase CYP3A4 metabolism of tacrolimus.

Effect
Immunosuppressive effects of tacrolimus on organ transplant recipients may decrease.

Nursing considerations
- Monitor tacrolimus level closely when rifamycin starts; it may decrease in as little as 2 days. Expected trough level is 6 to 10 mcg/L.
- Increase tacrolimus dosage to compensate for faster metabolism.
- Watch patient closely and check serum level when a rifamycin is stopped so dosage can be adjusted upward.
- Watch for signs of organ rejection or infection during rifamycin treatment.

tacrolimus ▶◀ St. John's wort

Prograf

Risk rating: 1
Severity: Major   Onset: Delayed   Likelihood: Probable

Cause
St. John's wort increases CYP3A4 metabolism of tacrolimus.

Effect
Tacrolimus level may decrease, increasing the risk of organ transplant rejection.

Nursing considerations
- Discourage use of tacrolimus with St. John's wort.
- Monitor tacrolimus level closely if patient takes St. John's wort. Dosage may need adjustment after St. John's wort is stopped.

■ It may take up to 2 weeks for this effect to fully dissipate after St. John's wort is stopped.
■ If patient takes tacrolimus, discourage use of any herbal product without consulting prescriber.

tacrolimus ▶◀ voriconazole
Prograf   Vfend

Risk rating: 2
Severity: Moderate   Onset: Delayed   Likelihood: Suspected

Cause
Voriconazole inhibits tacrolimus metabolism in the liver and GI tract.

Effect
Tacrolimus level and risk of adverse effects or toxicity may increase.

Nursing considerations
■ Monitor renal function and mental status closely when using these drugs together.
■ Check tacrolimus level often. Expected trough level is 6 to 10 mcg/L.
■ Tacrolimus dosage may need to be decreased.
■ This interaction may occur with other azole antifungals.
◣ALERT Watch for renal failure, nephrotoxicity, hyperkalemia, hyperglycemia, delirium, and other changes in mental status.

tadalafil ▶◀ nitrates
Cialis   amyl nitrite, isosorbide
                                dinitrate, isosorbide
                                mononitrate, nitroglycerin

Risk rating: 1
Severity: Major   Onset: Rapid   Likelihood: Suspected

Cause
Tadalafil potentiates the hypotensive effects of nitrates.

Effect
Risk of severe hypotension increases.

Nursing considerations
◣ ALERT Use of nitrates with tadalafil is contraindicated.
■ Carefully screen patient for tadalafil use before giving a nitrate. Even during an emergency, before giving a nitrate, find out if patient with chest pain has taken tadalafil during the previous 48 hours.

■ Monitor patient for orthostatic hypotension, dizziness, sweating, and headache.

---

telmisartan ▶◀ potassium-sparing diuretics
Micardis

amiloride, spironolactone, triamterene

Risk rating: 1
Severity: Major   **Onset: Delayed**   **Likelihood: Suspected**

Cause
Both angiotensin II receptor antagonists, such as telmisartan, and potassium-sparing diuretics may increase serum potassium level.

Effect
Risk of hyperkalemia may increase, especially among high-risk patients.

Nursing considerations
■ High-risk patients include elderly people and those with renal impairment, type 2 diabetes, or decreased renal perfusion; monitor these patients closely.
■ Check serum potassium, BUN, and creatinine levels regularly. If they increase, notify prescriber.
■ Advise patient to immediately report an irregular heartbeat, slow pulse, weakness, or other evidence of hyperkalemia.
■ Give patient a list of foods high in potassium; stress the need to eat them only in moderate amounts.

---

temazepam ▶◀ alcohol
Restoril

Risk rating: 2
Severity: Moderate   **Onset: Rapid**   **Likelihood: Established**

Cause
Alcohol inhibits hepatic enzymes, which decreases clearance and increases peak level of benzodiazepines, such as temazepam.

Effect
Combining a benzodiazepine and alcohol may have additive or synergistic effects.

Nursing considerations
■ Advise against consuming alcohol while taking a benzodiazepine.

■ Before benzodiazepine starts, assess patient thoroughly for history or evidence of alcohol use.
■ Watch for additive CNS effects, which may suggest benzodiazepine overdose.

---

terbinafine ━━▶◀━━ cyclosporine
Lamisil   Gengraf, Neoral, Sandimmune

Risk rating: 2
Severity: Moderate   Onset: Delayed   Likelihood: Suspected

Cause
Terbinafine may increase cyclosporine metabolism.

Effect
Cyclosporine level may decrease.

Nursing considerations
■ Monitor cyclosporine level.
■ Adjust cyclosporine dose as needed.
■ Closely monitor patient for signs and symptoms of rejection when terbinafine is started or stopped.

---

terbinafine ━━▶◀━━ tricyclic antidepressants
Lamisil   desipramine, imipramine, nortriptyline

Risk rating: 2
Severity: Moderate   Onset: Delayed   Likelihood: Suspected

Cause
Hepatic metabolism of tricyclic antidepressants (TCAs) may be inhibited.

Effect
Therapeutic and toxic effects of certain TCAs may increase.

Nursing considerations
■ Check for toxic TCA level, and report abnormal level.
■ TCA dosage may need to be decreased.
■ Adverse effects or toxicity may include vertigo, fatigue, loss of appetite, ataxia, muscle twitching, or trouble swallowing.
■ Terbinafine's inhibitory effects may take several weeks to dissipate after drug is stopped.
■ Describe signs and symptoms patient should look for.

tetracyclines ▶◀ aluminum salts

demeclocycline, doxycycline, minocycline, oxytetracycline, tetracycline

aluminum carbonate, aluminum hydroxide, magaldrate

Risk rating: 2
Severity: Moderate   Onset: Delayed   Likelihood: Probable

Cause
Formation of an insoluble chelate with aluminum may decrease tetracycline absorption.

Effect
Tetracycline level may decline more than 50%, reducing efficacy.

Nursing considerations
- Separate doses by at least 3 hours.
- If patient must take these drugs together, notify prescriber.
- Monitor patient for reduced anti-infective response, including infection flare-up, fever, and malaise.
- Other tetracyclines may interact with aluminum salts. If you suspect an interaction, consult prescriber or pharmacist.
- Help patient develop a plan to ensure proper dosage intervals.

tetracyclines ▶◀ calcium salts

demeclocycline, doxycycline, minocycline, oxytetracycline, tetracycline

calcium carbonate, calcium citrate, calcium gluconate, calcium lactate, tricalcium phosphate

Risk rating: 2
Severity: Moderate   Onset: Delayed   Likelihood: Probable

Cause
Calcium salts form an insoluble complex with tetracyclines that lowers tetracycline absorption.

Effect
Tetracycline level and anti-infective efficacy decrease.

Nursing considerations
- Separate tetracycline from calcium salt by at least 3 to 4 hours.
- Monitor efficacy of tetracycline in resolving infection. Notify prescriber if infection isn't responding to treatment.
- Doxycycline is somewhat less affected by this interaction.

■ Advise against taking tetracycline with dairy products or calcium-fortified orange juice or within 4 hours of a calcium supplement.

tetracyclines ➤◀ iron salts

demeclocycline, doxycycline, minocycline, oxytetracycline, tetracycline

ferrous fumarate, ferrous gluconate, ferrous sulfate, iron polysaccharide

Risk rating: 2
Severity: Moderate   **Onset: Delayed**   **Likelihood: Probable**

Cause
Tetracyclines form insoluble chelates with iron salts, which may reduce absorption of both substances.

Effect
Tetracycline and iron salt levels and effects may decrease.

Nursing considerations
◤ ALERT If possible, avoid giving tetracycline with iron salt.
■ Separate doses by 3 to 4 hours.
■ Monitor patient for expected response to tetracycline.
■ Assess patient for evidence of iron deficiency: fatigue, dyspnea, tachycardia, palpitations, dizziness, and orthostatic hypotension.
■ If you suspect an interaction, consult prescriber or pharmacist; an enteric-coated or sustained-release iron salt may reduce it.

tetracyclines ➤◀ magnesium salts

demeclocycline, doxycycline, minocycline, oxytetracycline, tetracycline

magaldrate, magnesium carbonate, magnesium citrate, magnesium gluconate, magnesium hydroxide, magnesium oxide, magnesium sulfate, magnesium trisilicate

Risk rating: 2
Severity: Moderate   **Onset: Delayed**   **Likelihood: Probable**

Cause
Magnesium salts form an insoluble complex with tetracyclines that lowers tetracycline absorption.

Effect
Tetracycline level and efficacy decrease.

Nursing considerations
■ Separate tetracycline from magnesium salt by at least 3 to 4 hours.
■ Monitor efficacy of tetracycline in resolving infection. Notify prescriber if infection isn't responding to treatment.
■ Teach patient to separate tetracycline dose from magnesium-based antacids, laxatives, and supplements by 3 to 4 hours.

---

tetracyclines ▶◀	penicillins
demeclocycline, doxycycline, minocycline, tetracycline	amoxicillin, ampicillin, carbenicillin, cloxacillin, dicloxacillin, nafcillin, oxacillin, penicillin G, penicillin V, piperacillin, ticarcillin

Risk rating: 1
Severity: Major   **Onset: Delayed**   **Likelihood: Suspected**

Cause
Tetracyclines may adversely affect the bactericidal activity of penicillins.

Effect
Penicillin efficacy may be reduced.

Nursing considerations
■ If possible, avoid giving tetracycline with penicillin.
■ Monitor patient closely for lack of penicillin effect.

---

theophyllines ▶◀	acyclovir
aminophylline, theophylline	Zovirax

Risk rating: 2
Severity: Moderate   **Onset: Delayed**   **Likelihood: Suspected**

Cause
Acyclovir may inhibit oxidative metabolism of theophyllines.

Effect
Theophylline level, adverse effects, and toxicity may increase.

Nursing considerations
■ Monitor serum theophylline level closely. Therapeutic range is 10 to 20 mcg/ml for adults and 5 to 15 mcg/ml for children.
■ Theophylline dosage may need to be decreased.

- Watch for increased adverse effects of theophylline, such as tachycardia, anorexia, nausea, vomiting, diarrhea, seizures, restlessness, irritability, and headache.
- Describe adverse effects of theophylline and signs of toxicity, and tell patient to report them immediately.

theophyllines ▶◀ barbiturates

aminophylline,
theophylline

amobarbital, butabarbital,
pentobarbital, phenobarbital,
primidone, secobarbital

Risk rating: 2
Severity: Moderate   **Onset: Delayed**   **Likelihood: Suspected**

Cause
Barbiturates may stimulate theophylline clearance by inducing the CYP pathway.

Effect
Theophylline level and efficacy may decrease.

Nursing considerations
- Monitor patient closely to determine theophylline efficacy.
- Monitor serum theophylline level regularly. Therapeutic range is 10 to 20 mcg/ml for adults and 5 to 15 mcg/ml for children.
- Theophylline dosage may need to be increased.

theophyllines ▶◀ beta blockers, nonselective

aminophylline,
theophylline

bisoprolol, carteolol,
penbutolol, pindolol,
propranolol, timolol

Risk rating: 2
Severity: Moderate   **Onset: Rapid**   **Likelihood: Probable**

Cause
Theophylline clearance may be reduced up to 50%.

Effect
Theophylline efficacy may decrease.

Nursing considerations
- Watch for decreased theophylline efficacy.

■ Monitor serum theophylline level closely, and notify prescriber about subtherapeutic level. Therapeutic range for theophylline is 10 to 20 mcg/ml for adults and 5 to 15 mcg/ml for children.
■ Selective beta blockers may be preferred for patients who take theophylline, but interaction still occurs with high doses of beta blocker.
■ Other beta blockers may interact with theophyllines. If you suspect an interaction, consult prescriber or pharmacist.

theophyllines ◄► cimetidine
aminophylline, theophylline   Tagamet

Risk rating: 2
Severity: **Moderate**   Onset: **Delayed**   Likelihood: **Established**

Cause
Cimetidine inhibits hepatic metabolism of theophyllines.

Effect
Serum theophylline level and risk of toxicity may increase.

Nursing considerations
■ Watch for evidence of toxicity, such as tachycardia, anorexia, nausea, vomiting, diarrhea, seizures, restlessness, irritability, and headache.
■ Monitor serum theophylline level closely. Therapeutic range is 10 to 20 mcg/ml for adults and 5 to 15 mcg/ml for children.
■ Theophylline dosage may need to be decreased by 20% to 40%.
■ Describe adverse effects of theophylline and signs of toxicity, and tell patient to report them immediately to prescriber.
■ Giving ranitidine or famotidine instead of cimetidine for gastric hypersecretion may decrease risk of this interaction.

theophyllines ◄► diltiazem
aminophylline, theophylline   Cardizem

Risk rating: 2
Severity: **Moderate**   Onset: **Delayed**   Likelihood: **Suspected**

Cause
Theophylline metabolism may be inhibited.

Effect
Serum theophylline level and risk of toxicity may increase.

Nursing considerations
■ Watch for evidence of toxicity, such as tachycardia, anorexia, nausea, vomiting, diarrhea, seizures, restlessness, irritability, and headache.

- Monitor serum theophylline level closely. Therapeutic range is 10 to 20 mcg/ml for adults and 5 to 15 mcg/ml for children.
- Describe adverse effects of theophylline and signs of toxicity, and tell patient to report them immediately to prescriber.

theophyllines ▶◀ disulfiram
aminophylline, theophylline   Antabuse

Risk rating: 2
Severity: Moderate   Onset: Delayed   Likelihood: Suspected

Cause
Disulfiram inhibits metabolism of theophylline.

Effect
Theophylline effects, including toxic effects, increase.

Nursing considerations
- Watch for evidence of toxicity, such as tachycardia, anorexia, nausea, vomiting, diarrhea, seizures, restlessness, irritability, and headache.
- Monitor serum theophylline level closely. Therapeutic range is 10 to 20 mcg/ml for adults and 5 to 15 mcg/ml for children.
- Disulfiram causes dose-dependent inhibition of theophylline; the theophylline dosage may need adjustment.
- Describe adverse effects of theophylline and signs of toxicity, and tell patient to report them immediately to prescriber.

theophyllines ▶◀ fluvoxamine
aminophylline, theophylline   Luvox

Risk rating: 2
Severity: Moderate   Onset: Delayed   Likelihood: Suspected

Cause
Fluvoxamine inhibits CYP1A2 metabolism of theophylline in the liver.

Effect
Theophylline level and risk of toxicity may increase.

Nursing considerations
- Monitor serum theophylline level closely. Therapeutic range is 10 to 20 mcg/ml for adults and 5 to 15 mcg/ml for children.
- If patient taking fluvoxamine starts taking theophylline, the theophylline dosage may be reduced by 33%.

■ Watch for evidence of toxicity, such as tachycardia, anorexia, nausea, vomiting, diarrhea, seizures, restlessness, irritability, and headache.
■ Describe adverse effects of theophylline and signs of toxicity, and tell patient to report them immediately to prescriber.

theophyllines ▶◀ macrolide antibiotics

aminophylline, theophylline

azithromycin, clarithromycin, erythromycin

Risk rating: 2
Severity: Moderate   Onset: Delayed   Likelihood: Established

Cause
Certain macrolides inhibit metabolism of theophylline. Theophylline increases renal clearance and decreases availability of oral erythromycin.

Effect
Theophylline level and risk of toxicity may increase. Erythromycin level may decrease.

Nursing considerations
■ Monitor serum theophylline level. Therapeutic range is 10 to 20 mcg/ml for adults and 5 to 15 mcg/ml for children.
■ Consult prescriber about possibility of using another antibiotic.
■ Watch for evidence of toxicity, such as tachycardia, anorexia, nausea, vomiting, diarrhea, seizures, restlessness, irritability, and headache.
■ Describe adverse effects of theophylline and signs of toxicity, and tell patient to report them immediately to prescriber.
■ If patient takes theophylline, watch for decreased erythromycin efficacy; tell prescriber promptly.

theophyllines ▶◀ mexiletine

aminophylline, theophylline

Mexitil

Risk rating: 2
Severity: Moderate   Onset: Delayed   Likelihood: Established

Cause
Mexiletine inhibits CYP metabolism of theophylline.

Effect
Serum theophylline level may increase, increasing risk of toxicity.

Nursing considerations
■ Monitor theophylline level closely. Therapeutic range is 10 to 20 mcg/ml for adults and 5 to 15 mcg/ml for children.
■ Interaction usually occurs within 2 days of combining these drugs. Theophylline dosage may be decreased when mexiletine starts.
■ Watch for evidence of toxicity, such as ventricular tachycardia, anorexia, nausea, vomiting, diarrhea, seizures, restlessness, irritability, and headache.
■ Describe adverse effects of theophylline and signs of toxicity, and tell patient to report them immediately to prescriber.

---

theophyllines ➤◀ nondepolarizing muscle relaxants
aminophylline,
theophylline

atracurium, mivacurium,
pancuronium, vecuronium

Risk rating: 2
Severity: Moderate   **Onset: Rapid**   **Likelihood: Suspected**

Cause
These drugs may act antagonistically.

Effect
Neuromuscular blockade may be reversed.

Nursing considerations
■ Monitor patient closely for lack of drug effect.
■ Dosage of nondepolarizing muscle relaxant may need adjustment.
■ This interaction is dose dependent.
■ Make sure patient is adequately sedated when receiving a nondepolarizing muscle relaxant.

---

theophyllines ➤◀ phenytoin
aminophylline,
theophylline

Dilantin

Risk rating: 2
Severity: Moderate   **Onset: Delayed**   **Likelihood: Probable**

Cause
Metabolism of both drugs increases.

Effect
Theophylline or phenytoin efficacy may decrease.

Nursing considerations
- Monitor levels of both drugs carefully. Expected phenytoin level is 10 to 20 mcg/ml. Expected theophylline level is 10 to 20 mcg/ml for adults and 5 to 15 mcg/ml for children.
- Assess patient for seizures and respiratory distress, and report findings to prescriber promptly; dosages may need adjustment.
- Interaction typically occurs within 5 days of combined therapy.

---

theophyllines ➤◀ rifamycins
aminophylline, theophylline   rifabutin, rifampin, rifapetine

Risk rating: 2
Severity: Moderate   Onset: Delayed   Likelihood: Established

Cause
Rifamycins may induce GI and hepatic metabolism of theophyllines.

Effect
Theophylline efficacy may decrease.

Nursing considerations
- Monitor theophylline level closely. Therapeutic range is 10 to 20 mcg/ml for adults and 5 to 15 mcg/ml for children.
- After a rifamycin is started, watch for increased pulmonary signs and symptoms.
- Tell patient to immediately report all concerns about drug efficacy to prescriber; dosage may need adjustment.

---

theophyllines ➤◀ thioamines
aminophylline, theophylline   methimazole, propylthiouracil

Risk rating: 2
Severity: Moderate   Onset: Delayed   Likelihood: Suspected

Cause
Thioamines increase theophylline clearance in hyperthyroid patients.

Effect
Theophylline level and effects decrease.

Nursing considerations
- Watch closely for decreased theophylline efficacy while abnormal thyroid status continues.
- ◤ ALERT Assess patient for return to euthyroid state, when interaction no longer occurs.

■ Explain that hyperthyroidism and hypothyroidism can affect theophylline efficacy and toxicity; tell patient to immediately report evidence of either one to prescriber.
■ To prevent this interaction, urge patients to have TSH and theophylline levels tested regularly.

theophyllines ➤◄ thyroid hormones
aminophylline, theophylline   levothyroxine, liothyronine, liotrix, thyroid

Risk rating: 2
Severity: Moderate   **Onset: Delayed**   **Likelihood: Suspected**

Cause
T_4 level is directly related to theophylline level. Patients who are hyperthyroid or hypothyroid may have varying interactions.

Effect
In hypothyroidism, theophylline metabolism decreases and serum level—and risk of toxicity—increase.

Nursing considerations
■ Monitor theophylline level and dosage carefully; adjust as needed to avoid toxicity. Therapeutic range is 10 to 20 mcg/ml for adults and 5 to 15 mcg/ml for children.
◤ **ALERT** Watch for increased adverse effects of theophylline, such as tachycardia, anorexia, nausea, vomiting, diarrhea, seizures, restlessness, irritability, and headache.
■ Once patient is euthyroid, theophylline clearance returns to normal.
■ Explain common side effects of theophylline and signs of toxicity, and tell patient to report them immediately to prescriber.

theophyllines ➤◄ ticlopidine
aminophylline, theophylline   Ticlid

Risk rating: 2
Severity: Moderate   **Onset: Delayed**   **Likelihood: Suspected**

Cause
Theophylline elimination is impaired.

Effect
Theophylline level and risk of toxicity may increase.

Nursing considerations
■ Use together cautiously. Monitor theophylline level and patient response closely.
■ Watch for evidence of theophylline toxicity, including nausea, vomiting, seizures, and arrhythmias.
■ If ticlopidine is stopped, theophylline dosage should be increased.
■ Urge patient to report decreasing theophylline effects.

---

theophyllines 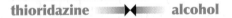 zileuton
aminophylline,   Zyflo
theophylline

Risk rating: 2
Severity: Moderate   Onset: Delayed   Likelihood: Probable

Cause
Zileuton may inhibit theophylline metabolism.

Effect
Theophylline level and risk of adverse effects may increase.

Nursing considerations
■ Monitor serum theophylline level closely. Therapeutic range is 10 to 20 mcg/ml for adults and 5 to 15 mcg/ml for children.
■ Watch for evidence of toxicity, such as tachycardia, anorexia, nausea, vomiting, diarrhea, seizures, restlessness, irritability, and headache.
■ If patient starts zileuton while already taking theophylline, theophylline dosage should decrease by 50%.
■ Explain common side effects of theophylline and signs of toxicity, and tell patient to report them immediately to prescriber.

---

thioridazine alcohol

Risk rating: 2
Severity: Moderate   Onset: Rapid   Likelihood: Probable

Cause
The mechanism of this interaction is unknown. These substances may produce CNS depression by working on different sites in the brain. Also, alcohol may lower resistance to neurotoxic effects of phenothiazines, such as thioridazine.

Effect
CNS depression may increase.

Nursing considerations
■ Watch for extrapyramidal reactions, such as dystonic reactions and acute akathisia or restlessness.
■ If patient takes a phenothiazine, warn that alcohol may worsen CNS depression and impair psychomotor skills.
■ Discourage alcohol consumption during phenothiazine therapy.

---

thioridazine ▬▶◀▬ **antiarrhythmics**
amiodarone, bretylium, disopyramide, procainamide, quinidine, sotalol

Risk rating: 1
Severity: Major   **Onset: Delayed**   **Likelihood: Suspected**

Cause
Thioridazine may have additive effects on prolongation of the QTc interval.

Effect
Risk of life-threatening arrhythmias may increase.

Nursing considerations
⚡ **ALERT** Use of these drugs together is contraindicated.
■ Life-threatening torsades de pointes may result.
■ Bradycardia, hypokalemia, and congenital prolongation of the QTc are added risk factors for torsades de pointes or sudden death.
■ Prolongation of the QTc interval depends on the dose of thioridazine, becoming more pronounced as the dose increases.

---

thioridazine ▬▶◀▬ **anticholinergics**
atropine, belladonna, benztropine, biperiden, dicyclomine, hyoscyamine, oxybutynin, propantheline, scopolamine

Risk rating: 2
Severity: Moderate   **Onset: Delayed**   **Likelihood: Suspected**

Cause
Anticholinergics may antagonize thioridazine and other phenothiazines. Also, phenothiazine metabolism may increase.

Effect
Phenothiazine efficacy may decrease.

Nursing considerations
- Data regarding this interaction conflict.
- Monitor patient for decreased phenothiazine efficacy.
- The phenothiazine dosage may need adjustment.
- Anticholinergic side effects may increase.
- Monitor patient for adynamic ileus, hyperpyrexia, hypoglycemia, and neurologic changes.

---

thioridazine 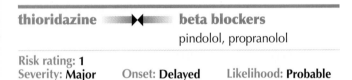 beta blockers
pindolol, propranolol

Risk rating: 1
Severity: Major   **Onset: Delayed**   **Likelihood: Probable**

Cause
Pindolol and propranolol inhibit thioridazine metabolism.

Effect
Effects of both drugs and the risk of serious adverse reactions may increase.

Nursing considerations
⚡ ALERT Use of thioridazine with pindolol or propranolol is contra-indicated.
- Assess patient for fatigue, lethargy, dizziness, nausea, heart failure, and agranulocytosis, all of which are adverse reactions to propranolol.
- Explain expected and adverse effects of these drugs and the risk of interaction.
- Other beta blockers may interact with thioridazine. If you suspect an interaction, consult prescriber or pharmacist.

---

thioridazine 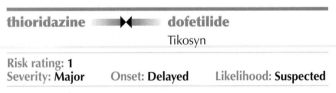 dofetilide
Tikosyn

Risk rating: 1
Severity: Major   **Onset: Delayed**   **Likelihood: Suspected**

Cause
Thioridazine and dofetilide may have additive effects on prolongation of the QTc interval.

Effect
Risk of life-threatening arrhythmias may increase.

Nursing considerations
⚠ **ALERT** Use of these drugs together is contraindicated.
■ Life-threatening torsades de pointes may result.
■ Bradycardia, hypokalemia, and congenital prolongation of the QTc are added risk factors for torsades de pointes or sudden death.
■ Prolongation of the QTc interval depends on the dose of thioridazine, becoming more pronounced as the dose increases.

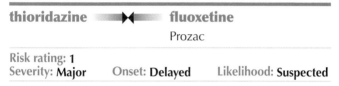

thioridazine ◼▶◀◼ fluoxetine
Prozac

Risk rating: 1
Severity: Major   **Onset: Delayed**   **Likelihood: Suspected**

Cause
Thioridazine metabolism may be inhibited by fluoxetine.

Effect
Risk of life-threatening arrhythmias may increase.

Nursing considerations
⚠ **ALERT** Use of these drugs together is contraindicated.
■ Life-threatening torsades de pointes may result.
■ Prolongation of QTc interval depends on the dose of thioridazine, becoming more pronounced as the dose increases.
■ The CYP2D6 pathway is implicated in the slowed metabolism of thioridazine when given with fluoxetine.

---

thioridazine ◼▶◀◼ fluvoxamine
Luvox

Risk rating: 1
Severity: Major   **Onset: Delayed**   **Likelihood: Suspected**

Cause
Thioridazine metabolism may be inhibited by fluvoxamine.

Effect
Risk of life-threatening arrhythmias and other adverse effects may increase.

Nursing considerations
⚠ **ALERT** Use of these drugs together is contraindicated.

- Life-threatening torsades de pointes may result.
- This interaction continues for more than 2 weeks after fluvoxamine is stopped.
- Other possible adverse effects include tardive dyskinesia, neuroleptic malignant syndrome, constipation, orthostatic hypotension, and urine retention.

---

thioridazine 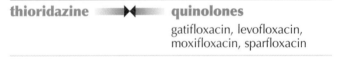 pimozide
Orap

Risk rating: 1
Severity: Major   **Onset: Delayed**   **Likelihood: Suspected**

Cause
Thioridazine may have additive effects on prolongation of the QTc interval.

Effect
Risk of life-threatening arrhythmias may increase.

Nursing considerations
▸ ALERT Use of these drugs together is contraindicated.
- Life-threatening torsades de pointes may result.
- Bradycardia, hypokalemia, and congenital prolongation of the QTc are added risk factors for torsades de pointes or sudden death.
- Prolongation of the QTc interval depends on the dose of thioridazine, becoming more pronounced as the dose increases.

---

thioridazine 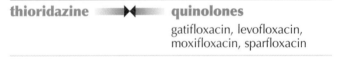 quinolones
gatifloxacin, levofloxacin,
moxifloxacin, sparfloxacin

Risk rating: 1
Severity: Major   **Onset: Delayed**   **Likelihood: Suspected**

Cause
The mechanism of this interaction is unknown.

Effect
Risk of life-threatening arrhythmias, including torsades de pointes, may increase.

Nursing considerations
▸ ALERT Sparfloxacin is contraindicated in patients taking drugs that prolong the QTc interval, including thioridazine and other phenothiazines.

- Avoid giving levofloxacin with thioridazine.
- Use gatifloxacin and moxifloxacin cautiously, with increased monitoring.
- Quinolones that don't prolong the QTc interval or that aren't metabolized by CYP3A4 isoenzymes may be better alternatives.

---

thyroid hormones ▶◀ cholestyramine

levothyroxine,
liothyronine,
liotrix, thyroid

LoCHOLEST, Prevalite,
Questran

Risk rating: 2
Severity: **Moderate**   Onset: **Delayed**   Likelihood: **Suspected**

Cause
Cholestyramine may prevent GI absorption of thyroid hormones.

Effect
Thyroid hormone effects may be lost; hypothyroidism may develop.

Nursing considerations
- Separate doses by 6 hours.
- Monitor patient for signs of hypothyroidism: weakness, fatigue, weight gain, coarse dry hair, rough skin, cold intolerance, muscle aches, constipation, depression, mental irritability, and memory loss.
- Monitor thyroid function tests during combined use (TSH, 0.2 to 5.4 microunits/ml; T_3, 80 to 200 nanograms/dl; T_4, 5.4 to 11.5 mcg/dl).
- Consult prescriber for an antihyperlipidemic drug as an alternative to cholestyramine.
- Other thyroid hormones may interact with cholestyramine. If you suspect an interaction, consult prescriber or pharmacist.

---

thyroid hormones ▶◀ estrogens

levothyroxine, liotrix

conjugated estrogens, esterified estrogens, estradiol, estrone, estropipate, ethinyl estradiol

Risk rating: 2
Severity: **Moderate**   Onset: **Delayed**   Likelihood: **Probable**

Cause
Estrogen increases serum level of thyroxine-binding globulin. Because thyroid hormone binds to the protein, T_3 and T_4 levels decrease, and TSH is secreted to compensate.

Effect
In hypothyroid women, decreased T_3 and T_4 levels and increased TSH level decrease the efficacy of thyroid hormone replacement.

Nursing considerations
■ Check serum TSH, T_3, and T_4 levels about 12 weeks after hypothyroid patient starts estrogen therapy. Therapeutic range for TSH is 0.2 to 5.4 microunits/ml; for T_3, 80 to 200 nanograms/dl; and for T_4, 5.4 to 11.5 mcg/dl.
■ Watch for evidence of hypothyroidism, including weakness, fatigue, weight gain, coarse dry hair, rough skin, cold intolerance, muscle aches, constipation, depression, irritability, and memory loss.
■ Adjust thyroid hormone dose as ordered.
■ Explain that thyroid hormone dose may need to be altered during estrogen therapy.
■ Tell patient to report evidence of hypothyroidism, such as fatigue, weight gain, cold intolerance, and constipation.

---

thyroid hormones ▶◀ theophyllines

levothyroxine,
liothyronine,
liotrix, thyroid

aminophylline, theophylline

Risk rating: **2**
Severity: **Moderate**   Onset: **Delayed**   Likelihood: **Suspected**

Cause
T_4 level is directly related to theophylline level. Patients who are hyperthyroid or hypothyroid may have varying interactions.

Effect
In hypothyroidism, theophylline metabolism decreases and serum level—and risk of toxicity—increase.

Nursing considerations
■ Monitor theophylline level and dosage carefully; adjust dosage as needed to avoid toxicity. Therapeutic range is 10 to 20 mcg/ml for adults and 5 to 15 mcg/ml for children.
■ Watch for increased adverse effects of theophylline, such as tachycardia, anorexia, nausea, vomiting, diarrhea, seizures, restlessness, irritability, and headache.
■ Once patient is euthyroid, theophylline clearance returns to normal.
■ Explain common adverse effects of theophylline and signs of toxicity, and tell patient to report them immediately to prescriber.

ticarcillin ▶◀ aminoglycosides

Ticar

amikacin, gentamicin, kanamycin, netilmicin, streptomycin, tobramycin

Risk rating: 2
Severity: Moderate   **Onset: Delayed**   **Likelihood: Probable**

Cause
The mechanism of this interaction is unknown.

Effect
Ticarcillin and other penicillins may inactivate certain aminoglycosides, decreasing their effects.

Nursing considerations
⚡ **ALERT** Check peak and trough aminoglycoside levels after third dose. For peak level, draw blood 30 minutes after I.V. or 60 minutes after I.M. dose. For trough level, draw blood just before a dose.
■ Monitor patient's renal function.
■ Other aminoglycosides may interact with penicillins. If you suspect an interaction, consult prescriber or pharmacist.
■ Penicillin affects gentamicin and tobramycin more than amikacin and netilmicin.

ticarcillin ▶◀ tetracyclines

Ticar

demeclocycline, doxycycline, minocycline, tetracycline

Risk rating: 1
Severity: Major   **Onset: Delayed**   **Likelihood: Suspected**

Cause
Tetracyclines may adversely affect the bactericidal activity of ticarcillin and other penicillins.

Effect
Ticarcillin efficacy may be reduced.

Nursing considerations
■ If possible, avoid giving tetracycline with penicillin.
■ Monitor patient closely for lack of penicillin effect.

ticlopidine ➤◄ hydantoins

Ticlid   ethotoin, fosphenytoin, phenytoin

Risk rating: 2
Severity: Moderate   Onset: Delayed   Likelihood: Probable

Cause
Ticlopidine may inhibit hepatic metabolism of hydantoins.

Effect
Hydantoin level and risk of adverse effects may increase.

Nursing considerations
■ Monitor serum hydantoin level. Therapeutic range for phenytoin is 10 to 20 mcg/ml.
■ Hydantoin level may increase gradually over a month, and hydantoin dosage may need adjustment.
■ If ticlopidine starts during hydantoin therapy, monitor patient for adverse CNS effects of hydantoins, including vertigo, ataxia, and somnolence. If ticlopidine stops during hydantoin therapy, watch for decreased anticonvulsant effect and increased seizure activity.

ticlopidine ➤◄ theophyllines

Ticlid   aminophylline, theophylline

Risk rating: 2
Severity: Moderate   Onset: Delayed   Likelihood: Suspected

Cause
Theophylline elimination is impaired.

Effect
Theophylline level and risk of toxicity may increase.

Nursing considerations
■ Combine cautiously. Monitor theophylline level and patient response.
■ Watch for evidence of theophylline toxicity, including nausea, vomiting, seizures, and arrhythmias.
■ If ticlopidine is stopped, theophylline dosage should be increased.
■ Urge patient to report decreased theophylline benefits.

timolol ━━━━►◄━━━━ cimetidine
Blocadren   Tagamet

Risk rating: 2
Severity: Moderate   **Onset: Rapid**   **Likelihood: Probable**

Cause
By inhibiting the CYP pathway, cimetidine reduces the first-pass metabolism of certain beta blockers, such as timolol.

Effect
Timolol clearance decreases and action increases.

Nursing considerations
- Monitor patient for severe bradycardia and hypotension.
- If interaction occurs, beta blocker dosage may be decreased.
- Teach patient to monitor pulse rate. If it's significantly lower than usual, tell him to withhold beta blocker and to contact prescriber.
- Instruct patient to change positions slowly to reduce effects of orthostatic hypotension.
- Other beta blockers may interact with cimetidine. If you suspect an interaction, consult prescriber or pharmacist.

timolol ━━━━►◄━━━━ epinephrine
Blocadren

Risk rating: 1
Severity: Major   **Onset: Rapid**   **Likelihood: Established**

Cause
Alpha-receptor effects of epinephrine supersede effects of timolol and other nonselective beta blockers, increasing vascular resistance.

Effect
Initial marked hypertensive effect is followed by reflex bradycardia.

Nursing considerations
⚡ **ALERT** Three days before planned use of epinephrine, stop the beta blocker. Or, if possible, don't use epinephrine.
- Monitor blood pressure and pulse closely. If interaction occurs, give I.V. chlorpromazine, hydralazine, aminophylline, or atropine if needed.
- Explain the risks of this interaction, and tell patient to carry medical identification at all times.
- Other beta blockers may interact with epinephrine. If you suspect an interaction, consult prescriber or pharmacist.

timolol ▶◀ ergot derivatives

Blocadren   dihydroergotamine, ergotamine

Risk rating: 2
Severity: Moderate   **Onset: Delayed**   **Likelihood: Suspected**

Cause
Vasocontriction and blockade of peripheral beta$_2$ receptors by the beta blocker timolol allows unopposed ergot action.

Effect
Vasoconstrictive effects of ergot derivatives increase, causing peripheral ischemia, cold extremities, and possible gangrene.

Nursing considerations
■ Watch for evidence of peripheral ischemia.
■ If needed, stop beta blocker and adjust ergot derivative.
■ Other ergot derivatives may interact with beta blockers. If you suspect an interaction, consult prescriber or pharmacist.

timolol ▶◀ NSAIDs

Blocadren   ibuprofen, indomethacin,
                                           naproxen, piroxicam

Risk rating: 2
Severity: Moderate   **Onset: Delayed**   **Likelihood: Probable**

Cause
NSAIDs may inhibit renal prostaglandin synthesis, allowing pressor systems to be unopposed.

Effect
Timolol and other beta blockers may not be able to lower blood pressure.

Nursing considerations
■ Avoid using these drugs together if possible.
■ Monitor blood pressure and other evidence of hypertension closely.
■ Consult prescriber about ways to minimize interaction, such as adjusting beta blocker dosage or switching to sulindac as the NSAID.
■ Explain the risks of using these drugs together, and teach patient how to monitor his blood pressure.
■ Other NSAIDs may interact with beta blockers. If you suspect an interaction, consult prescriber or pharmacist.

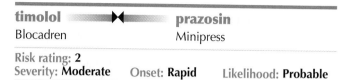

timolol ◄► prazosin
Blocadren   Minipress

Risk rating: 2
Severity: Moderate   **Onset: Rapid**   **Likelihood: Probable**

Cause
The mechanism of this interaction is unknown.

Effect
Effect of these drugs on orthostatic hypotension increases.

Nursing considerations
■ Assess patient's lying, sitting, and standing blood pressures closely, especially when combined therapy starts.
■ Adjust dosages of either drug based on patient effects.
■ To minimize effects of orthostatic hypotension, teach patient to change positions slowly.
■ Interaction is confirmed only with propranolol but also may occur with timolol and other beta blockers.

timolol ◄► quinidine
Blocadren

Risk rating: 2
Severity: Moderate   **Onset: Rapid**   **Likelihood: Suspected**

Cause
Quinidine may inhibit metabolism of certain beta blockers, such as timolol, in patients who are extensive metabolizers of debrisoquin.

Effect
Beta blocker effects may increase.

Nursing considerations
■ Monitor pulse and blood pressure more often during combined use.
■ If pulse slows or blood pressure falls, consult prescriber. Beta blocker dosage may need to be decreased.
■ Instruct patient to check blood pressure and pulse rate regularly.
■ If patient uses timolol eye drops, warn about possible systemic effects, including slow pulse and low blood pressure; urge patient to notify prescriber promptly if they occur.

timolol ◄►◄ salicylates

Blocadren

aspirin, bismuth subsalicylate, choline salicylate, magnesium salicylate, salsalate, sodium salicylate, sodium thiosalicylate

Risk rating: 2
Severity: Moderate   Onset: **Rapid**   Likelihood: **Suspected**

Cause
Salicylates inhibit synthesis of prostaglandins, which timolol and other beta blockers need to reduce blood pressure. In patients with heart failure, the mechanism of this interaction is unknown.

Effect
Beta blocker effects decrease.

Nursing considerations
■ Watch closely for signs of heart failure and hypertension, and notify prescriber if they occur.
■ Consult prescriber about switching patient to a different antihypertensive or antiplatelet drug.
■ Other beta blockers may interact with salicylates. If you suspect an interaction, consult prescriber or pharmacist.
■ Explain signs and symptoms of heart failure, and tell patient when to contact prescriber.

timolol ◄►◄ theophyllines

Blocadren

aminophylline, theophylline

Risk rating: 2
Severity: Moderate   Onset: **Rapid**   Likelihood: **Probable**

Cause
Theophylline clearance may be reduced up to 50%.

Effect
Theophylline efficacy may decrease.

Nursing considerations
■ When timolol or another nonselective beta blocker starts, watch for decreased theophylline efficacy.
■ Monitor theophylline level closely, and notify prescriber about subtherapeutic level. Therapeutic range for theophylline is 10 to 20 mcg/ml for adults and 5 to 15 mcg/ml for children.

- Selective beta blockers may be preferred for patients who take theophylline, but interaction still occurs with high doses of beta blocker.
- Other beta blockers may interact with theophyllines. If you suspect an interaction, consult prescriber or pharmacist.

timolol ◄► verapamil
Blocadren   Calan

Risk rating: 1
Severity: Major   **Onset: Rapid**   **Likelihood: Probable**

Cause
Verapamil may inhibit metabolism of beta blockers, such as timolol.

Effect
Effects of both drugs may increase.

Nursing considerations
- Combined use is common in hypertension with unstable angina.
- **ALERT** Risk of adverse effects increases, including heart failure, conduction disturbances, arrhythmias, and hypotension.
- Assess patient for adverse effects, including left ventricular dysfunction and AV conduction defects.
- Risk of interaction is greater when drugs are given I.V.
- Dosages of both drugs may need to be decreased.

tobramycin ◄► cephalosporins
cefazolin, cefoperazone, cefotaxime, cefotetan, cefoxitin, ceftazidime, ceftizoxime, ceftriaxone, cefuroxime, cephradine

Risk rating: 2
Severity: Moderate   **Onset: Delayed**   **Likelihood: Suspected**

Cause
The mechanism of this interaction is unknown.

Effect
Bactericidal activity may increase against some organisms, but the risk of nephrotoxicity also may increase.

Nursing considerations

◣ **ALERT** Check peak and trough tobramycin levels after third dose. For peak level, draw blood 30 minutes after I.V. or 60 minutes after I.M. dose. For trough level, draw blood just before a dose.

■ Assess BUN and creatinine levels.

■ Monitor urine output, and check urine for increased protein, cell, or cast levels.

■ If renal insufficiency develops, notify prescriber. Dosage may need to be reduced, or drug may need to be stopped.

■ Aminoglycosides other than tobramycin may interact with cephalosporins. If you suspect an interaction, consult prescriber or pharmacist.

---

tobramycin ━━━━▶◀━━━━ **loop diuretics**
bumetanide, ethacrynic acid, furosemide, torsemide

Risk rating: 1
Severity: Major   Onset: **Rapid**   Likelihood: **Suspected**

Cause
The mechanism of this interaction is unknown.

Effect
Synergistic ototoxicity may cause hearing loss of varying degrees, possibly permanent.

Nursing considerations

◣ **ALERT** Renal insufficiency increases the risk of ototoxicity.

■ Perform baseline and periodic hearing function tests.

■ Aminoglycosides other than tobramycin may interact with loop diuretics. If you suspect an interaction, consult prescriber or pharmacist.

■ Tell patient to immediately report ringing or roaring in the ears, muffled sounds, or any noticeable changes in hearing.

■ Advise family members to stay alert for evidence of hearing loss.

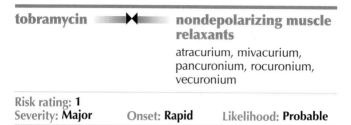

tobramycin ▶◀ nondepolarizing muscle relaxants

atracurium, mivacurium, pancuronium, rocuronium, vecuronium

Risk rating: 1
Severity: Major   **Onset: Rapid**   **Likelihood: Probable**

Cause
These drugs may be synergistic.

Effect
Effects of nondepolarizing muscle relaxants may increase.

Nursing considerations
- Give these drugs together only when needed.
- The nondepolarizing muscle relaxant dose may need adjustment based on neuromuscular response.
- Monitor patient for prolonged respiratory depression.
- Provide ventilatory support as needed.

tobramycin ▶◀ NSAIDs

diclofenac, etodolac, fenoprofen, flurbiprofen, ibuprofen, indomethacin, ketoprofen, ketorolac, meclofenamate, nabumetone, naproxen, oxaprozin, piroxicam, sulindac, tolmetin

Risk rating: 2
Severity: Moderate   **Onset: Delayed**   **Likelihood: Suspected**

Cause
NSAIDs may reduce glomerular filtration rate (GFR), causing tobramycin and other aminoglycosides to accumulate.

Effect
Aminoglycoside level in premature infants may increase.

Nursing considerations
- Before NSAID starts, aminoglycoside dose should be reduced.
- ◤ ALERT Check peak and trough tobramycin levels after third dose. For peak level, draw blood 30 minutes after I.V. or 60 minutes after I.M. dose. For trough level, draw blood just before a dose.

- Monitor patient's renal function.
- Although only indomethacin is known to interact with aminoglycosides, other NSAIDs probably do as well. If you suspect an interaction, consult prescriber or pharmacist.
- Other drugs cleared by GFR may have a similar interaction.

---

tobramycin ➤◄ penicillins

ampicillin, nafcillin, oxacillin, penicillin G, piperacillin, ticarcillin

Risk rating: 2
Severity: Moderate   Onset: Delayed   Likelihood: Probable

Cause
The mechanism of this interaction is unknown.

Effect
Penicillins may inactivate certain aminoglycosides, such as tobramycin, decreasing their effects.

Nursing considerations
⚡ ALERT Check peak and trough tobramycin levels after third dose. For peak level, draw blood 30 minutes after I.V. or 60 minutes after I.M. dose. For trough level, draw blood just before a dose.
- Monitor patient's renal function.

---

tolazamide ➤◄ alcohol

Tolinase

Risk rating: 2
Severity: Moderate   Onset: Rapid   Likelihood: Established

Cause
Chronic alcohol use may have several interactions with sulfonylureas, such as tolazamide.

Effect
Patients who take tolazamide may have a disulfiram-like reaction.

Nursing considerations
- Other sulfonylureas may cause these interactions.
- Naloxone may be used to antagonize a disulfiram-like reaction.

■ Tell patient who takes an oral antidiabetic to avoid ingesting more alcohol than an occasional single drink.

■ Urge patient to have regular follow-up blood tests to monitor diabetes and decrease episodes of hyperglycemia and hypoglycemia.

■ Describe the traits of a disulfiram-like reaction, including facial flushing and possible burning that spreads to the neck, headache, nausea, and tachycardia. Explain that it typically occurs within 20 minutes of alcohol intake and lasts for 1 to 2 hours.

tolazamide ◼▸◂ chloramphenicol
Tolinase   Chloromycetin

Risk rating: 2
Severity: Moderate   Onset: Delayed   Likelihood: Suspected

Cause
Chloramphenicol reduces hepatic clearance of sulfonylureas, such as tolazamide.

Effect
Because sulfonylurea level is prolonged, hypoglycemia may occur.

Nursing considerations
■ If patient takes a sulfonylurea, start chloramphenicol carefully, and monitor for signs and symptoms of hypoglycemia.

■ Describe signs and symptoms of hypoglycemia, including diaphoresis, fatigue, headache, hunger, irritability, malaise, nervousness, rapid heart rate, tension, and trembling.

■ Instruct patient to eat a small carbohydrate snack or meal if hypoglycemia develops, preferably after checking blood glucose level.

tolazamide ◼▸◂ diazoxide
Tolinase   Hyperstat, Proglycem

Risk rating: 2
Severity: Moderate   Onset: Delayed   Likelihood: Probable

Cause
Diazoxide may decrease insulin release or stimulate release of glucose and free fatty acids by various mechanisms.

Effect
Risk of hyperglycemia increases if patient stabilized on tolazamide or another sulfonylurea starts diazoxide.

Nursing considerations
■ Use these drugs together cautiously.
■ Monitor blood glucose level regularly, and consult prescriber about adjustments to either drug to maintain stable glucose level.
■ Tell patient to stay alert for evidence of high blood glucose level, such as increased fatigue, thirst, eating, or urination and possible blurred vision or dry skin and mucous membranes.

---

tolazamide ■◄►	MAO inhibitors
Tolinase	isocarboxazid, phenelzine, tranylcypromine

Risk rating: 2
Severity: Moderate   **Onset: Rapid**   **Likelihood: Suspected**

Cause
The mechanism of this interaction is unknown.

Effect
MAO inhibitors increase the hypoglycemic effects of sulfonylureas, such as tolazamide.

Nursing considerations
■ If patient takes a sulfonylurea, start the MAO inhibitor carefully, monitoring for signs and symptoms of hypoglycemia.
■ Consult prescriber about adjustments to either drug to control glucose level and mental status.
■ Describe signs and symptoms of hypoglycemia, including diaphoresis, fatigue, headache, hunger, irritability, malaise, nervousness, rapid heart rate, tension, and trembling.
■ Instruct patient to eat a small carbohydrate snack or meal if hypoglycemia develops, preferably after checking blood glucose level.

---

tolazamide ■◄►	rifamycins
Tolinase	rifabutin, rifampin, rifapentine

Risk rating: 2
Severity: Moderate   **Onset: Delayed**   **Likelihood: Probable**

Cause
Rifamycins may increase hepatic metabolism of certain sulfonylureas, such as tolazamide.

Effect
Risk of hyperglycemia increases.

Nursing considerations
■ Use these drugs together cautiously.
■ Monitor blood glucose level regularly, and consult prescriber about adjustments to either drug to maintain stable glucose level.
■ Tell patient to stay alert for evidence of high blood glucose level, such as increased fatigue, thirst, eating, or urination and possible blurred vision or dry skin and mucous membranes.

tolazamide ▬▬▬►◄▬▬▬ salicylates

Tolinase

aspirin, choline salicylate, magnesium salicylate, salsalate, sodium salicylate, sodium thiosalicylate

Risk rating: 2
Severity: Moderate   Onset: Delayed   Likelihood: Probable

Cause
Salicylates reduce glucose level and promote insulin secretion.

Effect
Hypoglycemic effects of sulfonylureas, such as tolazamide, increase.

Nursing considerations
■ Start salicylate carefully, monitoring patient for hypoglycemia.
■ Consult prescriber about possibly replacing a salicylate with acetaminophen or an NSAID.
■ Describe signs and symptoms of hypoglycemia, including diaphoresis, fatigue, headache, hunger, irritability, malaise, nervousness, rapid heart rate, tension, and trembling.
■ Instruct patient to eat a small carbohydrate snack or meal if hypoglycemia develops, preferably after checking blood glucose level.

tolazamide ▬▬▬►◄▬▬▬ sulfonamides

Tolinase

sulfasalazine, sulfisoxazole

Risk rating: 2
Severity: Moderate   Onset: Delayed   Likelihood: Suspected

Cause
Sulfonamides may hinder hepatic metabolism of sulfonylureas, such as tolazamide.

Effect
Prolonged sulfonylurea level increases risk of hypoglycemia.

Nursing considerations
■ Start sulfonamide carefully, monitoring patient for hypoglycemia. Consult prescriber about adjustments to either drug to maintain stable glucose level.
■ Glyburide doesn't interact and may be a good alternative to other sulfonylureas.
■ Describe signs and symptoms of hypoglycemia, including diaphoresis, fatigue, headache, hunger, irritability, malaise, nervousness, rapid heart rate, tension, and trembling.
■ Instruct patient to eat a small carbohydrate snack or meal if hypoglycemia develops, preferably after checking blood glucose level.

---

tolazamide ◼▶◀◼ thiazide diuretics

Tolinase

chlorothiazide, hydrochlorothiazide, indapamide, metolazone

Risk rating: 2
Severity: **Moderate**   Onset: **Delayed**   Likelihood: **Probable**

Cause
Thiazide diuretics may decrease insulin secretion and tissue sensitivity to insulin, and they may increase potassium loss.

Effect
Risk of hyperglycemia and hyponatremia may increase.

Nursing considerations
■ Use these drugs together cautiously.
■ Monitor patient's glucose level regularly, and consult prescriber about adjustments to either drug to maintain stable glucose level.
■ This interaction may occur several days to many months after dual therapy starts but is readily reversible when the diuretic stops.
■ Describe signs and symptoms of hypoglycemia, including diaphoresis, fatigue, headache, hunger, irritability, malaise, nervousness, rapid heart rate, tension, and trembling.
■ Instruct patient to eat a small carbohydrate snack or meal if hypoglycemia develops, preferably after checking blood glucose level.

tolmetin ◄►►◄ aminoglycosides

Tolectin

amikacin, gentamicin, kanamycin, streptomycin, tobramycin

Risk rating: 2
Severity: **Moderate**   Onset: **Delayed**   Likelihood: **Suspected**

Cause
Tolmetin and other NSAIDs may reduce glomerular filtration rate (GFR), causing aminoglycosides to accumulate.

Effect
Aminoglycoside level in premature infants may increase.

Nursing considerations
■ Before NSAID starts, aminoglycoside dose should be reduced.
■ ALERT Check peak and trough aminoglycoside levels after third dose. For peak level, draw blood 30 minutes after I.V. or 60 minutes after I.M. dose. For trough level, draw blood just before a dose.
■ Monitor patient's renal function.
■ Although only indomethacin is known to interact with aminoglycosides, other NSAIDs probably do as well. If you suspect an interaction, consult prescriber or pharmacist.
■ Other drugs cleared by GFR may have a similar interaction.

tolterodine ◄►►◄ azole antifungals

Detrol

fluconazole, itraconazole, ketoconazole

Risk rating: 2
Severity: **Moderate**   Onset: **Delayed**   Likelihood: **Suspected**

Cause
Azole antifungals inhibit CYP3A4, which is needed for tolterodine metabolism.

Effect
Tolterodine level, effects, and risk of adverse effects may increase.

Nursing considerations
■ Notify prescriber if patient takes both drugs; an alternative may be available.
■ Watch for evidence of tolterodine overdose, such as dry mouth, urine retention, constipation, dizziness, and headache.

■ Explain adverse tolterodine effects, and tell patient to report them promptly.
■ Other CYP3A4 inhibitors may interact with tolterodine. If you suspect an interaction, consult prescriber or pharmacist.

---

topiramate ▶◀ estrogens

Topamax

conjugated estrogens, esterified estrogens, estradiol, estrone, estropipate, ethinyl estradiol

Risk rating: 2
Severity: Moderate   Onset: Delayed   Likelihood: Suspected

Cause
Topiramate may increase estrogen metabolism.

Effect
Estrogen efficacy may decrease.

Nursing considerations
■ Watch for worsening of menopausal vasomotor symptoms, including hot flashes, diaphoresis, headache, nausea, palpitations, dizziness, and a skin-crawling sensation.
■ If patient takes topiramate, estrogen dosage may need to be increased; consult prescriber or pharmacist.
■ Tell patient that estrogen may be less effective when taken with topiramate. Suggest a nonhormonal contraceptive.
■ Urge patient to report loss of drug effect—such as spotting, breakthrough bleeding, and amenorrhea—or increased adverse effects.

---

torsemide ▶◀ aminoglycosides

Demadex

amikacin, gentamicin, kanamycin, neomycin, streptomycin, tobramycin

Risk rating: 1
Severity: Major   Onset: Rapid   Likelihood: Suspected

Cause
The mechanism of this interaction is unknown.

Effect
Synergistic ototoxicity may cause hearing loss of varying degrees, possibly permanent.

Nursing considerations

⚠ ALERT Renal insufficiency increases the risk of ototoxicity.

■ Perform baseline and periodic hearing function tests.

■ Other aminoglycosides may interact with loop diuretics, such as torsemide. If you suspect an interaction, consult prescriber.

■ Tell patient to immediately report ringing or roaring in the ears, muffled sounds, or any noticeable changes in hearing.

■ Advise family members to stay alert for evidence of hearing loss.

---

torsemide ▬▬►◄ thiazide diuretics

Demadex

chlorothiazide, hydrochlorothiazide, indapamide, methy-
clothiazide, metolazone, poly-
thiazide, trichlormethiazide

Risk rating: 2
Severity: Moderate   **Onset: Rapid**   **Likelihood: Probable**

Cause
The mechanism of this interaction is unclear.

Effect
Because these drugs work synergistically, they may cause profound diuresis and serious electrolyte abnormalities.

Nursing considerations
■ This combination may be used for therapeutic benefit.

■ Expect increased sodium, potassium, and chloride excretion and greater diuresis.

■ Monitor patient for dehydration and electrolyte abnormalities.

■ Carefully adjust drugs using small or intermittent doses.

---

trandolapril ▬▬►◄ indomethacin

Mavik

Indocin

Risk rating: 2
Severity: Moderate   **Onset: Rapid**   **Likelihood: Probable**

Cause
Indomethacin inhibits synthesis of prostaglandins, which trandolapril and other ACE inhibitors need to lower blood pressure.

Effect
ACE inhibitor's hypotensive effect is reduced.

Nursing considerations

⚠ ALERT Monitor blood pressure closely. Severe hypertension may persist until indomethacin is stopped.

■ If indomethacin can't be avoided, patient may need a different antihypertensive.

■ Other ACE inhibitors may interact with indomethacin. If you suspect an interaction, consult prescriber or pharmacist.

■ Remind patient that hypertension commonly causes no physical symptoms but sometimes may cause headache and dizziness.

---

trandolapril ▰▰►◄▰▰	potassium-sparing diuretics
Mavik	amiloride, spironolactone, triamterene

Risk rating: 1
Severity: Major   **Onset: Delayed**   **Likelihood: Probable**

Cause
The mechanism of this interaction is unknown.

Effect
Serum potassium level may increase.

Nursing considerations
■ Use cautiously in patients at high risk for hyperkalemia, especially those with renal impairment.

■ Monitor BUN, creatinine, and serum potassium levels as needed.

■ ACE inhibitors other than trandolapril may interact with potassium-sparing diuretics. If you suspect an interaction, consult prescriber.

■ Urge patient to immediately report an irregular heartbeat, a slow pulse, weakness, and other evidence of hyperkalemia.

---

trandolapril ▰▰►◄▰▰	salicylates
Mavik	aspirin, bismuth subsalicylate, choline salicylate, magnesium salicylate, salsalate, sodium salicylate

Risk rating: 2
Severity: Moderate   **Onset: Rapid**   **Likelihood: Suspected**

Cause
Salicylates inhibit synthesis of prostaglandins, which trandolapril and other ACE inhibitors need to lower blood pressure.

Effect
ACE inhibitor's hypotensive effect is reduced.

Nursing considerations
■ This interaction is more likely in people with hypertension, coronary artery disease, or heart failure.

---

tranylcypromine ▶◀ anorexiants
Parnate

amphetamine, benzphetamine, dextroamphetamine, methamphetamine, phentermine

Risk rating: 1
Severity: **Major**   Onset: **Rapid**   Likelihood: **Suspected**

Cause
This interaction probably stems from increased norepinephrine level at the synaptic cleft.

Effect
Anorexiant effects increase.

Nursing considerations
■ If possible, avoid giving these drugs together.
■ Headache and severe hypertension may occur rapidly if amphetamine is given with an MAO inhibitor, such as tranylcypromine.
⚠ ALERT Several deaths have resulted from hypertensive crisis and resulting cerebral hemorrhage.
■ Monitor patient for hypotension, hyperpyrexia, and seizures.
■ Hypertensive reaction may occur for several weeks after stopping an MAO inhibitor.

---

tranylcypromine ▶◀ atomoxetine
Parnate

Strattera

Risk rating: 1
Severity: **Major**   Onset: **Rapid**   Likelihood: **Suspected**

Cause
Level of monoamine in the brain may change.

Effect
Serious or fatal reaction resembling neuroleptic malignant syndrome may occur.

Nursing considerations

⚡ **ALERT** Use of atomoxetine and an MAO inhibitor together or within 2 weeks of each other is contraindicated.

■ Before starting atomoxetine, ask patient when he last took an MAO inhibitor. Before starting an MAO inhibitor, ask patient when he last took atomoxetine.

■ Monitor patient for hyperthermia, rapid changes in vital signs, rigidity, muscle twitching, and mental status changes.

---

tranylcypromine ➡◀ dextromethorphan

Parnate   Robitussin DM

Risk rating: 1
Severity: Major   **Onset: Rapid**   **Likelihood: Suspected**

Cause

MAO inhibitor may decrease serotonin metabolism. Dextromethorphan may decrease synaptic reuptake of serotonin.

Effect

Risk of serotonin syndrome increases.

Nursing considerations

■ If possible, avoid giving these drugs together.

⚡ **ALERT** Combined use may cause hyperpyrexia, abnormal muscle movement, hypotension, coma, and death.

■ If patient takes an MAO inhibitor, caution against taking OTC cough and cold medicines that contain dextromethorphan.

---

tranylcypromine ➡◀ foods that contain amines

Parnate

aged, fermented, and overripe foods and drinks: broad beans, caviar, fermented sausage, liver, pickled herring, red wine, some cheeses, yeast extract

Risk rating: 1
Severity: Major   **Onset: Rapid**   **Likelihood: Established**

Cause

MAO inhibition interferes with metabolism of tyramine and other amines in certain foods.

Effect
Risk of marked hypertension increases.

Nursing considerations
- Give patient a list of foods to avoid while taking an MAO inhibitor, such as tranylcypromine.
- Urge patient to avoid high-amine foods for 4 or more weeks after stopping an MAO inhibitor.
- ⚡ **ALERT** Monitor blood pressure closely because marked hypertension, hypertensive crisis, and hemorrhagic stroke are possible.
- Explain that dietary supplements containing yeast and chocolates containing cocoa may cause this interaction.

---

tranylcypromine ▰▶◀ levodopa
Parnate   Larodopa

Risk rating: 1
Severity: Major   **Onset: Rapid**   **Likelihood: Established**

Cause
Peripheral metabolism of levodopa-derived dopamine is inhibited, increasing level at dopamine receptors.

Effect
Risk of hypertensive reaction increases.

Nursing considerations
- If possible, avoid giving these drugs together.
- Interaction occurs within 1 hour and appears to be dose related.
- Monitor patient for flushing, light-headedness, and palpitations.
- Selegiline doesn't cause hypertensive reaction and may be used instead of tranylcypromine and other MAO inhibitors in patients taking levodopa.

---

tranylcypromine ▰▶◀ L-tryptophan
Parnate

Risk rating: 1
Severity: Major   **Onset: Rapid**   **Likelihood: Suspected**

Cause
Additive serotonergic effects may occur.

Effect
Risk of serotonin syndrome increases.

Nursing considerations
⚠ ALERT Combined use of these drugs is contraindicated.
■ They may cause CNS irritability, motor weakness, shivering, muscle twitching, and altered consciousness.

---

tranylcypromine ▶◀ meperidine
Parnate   Demerol

Risk rating: 1
Severity: Major   **Onset: Rapid**   **Likelihood: Probable**

Cause
The mechanism of this interaction is unknown.

Effect
Risk of severe adverse reactions increases.

Nursing considerations
■ If possible, avoid giving these drugs together.
■ Monitor patient; report agitation, seizures, diaphoresis, and fever.
⚠ ALERT Reaction may progress to coma, apnea, and death.
■ Reaction may occur several weeks after stopping the MAO inhibitor.
■ Give opioid analgesics other than meperidine cautiously. It isn't known if similar reactions occur.

---

tranylcypromine ▶◀ methylphenidates
Parnate   dexmethylphenidate,
                                 methylphenidate

Risk rating: 1
Severity: Major   **Onset: Delayed**   **Likelihood: Suspected**

Cause
The mechanism of this interaction is unknown.

Effect
Risk of hypertensive crisis increases.

Nursing considerations
⚠ ALERT Use of dexmethylphenidate with an MAO inhibitor, such as tranylcypromine, is contraindicated.
■ Don't use dexmethylphenidate within 14 days after stopping an MAO inhibitor.

- Monitor blood pressure closely.
- Teach patient and parent to monitor blood pressure at home.

---

tranylcypromine ➤◄ selective 5-HT₁ receptor agonists
Parnate

rizatriptan, sumatriptan, zolmitriptan

Risk rating: 1
Severity: Major   **Onset: Rapid**   **Likelihood: Suspected**

Cause
Tranylcypromine and other MAO inhibitors, subtype-A, may inhibit the metabolism of selective 5-HT₁ receptor agonists.

Effect
Selective 5-HT₁ receptor agonist level and risk of cardiac toxicity may increase.

Nursing considerations
❧ ALERT Use of certain selective 5-HT₁ receptor agonists with or within 2 weeks of stopping an MAO inhibitor is contraindicated.
- Naratriptan is less likely to interact with an MAO inhibitor.
- Cardiac toxicity may include coronary artery vasospasm and transient myocardial ischemia.

---

tranylcypromine ➤◄ serotonin reuptake inhibitors
Parnate

citalopram, escitalopram, fluoxetine, fluvoxamine, nefazodone, paroxetine, sertraline, venlafaxine

Risk rating: 1
Severity: Major   **Onset: Rapid**   **Likelihood: Probable**

Cause
Serotonin may accumulate rapidly in the CNS.

Effect
Risk of serotonin syndrome increases.

Nursing considerations
❧ ALERT Don't use these drugs together.

■ Allow 1 week after stopping nefazodone or venlafaxine (2 weeks after stopping citalopram, escitalopram, fluvoxamine, paroxetine, or sertraline; 5 weeks after stopping fluoxetine) before giving an MAO inhibitor, such as tranylcypromine.

■ Allow 2 weeks after stopping an MAO inhibitor before giving a serotonin reuptake inhibitor.

■ The selective MAO type-B inhibitor selegiline has been given with fluoxetine, paroxetine, or sertraline to patients with Parkinson's disease without negative effects.

■ Describe the traits of serotonin syndrome: CNS irritability, motor weakness, shivering, myoclonus, and altered consciousness.

■ Urge patient to promptly report adverse effects to prescriber.

---

tranylcypromine ▶◀ sulfonylureas

Parnate   acetohexamide, chlorpropamide, glipizide, glyburide, tolazamide, tolbutamide

Risk rating: 2
Severity: Moderate   **Onset: Rapid**   **Likelihood: Suspected**

Cause
The mechanism of this interaction is unknown.

Effect
Tranylcypromine and other MAO inhibitors increase the hypoglycemic effects of sulfonylureas.

Nursing considerations
■ Monitor patient for hypoglycemia.

■ Consult prescriber about adjustments to either drug to control glucose level and mental status.

■ Describe signs and symptoms of hypoglycemia, including diaphoresis, fatigue, headache, hunger, irritability, malaise, nervousness, rapid heart rate, tension, and trembling.

■ Instruct patient to eat a small carbohydrate snack or meal if hypoglycemia develops, preferably after checking blood glucose level.

tranylcypromine ▶◀ sympathomimetics

Parnate

dopamine, ephedrine, metaraminol, phenylephrine, pseudoephedrine

Risk rating: 1
Severity: Major   **Onset: Rapid**   **Likelihood: Established**

Cause
When MAO is inhibited, norepinephrine accumulates and is released by indirect and mixed-acting sympathomimetics, increasing the pressor response at receptor sites.

Effect
Risk of severe headaches, hypertension, high fever, and hypertensive crisis increases.

Nursing considerations
■ Avoid giving indirect or mixed-acting sympathomimetics with an MAO inhibitor, such as tranylcypromine.
■ Phentolamine can be administered to block epinephrine- and norepinephrine-induced vasoconstriction and reduce blood pressure.
■ Direct-acting sympathomimetics interact minimally.
◪ **ALERT** Warn patient that decongestants and other OTC medicines may cause this interaction.

tranylcypromine ▶◀ tricyclic antidepressants

Parnate

amitriptyline, amoxapine, clomipramine, desipramine, doxepin, imipramine, nortriptyline, trimipramine

Risk rating: 1
Severity: Major   **Onset: Rapid**   **Likelihood: Suspected**

Cause
The mechanism of this interaction is unknown.

Effect
Risk of hyperpyretic crisis, seizures, and death increase.

Nursing considerations
◪ **ALERT** Don't give a tricyclic antidepressant with or within 2 weeks of an MAO inhibitor, such as tranylcypromine.
■ Imipramine and clomipramine may be more likely to interact with MAO inhibitors.

■ Watch for adverse effects, including confusion, hyperexcitability, rigidity, seizures, increased temperature, increased pulse, increased respiration, sweating, mydriasis, flushing, headache, coma, and DIC.

---

triamcinolone ▸◂ barbiturates

Aristocort

amobarbital, butabarbital, pentobarbital, phenobarbital, primidone, secobarbital

Risk rating: 2
Severity: Moderate   Onset: Delayed   Likelihood: Established

Cause
Barbiturates induce liver enzymes, which stimulate metabolism of triamcinolone and other corticosteroids.

Effect
Corticosteroid effects may decrease.

Nursing considerations
■ If possible, avoid giving corticosteroids with barbiturates.
■ Watch for worsening symptoms when a barbiturate starts or stops.
■ Corticosteroid dosage may need to be increased.

---

triamcinolone ▸◂ cholinesterase inhibitors

Aristocort

ambenonium, edrophonium, neostigmine, pyridostigmine

Risk rating: 1
Severity: Major   Onset: Delayed   Likelihood: Probable

Cause
In myasthenia gravis, triamcinolone and other corticosteroids antagonize effects of cholinesterase inhibitors by an unknown mechanism.

Effect
Patient may develop severe muscular depression refractory to cholinesterase inhibitor.

Nursing considerations
■ Corticosteroids may have long-term benefits in myasthenia gravis.
■ Combined therapy may be attempted under strict supervision.
■ In myasthenia gravis, watch for severe muscle deterioration.
◪ ALERT Be prepared to provide respiratory support and mechanical ventilation if needed.

■ Consult prescriber or pharmacist about safe corticosteroid delivery to maximize improvement in muscle strength.

triamcinolone ▶◀ hydantoins

Aristocort

ethotoin, fosphenytoin, phenytoin

Risk rating: 2
Severity: Moderate   Onset: Delayed   Likelihood: Established

Cause
Hydantoins induce liver enzymes, which stimulate metabolism of triamcinolone and other corticosteroids.

Effect
Corticosteroid effects may decrease.

Nursing considerations
■ If possible, avoid giving corticosteroids with hydantoins.
■ Monitor patient for decreased corticosteroid effects. Also monitor phenytoin level, and adjust dosage of either drug as needed.
■ Corticosteroid effects may decrease within days of starting phenytoin and may stay decreased 3 weeks after it stops.
■ Dosage of either or both drugs may need to be increased.

triamcinolone ▶◀ rifamycins

Aristocort

rifabutin, rifampin, rifapentine

Risk rating: 1
Severity: Major   Onset: Delayed   Likelihood: Established

Cause
Rifamycins increase hepatic metabolism of triamcinolone and other corticosteroids.

Effect
Corticosteroid effects may decrease.

Nursing considerations
■ If possible, avoid giving corticosteroids with rifamycins.
■ Monitor patient for decreased corticosteroid effects, including loss of disease control.
■ Watch closely for symptom control after increasing rifamycin dose. Drug may need to be stopped to regain control of disease.

■ Corticosteroid effects may decrease within days of starting rifampin and may stay decreased 2 to 3 weeks after it stops.
■ Corticosteroid dose may need to be doubled after adding rifampin.

triamcinolone ➤◀ salicylates

Aristocort

aspirin, bismuth subsalicylate, choline salicylate, magnesium salicylate, salsalate, sodium salicylate, sodium thiosalicylate

Risk rating: 2
Severity: Moderate   Onset: Delayed   Likelihood: Probable

Cause
Triamcinolone and other corticosteroids stimulate hepatic metabolism of salicylates and may increase renal excretion.

Effect
Salicylate level and effects decrease.

Nursing considerations
■ Monitor salicylate level and efficacy; dosage may need adjustment.
◤ **ALERT** Giving a salicylate while tapering a corticosteroid may result in salicylate toxicity.
■ Watch for evidence of salicylate toxicity, including diaphoresis, nausea, vomiting, tinnitus, hyperventilation, and CNS depression.
■ Patient with renal impairment may be at greater risk.

triamterene ➤◀ ACE inhibitors

Dyrenium

benazepril, captopril, enalapril, fosinopril, lisinopril, moexipril, perindopril, quinapril, ramipril, trandolapril

Risk rating: 1
Severity: Major   Onset: Delayed   Likelihood: Probable

Cause
The mechanism of this interaction is unknown.

Effect
Serum potassium level may increase.

Nursing considerations
- Use cautiously in patients at high risk for hyperkalemia, especially those with renal impairment.
- Monitor BUN, creatinine, and serum potassium levels as needed.
- Other ACE inhibitors may interact with potassium-sparing diuretics, such as triamterene. If you suspect an interaction, consult prescriber or pharmacist.
- Urge patient to immediately report an irregular heartbeat, a slow pulse, weakness, and other evidence of hyperkalemia.

---

triamterene ▶◀ angiotensin II receptor antagonists

Dyrenium

candesartan, eprosartan, irbesartan, losartan, olmesartan, telmisartan, valsartan

Risk rating: 1
Severity: **Major**   Onset: **Delayed**   Likelihood: **Suspected**

Cause
Both angiotensin II receptor antagonists and potassium-sparing diuretics, such as triamterene, may increase serum potassium level.

Effect
Risk of hyperkalemia may increase, especially among high-risk patients.

Nursing considerations
- High-risk patients include elderly people and those with renal impairment, type 2 diabetes, or decreased renal perfusion; monitor these patients closely.
- Check serum potassium, BUN, and creatinine levels regularly. If they increase, notify prescriber.
- Advise patient to immediately report an irregular heartbeat, slow pulse, weakness, or other evidence of hyperkalemia.
- Give patient a list of foods high in potassium; stress the need to eat them only in moderate amounts.

triamterene ◄► potassium preparations

Dyrenium

potassium acetate, potassium bicarbonate, potassium chloride, potassium citrate, potassium gluconate, potassium iodine, potassium phosphate

Risk rating: 1
Severity: Major   **Onset: Delayed**   **Likelihood: Established**

Cause
This interaction reduces renal elimination of potassium ions.

Effect
Risk of severe hyperkalemia increases.

Nursing considerations
◼ **ALERT** Don't use this combination unless patient has severe hypokalemia that isn't responding to either drug class alone.
◼ To avoid hyperkalemia, monitor potassium level often.
◼ Tell patient to avoid high-potassium foods, such as citrus juices, bananas, spinach, broccoli, beans, potatoes, and salt substitutes.
◼ Urge patient to immediately report palpitations, chest pain, nausea, vomiting, paresthesias, muscle weakness, and other signs of potassium overload.

triazolam ◄► alcohol

Halcion

Risk rating: 2
Severity: Moderate   **Onset: Rapid**   **Likelihood: Established**

Cause
Alcohol inhibits hepatic enzymes, which decreases clearance and increases peak level of triazolam and other benzodiazepines.

Effect
Additive or synergistic effects may occur.

Nursing considerations
◼ Advise against consuming alcohol while taking a benzodiazepine.
◼ Before benzodiazepine therapy starts, assess patient thoroughly for history or evidence of alcohol use.
◼ Watch for additive CNS effects, which may suggest benzodiazepine overdose.

triazolam ▶◀ azole antifungals
Halcion

fluconazole, itraconazole,
ketoconazole, miconazole

Risk rating: 2
Severity: Moderate   **Onset: Rapid**   **Likelihood: Established**

Cause
Azole antifungals decrease CYP3A4 metabolism of certain benzodiazepines, such as triazolam.

Effect
Benzodiazepine effects are increased and prolonged.

Nursing considerations
◤ **ALERT** Use of triazolam with itraconazole or ketoconazole is con-
traindicated.
■ If patient takes fluconazole or miconazole, consult prescriber about
giving a lower benzodiazepine dose or a drug not metabolized by
CYP3A4, such as temazepam or lorazepam.
■ Caution that the effects of this interaction may last several days after
stopping the azole antifungal.
■ Explain that taking these drugs together may increase sedative ef-
fects; tell patient to report such effects promptly.
■ Explain alternative methods of inducing sleep or relieving anxiety.
■ Various benzodiazepine–azole antifungal combinations may inter-
act. If you suspect an interaction, consult prescriber or pharmacist.

triazolam ▶◀ grapefruit juice
Halcion

Risk rating: 2
Severity: Moderate   **Onset: Rapid**   **Likelihood: Suspected**

Cause
Grapefruit juice inhibits first-pass CYP3A4 metabolism of certain
benzodiazepines, such as triazolam.

Effect
Benzodiazepine onset is delayed and effects are increased.

Nursing considerations
◤ **ALERT** Tell patient not to take drug with grapefruit juice.
■ If he does, explain that oversedation may last up to 72 hours.
■ This interaction is increased in patients with cirrhosis of the liver.

■ Instruct patient to tell prescriber about increased sedation or trouble walking or using limbs.

---

triazolam ▶◀ **macrolide antibiotics**

Halcion   clarithromycin, erythromycin

Risk rating: 2
Severity: Moderate   **Onset: Rapid**   **Likelihood: Suspected**

Cause
Macrolide antibiotics may decrease metabolism of certain benzodiazepines, such as triazolam.

Effect
Sedative effects of benzodiazepines may be increased or prolonged.

Nursing considerations
■ Consult prescriber about decreasing benzodiazepine dosage during antibiotic therapy.
■ Urge patient to promptly report oversedation.
■ Lorazepam, oxazepam, and temazepam probably don't interact with macrolide antibiotics; substitution for triazolam may be possible.

---

triazolam ▶◀ **modafinil**

Halcion   Provigil

Risk rating: 2
Severity: Moderate   **Onset: Delayed**   **Likelihood: Suspected**

Cause
Modafinil may induce the GI and hepatic (CYP3A4/5) metabolism of triazolam.

Effect
Triazolam level and effects may decrease.

Nursing considerations
■ Observe patient for quality and quantity of sleep.
■ Triazolam dosage may need to be adjusted.
■ Discuss the possible effects of this combination on the sleep-wake cycle.

triazolam ━━━━►◄━━━━ nonnucleoside reverse-transcriptase inhibitors

Halcion

delavirdine, efavirenz

Risk rating: 2
Severity: Moderate   **Onset: Delayed**   **Likelihood: Suspected**

Cause
Nonnucleoside reverse-transcriptase inhibitors may inhibit CYP3A4 metabolism of certain benzodiazepines, such as triazolam.

Effect
Sedative effects of benzodiazepines may be increased or prolonged.

Nursing considerations
◼ **ALERT** Don't combine triazolam with delavirdine or efavirenz.
- Explain the risk of oversedation and respiratory depression.
- Urge patient to promptly report any suspected interaction.
- Other benzodiazepines and nonnucleoside reverse-transcriptase inhibitors may interact. If you suspect an interaction, consult prescriber or pharmacist.

triazolam ━━━━►◄━━━━ protease inhibitors

Halcion

amprenavir, atazanavir, indinavir, lopinavir-ritonavir, nelfinavir, ritonavir, saquinavir

Risk rating: 2
Severity: Moderate   **Onset: Delayed**   **Likelihood: Suspected**

Cause
Protease inhibitors may inhibit CYP3A4 metabolism of certain benzodiazepines, such as triazolam.

Effect
Sedative effects of benzodiazepines may be increased or prolonged.

Nursing considerations
◼ **ALERT** Use of triazolam with a protease inhibitor is contraindicated.
- If patient takes any benzodiazepine–protease inhibitor combination, notify prescriber. Interaction also involves other drugs in the class.
- Watch for evidence of oversedation and respiratory depression.
- Explain the risks of using these drugs together.

triazolam ▶◀ rifamycins
Halcion | rifabutin, rifampin, rifapentine

Risk rating: 2
Severity: Moderate   Onset: Delayed   Likelihood: Suspected

Cause
Rifamycins may increase CYP3A4 metabolism of benzodiazepines, such as triazolam.

Effect
Antianxiety, sedative, and sleep-inducing effects may decrease.

Nursing considerations
- Watch for expected benzodiazepine effects and lack of efficacy.
- If benzodiazepine efficacy decreases, dosage may be changed.
- Other benzodiazepines may interact with rifamycins. If you suspect an interaction, consult prescriber or pharmacist.
- For insomnia, temazepam may be more effective than triazolam because it doesn't undergo CYP3A4 metabolism.

trimethoprim ▶◀ methotrexate
Proloprim | Rheumatrex, Trexall

Risk rating: 1
Severity: Major   Onset: Delayed   Likelihood: Suspected

Cause
Combination may have a synergistic effect on folate metabolism.

Effect
Risk of methotrexate toxicity increases.

Nursing considerations
- Avoid using methotrexate with trimethoprim if possible.
- **⚑ ALERT** Monitor patient for methotrexate-induced bone marrow suppression and megaloblastic anemia.
- Consider leucovorin to treat megaloblastic anemia and neutropenia resulting from folic acid deficiency.

trimethoprim, ▶◀ dofetilide
trimethoprim-sulfamethoxazole
Tikosyn

Proloprim, Septra

Risk rating: 1
Severity: **Major**   Onset: **Delayed**   Likelihood: **Suspected**

Cause
Dofetilide renal elimination may be inhibited.

Effect
Dofetilide level and risk of ventricular arrhythmias, including torsades de pointes, increase.

Nursing considerations
■ **ALERT** Use of dofetilide with trimethoprim or trimethoprim-sulfamethoxazole is contraindicated.

■ Monitor ECG for excessive prolongation of the QTc interval or the development of ventricular arrhythmias.

■ Monitor renal function and the QTc interval every 3 months during dofetilide therapy.

■ Monitor patient for prolonged diarrhea, sweating, and vomiting during dofetilide therapy. Alert prescriber because electrolyte imbalance may increase the risk of arrhythmias.

■ Consult prescriber about alternative anti-infective therapy.

trimipramine ▶◀ cimetidine
Surmontil   Tagamet

Risk rating: 2
Severity: **Moderate**   Onset: **Rapid**   Likelihood: **Probable**

Cause
Cimetidine may interfere with metabolism of tricyclic antidepressants (TCAs), such as trimipramine.

Effect
TCA level and bioavailability increase.

Nursing considerations
■ When starting or stopping cimetidine, monitor serum TCA level and adjust dosage as needed.

■ If TCA level or effect increases, dosage may need to be decreased.

■ If needed, consult prescriber about switching from cimetidine to ranitidine.

■ Urge patient and family to watch for and report increased anti-cholinergic effects, dizziness, drowsiness, and psychosis.

---

trimipramine ◄►◄ fluoxetine
Surmontil   Prozac, Sarafem

Risk rating: 2
Severity: Moderate   **Onset: Delayed**   **Likelihood: Probable**

Cause
Fluoxetine may inhibit hepatic metabolism of tricyclic antidepressants (TCAs), such as trimipramine.

Effect
Serum TCA level and toxicity may increase.

Nursing considerations
■ Monitor serum TCA level and watch closely for evidence of toxicity, such as increased anticholinergic effects, delirium, dizziness, drowsiness, and psychosis.
■ Report evidence of increased TCA level or toxicity; dosage may need to be decreased.
■ If TCA starts when patient already takes fluoxetine, TCA dosage may need to be decreased by up to 75% to avoid interaction.
■ Inhibitory effects of fluoxetine may take several weeks to dissipate after drug is stopped.
■ Other TCAs may interact with fluoxetine. If you suspect an interaction, consult prescriber or pharmacist.

---

trimipramine ◄►◄ fluvoxamine
Surmontil   Luvox

Risk rating: 2
Severity: Moderate   **Onset: Delayed**   **Likelihood: Probable**

Cause
Fluvoxamine may inhibit oxidative metabolism of tricyclic antidepressants (TCAs), such as trimipramine, via the CYP2D6 pathway.

Effect
TCA level and risk of toxicity increase.

Nursing considerations
■ If combined use can't be avoided, TCA dosage may be decreased.
■ When starting or stopping fluvoxamine, monitor serum TCA level.
■ Report evidence of toxicity or increased TCA level.

- Inhibitory effects of fluvoxamine may take up to 2 weeks to dissipate after drug is stopped.
- Using desipramine instead of trimipramine may avoid this interaction.
- Urge patient and family to watch for and report increased anticholinergic effects, dizziness, drowsiness, and psychosis.

---

trimipramine ▶◀ MAO inhibitors
Surmontil

isocarboxazid, phenelzine, tranylcypromine

Risk rating: 1
Severity: Major **Onset: Rapid** **Likelihood: Suspected**

Cause
The mechanism of this interaction is unknown.

Effect
Risk of hyperpyretic crisis, seizures, and death increase.

Nursing considerations
⚑ ALERT Don't give a tricyclic antidepressant, such as trimipramine, with or within 2 weeks of an MAO inhibitor.
- Watch for adverse effects, including confusion, hyperexcitability, rigidity, seizures, increased temperature, increased pulse, increased respiration, sweating, mydriasis, flushing, headache, coma, and DIC.

---

trimipramine ▶◀ quinolones
Surmontil

gatifloxacin, levofloxacin, moxifloxacin, sparfloxacin

Risk rating: 1
Severity: Major **Onset: Delayed** **Likelihood: Suspected**

Cause
The mechanism of this interaction is unknown.

Effect
Life-threatening arrhythmias, including torsades de pointes, may increase when certain of these drugs are used together.

Nursing considerations
⚑ ALERT Sparfloxacin is contraindicated in patients taking a tricyclic antidepressant (TCA), such as trimipramine, because the QTc interval may be prolonged.
⚑ ALERT Avoid giving levofloxacin with a TCA.

- Use gatifloxacin and moxifloxacin cautiously with TCAs.
- If possible, use other quinolone antibiotics that don't prolong the QTc interval or aren't metabolized by the CYP3A4 isoenzyme.

---

trimipramine ➤◄ rifamycins
Surmontil   rifabutin, rifampin

Risk rating: 2
Severity: Moderate   **Onset: Delayed**   **Likelihood: Suspected**

Cause
Metabolism of tricyclic antidepressants (TCAs), such as trimipramine, in the liver may increase.

Effect
TCA level and efficacy may decrease.

Nursing considerations
- When starting, stopping, or changing the dosage of a rifamycin, monitor serum TCA level to maintain therapeutic range.
- Watch for resolution of depression as TCA dosage is adjusted to therapeutic level during rifamycin therapy.
- Urge patient and family to watch for adverse reactions, including increased drowsiness and dizziness, for several weeks after rifamycin stops. Tell them to notify prescriber promptly.
- Other TCAs may interact with rifamycins. If you suspect an interaction, consult prescriber or pharmacist.

---

trimipramine ➤◄ sertraline
Surmontil   Zoloft

Risk rating: 2
Severity: Moderate   **Onset: Delayed**   **Likelihood: Suspected**

Cause
Hepatic metabolism of a tricyclic antidepressant (TCA), such as trimipramine, by CYP2D6 may be inhibited.

Effect
Therapeutic and toxic effects of certain TCAs may increase.

Nursing considerations
- If possible, avoid this drug combination.
- Watch for evidence of TCA toxicity and serotonin syndrome.
- Signs of serotonin syndrome include delirium, bizarre movements, and tachycardia.

- Monitor TCA level when starting or stopping sertraline.
- If abnormalities occur, decrease TCA dosage or stop drug.

trimipramine ◄►► sympathomimetics

Surmontil

direct: dobutamine, epinephrine, norepinephrine, phenylephrine
mixed: dopamine, ephedrine, metaraminol

Risk rating: 2
Severity: Moderate   **Onset: Rapid**   **Likelihood: Established**

Cause
Tricyclic antidepressants (TCAs), such as trimipramine, increase the effects of direct-acting sympathomimetics and decrease the effects of indirect-acting sympathomimetics.

Effect
When sympathomimetic effects increase, the risk of hypertension and arrhythmias increases. When sympathomimetic effects decrease, blood pressure control decreases.

Nursing considerations
- If possible, avoid using these drugs together.
- Watch patient closely for hypertension and heart rhythm changes; they may warrant reduction of sympathomimetic dosage.
- If patient takes a mixed-acting sympathomimetic, watch for negative effects; dosage may need to be altered.
- Other TCAs and sympathomimetics may interact. If you suspect an interaction, consult prescriber or pharmacist.

trimipramine ◄►► valproic acid

Surmontil

divalproex sodium, valproate sodium, valproic acid

Risk rating: 2
Severity: Moderate   **Onset: Delayed**   **Likelihood: Suspected**

Cause
Valproic acid may inhibit hepatic metabolism of tricyclic antidepressants (TCAs), such as trimipramine.

Effect
TCA level and adverse effects may increase.

Nursing considerations
■ Use these drugs together cautiously.
■ If patient is stable on valproic acid, start TCA at reduced dosage and adjust upward slowly to address symptoms and serum level.
■ If patient is stable on a TCA, monitor serum level and patient status closely when starting or stopping valproic acid.
■ Explain signs and symptoms to watch for.
■ Other TCAs may interact with valproic acid. If you suspect an interaction, consult prescriber or pharmacist.

---

tromethamine ▶◀ anorexiants

Tham

amphetamine,
dextroamphetamine,
methamphetamine

Risk rating: 2
Severity: Moderate   **Onset: Rapid**   **Likelihood: Established**

Cause
When tromethamine alkalinizes the urine, amphetamine anorexiant clearance is prolonged.

Effect
In amphetamine overdose, the toxic period will be extended, increasing the risk of injury.

Nursing considerations
🄽 ALERT Avoid drugs that may alkalinize the urine, particularly during amphetamine overdose.
■ Watch for evidence of tromethamine toxicity, such as dermatoses, marked insomnia, irritability, hyperactivity, and personality changes.

---

valproic acid ▶◀ barbiturates

divalproex sodium,
valproic acid

phenobarbital, primidone

Risk rating: 2
Severity: Moderate   **Onset: Delayed**   **Likelihood: Established**

Cause
Barbiturate metabolism is decreased by valproic acid.

Effect

Barbiturate level and risk of adverse effects increase.

Nursing considerations

■ Monitor serum barbiturate level and patient status when starting or stopping valproic acid. Barbiturate level may need to be decreased.

■ Barbiturate toxicity may include drowsiness, lethargy, bradycardia, respiratory depression or apnea, angioedema, and rashes, some life-threatening.

■ Other barbiturates may interact with valproic acid; monitor patient closely.

■ Interaction may be more likely in children than adults.

■ Explain signs and symptoms to watch for.

---

valproic acid ▶◀ carbamazepine

divalproex sodium,
valproic acid

Carbatrol, Epitol, Equetro,
Tegretol

Risk rating: 2
Severity: Moderate   Onset: Delayed   Likelihood: Established

Cause

Metabolism of valproic acid may be altered by carbamazepine. Conversion of valproic acid to a hepatotoxic and teratogenic metabolite may increase.

Effect

Valproic acid level decreases, with possible loss of seizure control. Also, carbamazepine level may change.

Nursing considerations

■ These drugs have been used safely together in many patients to manage epilepsy and psychiatric disorders.

■ Monitor seizure control and toxicity for at least 1 month after starting or stopping combined use.

■ Check levels of both drugs during use and for 1 month after either drug is stopped.

■ Although rare, pancreatitis and acute psychosis may arise because of slow excretion after combined use has stopped.

valproic acid ➤◀ cholestyramine

divalproex sodium,
valproate sodium,
valproic acid

LoCHOLEST, Prevalite,
Questran

Risk rating: 2
Severity: Moderate   **Onset: Rapid**   **Likelihood: Suspected**

Cause
Cholestyramine may prevent GI absorption of valproic acid.

Effect
Valproic acid effects may decrease.

Nursing considerations
- Give valproic acid at least 3 hours before or after cholestyramine.
- Watch for loss of therapeutic effects (loss of seizure control).
- Valproic acid dosage may need adjustment during combined use.
- Consult prescriber about other antihyperlipidemic drugs as alternatives to cholestyramine.

valproic acid ➤◀ felbamate

divalproex sodium,
valproic acid

Felbatol

Risk rating: 2
Severity: Moderate   **Onset: Delayed**   **Likelihood: Probable**

Cause
Felbamate inhibits metabolism of valproic acid.

Effect
Valproic acid level and risk of toxicity may increase.

Nursing considerations
- Monitor serum valproic acid level when starting or stopping felbamate or adjusting its dose. Valproic acid dosage may need adjustment.
- If patient takes valproic acid, start felbamate slowly if possible.
- If felbamate must start quickly, valproic acid dosage may need to be reduced. Watch patient closely.
- Watch for valproic acid toxicity: sedation, nausea, vomiting, pancreatitis, hepatitis, hemorrhage, emotional changes, and serious rash.
- Teach signs and symptoms to watch for.

valproic acid ━━▶◀━━ lamotrigine

divalproex sodium,   Lamictal
valproic acid

Risk rating: 2
Severity: Moderate   **Onset: Delayed**   **Likelihood: Probable**

Cause
Valproic acid may inhibit lamotrigine metabolism.

Effect
Both drugs may have increased effects and toxicity.

Nursing considerations
■ Observe patient closely for Stevens-Johnson rash, disabling tremor, and other signs of toxicity when starting the second anticonvulsant.
■ Monitor serum valproic acid and lamotrigine levels, and report increasing level of either drug.
■ Explain that combined use may improve seizure control; instruct patient to be alert for adverse effects and toxicity.
■ Lamotrigine level decreases readily when valproic acid is stopped.

valproic acid ━━▶◀━━ phenytoin

divalproex sodium,   Dilantin
valproic acid

Risk rating: 2
Severity: Moderate   **Onset: Delayed**   **Likelihood: Suspected**

Cause
Valproic acid metabolism increases; phenytoin metabolism decreases.

Effect
Phenytoin effects may increase. Valproic acid effects may decrease. Phenytoin toxicity may occur despite therapeutic total serum level.

Nursing considerations
■ Watch for altered seizure control and evidence of toxicity: tremor, drowsiness, ataxia, nystagmus, slurred speech, and personality changes.
■ Monitor serum levels of free phenytoin and valproic acid. The amount of free phenytoin may be more important that the therapeutic range of 10 to 20 mcg/ml.
■ Be prepared to alter the dosage of either drug as needed.
■ Other hydantoins may interact with valproic acid. If you suspect an interaction, consult prescriber or pharmacist.

valproic acid ━━━▶◀━━━ salicylates

Depakene

aspirin, bismuth subsalicylate, choline salicylate, magnesium salicylate, salsalate, sodium salicylate, sodium thiosalicylate

Risk rating: 2
Severity: Moderate   Onset: Delayed   Likelihood: Suspected

Cause
Salicylates displace valproic acid from its usual binding sites and may alter valproic acid metabolic pathways.

Effect
Toxicity of valproic acid may increase.

Nursing considerations
- Check serum free fraction and serum valproic acid level.
- Hepatotoxic metabolites of valproic acid may be more likely to form.
- Watch for evidence of valproic acid toxicity, such as tremor, drowsiness, ataxia, nystagmus, and personality changes.
- Explain risks of combined use and signs of toxicity.

valproic acid ━━━▶◀━━━ tricyclic antidepressants

divalproex sodium, valproate sodium, valproic acid

amitriptyline, amoxapine, clomipramine, desipramine, doxepin, imipramine, nortriptyline, trimipramine

Risk rating: 2
Severity: Moderate   Onset: Delayed   Likelihood: Suspected

Cause
Valproic acid may inhibit hepatic metabolism of tricyclic antidepressants (TCAs).

Effect
Level and adverse effects of TCA may increase.

Nursing considerations
- Use these drugs together cautiously.
- If patient is stable on valproic acid, start a TCA at reduced dosage and adjust upward slowly to address symptoms and serum level.
- If patient is stable on a TCA, monitor serum level and patient status closely when starting or stopping valproic acid.

- Explain signs and symptoms to watch for.
- Other TCAs may interact with valproic acid. If you suspect an interaction, consult prescriber or pharmacist.

---

valsartan ━━▶◀━━ potassium-sparing diuretics
Diovan

amiloride, spironolactone, triamterene

Risk rating: 1
Severity: Major   **Onset: Delayed**   **Likelihood: Suspected**

Cause
Angiotensin II receptor antagonists, such as valsartan, and potassium-sparing diuretics may increase serum potassium level.

Effect
Risk of hyperkalemia may increase, especially in high-risk patients.

Nursing considerations
- High-risk patients include elderly people and those with renal impairment, type 2 diabetes, or decreased renal perfusion; monitor these patients closely.
- Check serum potassium, BUN, and creatinine levels regularly. If they increase, notify prescriber.
- Advise patient to immediately report an irregular heartbeat, slow pulse, weakness, or other evidence of hyperkalemia.
- Give patient a list of foods high in potassium; stress the need to eat them only in moderate amounts.

---

vancomycin ━━▶◀━━ nondepolarizing muscle relaxants
Vancocin

atracurium, pancuronium, vecuronium

Risk rating: 2
Severity: Moderate   **Onset: Rapid**   **Likelihood: Probable**

Cause
Vancomycin and other polypeptide antibiotics may act synergistically with nondepolarizing muscle relaxants.

Effect
Neuromuscular blockade may increase.

Nursing considerations
- If possible, avoid using polypeptide antibiotics with nondepolarizing muscle relaxants.
- Monitor neuromuscular function closely.
- Dosage of nondepolarizing muscle relaxant may need adjustment.
- Provide ventilatory support, as needed.
- Make sure patient is adequately sedated when receiving a nondepolarizing muscle relaxant.

---

vardenafil ▶◀ **antiarrhythmics**

Levitra   amiodarone, bretylium, disopyramide, moricizine, procainamide, sotalol

Risk rating: 1
Severity: Major   **Onset: Rapid**   **Likelihood: Suspected**

Cause
The mechanism of this interaction is unknown.

Effect
QTc interval may be prolonged, particularly in patients with previous QT-interval prolongation, increasing the risk of such life-threatening arrhythmias as torsades de pointes.

Nursing considerations
⚠ ALERT Use of vardenafil with a class IA or class III antiarrhythmic is contraindicated.
- Monitor ECG before and during vardenafil use.
- Urge patient to report light-headedness, faintness, palpitations, and chest pain or pressure while taking vardenafil.
- To reduce risk of adverse effects, patients age 65 and older should start with 5 mg vardenafil, half the usual starting dose.

---

vardenafil ▶◀ **nitrates**

Levitra   amyl nitrite, isosorbide dinitrate, isosorbide mononitrate, nitroglycerin

Risk rating: 1
Severity: Major   **Onset: Rapid**   **Likelihood: Suspected**

Cause
Vardenafil potentiates the hypotensive effects of nitrates.

Effect
Risk of severe hypotension increases.

Nursing considerations
⚠ **ALERT** Use of vardenafil with nitrates or nitric oxide donors is contraindicated.
- Carefully screen patient for vardenafil use before giving a nitrate.
- Watch for orthostatic hypotension, dizziness, sweating, and headache.
- This interaction may not occur if vardenafil was taken 24 hours or more before patient receives a nitrate.

---

vecuronium ▶◀ **aminoglycosides**
amikacin, gentamicin, kanamycin, neomycin, streptomycin, tobramycin

Risk rating: 1
Severity: Major   **Onset: Rapid**   **Likelihood: Probable**

Cause
These drugs may be synergistic.

Effect
Effects of nondepolarizing muscle relaxants, such as vecuronium, may increase.

Nursing considerations
- Give these drugs together only when needed.
- The nondepolarizing muscle relaxant dose may need adjustment based on neuromuscular response.
- Monitor patient for prolonged respiratory depression.
- Provide ventilatory support as needed.

---

vecuronium ▶◀ **carbamazepine**
Carbatrol, Epitol, Equetro, Tegretol

Risk rating: 2
Severity: Moderate   **Onset: Rapid**   **Likelihood: Probable**

Cause
The mechanism of this interaction is unknown.

Effect
Effects or duration of a nondepolarizing muscle relaxant, such as vecuronium, may decrease.

Nursing considerations
- Monitor patient for decreased efficacy of muscle relaxant.
- Dosage of nondepolarizing muscle relaxant may be increased.
- Make sure patient is adequately sedated when receiving a nondepolarizing muscle relaxant.

---

vecuronium ▸◂ clindamycin
Cleocin

Risk rating: 2
Severity: Moderate   **Onset: Rapid**   **Likelihood: Suspected**

Cause
Clindamycin may potentiate the actions of nondepolarizing muscle relaxants, such as vecuronium.

Effect
Vecuronium effects may increase.

Nursing considerations
- If possible, avoid using clindamycin or other lincosamides with a nondepolarizing muscle relaxant.
- Monitor patient for respiratory depression, which may be profound.
- Provide ventilatory support as needed.
- Cholinesterase inhibitors or calcium may help reverse drug effects.
- Make sure patient is adequately sedated when receiving a nondepolarizing muscle relaxant.

---

vecuronium ▸◂ magnesium sulfate

Risk rating: 2
Severity: Moderate   **Onset: Rapid**   **Likelihood: Suspected**

Cause
Magnesium probably potentiates the action of nondepolarizing muscle relaxants, such as vecuronium.

Effect
Vecuronium effects may increase.

Nursing considerations
- Use these drugs together cautiously.
- The nondepolarizing muscle relaxant dosage may need adjustment.
- Monitor patient for respiratory depression, which may be profound.
- Provide ventilatory support as needed.
- Make sure patient is adequately sedated when receiving a nondepolarizing muscle relaxant.

---

vecuronium ━━━▶◀━━━ phenytoin
Dilantin

Risk rating: 2
Severity: Moderate   **Onset: Rapid**   **Likelihood: Probable**

Cause
Phenytoin effects at prejunctional sites are similar to those of nondepolarizing muscle relaxants, such as vecuronium.

Effect
Nondepolarizing muscle relaxant effects or duration may decrease.

Nursing considerations
- Monitor patient for decreased efficacy of the muscle relaxant.
- Dosage of nondepolarizing muscle relaxant may be increased.
- Atracurium may be a suitable alternative to vecuronium because this interaction may not occur in all patients.
- Make sure patient is adequately sedated when receiving a nondepolarizing muscle relaxant.

---

vecuronium ━━━▶◀━━━ polypeptide antibiotics
bacitracin, polymyxin B, vancomycin

Risk rating: 2
Severity: Moderate   **Onset: Rapid**   **Likelihood: Probable**

Cause
Polypeptide antibiotics may act synergistically with nondepolarizing muscle relaxants, such as vecuronium.

Effect
Neuromuscular blockade may increase.

Nursing considerations
- If possible, avoid using polypeptide antibiotics with nondepolarizing muscle relaxants.

- Monitor neuromuscular function closely.
- Dosage of nondepolarizing muscle relaxant may need adjustment.
- Provide ventilatory support, as needed.
- Make sure patient is adequately sedated when receiving a nondepolarizing muscle relaxant.

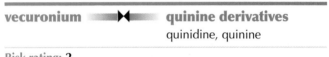

vecuronium ➤◄ quinine derivatives
quinidine, quinine

Risk rating: 2
Severity: Moderate   **Onset: Rapid**   **Likelihood: Suspected**

Cause
Quinine derivatives may act synergistically with nondepolarizing muscle relaxants, such as vecuronium.

Effect
Intensity and duration of neuromuscular blockade may increase.

Nursing considerations
⚡ ALERT This interaction may be life-threatening. Monitor neuromuscular function closely.
- Dosage of nondepolarizing muscle relaxant may need adjustment.
- Provide ventilatory support, as needed.
- Make sure patient is adequately sedated when receiving a nondepolarizing muscle relaxant.

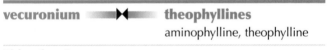

vecuronium ➤◄ theophyllines
aminophylline, theophylline

Risk rating: 2
Severity: Moderate   **Onset: Rapid**   **Likelihood: Suspected**

Cause
These drugs may act antagonistically.

Effect
Neuromuscular blockade may be reversed.

Nursing considerations
- Monitor patient closely for lack of drug effect.
- Dosage of nondepolarizing muscle relaxant may need adjustment.
- This interaction is dose dependent.
- Make sure patient is adequately sedated when receiving a nondepolarizing muscle relaxant.

vecuronium 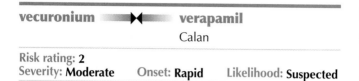 verapamil
Calan

Risk rating: 2
Severity: Moderate   **Onset: Rapid**   **Likelihood: Suspected**

Cause
This interaction may stem from a blockade of calcium channels in the skeletal muscle.

Effect
Effects of nondepolarizing muscle relaxants, such as vecuronium, may increase.

Nursing considerations
- If possible, avoid using verapamil and nondepolarizing muscle relaxants together.
- Monitor patient for prolonged respiratory depression.
- Provide ventilatory support, as needed.
- Dosage of nondepolarizing muscle relaxant may be decreased.

venlafaxine ◀▶ MAO inhibitors
Effexor

isocarboxazid, phenelzine, selegiline, tranylcypromine

Risk rating: 1
Severity: Major   **Onset: Rapid**   **Likelihood: Probable**

Cause
Serotonin may accumulate rapidly in the CNS.

Effect
Risk of serotonin syndrome increases.

Nursing considerations
- ⚡ **ALERT** Don't use these drugs together.
- Allow 1 week after stopping venlafaxine before giving an MAO inhibitor.
- The selective MAO type-B inhibitor selegiline has been given with fluoxetine, paroxetine, or sertraline to patients with Parkinson's disease without negative effects.
- Describe the traits of serotonin syndrome, including CNS irritability, motor weakness, shivering, myoclonus, and altered consciousness.
- Urge patient to promptly report adverse effects to prescriber.

venlafaxine ▶◀ selective 5-HT₁ receptor agonists

Effexor

almotriptan, eletriptan, frovatriptan, naratriptan, rizatriptan, sumatriptan, zolmitriptan

Risk rating: 1
Severity: Major   **Onset: Rapid**   **Likelihood: Suspected**

Cause
Serotonin may accumulate rapidly in the CNS.

Effect
Risk of serotonin syndrome increases.

Nursing considerations
⚠ **ALERT** If possible, avoid combined use of these drugs.
- Start with lowest doses possible, and assess patient closely.
- Stop the selective 5-HT₁ receptor agonist at the first sign of interaction, and start an antiserotonergic.
- Describe the traits of serotonin syndrome: CNS irritability, motor weakness, shivering, muscle twitching, and altered consciousness.
- Explain that serotonin syndrome can be fatal if not treated immediately.

---

venlafaxine ▶◀ sibutramine

Effexor

Meridia

Risk rating: 1
Severity: Major   **Onset: Rapid**   **Likelihood: Suspected**

Cause
Serotonin may accumulate rapidly in the CNS.

Effect
Risk of serotonin syndrome increases.

Nursing considerations
⚠ **ALERT** If possible, don't give these drugs together.
- Watch carefully for adverse effects; they need immediate attention.
- Describe the traits of serotonin syndrome: CNS irritability, motor weakness, shivering, muscle twitching, and altered consciousness.
- Explain that serotonin syndrome can be fatal if not treated immediately.

venlafaxine ━━▶◀━━ St. John's wort
Effexor

Risk rating: 2
Severity: Moderate   **Onset: Rapid**   **Likelihood: Suspected**

Cause
St. John's wort may cause additive inhibition of serotonin reuptake.

Effect
Sedative-hypnotic effects of serotonin reuptake inhibitors, such as venlafaxine, may increase.

Nursing considerations
◤ ALERT Discourage use of a serotonin reuptake inhibitor with St. John's wort.
- In addition to oversedation, mild serotonin-like symptoms may occur, including anxiety, dizziness, nausea, restlessness, and vomiting.
- Inform patient about the dangers of this combination.
- Urge patient to consult prescriber before taking any herb.

verapamil ━━▶◀━━ beta blockers
Calan

acebutolol, atenolol, betaxolol, bisoprolol, carteolol, esmolol, metoprolol, nadolol, penbutolol, pindolol, propranolol, sotalol, timolol

Risk rating: 1
Severity: Major   **Onset: Rapid**   **Likelihood: Probable**

Cause
Verapamil may inhibit metabolism of beta blockers.

Effect
Effects of both drugs may increase.

Nursing considerations
- Combined use is common in hypertension with unstable angina.
◤ ALERT Risk of adverse effects increases, including heart failure, conduction disturbances, arrhythmias, and hypotension.
- Assess patient for adverse effects, including left ventricular dysfunction and AV conduction defects.
- Risk of interaction is greater when drugs are given I.V.
- Dosages of both drugs may need to be decreased.

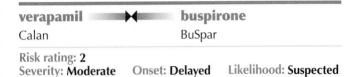

verapamil ►◄ buspirone
Calan   BuSpar

Risk rating: 2
Severity: Moderate   **Onset: Delayed**   **Likelihood: Suspected**

Cause
Buspirone level may increase from reduced CYP3A4 metabolism.

Effect
Buspirone level and adverse effects may increase.

Nursing considerations
■ Watch closely if verapamil is started or stopped or if its dosage is changed.
■ Watch for evidence of buspirone toxicity, including increased CNS effects (dizziness, drowsiness, headache), vomiting, and diarrhea.
■ Buspirone dose may need to be adjusted.
■ An antianxiety drug not metabolized by CYP3A4 (such as lorazepam) should be considered if patient takes verapamil.
■ Calcium channel blockers other than verapamil may interact with buspirone. If you suspect an interaction, consult prescriber or pharmacist.
■ Dihydropyridine calcium channel blockers that don't inhibit CYP3A4 metabolism (such as amlodipine and felodipine) probably don't disrupt buspirone metabolism. Consult prescriber.

verapamil ►◄ calcium salts
Calan   calcium acetate, calcium
                              carbonate, calcium chloride,
                              calcium citrate, calcium
                              gluceptate, calcium gluconate,
                              calcium lactate, tricalcium
                              phosphate

Risk rating: 2
Severity: Moderate   **Onset: Rapid**   **Likelihood: Suspected**

Cause
Calcium salts antagonize certain of verapamil's effects.

Effect
Calcium can reverse changes in cardiac output, blood pressure, and AV intervals without slowing the sinus rate or causing AV block.

Nursing considerations
■ Calcium can be useful in verapamil overdose and in reversing or preventing hypotension when verapamil starts.
■ The beneficial effects of calcium with verapamil are dose dependent. If too much calcium is used, verapamil may be ineffective.
■ Obtain a complete drug history to detect calcium consumption in any patient who takes verapamil.
■ Teach patient taking verapamil to always consult prescriber before consuming anything that contains calcium.

---

verapamil ■■■■►◄■■■■ carbamazepine
Calan   Carbatrol, Epitol, Equetro, Tegretol

Risk rating: 2
Severity: Moderate   Onset: Delayed   Likelihood: Suspected

Cause
Verapamil may decrease hepatic metabolism of carbamazepine.

Effect
Carbamazepine level and toxic effects may increase.

Nursing considerations
■ Monitor carbamazepine level; therapeutic range is 4 to 12 mcg/ml.
■ Watch for evidence of carbamazepine toxicity: dizziness, ataxia, respiratory depression, tachycardia, arrhythmias, blood pressure changes, impaired consciousness, abnormal reflexes, nystagmus, seizures, nausea, vomiting, and urine retention.
■ Carbamazepine dose may need to be reduced by 40% to 50%.
■ If verapamil is stopped, watch for loss of carbamazepine effect.
■ Calcium channel blockers other than verapamil may interact with carbamazepine. If you suspect an interaction, consult prescriber or pharmacist.

---

verapamil ■■■■►◄■■■■ digoxin
Calan   Lanoxin

Risk rating: 1
Severity: Major   Onset: Delayed   Likelihood: Established

Cause
Verapamil decreases digoxin elimination. Verapamil and digoxin have additive effects in decreasing AV conduction.

Effect
Digoxin level, effects, and risk of toxicity may increase.

Nursing considerations
- Monitor digoxin level. Therapeutic range is 0.8 to 2 nanograms/ml.
- Watch for evidence of digoxin toxicity, including arrhythmias (bradycardia, AV block, and ventricular ectopy), lethargy, drowsiness, confusion, hallucinations, headaches, syncope, visual disturbances, nausea, anorexia, vomiting, and diarrhea.
- Digoxin dosage may need reduction.
- Advise patient to report adverse reactions, such as nausea, vomiting, diarrhea, appetite loss, and visual disturbances, which may be early indicators of toxicity.

---

verapamil 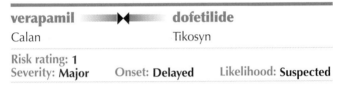	dofetilide
Calan	Tikosyn

Risk rating: 1
Severity: **Major**   Onset: **Delayed**   Likelihood: **Suspected**

Cause
Verapamil may increase dofetilide absorption.

Effect
Dofetilide level and risk of ventricular arrhythmias, including torsades de pointes, may increase.

Nursing considerations
⚡ ALERT Use of dofetilide with verapamil is contraindicated.
- Monitor ECG for excessive prolongation of the QTc interval and development of ventricular arrhythmias.
- Monitor renal function and QTc interval every 3 months during dofetilide therapy.

---

verapamil	HMG-CoA reductase inhibitors
Calan	atorvastatin, lovastatin, simvastatin

Risk rating: 2
Severity: **Moderate**   Onset: **Delayed**   Likelihood: **Probable**

Cause
CYP3A4 metabolism of certain HMG-CoA reductase inhibitors may decrease.

Effect
HMG-CoA reductase inhibitor level and risk of adverse effects may increase.

Nursing considerations
- Avoid giving an HMG-CoA reductase inhibitor with verapamil.
- Consult prescriber; HMG-CoA reductase inhibitor dosage may be decreased.
- **⚑ ALERT** Watch for evidence of rhabdomyolysis, including fatigue; muscle aches and weakness; joint pain; dark, red, or cola-colored urine; weight gain; seizures; and greatly increased serum CK level.
- Fluvastatin and pravastatin are metabolized by other enzymes and may be better choices for combined use with verapamil.
- Urge patient to report muscle pain, tenderness, or weakness.

---

verapamil ➤◀ nondepolarizing muscle relaxants
Calan

atracurium, mivacurium, pancuronium, vecuronium

Risk rating: 2
Severity: Moderate   **Onset: Rapid**   **Likelihood: Suspected**

Cause
This interaction may stem from a blockade of calcium channels in the skeletal muscle.

Effect
Nondepolarizing muscle relaxant effects may increase.

Nursing considerations
- Avoid using verapamil with nondepolarizing muscle relaxants.
- Monitor patient for prolonged respiratory depression.
- Provide ventilatory support, as needed.
- The dosage of nondepolarizing muscle relaxant may need to be decreased.

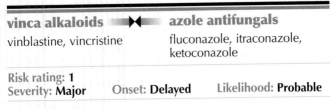

vinca alkaloids ➤◄ azole antifungals

vinblastine, vincristine

fluconazole, itraconazole, ketoconazole

Risk rating: 1
Severity: Major   **Onset: Delayed**   **Likelihood: Probable**

Cause
Azole antifungals inhibit CYP3A4, which is needed for vinca alkaloid metabolism.

Effect
Risk of vinca alkaloid toxicity increases.

Nursing considerations
- If possible, avoid giving these drugs together.
- ⚡ **ALERT** The risk of serious toxicity is increased with itraconazole.
- Watch for evidence of toxicity, such as constipation, myalgia, hypertension, hyponatremia, and neutropenia.
- Explain adverse vinca alkaloid effects; tell patient to report them.
- Stop azole antifungal as soon as possible.

voriconazole ➤◄ carbamazepine

Vfend

Carbatrol, Epitol, Equetro, Tegretol

Risk rating: 1
Severity: Major   **Onset: Delayed**   **Likelihood: Suspected**

Cause
Carbamazepine may increase CYP3A4 metabolism of voriconazole.

Effect
Voriconazole effects may decrease.

Nursing considerations
- ⚡ **ALERT** Use of these drugs together is contraindicated.
- Instruct patient to avoid carbamazepine while taking voriconazole; consult prescriber about alternative therapies.

voriconazole ━━►◄━━ cisapride
Vfend   Propulsid

Risk rating: 1
Severity: Major   **Onset: Delayed**   **Likelihood: Suspected**

Cause
Voriconazole may inhibit hepatic metabolism of cisapride.

Effect
Risk of life-threatening arrhythmias, including torsades de pointes, may increase.

Nursing considerations
⚠ **ALERT** Use of cisapride with voriconazole is contraindicated.
⚠ **ALERT** Because of the risk of serious arrhythmias and death, cisapride is available in the U.S. only through an investigational limited access program.
■ Patients receiving cisapride may have prolonged QT interval, torsades de pointes, cardiac arrest, and sudden death.
■ Cisapride is metabolized mainly by CYP3A4. Drugs that inhibit this enzyme may increase cisapride level, leading to QT prolongation and serious arrhythmias.

voriconazole ━━►◄━━ ergot derivatives
Vfend   dihydroergotamine, ergotamine

Risk rating: 1
Severity: Major   **Onset: Delayed**   **Likelihood: Suspected**

Cause
Voriconazole may inhibit CYP3A4 metabolism of ergot derivatives.

Effect
Risk of ergot toxicity many increase.

Nursing considerations
⚠ **ALERT** Use of these drugs together is contraindicated.
■ Signs of ergot toxicity include peripheral vasospasm and ischemia of the extremities.
■ Instruct patient to avoid taking ergot derivatives, as for migraine, while taking voriconazole.

voriconazole ━━▶◀━━ HMG-CoA reductase inhibitors

Vfend

atorvastatin, fluvastatin, lovastatin, pravastatin, rosuvastatin, simvastatin

Risk rating: 2
Severity: Moderate   **Onset: Rapid**   **Likelihood: Probable**

Cause
Voriconazole and other azole antifungals may inhibit hepatic metabolism of HMG-CoA reductase inhibitors.

Effect
HMG-CoA reductase inhibitor level and adverse effects may increase.

Nursing considerations
- If possible, avoid use together.
- HMG-CoA reductase inhibitor dosage may need to be decreased.
- Monitor serum cholesterol and lipid levels.
- ⚡ ALERT Assess patient for evidence of rhabdomyolysis, including fatigue; muscle aches and weakness; joint pain; dark, red, or cola-colored urine; weight gain; seizures; and greatly increased CK level.
- Pravastatin is least affected by this interaction and may be preferable for use with an azole antifungal, if needed.

voriconazole ━━▶◀━━ phenobarbital

Vfend

Risk rating: 1
Severity: Major   **Onset: Delayed**   **Likelihood: Suspected**

Cause
Long-acting barbiturates, such as phenobarbital, may increase CYP3A4 metabolism of voriconazole.

Effect
Voriconazole level and efficacy may decrease.

Nursing considerations
- ⚡ ALERT Use of these drugs together is contraindicated.
- Voriconazole efficacy in treating fungal infections may decrease.
- Other barbiturates and voriconazole may interact. If you suspect an interaction, consult prescriber or pharmacist.

voriconazole ▶◀ sirolimus
Vfend   Rapamune

Risk rating: 2
Severity: Moderate   Onset: Delayed   Likelihood: Probable

Cause
Voriconazole may increase CYP3A4 metabolism of sirolimus.

Effect
Sirolimus level and adverse effects may increase.

Nursing considerations
⚠ **ALERT** Use of these drugs together is contraindicated.
■ The immunosuppressant benefits of sirolimus may be compromised by increased side effects, such as heart failure, toxic nephropathy, thrombocytopenia with hemorrhage, sepsis, and lung edema.

warfarin ▶◀ acetaminophen
Coumadin   Acephen, Neopap, Tylenol

Risk rating: 2
Severity: Moderate   Onset: Delayed   Likelihood: Suspected

Cause
Acetaminophen or one of its metabolites may enhance vitamin K antagonism.

Effect
Antithrombotic effect of warfarin may increase.

Nursing considerations
⚠ **ALERT** Effects of this interaction seem to be dose related. Daily acetaminophen use at 325 to 650 mg causes a 3.5-fold INR elevation. Daily use of 1,250 mg increases this risk 10-fold.
■ This interaction may be of little significance with low-dose acetaminophen or up to six 325-mg tablets weekly.
■ Monitor coagulation values once or twice weekly when starting or stopping acetaminophen.
■ Other risk factors may be present that place patient at higher risk, including diarrheal illness or medical conditions that affect acetaminophen metabolism.
■ Tell patient to report unusual bruising or bleeding.
■ Remind patient that warfarin interacts with many drugs and that he should report any change in drug regimen.

warfarin ▬▶◀▬ alteplase
Coumadin   Activase, tPA

Risk rating: 1
Severity: Major   **Onset: Rapid**   **Likelihood: Suspected**

Cause
Combined effect of this interaction may be greater than the sum of each individual effect.

Effect
Risk of serious bleeding increases.

Nursing considerations
⚡ **ALERT** Using alteplase in patient with acute ischemic stroke is contraindicated if patient has a bleeding diathesis, including use of oral anticoagulants. Doing so increases the risk of bleeding and may cause disability or death.
■ Oral anticoagulants other than warfarin may interact with alteplase. Consult prescriber or pharmacist.
■ Alert prescriber that patient takes warfarin.
■ Tell patient to report unusual bruising or bleeding.
■ Remind patient that warfarin interacts with many drugs and that he should report any change in drug regimen.

warfarin ▬▶◀▬ amiodarone
Coumadin   Cordarone, Pacerone

Risk rating: 1
Severity: Major   **Onset: Delayed**   **Likelihood: Established**

Cause
Amiodarone inhibits CYP1A2 and CYP2C9 metabolism of warfarin.

Effect
Anticoagulant effects increase.

Nursing considerations
■ Monitor patient closely for bleeding. Urge compliance with required blood tests.
⚡ **ALERT** Check INR closely during the first 6 to 8 weeks of amiodarone use. Warfarin dose reduction depends on escalating amiodarone dose. Typically, warfarin needs a 30% to 50% reduction.
■ If amiodarone is stopped, effects of interaction may persist up to 4 months, requiring continual warfarin adjustment.
■ Tell patient to report unusual bruising or bleeding.

■ Remind patient that warfarin interacts with many drugs and that he should report any change in drug regimen.

---

warfarin ◀▶ **androgens (17-alkyl)**

Coumadin

danazol, fluoxymesterone, methyltestosterone, oxandrolone

Risk rating: 1
Severity: Major   **Onset: Delayed**   **Likelihood: Probable**

Cause
The mechanism of this interaction is unknown.

Effect
Anticoagulant effects increase.

Nursing considerations
■ If possible, avoid this combination.
■ Monitor coagulation values carefully. Warfarin dosage will be decreased.
■ Tell patient to report unusual bruising or bleeding.
■ Remind patient that warfarin interacts with many drugs and that he should report any change in drug regimen.

---

warfarin ◀▶ **antineoplastics**

Coumadin

capecitabine, carboplatin, cyclophosphamide, etoposide, fluorouracil, gemcitabine, paclitaxel

Risk rating: 2
Severity: Moderate   **Onset: Delayed**   **Likelihood: Suspected**

Cause
Warfarin metabolism, clotting factor synthesis, and possibly protein displacement may be inhibited.

Effect
Anticoagulant effects increase.

Nursing considerations
■ Monitor PT and INR closely during and after chemotherapy.
■ Tell patient to report unusual bruising or bleeding.
■ Remind patient that warfarin interacts with many drugs and that he should report any change in drug regimen.

warfarin 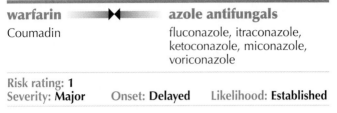 azole antifungals

Coumadin

fluconazole, itraconazole, ketoconazole, miconazole, voriconazole

Risk rating: 1
Severity: Major   **Onset: Delayed**   **Likelihood: Established**

Cause
Warfarin metabolism is inhibited.

Effect
Anticoagulant effects may increase.

Nursing considerations
- Monitor PT and INR at least every 2 days.
- Patients with renal insufficiency may be at greater risk.
- Although all azole antifungals interact with warfarin, some interactions may be more significant than others.
- Watch for evidence of bleeding.
- Tell patient to report unusual bruising or bleeding.
- Remind patient that warfarin interacts with many drugs and that he should report any change in drug regimen.

warfarin 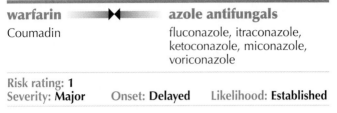 barbiturates

Coumadin

amobarbital, butabarbital, pentobarbital, phenobarbital, primidone, secobarbital

Risk rating: 1
Severity: Major   **Onset: Delayed**   **Likelihood: Established**

Cause
Microsomal enzymes in the liver may be induced, increasing the rate of warfarin clearance.

Effect
Anticoagulant effects may decrease.

Nursing considerations
- Patient may be switched from a barbiturate to a benzodiazepine if appropriate.
- Monitor patient for inadequate response to warfarin.
- If patient's INR is stabilized while taking a barbiturate, monitor it closely when the barbiturate stops—the warfarin dose may need to be reduced to avoid serious bleeding.

■ Urge patient to keep all follow-up medical appointments for monitoring and dosage adjustments. Monitoring may take several weeks.
■ Tell patient to report unusual bruising or bleeding.
■ Remind patient that warfarin interacts with many drugs and that he should report any change in drug regimen.

---

warfarin ▶◀ carbamazepine

Coumadin

Carbatrol, Epitol, Equetro, Tegretol

Risk rating: 2
Severity: Moderate   Onset: Delayed   Likelihood: Suspected

Cause
Carbamazepine may increase hepatic metabolism of warfarin.

Effect
Anticoagulant effects decrease.

Nursing considerations
■ Monitor PT and INR when starting, changing, or stopping carbamazepine therapy in patient who takes warfarin.
■ Maintain INR at 2 to 3 for an acute MI, atrial fibrillation, treatment of pulmonary embolism, prevention of systemic embolism, tissue heart valves, valvular heart disease, or prophylaxis or treatment of venous thrombosis. Maintain INR at 3 to 4.5 for mechanical prosthetic valves or recurrent systemic embolism.
■ Warfarin dose may need to be adjusted.
■ Tell patient to report unusual bruising or bleeding.
■ Remind patient that warfarin interacts with many drugs and that he should report any change in drug regimen.

---

warfarin ▶◀ cephalosporins

Coumadin

cefazolin, cefoperazone, cefotetan, cefoxitin, ceftriaxone

Risk rating: 2
Severity: Moderate   Onset: Delayed   Likelihood: Suspected

Cause
The mechanism of this interaction is unknown.

Effect
Anticoagulant effects increase.

Nursing considerations
- If given with a parenteral cephalosporin, warfarin dose may need to be reduced.
- Monitor PT and INR closely.
- Patients with renal insufficiency may be at greater risk.
- Monitor patient for signs of bleeding.
- Tell patient to report unusual bruising or bleeding.
- Remind patient that warfarin interacts with many drugs and that he should report any change in drug regimen.

---

warfarin ▸◂	cholestyramine
Coumadin	LoCHOLEST, Prevalite, Questran

Risk rating: 2
Severity: **Moderate**   Onset: **Delayed**   Likelihood: **Probable**

Cause
Warfarin absorption may decrease and elimination increase.

Effect
Anticoagulant effects may decrease.

Nursing considerations
- Tell patient to separate warfarin dose from cholestyramine by at least 3 hours.
- Advise patient of the risks of reduced anticoagulant effects.
- Help patient develop a plan to ensure proper dosage intervals.
- Tell patient to report unusual bruising or bleeding.
- Remind patient that warfarin interacts with many drugs and that he should report any change in drug regimen.

---

warfarin ▸◂	cimetidine
Coumadin	Tagamet

Risk rating: 1
Severity: **Major**   Onset: **Delayed**   Likelihood: **Established**

Cause
Hepatic metabolism of warfarin is inhibited.

Effect
Anticoagulant effects increase.

Nursing considerations
■ Suggest the use of an H_2 antagonist other than cimetidine because famotidine, ranitidine, and nizatidine are unlikely to interact with warfarin.
■ Avoid using these drugs together. If unavoidable, monitor coagulation values closely.
■ Tell patient to report unusual bruising or bleeding.
■ Remind patient that warfarin interacts with many drugs and that he should report any change in drug regimen.

---

warfarin 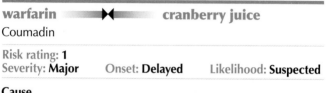 cranberry juice
Coumadin

Risk rating: 1
Severity: **Major**   Onset: **Delayed**   Likelihood: **Suspected**

Cause
The mechanism of this interaction is unknown.

Effect
Risk of serious bleeding increases.

Nursing considerations
■ Tell patient to take warfarin with liquid other than cranberry juice.
■ If warfarin dose has been stabilized with patient consuming cranberry juice, patient's coagulation status may need to be monitored if he switches to another beverage.
■ Tell patient to report unusual bruising or bleeding.
■ Remind patient that warfarin interacts with many drugs and that he should report any change in drug regimen.

---

warfarin danshen
Coumadin

Risk rating: 2
Severity: **Moderate**   Onset: **Delayed**   Likelihood: **Suspected**

Cause
The mechanism of this interaction is unknown.

Effect
Risk of bleeding may increase.

Nursing considerations
■ Monitor coagulation values.
■ Monitor patient for signs of bleeding.

- Caution patient to consult prescriber before taking OTC drugs or herbal supplements.
- Tell patient to report unusual bruising or bleeding.

---

warfarin ▶◀ disulfiram
Coumadin Antabuse

Risk rating: 2
Severity: Moderate **Onset: Delayed** **Likelihood: Probable**

Cause
The mechanism of this interaction is unknown.

Effect
Anticoagulant effects may increase.

Nursing considerations
- Monitor coagulation values.
- Disulfiram's effects on warfarin may be dose dependent. If disulfiram dose decreases, warfarin dose may need to be increased.
- Monitor patient for signs of bleeding.
- Tell patient to report unusual bruising or bleeding.
- Remind patient that warfarin interacts with many drugs and that he should report any change in drug regimen.

---

warfarin ▶◀ fibric acids
Coumadin clofibrate, fenofibrate, gemfibrozil

Risk rating: 1
Severity: Major **Onset: Delayed** **Likelihood: Established**

Cause
Coagulation factor synthesis may be altered.

Effect
Hypoprothrombinemic effects of warfarin may increase.

Nursing considerations
- Avoid use together if possible. If unavoidable, INR should be checked often.
- **◣ ALERT** Plasma warfarin level isn't affected by this interaction, but INR will increase. Hemorrhage and death may occur.
- Tell patient to report unusual bruising or bleeding.
- Remind patient that warfarin interacts with many drugs and that he should report any change in drug regimen.

■ Advise patient to keep all follow-up medical appointments for proper monitoring and dosage adjustments.

---

warfarin ◄► **HMG-CoA reductase inhibitors**
Coumadin

fluvastatin, lovastatin, simvastatin

Risk rating: 2
Severity: Moderate   **Onset: Delayed**   **Likelihood: Suspected**

Cause
Hepatic metabolism of warfarin may be inhibited.

Effect
Anticoagulant effects may increase.

Nursing considerations
■ Monitor PT and INR closely when starting or stopping an HMG-CoA inhibitor.
■ Atorvastatin and pravastatin don't appear to have this interaction with warfarin.
■ Tell patient to report unusual bruising or bleeding.
■ Remind patient that warfarin interacts with many drugs and that he should report any change in drug regimen.
■ Advise patient to keep all follow-up medical appointments for proper monitoring and dosage adjustments.

---

warfarin ◄► **macrolide antibiotics**
Coumadin

azithromycin, clarithromycin, erythromycin

Risk rating: 1
Severity: Major   **Onset: Delayed**   **Likelihood: Probable**

Cause
Warfarin clearance is reduced.

Effect
Anticoagulant effects and risk of bleeding increase.

Nursing considerations
■ Monitor PT and INR closely during when starting or stopping a macrolide antibiotic. The PT may be prolonged within a few days.
■ Warfarin dose adjustment may continue for several days after antibiotic therapy stops.

- Treat excessive anticoagulation with vitamin K.
- Tell patient to report unusual bruising or bleeding.
- Remind patient that warfarin interacts with many drugs and that he should report any change in drug regimen.
- Advise patient to keep all follow-up medical appointments for proper monitoring and dosage adjustments.

---

warfarin ▶◀ metronidazole
Coumadin   Flagyl

Risk rating: 1
Severity: Major   **Onset: Delayed**   **Likelihood: Established**

Cause
May decrease hepatic metabolism of warfarin.

Effect
Anticoagulant effects and risk of bleeding increase.

Nursing considerations
- Monitor patient for signs of bleeding.
- Warfarin dose may need to be reduced during metronidazole use.
- Tell patient to report unusual bruising or bleeding.
- Remind patient that warfarin interacts with many drugs and that he should report any change in drug regimen.

---

warfarin ▶◀ NSAIDs
Coumadin   diclofenac, etodolac, fenopro-
                                      fen, flurbiprofen, ibuprofen,
                                      indomethacin, ketoprofen,
                                      ketorolac, nabumetone,
                                      naproxen, oxaprozin,
                                      piroxicam, sulindac, tolmetin

Risk rating: 1
Severity: Major   **Onset: Delayed**   **Likelihood: Probable**

Cause
Platelet function is decreased and GI irritation increased.

Effect
Anticoagulant effects and risk of bleeding increase.

Nursing considerations
- Monitor PT and INR closely during combined use and when starting or stopping an NSAID.

- Tell patient to report unusual bruising or bleeding.
- Remind patient that warfarin interacts with many drugs and that he should report any change in drug regimen.
- Advise patient to keep all follow-up medical appointments for proper monitoring and dosage adjustments.

warfarin ◄►► penicillins
Coumadin

ampicillin, dicloxacillin, nafcillin, oxacillin, penicillin G, piperacillin, ticarcillin

Risk rating: 2
Severity: Major   **Onset: Delayed**   **Likelihood: Suspected**

Cause
Warfarin induces hypoprothrombinemia, and penicillin inhibits platelet aggregation.

Effect
Bleeding time is prolonged.

Nursing considerations
- Monitor PT and INR closely during combined use.
- Risk of interaction increases with large doses of I.V. penicillins. Nafcillin and dicloxacillin may cause warfarin resistance.
- Monitor coagulation values before starting nafcillin or dicloxacillin and for at least 3 weeks after stopping to check for warfarin resistance.
- Tell patient to report unusual bruising or bleeding.
- Remind patient that warfarin interacts with many drugs and that he should report any change in drug regimen.
- Advise patient to keep all follow-up medical appointments for proper monitoring and dosage adjustments.

warfarin ◄►► quinine derivatives
Coumadin   quinidine, quinine

Risk rating: 1
Severity: Major   **Onset: Delayed**   **Likelihood: Suspected**

Cause
Quinidine derivatives may inhibit clotting factors synthesized in the liver.

Effect
Anticoagulant effects and risk of bleeding may increase.

Nursing considerations
- Monitor PT and INR closely.
- Tell patient to report unusual bruising or bleeding.
- Remind patient that warfarin interacts with many drugs and that he should report any change in drug regimen.

---

warfarin ━━━━▶◀━━━━ **quinolones**
Coumadin   ciprofloxacin, levofloxacin, norfloxacin, ofloxacin

Risk rating: **2**
Severity: **Moderate**   Onset: **Delayed**   Likelihood: **Suspected**

Cause
The mechanism of this interaction is unknown.

Effect
Anticoagulant effects may increase.

Nursing considerations
- Monitor PT and INR closely.
- Tell patient to report unusual bruising or bleeding.
- Remind patient that warfarin interacts with many drugs and that he should report any change in drug regimen.

---

warfarin ━━━━▶◀━━━━ **rifamycins**
Coumadin   rifabutin, rifampin, rifapentine

Risk rating: **2**
Severity: **Moderate**   Onset: **Delayed**   Likelihood: **Established**

Cause
Hepatic metabolism of warfarin is increased by rifamycins.

Effect
Anticoagulant effects decrease.

Nursing considerations
- Monitor patient for inadequate response to warfarin.
- Warfarin dose may need to be increased during rifamycin therapy; monitor PT and INR often.
- Blood tests may be needed for several weeks after stopping a rifamycin.

- Tell patient to report unusual bruising or bleeding.
- Remind patient that warfarin interacts with many drugs and that he should report any change in drug regimen.
- Explain importance of following up with prescriber for proper monitoring and dosage adjustments.

---

warfarin ▶◀ salicylates
Coumadin   aspirin, methyl salicylate

Risk rating: 1
Severity: Major   **Onset: Delayed**   **Likelihood: Established**

Cause
Anticoagulant activity increases; platelet aggregation decreases.

Effect
Risk of significant bleeding may increase.

Nursing considerations
- Use together should be avoided.
- Monitor coagulation values closely.
- Aspirin doses of 500 mg or more daily increase risk of bleeding.
- Explain that interaction can happen with topical and oral salicylates.
- Tell patient to report unusual bruising or bleeding.
- Remind patient that warfarin interacts with many drugs and that he should report any change in drug regimen.
- ⚡ ALERT Warfarin dose should adjusted when aspirin is stopped.

---

warfarin ▶◀ sulfinpyrazone
Coumadin   Anturane

Risk rating: 1
Severity: Major   **Onset: Delayed**   **Likelihood: Established**

Cause
Hepatic metabolism of warfarin decreases.

Effect
Warfarin level, effects, and risk of bleeding may increase.

Nursing considerations
- Monitor coagulation values closely.
- ⚡ ALERT Warfarin dose may decrease when sulfinpyrazone is started and increased when sulfinpyrazone is stopped.
- Tell patient to report unusual bruising or bleeding.

■ Remind patient that warfarin interacts with many other drugs and that he should report any changes in drug regimen.

---

warfarin ▶◀	sulfonamides
Coumadin	sulfasalazine, sulfisoxazole trimethoprim-sulfamethoxazole

Risk rating: 1
Severity: Major   **Onset: Delayed**   **Likelihood: Established**

Cause
Hepatic metabolism of warfarin may be inhibited.

Effect
Warfarin level, effects, and risk of bleeding may increase.

Nursing considerations
■ Monitor coagulation values closely.
■ Tell patient to report unusual bruising or bleeding.
■ Remind patient that warfarin interacts with many other drugs and that he should report any change in drug regimen.

---

warfarin ▶◀	thioamines
Coumadin	methimazole, propylthiouracil

Risk rating: 1
Severity: Major   **Onset: Delayed**   **Likelihood: Suspected**

Cause
The mechanism of this interaction is unknown.

Effect
Anticoagulant effects may be altered.

Nursing considerations
■ Monitor coagulation values closely.
■ Monitor patient for inadequate response to anticoagulant.
■ Tell patient to report unusual bruising or bleeding.
■ Remind patient that warfarin interacts with many other drugs and that he should report any change in drug regimen.

warfarin ▶◀ thyroid hormones

Coumadin

levothyroxine, liothyronine, liotrix, thyroid

Risk rating: 1
Severity: Major   **Onset: Delayed**   **Likelihood: Probable**

Cause
Thyroid hormones increase the breakdown of vitamin K–dependent clotting factors.

Effect
Anticoagulant effects and risk of bleeding may increase.

Nursing considerations
- Monitor coagulation values carefully.
- A lower warfarin dose may be needed.
- If patient's anticoagulant values are stabilized during combined therapy and the thyroid hormones are stopped, warfarin dose may need to be increased.
- Tell patient to report unusual bruising or bleeding.
- Remind patient that warfarin interacts with many drugs and that he should report any change in drug regimen.

warfarin ▶◀ vitamin E

Coumadin

Risk rating: 1
Severity: Major   **Onset: Delayed**   **Likelihood: Suspected**

Cause
Vitamin E may interfere with vitamin K–dependent clotting factors.

Effect
Anticoagulant effects may increase.

Nursing considerations
- Monitor coagulation values carefully.
- A lower warfarin dose may be needed if patient is taking vitamin E.
- Less than 400 mg of vitamin E daily may not affect anticoagulation.
- Tell patient to report unusual bruising or bleeding.
- Remind patient that warfarin interacts with many drugs and that he should report any change in drug regimen.

warfarin ▸◂ vitamin K
Coumadin

Risk rating: 2
Severity: **Moderate**   Onset: **Delayed**   Likelihood: **Established**

Cause
Warfarin interferes with activation of vitamin K–dependent clotting factors in blood, an action overcome by vitamin K.

Effect
Anticoagulant effects are reversed and risk of thrombus is increased.

Nursing considerations
- Monitor PT and INR closely.
- Tell patient to avoid or minimize variations in vitamin K consumption, including green, leafy vegetables, green tea, and supplements.
- ⚡ ALERT Watch for signs of thrombus formation, including dyspnea, mottled extremities, and impaired thinking or coordination.
- Tell patient to report a change in dietary habits if he has been stabilized on warfarin. Coagulation values may have to be monitored and warfarin dose adjusted.
- Tell patient to report unusual bruising or bleeding.
- Remind patient that warfarin interacts with many drugs and that he should report any change in drug regimen.

zidovudine ▸◂ ganciclovir
AZT, Retrovir   Cytovene

Risk rating: 1
Severity: **Major**   Onset: **Delayed**   Likelihood: **Probable**

Cause
Ganciclovir may increase zidovudine level.

Effect
Risk of severe hematologic toxicities, including anemia, neutropenia, and leukopenia, increases.

Nursing considerations
- Use together should be avoided. Foscarnet (Foscavir) may be an adequate substitute for ganciclovir.
- Monitor CBC with differential.
- Use together may warrant reduction of ganciclovir dosage.

■ Explain that adverse hematologic effects may not appear for 3 to 5 weeks; tell patient to report symptoms of infection, such as fever, sore throat, and unexplained tiredness.

zidovudine ━━━━►◄━━━━ probenecid
AZT, Retrovir

Risk rating: 2
Severity: Moderate   **Onset: Delayed**   **Likelihood: Suspected**

Cause
Zidovudine glucuronidation decreases and level increases.

Effect
Risk of rash increases, possibly with malaise, myalgia, and fever.

Nursing considerations
■ Monitor patient for rash.
■ Zidovudine dosage interval may need to be doubled.
■ Tell patient to report muscle aches, fever, and general illness.

zileuton ━━━━►◄━━━━ theophyllines
Zyflo   aminophylline, theophylline

Risk rating: 2
Severity: Moderate   **Onset: Delayed**   **Likelihood: Probable**

Cause
Zileuton may inhibit theophylline metabolism.

Effect
Theophylline level and risk of adverse effects may increase.

Nursing considerations
■ Monitor theophylline level closely. Therapeutic range is 10 to 20 mcg/ml for adults and 5 to 15 mcg/ml for children.
■ Watch for evidence of toxicity, such as tachycardia, anorexia, nausea, vomiting, diarrhea, seizures, restlessness, irritability, and headache.
■ If patient starts zileuton while taking theophylline, theophylline dosage should decrease by 50%.
■ Explain common adverse effects of theophylline and signs of toxicity, and tell patient to report them immediately to prescriber.

ziprasidone ▶◀ antiarrhythmics

Geodon

amiodarone, bretylium,
disopyramide, procainamide,
quinidine, sotalol

Risk rating: 1
Severity: **Major**   Onset: **Delayed**   Likelihood: **Suspected**

Cause
The mechanism of this interaction is unknown.

Effect
Risk of life-threatening arrhythmias, including torsades de pointes,
increases.

Nursing considerations
◤ ALERT Use of ziprasidone with certain antiarrhythmics is contrain-
dicated.
■ Monitor patient for other risk factors for torsades de pointes, in-
cluding bradycardia, hypokalemia, and hypomagnesemia.
■ Ask patient if he or anyone in his family has a history of prolonged
QT interval or arrhythmias.
■ Monitor patient for bradycardia.
■ Measure the QTc interval at baseline and throughout therapy.

ziprasidone ▶◀ arsenic trioxide

Geodon

Trisenox

Risk rating: 1
Severity: **Major**   Onset: **Delayed**   Likelihood: **Suspected**

Cause
The mechanism of this interaction is unknown.

Effect
Risk of life-threatening arrhythmias, including torsades de pointes,
increases.

Nursing considerations
◤ ALERT Use of ziprasidone with arsenic trioxide is contraindicated.
■ Monitor patient for other risk factors for torsades de pointes, in-
cluding bradycardia, hypokalemia, and hypomagnesemia.
■ Ask patient if he or anyone in his family has a history of prolonged
QT interval or arrhythmias.
■ Monitor patient for bradycardia.
■ Measure the QTc interval at baseline and throughout therapy.

ziprasidone ━━━◄►━━━ dofetilide
Geodon   Tikosyn

Risk rating: 1
Severity: Major   **Onset: Delayed**   **Likelihood: Suspected**

Cause
Interaction may cause additive prolongation of the QTc interval.

Effect
Risk of ventricular arrhythmias, including torsades de pointes, increases.

Nursing considerations
◼ **ALERT** Use of dofetilide with ziprasidone is contraindicated.
◼ Monitor ECG for excessive prolongation of QTc interval and development of ventricular arrhythmias.
◼ Monitor renal function and QTc interval every 3 months during dofetilide therapy.
◼ If patient takes dofetilide, consult prescriber or pharmacist about antipsychotic other than ziprasidone.
◼ Urge patient to tell prescriber about increased adverse effects.

ziprasidone ━━━◄►━━━ dolasetron
Geodon   Anzemet

Risk rating: 1
Severity: Major   **Onset: Delayed**   **Likelihood: Suspected**

Cause
The mechanism of this interaction is unknown.

Effect
Risk of life-threatening arrhythmias, including torsades de pointes, increases.

Nursing considerations
◼ **ALERT** Use of ziprasidone with dolasetron is contraindicated.
◼ Ask patient if he or anyone in his family has a history of prolonged QT interval or arrhythmias.
◼ Monitor patient for other risk factors for torsades de pointes, including bradycardia, hypokalemia, and hypomagnesemia.
◼ Measure the QTc interval at baseline and throughout therapy.
◼ Monitor patient for bradycardia.

ziprasidone ━━━▶◀━━━ droperidol
Geodon   Inapsine

Risk rating: 1
Severity: Major   **Onset: Delayed**   **Likelihood: Suspected**

Cause
The mechanism of this interaction is unknown.

Effect
Risk of life-threatening arrhythmias, including torsades de pointes, increases.

Nursing considerations
◤ ALERT Use of ziprasidone with droperidol is contraindicated.
■ Ask patient if he or anyone in his family has a history of prolonged QT interval or arrhythmias.
■ Monitor patient for other risk factors for torsades de pointes, including bradycardia, hypokalemia, and hypomagnesemia.
■ Monitor patient for bradycardia.
■ Measure the QTc interval at baseline and throughout therapy.

ziprasidone ━━━▶◀━━━ phenothiazines
Geodon   chlorpromazine, mesoridazine, thioridazine

Risk rating: 1
Severity: Major   **Onset: Delayed**   **Likelihood: Suspected**

Cause
The mechanism of this interaction is unknown.

Effect
Risk of life-threatening arrhythmias, including torsades de pointes, increases.

Nursing considerations
◤ ALERT Use of ziprasidone with a phenothiazine is contraindicated.
■ Monitor patient for other risk factors for torsades de pointes, including bradycardia, hypokalemia, and hypomagnesemia.
■ Ask patient if he or anyone in his family has a history of prolonged QT interval or arrhythmias.
■ Monitor patient for bradycardia.
■ Measure the QTc interval at baseline and throughout therapy.

ziprasidone 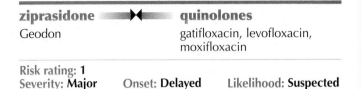 quinolones

Geodon

gatifloxacin, levofloxacin, moxifloxacin

Risk rating: 1
Severity: Major   **Onset: Delayed**   **Likelihood: Suspected**

Cause
The mechanism of this interaction is unknown.

Effect
Risk of life-threatening arrhythmias, including torsades de pointes, increases.

Nursing considerations
◼ **ALERT** Use of ziprasidone with a quinolone is contraindicated.
■ Monitor patient for other risk factors for torsades de pointes, including bradycardia, hypokalemia, and hypomagnesemia.
■ Ask patient if he or anyone in his family has a history of prolonged QT interval or arrhythmias.
■ Monitor patient for bradycardia.
■ Measure the QTc interval at baseline and throughout therapy.

ziprasidone 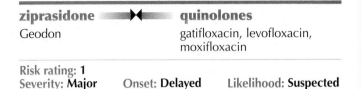 tacrolimus

Geodon

Prograf

Risk rating: 1
Severity: Major   **Onset: Delayed**   **Likelihood: Suspected**

Cause
The mechanism of this interaction is unknown.

Effect
Risk of life-threatening arrhythmias, including torsades de pointes, increases.

Nursing considerations
◼ **ALERT** Use of ziprasidone with tacrolimus is contraindicated.
■ Monitor patient for other risk factors for torsades de pointes, including bradycardia, hypokalemia, and hypomagnesemia.
■ Ask patient if he or anyone in his family has a history of prolonged QT interval or arrhythmias.
■ Monitor patient for bradycardia.
■ Measure the QTc interval at baseline and throughout therapy.

zolmitriptan ━━━▶◀━━━ ergot derivatives
Zomig   dihydroergotamine, ergotamine

Risk rating: 1
Severity: **Major**   Onset: **Rapid**   Likelihood: **Suspected**

Cause
Combined use may have additive effects.

Effect
Risk of vasospastic effects increases.

Nursing considerations
⚑ ALERT Use of these drugs within 24 hours of each other is contra-indicated.
■ Combined use may cause severe vasospastic effects, including sustained coronary artery vasospasm that triggers MI.
⚑ ALERT Use of two selective 5-HT$_1$ receptor agonists within 24 hours of each other is contraindicated. Warn patient not to mix migraine headache drugs within 24 hours of each other, but to call prescriber if a drug isn't effective.

zolmitriptan ━━━▶◀━━━ MAO inhibitors
Zomig   isocarboxazid, phenelzine,
                         tranylcypromine

Risk rating: 1
Severity: **Major**   Onset: **Rapid**   Likelihood: **Suspected**

Cause
MAO inhibitors, subtype-A, may inhibit metabolism of selective 5-HT$_1$ receptor agonists, such as zolmitriptan.

Effect
Zolmitriptan level and risk of cardiac toxicity may increase.

Nursing considerations
⚑ ALERT Use of certain selective 5-HT$_1$ receptor agonists with or within 2 weeks of stopping an MAO inhibitor is contraindicated.
■ If these drugs must be used together, naratriptan is less likely than zolmitriptan to interact with an MAO inhibitor.
■ Cardiac toxicity may include coronary artery vasospasm and transient myocardial ischemia.

zolmitriptan ▶◀ serotonin reuptake inhibitors

Zomig

citalopram, fluoxetine, fluvoxamine, nefazodone, paroxetine, sertraline, venlafaxine

Risk rating: 1
Severity: Major   **Onset: Rapid**   **Likelihood: Suspected**

Cause
Serotonin may accumulate rapidly in the CNS.

Effect
Risk of serotonin syndrome increases.

Nursing considerations
◼ **ALERT** If possible, avoid combined use of these drugs.
◼ Start with lowest dosages possible, and assess patient closely.
◼ Stop the selective $5\text{-}HT_1$ receptor agonist at the first sign of interaction, and start an antiserotonergic.
◼ In some patients, migraine frequency may increase and antimigraine drug efficacy may decrease when a serotonin reuptake inhibitor is started.
◼ **ALERT** Describe the traits of serotonin syndrome, including headache, dizziness, vomiting, coma, and death.

---

zolmitriptan ▶◀ sibutramine

Zomig   Meridia

Risk rating: 1
Severity: Major   **Onset: Rapid**   **Likelihood: Suspected**

Cause
Sibutramine inhibits serotonin reuptake, which may have additive effects with selective $5\text{-}HT_1$ receptor agonists, such as zolmitriptan.

Effect
Risk of serotonin syndrome increases.

Nursing considerations
◼ **ALERT** If possible, avoid giving these drugs together.
◼ Adverse effects may require immediate medical attention.
◼ Stop the selective $5\text{-}HT_1$ receptor agonist at the first sign of interaction, and start an antiserotonergic drug.
◼ Describe the traits of serotonin syndrome, including headaches, dizzines, shivering, coma, and death.